NUTRITIONAL IMPROVEMENT OF FOOD AND FEED PROTEINS

ADVANCES IN EXPERIMENTAL MEDICINE AND BIOLOGY

Recent Volumes in this Series

NUTRITIONAL
IMPROVEMENT
OF FOOD AND
FEED PROTEINS

Edited by

Mendel Friedman

Western Regional Research Laboratory
Science and Education Administration
U.S. Department of Agriculture
Berkeley, California

PLENUM PRESS • NEW YORK AND LONDON

Library of Congress Cataloging in Publication Data

Symposium on Improvement of Protein Nutritive Quality of Foods and Feeds,
    Chicago, 1977.
    Nutritional improvement of food and feed proteins.

    (Advances in experimental medicine and biology; 105)
    Sponsored by the Protein Subdivision of the Division of Agricultural and Foods
Chemistry of the American Chemical Society.
    Includes index.
    1. Proteins in human nutrition—Congresses. 2. Proteins in animal nutrition—Con-
gresses. 3. Amino acids in human nutrition—Congresses. 4. Amino acids in animal
nutrition—Congresses. I. Friedman, Mendel. II. American Chemical Society. Division
of Agricultural and Foods Chemistry. Protein Subdivision. III. Title. IV. Series.
[DNLM: 1. Dietary proteins. 2. Plant proteins. 3. Amino acids. 4. Food, Fortified.
5. Nutrition. W1 AD559 v. 105/QU55.3 N976]
TX553.P7S8 1977   641.1'2   78-17278
ISBN 0-306-40026-X

Proceedings of the Symposium on Improvement of Protein Nutritive Quality
of Foods and Feeds, sponsored by the Protein Subdivision of the Division of Agricultural
and Food Chemistry of the American Chemical Society, Chicago, Illinois,
August 29—September 2, 1977, with additional invited contributions.

© 1978 Plenum Press, New York
A Division of Plenum Publishing Corporation
227 West 17th Street, New York, N.Y. 10011

Printed in the United States of America

Preface

The nutritional quality of a protein depends on the proportion of its amino acids-especially the essential amino acids-their physio-logical availability, and the specific requirements of the consumer. Availability varies and depends on protein source, interaction with other dietary components, and the consumer's age and physiological state.

In many foods, especially those from plants, low levels of various essential amino acids limits their nutritive value. This is particularly important for cereals (which may be inadequate in the essential amino acids isoleucine, lysine, threonine, and tryto-phan) and legumes (which are often poor sources of methionine). Moreover, these commodities are principle sources of protein for much of the earth's rapidly growing population.

At the current annual growth rate of about 2 percent, the world population of about 4 billion will increase to 6.5 billion by the year 2000 and to 17 billion by the year 2050. Five hundred million people are presently estimated to suffer protein malnutrition, with about fifteen thousand daily deaths. The ratio of malnourished to adequately nourished will almost surely increase. For these reasons, and especially in view of the limited availability of high quality (largely animal) protein to feed present and future populations, improvement of food and feed quality is especially important.

The key questions in my mind are "What may or will happen if we do not develop new and improved food and feed sources? What are the consequences of population pressures for our future well-being?" In his analysis of the subject, Robert R. Heilbronner (*An Inquiry into the Human Prospect*, W. W. Norton, 1975) foresees dire prospects which include: (a) rule of the world by military-socialist dictatorships; (b) seizures of weak nations by strong ones; (c) use of nuclear blackmail by underdeveloped countries to transfer wealth; and (d) deterioration of the environment, whereby exponential-ly growing emission of man-made heat will cause drastic climactic changes and major decreases in industrial and agricultural production. In a related analysis (*Engineering Science*, pp. 22-36, 1956), Sir

Charles Darwin also suggests that man will come to a 'semi-bestial'
existence (his grandfather did not have this type of 'evolution'
in mind when he wrote *Origin of Species* and *The Descent of Man*).
Although Fred Hoyle (*ibid.*, pp. 8-10) and Robert Heilbronner suggest
that human negative feed-back processes will exercise a dampening
effect on the impending crisis, such feed-backs may not suffice to
prevent it.   (A result of important feed-back processes is the
differential growth rate of the world's population. Western Europe,
the United States, and apparently also the Peoples Republic of China,
seem to be approaching true zero growth, in contrast to Latin America,
Africa, and most other parts of Asia, which are growing by 2 to 3
percent annually).

    We are, therefore, challenged to respond to humanity's common
danger. I feel that as scientists interested in proteins in all
aspects, we are indeed responding to this challenge. Aside from
limiting population growth, which is a sociological and political
problem, our work as agronomists, plant breeders, animal scientists,
food chemists, food technologists, nutritionists, dieticians, physicians, toxicologists, agricultural economists, and industrialists
can help avoid and alleviate shortages of high quality foods and
feeds and thus counter and mitigate some of the more serious threats
to the quality of life for ourselves and our descendants. Our objective should be to improve the quality and quantity of available
food and feed sources by all feasible methods. Much new chemistry
and engineering is needed to support genetics and agronomy. Food
fortification and supplementation need better guidance based on research. Deleterious side reactions in food storage and processing
need to be eliminated or minimized. Ways to measure protein nutritional quality based on information from chemical, biochemical,
microbiological, animal, and human studies need to be correlated and
optimized. New protein food sources need to be developed; related
toxicological and nutritional problems need solutions.

    Because I feel that the most important function of a symposium
is dissemination of insights and catalysis of progress by bringing
together ideas and experiences needed for synergistic interaction
among different, yet related disciplines, in organizing the Symposium
on "Improvement of Protein Nutritive Quality of Foods and Feeds"
(sponsored by the Protein Subdivision of the Division of Agricultural
and Food Chemistry of the American Chemical Society, Chicago, Illinois, August 29-September 2, 1977), I invited papers discussing one
or more of the following topics: (1) Improvement of protein quality
by genetic methods; (2) Fortification of foods and feeds with essential amino acids, amino acid analogs, or derivatives; (3) Enrichment
of foods and feeds with protein supplements; (4) Use of special processes such as the plastein reaction to maximize protein quality and
utilization; (5) Use of protected amino acids and proteins in ruminant feeds to increase meat, milk, and wool production; (6) Chemical
and microbiological syntheses of essential amino acids; (7) Interac-

tions of supplemental amino acids or proteins with other food
ingredients during storage and processing and ways to minimize
such undesirable interactions; (8) Economic aspects, including
calculation of least cost-optimum quality supplemented foods
and feeds; (9) Animal and human feeding tests of nutritional
availability of amino acids or proteins in supplements; and (10)
Safety of supplemented or specially processed foods and feeds,
including amino acid antagonisms *in vivo*.

In addition, many scientists accepted invitations to contribute
papers to this volume. Indeed more than half the papers are
specially written, invited contributions. This book is, therefore,
a hybrid between a symposium proceedings and a collection of invited
contributions.

This volume brings together outstanding international authors
from ten countries, who, in forty papers, thoroughly discuss
various ways to improve foods and feeds. Though an adequate
summary is not possible in a preface, I wish to call special
attention to several manuscripts. First, F. Monckeberg and
C. O. Chichester describe in a particularly enlightening way
the interdependent efforts among several scientific disciplines,
government agencies, and industry to successfully develop a fortified food formula for children in Chile. Related discussions of
nutrition intervention programs in Guatemala are ably presented
by R. Bressani, L. G. Elias, and J. E. Braham, and in India, by
R. P. Devadas. These papers and related ones by A. A. Betschart
on bread fortification and by V. H. Holsinger on beverage fortification will serve well those planning to commercialize fortified,
supplemented, or complemented solid and liquid foods for human
consumption. A note of caution is, however, needed. As H. N.
Munro points out, excessive intake of certain free amino acids
in (fortified) foods can have undesirable physiological consequences. The methods for predicting protein quality described in
three papers by J. M. McLaughlan, A. A. Woodham, and N. J. Benevenga and D. G. Cieslak are also noteworthy because the ideal
method for protein quality evaluation has been so elusive.
Another immediate concern is the current widespread interest
among nutritionists and consumers about the role of plant fiber
in human nutrition. I am therefore pleased that G. A. Spiller
has contributed a critical overview of this subject, co-authored
by Joan Gates. This attempt to define the problem precisely will
undoubtedly stimulate further nutritional and medical progress.
Finally, the comprehensive paper by S. G. Platt and J. A. Bassham
on the potential for controlling photosynthesis to increase protein
production offers great promise for more efficient photosynthesis,
the ultimate source of our indispensible food and feed protein.

The papers are being published by Plenum under the title
NUTRITIONAL IMPROVEMENT OF FOOD AND FEED PROTEINS as a volume in

the series Advances in Experimental Medicine and Biology. This
book is intended to complement the previously published *Chemistry
and Biochemistry of the Sulfhydryl Group in Amino Acids, Peptide,
and Proteins* (Pergamon, 1973); *Protein-Metal Interactions* (Plenum,
1974); *Protein Nutritional Quality of Foods and Feeds. Part 1:
Assay Methods--Biological, Biochemical, and Chemical* (Dekker, 1975);
*Protein Nutritional Quality of Foods and Feeds. Part 2: Quality
Factors--Plant Breeding, Composition, Processing, and Antinutrients*
(Dekker, 1975); *Protein Crosslinking: Biochemical and Molecular
Aspects* (Plenum, 1977); *Protein Crosslinking: Nutritional and
Medical Consequences* (Plenum, 1977). (I wrote the sulfhydryl
book and edited the others). I hope that these books will be
a valuable resource for further progress in protein chemistry,
agriculture, food science, animal and human nutrition, biochemistry,
and medicine; areas of world-wide urgency.

I am particularly grateful to all contributors for excellent
cooperation, to Wilfred H. Ward for constructive contributions to
several manuscripts, to my son, Kenneth A. Friedman, for his help
in preparing the index, and to Miles Laboratories and Gerber
Baby Products for financial assistance.

I dedicate this book to my parents, Rachel and Efroim
Frydman, who nurtured their children with love under extraordinary
circumstances.

Mendel Friedman
Moraga, California
July 1978

*The earth is full of the fruit of Thy works.
Thou causest grass to spring up for cattle,
And herbs for the service of man.
Thou bringest forth bread out of the earth
To sustain man's life,
And wine to gladden his heart.*

Psalm 104: 28-33

Contents

POSITION PAPER ON RDA FOR PROTEIN FOR CHILDREN

R. P. Abernathy and S. J. Ritchey

Purdue University and VPI & SU

W. Lafayette, IN and Blacksburg, VA

ABSTRACT

The Recommended Dietary Allowances (RDA) by the National
Academy of Sciences are revised approximately every five years.
The RDA are compromise opinions of highly qualified nutritional
scientists based on interpretations of available data. As with
any interpretations and opinions not founded on definitive information, they are subject to challenges. The RDA for protein for 7-
to 9-year-old children have been adjusted downward from 60 g in
1958 to 36 g in 1974, a 40% reduction. Data from our laboratories
have shown positive apparent nitrogen balances on intakes as low
as 18 g daily when no allowances were made for integumental and
other nitrogen losses, however, based on accumulative data over
several years we calculate the protein requirement to be 45 g daily
from a typical American diet. If a safety factor of 30% is added
the allowance would become 58.5 g. Currently the RDA for protein
for the 7- to 10-year-old child supplies 6% of the RDA for Calories
which contrasts to 8.30 and 9.20% for adult males and females,
respectively. For comparison, energy from protein as a percentage
of total energy for some common foods are: white bread, 12%; corn
meal 10%; white rice 7%; and wheat flour 13%.

INTRODUCTION

Approximately every five years the Food and Nutrition Board
of the National Academy of Sciences revises the Recommended Dietary
Allowances. The Board, composed of active nutritional scientists,
utilizes existing literature concerned with nutritional needs of
various age groups. The RDA reflect the best estimates of nutrient

intakes which will meet the needs of practically all healthy
persons.

That these best estimates are often crude and perhaps influenced by personal bias of the current Board members is attested to
by the fact that the RDA may change very dramatically in only a
few years even in the absence of any significant new data on actual
requirements for a given nutrient. For example, the RDA for vitamin
E for the adult was decreased from 30 IU in 1968 to 15 IU per day
in 1974 with very little new data on actual requirements.

The RDA for protein for 7- to 10-year-old children (Table 1)
decreased from 60 g per day in 1958 to 36 g in 1974, a 40% drop
(NRC, 1958 and NRC, 1974). This decrease in the RDA is the subject
of this paper. We are suggesting that the 1974 RDA for protein for
7- to 10-year-old children is too low.

Obviously, the Food and Nutrition Boards for the last two
revisions believed that the previous RDA for young school age
children were too high. Current protein allowances, except for
infants, are based on theoretical calculations assuming an average
requirement for maintenance of 0.47 g of protein per kilogram of
body weight per day as estimated by nitrogen balance technique.
This value is increased by 30% to cover individual variation and
by another 33% to correct for an average of 75% efficiency of
utilization making the recommended allowance for maintenance 0.8 g
of protein per kilogram of body weight per day. An allowance for
growth, also corrected for inefficient utilization, is added. In
the case of the 7- to 10-year-old child, the value, as corrected,
is 0.4 g per kilogram per day; thus, the recommended allowance is
1.2 g of protein per kilogram of body weight or 36 g of protein
daily for a 30 kilogram child. This value is in line with the
FAO/WHO recommended intake of 25 g of protein per day as egg or
milk protein for 7- to 9-year-old children (FAO/WHO, 1973).
Twenty-five grams when corrected for 75% efficiency of utilization
would become 34 g per day for the 28.1 kg child used as a reference
by the FAO/WHO group.

Though the RDA and FAO/WHO values agree closely, there are
important questions about the recommended allowances. First, these
recommended allowances are not based on research data with children, but are extrapolations from data obtained with adults. The
Food and Nutrition Board, as well as the FAO/WHO Expert Panel,
considered existing data available for children but were faced with
widely varying estimates of requirements ranging from 0.7 to 3.5 g
of protein per kilogram of body weight (Irwin and Hegsted, 1971).
Secondly, a diet recommended for the growing child should be
adequate in protein concentration for non-growing adult men and
women. Thirdly, our research data, as we interpret them, are not

TABLE 1

Changes in the RDA for Protein for School Age Children Since 1958

Date	Ages Years	Protein g/day
1958	7-9	60
1964	6-9	52
1968	6-8	35
	8-10	40
1974	7-10	36

supportive of the current RDA (Abernathy et al., 1966, Abernathy and Ritchey, 1972, Korslund et al., 1976), and fourthly, other qualified researchers also have proposed that the recommended allowances for adults and children be adjusted (Swaminathan et al., 1970, 1971, Swaminathan and Parpia, 1971).

Table 2 shows the 1974 Recommended Dietary Allowances for protein expressed as grams of protein per 100 kcal and energy from protein expressed as a percentage of total calories. The recommended protein concentration decreases from infancy reaching lowest level of 6% of calories at 7 to 10 years of age, then increases again reaching the highest level in the age group, 51 and above. Even though the allowances were set only after extensive debate, it almost looks as if they were proposed by meat loving adults who believe children should be allowed to come to the table only after their elders have consumed their meals. The percentages of energy from protein in cereal grains, potatoes and green leafy vegetables are higher than the level recommended for children. For comparison to the level recommended for 7- to 10-year-old children of 6%, the percentages of energy of protein from some common, non-protein-rich foods are: sweet corn, 14.6; corn flour, 8.5; corn grits, 8.3; boiled potato, 11.0; French fried potatoes, 6.3; sweet potatoes and yams, 6.0 to 8.3; white bread, 12.9; whole wheat bread, 17.3; rye, 14.5; polished rice, 7.3; green leafy vegetables 20-50; and ice cream with 10% fat, 9.3.

NITROGEN BALANCES

We have conducted a large number of nitrogen balance studies with healthy 7- to 9-year-old children with protein intakes from commonly consumed foods ranging from 18 to 88 grams per day

TABLE 2

1974 RDA for Protein

Age years	Energy kcal	Protein g	g Protein/ 100 kcal	% of energy from protein
1–3	1300	23	1.77	7.07
4–6	1800	30	1.67	6.67
7–10	2400	36	1.50	6.00
Males				
11–14	2800	44	1.57	6.28
15–22	3000	54	1.80	7.20
23–50	2700	56	2.07	8.30
51+	2400	56	2.33	9.33
Females				
11–14	2400	44	1.83	7.33
15–18	2100	48	2.29	9.14
19–22	2100	46	2.19	8.76
23–50	2000	46	2.30	9.20
51+	1800	46	2.56	10.22

(Abernathy et al., 1966, 1970, 1972, Spence et al., 1972, Howat et al., 1975, Meiners et al., 1977). These studies varied in length from 18 to 64 days. The subjects were all judged to be healthy and free from intestinal parasites, except for pin worms which were observed and treated in a few girls. The diets were ordinary foods which supplied 1800 to 2400 kcal daily depending on the size of subjects. Any subject losing weight or in negative nitrogen balance was given additional energy in increments of 200 kcal per day and/or increments or protein if necessary. The food was provided in three meals and two snacks daily.

A summarization of nitrogen balance data from several of these studies is presented in Table 3. The percentage of total protein from animal sources ranged from 0 to 75%. The essential amino acid levels were in the range of that seen in common foods patterns of school children in the United States with lysine, sulfur containing amino acids or tryptophan being the most limiting (Abernathy et al., 1966). Except for low levels of riboflavin and

TABLE 3

Observed and Predicted Nitrogen Retention at Several
Levels of Nitrogen Intake

(mg./kg. body weight/day)

Animal Protein (% of total)	Mean Nitrogen Intake X	Mean Nitrogen Absorbed (apparent)	Mean Nitrogen Retention	
			Observed Y	Predicted Y^1
74	432	401 (392–414)[2]	35 (27–44)[2]	50
72	430	400 (391–414)	48 (37–55)	50
70	356	323 (245–416)	52 (38–76)	47
60	319	284 (276–299)	50 (44–53)	45
75	300	268 (254–278)	43 (34–59)	44
67	217	188 (166–211)	37 (20–55)	35
72	204	185 (179–192)	29 (19–37)	33
0	225	177 (168–188)	26 (15–34)	36
0	218	168 (137–199)	30 (13–42)	35
45	128	103 (88–122)	25 (13–43)	20
0	135	99 (86–106)	18 (8–26)	21
0^3	128	89 (83–96)	7 (4–11)	20
30	104	78 (64–91)	16 (11–25)	15

1 – $Y = -9.10 + 0.267X - 0.0003038X^2$ prediction equation
2 – range
3 – Diet low in riboflavin and niacin

niacin in one study, the other nutrients were provided at levels
approximately the RDA.

There was a highly significant linear relationship between
nitrogen intake and apparent nitrogen retention, however, the best
fit of the data was a slightly currilinear regression, ($Y = -9.10
+ 0.276 X 0.0003038X^2$), where Y is apparent nitrogen retention
and X is nitrogen intake, both in milligrams per kilograms of body
weight. About 64% of the variation in retension data was accounted
for by this regression.

The next steps then are to determine whether or not these
data are representative of nitrogen retentions in the general population and if so which of the retention values represent the actual
requirements. When diet simulating that of low-income families
were fed, nitrogen retention was lower. The retention was not
improved by supplementation of the most limiting amino acid or
zinc (Abernathy et al., 1972 and Meiners et al., 1977). Therefore,
the data from which the regression was calculated probably were
near maximal for healthy children consuming typical American foods
at similar protein intakes. This is especially true at the lower
intake levels where supplements of energy and protein were given to
those who retained less than 0.3 g nitrogen or about 10 mg per
kilogram daily, the amount calculated to be required to cover needs
for growth.

Nitrogen retention values in our studies were generally higher
than reported for American children by Macy (1946), but were similar
to or lower than values reported in undernourished children from
other countries (Luyken and Luyken-Koning, 1960). Luyken and
Luyken-Koning reported nitrogen retentions of 45 and 64 mg per kg
per day for undernourished Bushnegro and Japanese children fed
diets supplying 256 and 314 mg of nitrogen per kg per day respectively. Nitrogen retentions reported by Stearns et al., 1958 and
Ziegler et al., 1977, for 7- to 11-year-old children whose intakes
ranged from 227 to 385 mg per kg were generally lower than our
values. At higher nitrogen intakes, their subjects retained as
much or more nitrogen than our subjects did.

It is obvious from our data and from that of most other
researchers that apparent nitrogen retentions are often much higher
than the amount which can be deposited in the body. These high
apparent retentions make maximum retention unreliable for use in
estimation of protein requirements unless corrected for skin and
gaseous losses. The nitrogen retention technique almost always
overestimates actual retentions because of small amounts of urinary
and fecal nitrogen are not collected for assays and gaseous and
skin losses are not measured. These losses are not constant but
tend to increase with increasing protein intakes and are affected
by other factors such as temperature and nature of the diet. In
spite of these limitations we believe that the nitrogen balance
technique can provide important data from which estimations of
recommended allowances can be made.

                        CALCULATED REQUIREMENTS

The recommended allowances for protein in the 1968 revision
of the RDA (NRC, 1968) were calculated by using the following
formula: R = U + F + S + G (Table 4) where R = nitrogen requirement; U = loss of endogenous nitrogen in the urine; F = loss of

endogenous nitrogen in the feces; S = skin, sweat and integumental nitrogen loss; and G = nitrogen requirements for growth. The total nitrogen needed to be retained by the body can be estimated by adding these values. The regression calculated from our regional studies can be used to estimate the level of dietary protein which would provide for these needs. In the nitrogen balance procedure. U and F do not need to be calculated as they are included in urinary and fecal nitrogen, thus have been met before apparent nitrogen balances are calculated. Apparent nitrogen retention needs to be large enough to cover S and G. The need for growth for the 7- to 10-year-old child can be calculated to approximately 0.3 g per day or 10-12 mg of nitrogen per kilogram of body weight per day by calculating average weight gain and assuming 18 to 20% of the gain is body protein. The amount for S is more difficult to estimate. The 1968 edition of the Recommended Dietary Allowance used a value of 0.8 mg of nitrogen per basal kilocalorie or approximately 0.8 g per day for this age group. Average sweat nitrogen losses in our studies for various groups ranged from 0.235 to 0.375 g daily (Spence et al., 1972). If the losses by hair, nails, gases and other areas as well as the sweat nitrogen losses are included, a value of 0.8 g per day may be a reasonable estimate. This value probably is large enough to also cover small losses of urinary and fecal losses associated with incomplete collections. By adding the values for G of 0.3 g and for S of 0.8 g and dividing by average weight, the amount needed for S and G is 39.3 mg per kg of body weight. By using the regression equation calculated from our earlier studies (Abernathy et al., 1966) $Y = -9.10 + 0.267X - 0.0003038X^2$ where Y is apparent nitrogen balance and X is intake both expressed as mg of N per kg of body weight, the intake required to meet this need is 256 mg per kg or 44.8 of protein per day for a 28 kg child. If a safety factor of 30% is included, the recommended allowance

TABLE 4

Method of Calculating Protein Requirements

R = U + F + S + G

R = Nitrogen requirement

U = Endogenous nitrogen in urine

F = Endogenous nitrogen in feces

S = Sweat, skin and integumental loss

G = Requirement for growth

---

would become 58 g or 9.7% of the dietary calories as protein. Even
if the value for S is reduced from 0.8 g to a conservative 0.5 g,
the average intake to meet the reduced needs would be 176 mg of
nitrogen per kilogram of body weight or 34 g per day for a 28 kg
child which would become 44 g per day when increased to cover
individual variation. We therefore believe the Recommended Dietary
Allowance for protein for the 7- to 10-year-old child should be
between 44 and 58 g per day, which would provide 7.3 to 9.7 per
cent of the calories as protein instead of 6.0 per cent recommended
presently by the current Recommended Dietary Allowance. For
practical purposes a change in the allowance in the United States
would make little difference as nearly all children are consuming
far in excess of the RDA. If these same allowances were used in
the developing countries, the need for additional protein foods
would be minimal as the cereal grains provide levels to meet the
proposed needs. Protein supplements would be for improvement in
quality rather than increasing intake if energy needs were met
through common foods. If energy needs are not met, the protein
requirements would increase as more of the protein would be
shifted for energy uses.

CONCLUSIONS

Based on our studies and on assumptions that skin and gaseous
losses plus other small losses associated with the nitrogen balance
are within the range of 0.5 to 0.8 mg of nitrogen per basal calorie,
the protein requirement for the average 7- to 10-year-old child is
estimated to be between 34 and 44 g daily. When corrected for
individual variation, the recommended allowances would become 44
to 58 g daily. Because the children in our studies ate 3 meals
plus 2 snacks per day throughout the studies, we believe apparent
nitrogen retentions were higher than would be retained at the same
level of protein by an average child with irregular eating patterns.
Also, we were unable to demonstrate a beneficial effect of supplementation of some of our diets with lysine, methionine and threonine or zinc. For the reasons outlined above we suggest the next
revision of the Recommended Dietary Allowance of the National
Academy of Sciences show higher protein allowances for children.

REFERENCES

Abernathy, R.P., Speirs, M., Engel, R.W. and Moore, M.E. (1966).
    Effect of several levels of dietary amino acids and amino
    acids on nitrogen balance in preadolescent girls. Am. J.
    Clin. Nutrition, 19, 407-414.

Abernathy, R.P., Ritchey, S.J., Korslund, M.K., Gorman, J.C. and
    Price, N.O. (1970). Nitrogen balance studies with children
    fed foods representing diets of low-income southern families.
    Am. J. Clin. Nutrition, 23, 408-412.

Abernathy, R.P., Ritchey, S.J. and Gorman, J.C. (1972). Lack of response to amino acid supplements by preadolescent girls. Am. J. Clin. Nutrition, 25, 980-982.

Abernathy, R.P. and Ritchey, S.J. (1972). Protein requirements of preadolescent girls. J. Home Econ., 64, 56-58.

FAO/WHO. (1973). Energy and protein requirements. WHO Report Series No. 522, Geneva; FAO Nutrition Meetings Report Series No. 52, Rome.

Howat, P.M., Korslund, M., Abernathy, R.P. and Ritchey, S.J. (1977). Sweat nitrogen losses by and nitrogen balance of preadolescent girls consuming three levels of dietary protein. Am. J. Clin. Nutrition, 28, 879-882.

Irwin, M.I. and Hegsted, D.M. (1971). A conspectus of research on protein requirements of man. J. Nutrition, 101, 385-430.

Korslund, M.K., Leung, E.Y., Meiners, C.R., Crews, M.G., Taper, J., Abernathy, R.P. and Ritchey, S.J. (1976). The effect of sweat nitrogen losses in evaluating protein utilization by preadolescent children. Am. J. Clin. Nutrition, 29, 600-603.

Macy, I.G. (1946). Nutrition and chemical growth in childhood. Vol. II, Original data. Charles C. Thomas. Springfield, Illinois.

Meiners, C.R., Taper, L.J., Korslund, M.K. and Ritchey, S.J. (1977). The relationship of zinc to protein utilization in the pre-adolescent child. Am. J. Clin. Nutrition, 30, 879-882.

Luyken, R. and Luyken-Koning, F.W.M. (1960). Studies on the physiology of nutrition in Surinam. IV. Nitrogen balance studies. Trop. Georgr. Med., 12, 303-307.

National Research Council, (1958). Recommended Dietary Allowances, 5th ed. National Academy of Sciences, Washington, D.C.

National Research Council (1968). Recommended Dietary Allowances, 7th ed. National Academy of Sciences, Washington, D.C.

National Research Council (1974). Recommended Dietary Allowances, 8th ed. National Academy of Sciences, Washington, D.C.

Spence, M.R., Abernathy, R.P. and Ritchey, S.J. (1972). Excretion of nitrogen in sweat by preadolescent girls consuming low protein diets. Am. J. Clin. Nutrition, 25, 275-278.

Sterns, G., Newman, K.J., McKinley, J.B. and Jeans, P.C. (1958).
    The protein requirements of children from one to ten years of
    age. Ann. N.Y. Acad. Sci., 69, 857–868.

Swaminathan, M. (1970). Protein requirements – a critical evalua-
    tion of the FAO/WHO expert group recommendations. Nutrition
    Rpts. Intern., Z., 153–171.

Swaminathan, M. (1971). A note on the factorial method for calcu-
    lating protein requirements for human subjects. Nutrition
    Repts. Intern., 3, 277–281.

Swaminathan, M. and Parpia, H.A. (1971). Human calorie and protein
    requirements. Nutrition Rpts. Intern., 3, 327–349.

Ziegler, E.E., O'Donnell, A.M., Stearns, G., Nelson, S.E.,
    Burmeister, L.F. and Fomon, S.J. (1977). Nitrogen balance
    studies with normal children. Am. J. Clin. Nutrition, 30,
    939–946.

2

CHILEAN EXPERIENCE WITH FORTIFIED CHILDREN'S FORMULAS

Fernando Monckeberg*   and C. O. Chichester**

*Departmento de Nutricion y Tecnologia de los Alimentos,
Universidad de Chile, Santiago, Chile (Associated Institution of the United Nations University)
**Department of Food and Resource Chemistry, University
of Rhode Island, Kingston, Rhode Island

INTRODUCTION

In southern Latin America, as well as in other regions of the
world where serious malnutrition exists, the problem is particularly acute among infants and preschool children. In Chile, in 1968,
almost 30% of the children less than one year old showed some degree
of malnutrition. This percentage increased gradually with age; by
six years, almost 60% of the children were malnourished.

During the last 15 years, different governments aware of the
severity of this problem have undertaken various nutrition intervention programs, specifically targeted to prevent malnutrition in
preschool children. In 1974, considering the complexity of the
problem, the National Food and Nutrition Council (CONPAN) was established; the main objective was to develop a national food and
nutrition policy. This planning and coordinating body acts at the
highest level. It is composed of the Ministers of all state agencies that directly or indirectly affect the food system (Ministries
of Planning, Education, Agriculture, Economy, and Labor). CONPAN
prepared a national food and nutrition policy with a set of well-
defined objectives. Its first priority was preventing malnutrition
in infants and preschool children. The target groups were pregnant
and lactating women, infants, and preschoolers. To attain this
goal, various nutrition intervention programs were designed and
implemented. One of these was free distribution of food for these
groups. For pregnant and lactating women, powdered milk was distributed in the amount of four thousand tons yearly to 65% of all
mothers. For children less than two years of age, 16 million Kg
of powdered milk with a fat content of 26% was distributed, reaching

90% of this target group. For children two to six, 17 million Kg of fortified formulas were distributed, reaching 85% of all children of this age group.

The different steps followed to implement this children's fortified formula program on a national scale are presented in this paper. Sharing this knowledge is important because of the success reached after several years of research and three years of full scale national implementation.

DESCRIPTION OF ACTIVITIES

Research on various fortified formulas intended to prevent children's malnutrition is copiously documented. Yet very few findings have been successfully implemented to a significant degree. Laboratory research and pilot project studies may show many nutritional advantages in addition to technological feasibility, but these are not enough to assure success. Many collateral studies and a strategy that permits successful implementation are also necessary:

a) First, a well defined policy strategy is required that will convince decision makers on the need and usefulness of such a program.
b) In a non-state-planned economy, certainty of economic success is a basic requirement in order to elicit investments needed for production.
c) Clear and precise knowledge of dietary habits and beliefs of the target population is a primary need in order to maximize acceptability of the products designed.
d) Finally, a carefully designed marketing strategy is needed to assure a demand for the product, which ideally will become a felt need, thus securing the continuity of the program.

Without doubt, this complex process requires leadership and a coordinated multidisciplinary team effort (nutritionists, food technologists and engineers, marketing specialists, social scientists, etc.). The investigator who works in a team submerged in the environment of a laboratory is not prepared for this; it soon becomes clear that laboratory results or even a pilot project trial represent only the first steps toward elaborating a formula. Efforts toward implementation at a national level often fail.

All the previously described variables were carefully studied by a group of investigators from the Instituto de Nutricion y Tecnologia de Alimentos de la Universidad de Chile (INTA) in collaboration with the Department of Food Science and Technology, Nutrition, and Dietetics of the University of Rhode Island. This study comprised the following steps:

- Study of habits and beliefs about foods
- Development of a formula
- Acceptability tests of the product in the general population
- Promotion efforts to achieve a policy decision
- Implementation of industrial production
- Management of the system by the National Food and Nutrition Council

STUDY OF HABITS AND BELIEFS ABOUT FOOD

The first necessary step is to study the food habits and beliefs of a social group in order to achieve the ultimate goal of consumption of the test food by preschool children. For example, it is important to know the acceptability of a test food by the children. However, it is perhaps even more important to know the acceptability of the food to their mothers or guardians. A food could be made perfectly acceptable to a child, but if the mother does not consider it adequate, the chance of it reaching the child is very little. Furthermore, it is also important to know the food habits of adults, so that they will not preempt food distributed specifically for children.

To study the feeding habits of the population, the province of Curicó was selected. Curicó is considered typical of the central zone of Chile in which 80% of the population of the country is concentrated. Five hundred families were selected for this study; half representing the urban population and the other half, the rural population. The following conclusions were obtained by analyzing answers to a questionaire sent to each family (CONPAN, 1976).

A. In both rural and urban zones, breast feeding was extraordinary short; on the average, at 3 months of age, only 20% of the infants were receiving mother's milk.

B. To replace mother's milk, cow's milk was given (usually powdered milk distributed by the National Health Service of the Chilean Government). At some time between the third and fifth month, most mothers added some kind of flour to the milk because they believed that for this age milk was not an adequate food. A few added toasted wheat flour. The majority of mothers, however, bought one of various commercial products composed of wheat flour or corn flour plus some vitamins. This habit was observed in almost 96% of the families at all socio-economic levels. The habit is so popular that most stated that the product they added to the milk was more important than the milk itself. If given the alternative of eliminating one of the two ingredients, they would eliminate milk, not flour. If asked, however, which one they preferred to be distributed by the National Health Service, milk or flour, the majority preferred milk. Further analysis showed that this preference was due to the fact that milk could be consumed by all members of the family. This was not true for the flour, because mothers believed that the commercial product based on flour plus vitamins was only for children. It was also noted that almost all mothers stated that their children liked the taste of toasted wheat flour.

C. Between 9 months and 1 year of age, most children ate solids twice a day in a diet like that the rest of the family. In addition, twice a day they drank cow's milk, or flour, or a mixture of both. Seventy per cent of these diets were insufficient in protein, mainly in animal protein, in terms of the requirements for this age group.

D. When asked which brand of flour mix they preferred among available products, the mothers indicated a preference for the most expensive ones, those with better packaging and higher prestige. When asked which flour they preferred, most mothers indicated that their children liked the taste of chocolate and toasted wheat flour.

E. When asked whether their children were well nourished or undernourished, 97% of the mothers answered that their children were well nourished (65% were really undernourished) and indicated that this question irritated them. On the other hand, when they were asked if a neighbor's child was well nourished or undernourished, 52% replied that the neighbor's child was undernourished.

F. The mothers were asked why the flours were good for children. Their answers were usually the same: because their children grew strong and healthy, because they developed strong bones, because they gained more weight, or because the product had vitamins.

Very valuable information was obtained from this study of the habits and beliefs of a typical population. This was used in developing the successful program.

BASIC STUDIES OF THE PRODUCT

Obviously it was important to utilize the habit of consuming flours, together with the belief that these have high nutritive value. As we have indicated, the mothers believed that at 4 months of age, children should be given something added to milk to make it more nutritious.

The product to be developed should have the following

characteristics:
a) It should provide adequate proteins, considering quality as well as quantity. It should also be adequate in calories.
b) The carbohydrates should be perfectly digestible and produce no gastrointestinal disorders.
c) It should be low in lactose, since studies carried out in the Chilean population show a high prevalence of lactose intolerance. At 4 years of age, 40% of Chilean children are lactose-intolerant.
d) The powdered product must be easily dispersed in water.
e) It should be consumed by the child and not diverted to other uses.
f) The principal ingredients for the mixture must be produced in Chile or at least potentially produced locally.
g) The cost of the new product must be lower than powdered milk.

In accordance with these considerations, a formula was eventually designed consisting of powdered milk (25%) and a vegetable flour mixture (wheat-soy blend, 75%). This mix would accomplish two objectives: the mother would receive, in agreement with her beliefs, a milk enriched with flour in a form ready to feed the child. Secondly, by providing milk mixed with flour, the possibility of adult consumption was reduced in accordance with the population's habit of considering this food solely for children and not to be utilized in other ways. A formula containing only 25% milk would have a decreased lactose load and at the same time its cost would be lower than that of milk.

The first research efforts were carried out with a wheat-soy blend (WSB) without added milk (Monckeberg et al., 1975):

        73.3% Bulgur wheat
        20.0% Defatted soy flour
        4.0% Soy oil
        2.4% Vitamins and minerals.

The Net Protein Utilization (NPU) of this mix, determined in rats by the Miller and Bender method (1955), was 62, which is lower than that obtained for casein under the same conditions (NPU = 70).

The quality of the mix was also studied in infants about 2 months old. The objective of the test was to study the biological value and digestibility of the protein in humans. Small infants were chosen because their rate of growth is higher and their need for good quality protein is greater. At the same time, digestibility and gastrointestinal intolerance can be critical in these small infants. These conditions for evaluating a protein mixture constitute the most exacting test that can be conducted. Four children, between 1 and 4 months old, were fed exclusively with WSB plus corn oil and a mixture of vitamins and minerals to preclude any possible deficit in the diet. A control group of three children of similar age received cow's milk. Both formulas provided

similar caloric, protein, and fat content per unit of volume. The
results were not satisfactory. Children who received WSB, in spite
of protein intakes higher than 4.5 grams of protein per kilo per day,
did not gain weight satisfactorily. The tests were suspended after
ten days and milk was reinstituted.

From these studies we concluded that the protein quality of a
mixture of soy and wheat flour had an acceptable biological value
but not an optimum NPU (62) and that it was not capable of promoting
normal growth if used as the sole source of protein for infants
receiving up to 4.5 grams of protein per kilo per day. The digestibility of the protein mix was also not optimal in these children.
Acceptance by preschool children was good, but those who prepared it
complained that the product did not dissolve well so that sedimentation was very rapid. In addition, the formula was grainy and
felt like sand in the mouth. To improve it, the following modification had to be made:

1.- Addition of 25% milk powder, thus considerably increasing the
    amino acid score.
2.- Treatment of the WSB by an extrusion process to create a product
    dispersed more easily in water and remained suspended. The be-
    nefits of the extrusion process were two-fold: the mixture lost
    much of its grainy texture and, since the process hydrolyzed the
    starch to dextrans and disaccharides, the carbohydrate digesti-
    bility of the mixture was increased significantly.
    The optimal processing conditions used in our experimental
    (Wenger x 25) extruder were as follows:

                    - retention time, 10 to 20 seconds
                    - maximum temperature, 115 to 120°C
                    - inlet moisture, 24%.

The extruded product was dried and ground to 80 mesh.

3.- Addition of 5% cocoa to the mixture to give it a chocolate fla-
    vor. The name "Fortesan" was given to the new formula:

                    - 70% WSB/extruded
                    - 25% powdered milk
                    - 5% powdered cocoa
                    - vitamins and minerals.

By chemical analysis, the formula had the following composition:

                    23% protein
                     4% fat
                     6.6% ash
                    (345 calories per 100 grams)

The vitamin content of Fortesan (100 grams) is as follows:

$$
\begin{array}{lll}
\text{Vitamin B}_1 & 0.57 & \text{mg} \\
\text{Vitamin B}_2 & 0.80 & \text{mg} \\
\text{Vitamin B}_6 & 0.12 & \text{mg} \\
\text{Vitamin B}_{12} & \text{traces} & \\
\text{Vitamin A} & 1.170 & \text{IU} \\
\text{Vitamin D} & 140 & \text{IU} \\
\text{Vitamin E} & 1.0 & \text{IU} \\
\text{Niacin} & 4.2 & \text{mg}
\end{array}
$$

The mineral content of Fortesan (100 grams) is as follows:

Calcium	800	mg
Phosphorus	450	mg
Iron	7.4	mg
Iodine	38	mg

This formula was easy to prepare in tepid water and it remained suspended in water for more than 8 hours. The flavor was a mixture of those of toasted wheat flour and chocolate.

STUDY OF THE BIOLOGICAL QUALITY OF FORTESAN IN RATS

The PER value of Fortesan determined by Campbell's method (Campbell, 1957) and the NPU according to Miller and Bender (1955) at a level of 10% protein calories, compare as follows to a casein control:

Fortesan	2.65 (PER)	70	(NPU)
Casein	2.87 (PER)	72	(NPU)

From these results it is evident that the biological value of Fortesan was similar to that of casein.

STUDY OF THE BIOLOGICAL QUALITY OF FORTESAN IN INFANTS

Eight normal infants were selected for study, with ages ranging between 2 and 4 months. During the study they were hospitalized in a Metabolic Unit for 20 days, when they were fed with Fortesan as the only source of protein, prepared in the following manner:

For each 100 ml: Fortesan	10	g
Sugar	10	g
Corn oil	2	g

This mixture gives 91 calories per 100 ml. The infants received 130 calories per kilo per day and 3 grams of protein per kilo per day for the 20 day period. At the beginning and end of the experiment, the following tests were made: urine analysis, urine culture, complete blood count, total serum proteins, carotenemia, sedimentation rate, and flocculation test.

Both at the beginning and end of the experiment, all the laboratory examinations showed normal values. In <u>Figure 1</u>, the weight
curves of the eight infants suggest that weight gains were normal
or better than normal. During the 20 day period, growth averaged
1.4 cm, which is also normal for this age group. Acceptability was
good, no digestive disorders were noted, and the infants had normal
stools throughout the study.

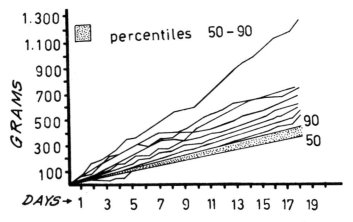

FIG. 1. Weight increment of eight normal children fed Fortesan as
the only protein source.

A second experiment was performed with severely undernourished,
marasmic infants. This type of infant is very hard to treat, even
with milk, because of its disturbed metabolism. This makes adequate
utilization of the various nutrients difficult, so that the children
are highly susceptible to digestive disturbances. These patients
experience difficulties in intestinal absorption of lactose and also
fats. The test of Fortesan in treating infants with severe marasmic
malnutrition was interesting because, if this formula were capable
of "curing" such an infant, it would mean that its digestibility
was very good and that the protein was of good quality.

Eight infants were chosen, with ages between 4 and 11 months,
who showed signs of severe malnutrition with weight 60% less than
normal for their ages. Weights at the time of the experiment ranged
from 2.7 to 5.1 kilograms. The experiment began with administration

of skimmed milk to which rape seed oil and sunflower oil were added during a period of 15 days. At the end of 15 days, all of the infants received Fortesan to which corn oil had been added. While they received cow's milk or Fortesan, metabolic balances of 5 days duration were performed.

The Fortesan was prepared as shown in Table 1. This mixture or milk was administered ad libitum during the entire period of 15 days; the total volume ingested varied between 130 and 150 ml per kilo per day. The caloric intake was approximately 130 calories per kilo per day and the protein intake was about 4.1 grams per kilo per day.

TABLE 1

Preparation of Fortesan (100 ml)

ITEM	GRAMS	PROTEIN	FATS	CARBOHYDRATES	CALORIES
Fortesan mixture	12.0	2.9	0.2	7.0	--
Corn oil	3.5	--	3.5	--	--
Maltose dextrose	6.0	--	--	6.0	--
Total		2.9	3.7	13.0	97

Both diets, the control diet (milk) and Fortesan, had excellent acceptability. The average weight gain during the control period was 6.7 grams per kilo per day for the control diet, and 5.7 grams per kilo per day with Fortesan. The difference is not significant; in both cases the weight gains could be considered good for this type of patient.

The results of nitrogen balance studies can be seen in Table 2.

TABLE 2

Nitrogen Balance Study of Fortesan and Control Diet

ITEM	CONTROL DIET	FORTESAN
	mg N per kilo per day	
Nitrogen ingestion	528	610
Fecal nitrogen excretion	110	133
Nitrogen absorbed	418 (79%)	477 (78%)
Urinary nitrogen excretion	333	300
Nitrogen retained	85 (16%)	177 (29%)

Protein utilization can be determined by expressing retained nitrogen as a percentage of absorbed nitrogen. Twenty per cent was utilized during the control diet (skimmed milk) and 37% was utilized
on Fortesan. The difference in nitrogen utilization is statistically
significant (p < 0.001).

     The results of fat balance studies can be seen in Table 3.
In the group fed Fortesan, one observes better absorption of fats
and a higher percentage of retained fat. One cannot draw a definite
conclusion from this difference, since the oils used in the control
group (rape seed oil and sunflower oil) were different from the oil
used with Fortesan (corn oil). Note, however, that better absorption of fat did occur in those who received Fortesan. The results
of this experiment indicate that Fortesan is a good mixture that
can be tolerated and digested by undernourished infants. The percentage of nitrogen retained was higher when Fortesan was fed than
observed during milk feeding. This test demonstrates the excellent
quality of Fortesan as a protein and energy source.

TABLE 3

Fat Balance Study of Fortesan and Control Diet

ITEM	CONTROL DIET	FORTESAN
	g per kilo per day	
Fat ingestion	4.9	4.6
Fat excretion	1.0	0.31
Fat absorbed	3.9	4.2
Percentage of absorption	80%	93%

ACCEPTABILITY TEST OF FORTESAN IN THE GENERAL POPULATION

     An acceptability test for Fortesan in the province of Curicó
was conducted for 9 months. Approximately 1,400 children from one
to six years old were selected to receive Fortesan, while a control
group of 350 children of the same age group received a similar quantity of powdered milk (12% fat). Fortesan was distributed in 8
primary health centers of the National Health Service (NHS) and
the skimmed milk in three other centers of the NHS. Every 40 days
the children were examined, weighed, and measured in those places
where the Fortesan or milk was distributed. The mothers received
two boxes of Fortesan (1 Kg. each), with instructions for preparation. Taking advantage of the occasion, the mothers of both programs discussed infant nutrition and related topics on distribution
day. A program of house visits was developed to assure that the
mothers were following instructions properly with respect to

preparation and use of Fortesan or milk and to provide additional information on nutrition and hygiene. At the end of the experiment, tests were performed on blood samples from two groups (serum proteins, hematocrit, hemoglobin) to determine if significant differences appeared between groups receiving Fortesan or milk for 9 months.

The compliance of mothers receiving Fortesan to the eight scheduled test sessions was 87%; for mothers receiving milk, compliance was 84%. During these visits, mothers were given the respective infant food. These results show the high acceptability of both products during the 9 month study period.

Table 4 shows the six-month weight and length increments for children receiving Fortesan or powdered milk. The differences between the two groups are statistically significant in favor of Fortesan. This result is probably due to Fortesan being mainly consumed by children, but the powdered milk, by the entire family. With respect to blood tests performed, no significant differences were observed between the groups; the values varied within the normal range.

TABLE 4

Mean Weight and Length, Six Month Increment for Children

Receiving Fortesan and Powdered Milk

TYPE OF INFANT FOOD	WEIGHT GAIN (g)	LENGTH INCREMENT (cm)
Fortesan	1230	4.52
Powdered milk	1056	3.01
Student's t test p	<0.001	<0.001

An interesting observation was the significant difference observed between the number of diarrheal episodes in the two groups. For the 9-month observation period, the group receiving Fortesan had a mean of 0.8 ± 0.52 episodes per child and the milk group had 3.6 ± 1.1. This lower incidence for the Fortesan group was significant at the $p < 0.001$ level. This difference may be attributed to the lower lactose content in Fortesan since other variables such as environmental sanitation and socioeconomic status were carefully controlled and were not different between the groups. The significant difference in diarrheal episodes could also help to explain the greater weight gains in the Fortesan group.

Before this study was finished, the families were surveyed in order to ascertain their opinions of Fortesan. When mothers were asked what they did with the Fortesan they received, 88% answered

that they gave it to their child and he liked it. The remaining 12%
said that they received it but did not give it to their children
because they did not like it or it gave them diarrhea. Most mothers,
63%, preferred giving Fortesan as a hot beverage; 12% preferred it
as a cold drink, and smaller groups as porridge, either hot, 20%,
or cold, 5%. Asked if their husbands took Fortesan, 25% said, "Yes",
at least occasionally". This figure is less than the 58% reported
in the milk group.

When asked about the flavors their children liked, 70% answered, "Toasted wheat flour" and 6% said, "Chocolate". Ninety per
cent of mothers said they had no difficulties in preparing Fortesan;
that it was easy to dissolve. If asked about the appropriateness
of the package, 98% said it was appropriate. Their estimated price
for Fortesan was similar to the market price of like products made
by Nestle (in Chile, Nestle had a virtual monopoly of infant
feeding products).

Mothers were also asked what infant food they would give their
child if Fortesan were not available. Forty five per cent answered
they would give milk, 17% said Milo (a Nestle product with 9% protein), 12% preferred toasted wheat flour, and 10% would give tea.
When asked what product would be their choice if all were distributed free of charge by the National Health Service, 32% said Fortesan, 26% answered Nido milk (Nestle's powdered milk), and 14% said
they would choose Milo. It should be pointed out that Nestle's
Milo is very similar to Fortesan but is widely publicized by radio
and television.

In summary, the long term acceptability of Fortesan during
this 9 month study was very satisfactory. We believe this favorable result is due to the quality of the product, its presentation,
and also to the fact that Fortesan was formulated in accordance
with the dietary habits and beliefs of Chilean mothers.

PROMOTION TO ACHIEVE A POLICY DECISION

To obtain support from a government for nutrition programs and
efficient policies is not easy. Support can only be obtained when
such programs provide political benefits and demand minimal investments. One should not forget that the first priority of any government is to remain in power. Only by keeping this basic fact in
mind can support for a nutrition program be obtained. This should
be taken into consideration by scientists working on applied nutrition as well as planners. To be realistic, one must calculate not
only the nutritional and economic cost-benefit relations of a specific intervention program, but also the political costs and benefits. In practice, this political aspect represents the fundamental basis that decides, one way or another, support by any government. It is noteworthy as an example that almost all countries

that have implemented efficient school feeding or supplementary food programs, have done so as political decisions based on political, not on nutritional benefits derived from these programs. Very few have implemented programs to promote breast feeding, nutrition education, or other programs that could be better nutritionally but do not provide quick, significant political dividends. Thus, after nutritional and economic cost-benefits have been optimized, the problem becomes one of making the program attractive for possible political benefits.

The first step is long and should also be aimed at creating awareness of the malnutrition among preschool children, not only by politicians or others seeking power, but mainly at the community level. Only when the community is fully conscious of the problem, will a force develop that the power seeker or politician can try to exploit. Several ways are available for educating the community, but undoubtedly the most efficient is the use of social communication systems. Those who undertake this responsibility should abandon all commitments or participation in political activities or movements.

On the other hand, in addition to a strong community awareness alternative solutions to the problem must be offered with stress on their technical imperatives. This latter aspect is important because if expectations are raised without understanding the facts, increased awareness of the nutrition problem will probably lead to equivocal actions with strong political motivation but with little impact on the nutritional problem. This task is complex and filled with risks, because the government that happens to be in charge will not be sympathetic to constant publicity given to a serious problem such as infant malnutrition. Whoever undertakes this responsibility runs the risk of being considered an enemy of the government, but this risk can be lessened by refusal to be utilized by politicians who oppose the political system in power.

These comments are based mainly on the experiences of one of the authors of this paper in Chile over the last 20 years. It is perfectly possible that the strategy in other countries and under different political systems should be quite different.

In the case of Chile, the following steps occurred. During the last few years, by various means of social communications, a national awareness of the nutritional problems of preschool children was created. At times, the measures taken have been guided by political imperatives than by real, significant nutritional motives. Nevertheless, in the long run this tendency has been corrected. During 1970, presidential elections were held in Chile. Awareness reached such a degree that all three candidates had, as cornerstones to their political campaigns, programs aimed at preventing malnutrition in children.

If support by a government is achieved and if its decision is
to carry out this or any other program in a technical way, all
efforts should be aimed at implementing and assuring the continuity
of this effort. This step is also very risky for those with a responsibility of bringing the program into practice. Every government has its supporters and adversaries within and beyond national
boundaries. Necessarily the program will be identified with the
government. The technical staff working in the program will be
compromised in some measure. The important thing on this issue is
to achieve a balance between the degree of compromise and one's
moral responsibility as a technical expert.

IMPLEMENTATION OF INDUSTRIAL PRODUCTION

Once the political support from the government has been achieved, the norms and regulations required for production, marketing,
and distribution of the product should be dictated by the government.
Will the product be placed in the open market? Will it be distributed
free or partly subsidized? The government must also decide who
will manufacture the product. Will it be made by state-owned or
privately owned enterprises? Finally, will the channels for distribution be the established commercial ones or will some state agency
be used?

In the case of Chile, all of these questions have been decided:
a) the products are distributed free of charge, b) distribution is
handled by the National Health Service and coordinated with the entire health sector policy (Chile has a socialized medical system
initiated 25 years ago. The National Health Service has 300 hos-
pitals and 1520 primary Health Care Centers. Nearly 90% of all
physicians are employed by the National Health Service or other
State Health agencies), and c) production is carried out by private
enterprises.

After deciding that the products should be manufactured by
private enterprises, the government must develop a strategy to
achieve support of the private sector. Although it may appear
obvious, a reminder is needed that the basic motivation that guides
private enterprises is the potential profit from a given investment.
Considering this fact, to secure their support, an adequate return
from invested capital must be assured.

In the case of Chile, the support of numerous local enterprises
has been achieved. Based on the advantages of a secure, state-
supported demand for the product within the framework of a free
market where supply and demand are balanced, potential investors
were assured that the state's annual budget of $50 million for
supplementary infant feeding programs would be disbursed in accordance with open bidding for contracts to supply the products to
be purchased. This is evidently an important step, but within the

constraints of a developing country's economic system, this is not enough. Other prerequisites are also crucial.

a) First, potential investors basically distrust the capacity of the state to maintain such a program long enough to justify their investment. A credibility gap exists that in some situations cannot be bridged. To overcome this obstacle, two alternatives can be used. The state may either grant more profitable franchises through taxes or otherwise, to make investment more attractive, or collaborate with a credible technical team that has the respect of investors. This credibility must be technical, executive, and moral. Technical credibility depends on the ability of the technical team to offer not only a secure market for the product, but also advice on appropriate technology. Moreover, the team must provide industrial scale feasibility studies for the manufacture of the specific product and also of other products, for internal consumption or for export, that can be made with the same basic investment. The idea is to convince investors to develop a food industry using, as a starting point or as a security margin, the assured government demand.

Finally, investors must be convinced that the government's technical team has sufficient executive power to operate effectively and exercises this power with the moral authority the task demands.

In the case of Chile, even without new benefits, enough credibility has been achieved that several investors have installed or reconditioned necessary manufacturing facilities.

b) The collaboration of the state's technical team should go even further. It should help to obtain internal or external loans needed for investment under the best possible conditions.

c) Finally, possible interferences such as food donations from agricultural surpluses in other countries (WSB, CSM—corn-soy-milk, etc.) must be eliminated. By accepting such apparently attractive donations, national solutions are usually delayed. In the case of Chile, this problem was handled by accepting and even promoting such donations, but utilising them as raw materials for manufacturing the definitive product. We requested from AID (Agency for International Development, USA) that the WSB and/or CSM to be donated be given to those industries which had won the bidding and that they utilize these as raw material, subtracting these contributions from the final cost. By this mechanism, donations would not only not inhibit development of a national solution but, on the contrary, would stimulate it by reducing the costs of the program.

MANAGEMENT OF THE SYSTEM BY THE NATIONAL

FOOD AND NUTRITION COUNCIL

The success of the program depends not only on logistic efficiency but also on the prestige it achieves. Fortunately, in the
case of Chile, we had the necessary infrastructure to store and dis-
tribute these foods even in the farthest corners of the country.
This infrastructure is based on the National Health Service, which
has storage and distribution facilities in 1,600 locations throughout the nation. These are the primary care Health Centers, the
staffs of which include 600 nutritionists carrying out educational
and promotional efforts.

But all of this is not enough if the product distributed lacks
prestige in the eyes of the recipient. If the product is to be distributed free of charge, that in itself can make it less prestigious.
The normal attitude of the beneficiary is to believe that if something is free, it must be second-rate. This inference must be avoided at all costs. It is necessary to eliminate the concept of a
product designed to "feed the poor". This purpose can be perfectly
achieved by using certain tricks.

a) The product must be of excellent quality, with flavors that please
   children, and at the same time be easy to prepare and dissolve
   in water.

b) The product should have an excellent presentation and package;
   this will make it attractive, just like any product in the
   conventional market.

c) Advertisement of the product should be based, not on the preven-
   tion of malnutrition, but on the contrary, on the positive advantages of the product. Nobody likes to accept that he belongs to
   the lowest strata of society. In summary, the product will
   succeed if in the perception of the recipient, it will elevate
   his social status. If, on the contrary, it appears to lower his
   social status, rejection will be immediate.

d) The product must also succeed in the middle income group; only
   then can it be accepted by the low income group that is our
   true target. These facts being realized, industries were com-
   pelled to place the product on the open market before they became
   eligible to take part in the National Health Service bidding.
   Moreover, the decision on the bids are based not only on the
   price of the proposal but also on the share that the product has
   in the open market. In other words, if, for example, a given
   product sells 0.5 ton in the open market and this represents 70%
   of the total demand in the open market, and if the state needs
   17 thousand tons for its program, it will purchase 70% of 17

thousand tons of that product. This means that the various industries will put tremendous effort into competing for the open market, improving the quality and advertisement of their product to gain a greater share of the open market. In the final analysis, the program gains prestige in the low income group since the product is accepted by the middle income group. This trick is responsible to a significant degree for the success of the program and eliminates the concept of "food for the poor".

e) It is very useful to tie distribution of these products to the overall health program. The distribution of food is a great incentive to a mother for taking her child to the primary health center, where he will have his well-baby check-up by a physician and receive immunizations and the mother will be exposed to educational and other programs.

SUMMARY

In this paper we have described all the steps needed to develop an efficient program for distributing children's fortified formulas. The easiest steps are to develop the formulas on an experimental and laboratory basis. The real obstacles lie in implementation at the national level.

All that has been described applies to experience in Chile, which we consider very successful because of the acceptance of the program as well as spectacular advances in preventing malnutrition. The figures for 1977 show that combining all degrees of malnutrition in the under six age group, the prevalence is now 12.2% compared to nearly 60% found 10 years ago. This progress is due, not only to the specific program, but also to the many others that constitute the national food and nutrition policy (CONPAN, 1976).

This success is due to the persistent, skilled effort of many professional and technical staff members. It is impractical to acknowledge all individual contributions here. The National Food and Nutrition Council, the National Health Service, Universities, Research Bodies, and private enterprizes have all contributed to this joint effort.

The purpose of this presentation is that this experience may benefit other countries with similar problems.

ACKNOWLEDGMENT

We thank the Agency for International Development (AID) for financial assistance.

REFERENCES

Araya, M., Lacassie, I., Contreras, I., Brunser, O., Rona, R., Salinas, J., Jaque, G., Ojeda, E., Aguayo, M. and Monckeberg, F. (1972). Lactose intolerance incidence in Chile and conditioning factors. Proceedings of the 9th International Congress of Nutrition, Mexico.

Campbell, J. A. (1957). In "FAO Committee on Protein Requirements, Food and Agriculture Organization of the United Nations, Rome, Italy, Volume 16, Nutrition Studies".

CONPAN (1976). Food and Nutrition Policy in Chile. Documento de CONPAN, Ahumada 236, 7º piso, Santiago, Chile.

Miller, D. S. and Bender A. E. (1955). The determination of net protein utilization by a shortened method. Brit. J. Nutr., 9, 382.

Monckeberg, F., Donoso, G. and Valiente, A. (1967). Análysis y commentarios de la encuesta nutritiva y de las condiciones de vida de la población infantil de la provincia de Curicó. Rev. Child. Ped., 38, 522.

Monckeberg, F., Yanez, E., Ballester, D., Chichester, C. O. and Lee, Tung-Ching. (1975). Effects of processing on the nutritive value of WSB-skim milk mixtures for infants. In "Protein Nutritional Quality of Foods and Feeds", Part 2, M. Friedman (Ed.), Marcel Dekker, New York, pp. 417-431.

3

IMPROVEMENT OF THE PROTEIN QUALITY OF CORN WITH SOYBEAN
PROTEIN

Ricardo Bressani, Luiz G. Elías and
J. Edgar Braham

Division of Agricultural and Food Sciences

Institute of Nutrition of Central America
and Panama (INCAP), P.O. Box 1188, Guatemala,
Central America.

ABSTRACT

In most Central American countries, lime-treated
corn provides 31% of the total protein and 45% of the
energy intake, and beans 24% of the protein and 12%
of the calories. Such diet is low in protein quality and quantity, as well as in energy. To overcome
these deficiencies, corn can be supplemented either
with its limiting amino acids, lysine and tryptophan,
or, better still, with whole soybeans which improve
not only the amount and quality of the protein consumed
but, because of their high oil content, the energy intake as well. In addition, animal experiments have
shown that for maximum utilization of these nutrients,
adequate vitamin and mineral intake is indispensable.

At a level of 15 parts of whole soybean or 8 parts
soybean-derived products, to 85-92 parts of corn there
were no significant changes in the rheological or organoleptic characteristics of the tortilla prepared there
of. Higher levels of soybean products, however, may
affect the consistency of the lime-treated corn dough
and, therefore, the tortilla acceptability. Since corn
is usually cooked, but not ground, at home, the soybean

supplement can be successfully added at the wet-milling
stage of dough preparation or whole soybeans and corn
may be cooked together, when a nutritional intervention
is desired at the village level. At an industrial scale,
if whole soybeans are used, they may be cooked together
with corn, and if soy flour is used, this can be mixed
at the end of the process when the cooked corn is ground
to a flour.

A flow diagram for supplementing corn with 15% whole
soybeans is presented. If interventions of this nature
are to be successful, there is need for increasing the
prestige of corn-based foods, as well as of nutrition
education programs in these populations.

INTRODUCTION

The importance of cereal grains in the nutrition of
millions of people around the world is a well recognized
fact. Because of their relatively high intake in the
developing countries, cereal grains can not be considered only as energy sources, since they also provide significant amounts of protein. However, it is also of
general knowledge that cereal grains have a low protein
concentration of a quality limited by deficiencies of
certain essential amino acids, mainly lysine. The above
statements are the reason for the intensive research
efforts that are being made to improve the protein
quality of cereal grains either by genetic means or
through agronomic interventions. Extraordinary results
have already been obtained, although in some cases
other desirable attributes of the cereal crop such as
yield and physical characteristics still have to be
improved. In the meantime, while the goal for increased
productivity is being fulfilled, the protein quality
remains the same. Because of well-defined sociological
trends in developing countries, it can be stated that
in future years more and more people will depend on
industrialized food products. It would appear, therefore, that a logical and efficient way of improving
the protein quality of these foods would be by supplementation procedures.

THE NUTRITIONAL QUALITY OF TYPICAL DIETS CONSUMED IN SOME LATIN AMERICAN COUNTRIES

To start the description of the work concerning improvement of the nutritional quality of corn in the form of the traditional tortilla consumed in several Latin American countries, consideration of the type of diet ingested by the rural population of these countries seems adequate. Since preschool children are more affected by the lack of a balanced and ample nutrient intake, the diet ordinarily consumed by this population group will be discussed first.

The data shown in Table 1 were obtained by means of dietary surveys. The values represent the weight of foods as consumed. As they indicate, consumption includes on the average 13 food items, with cereal grains making up 42% of their total weight. The starchy-type foods represent 19%; beans (Phaseolus vulgaris) about 15%; vegetables, around 6.5% and animal food products approximately 4% not including meat broth. Since the data represent average values from a relatively large group of children, it is obvious that some of them probably do not have access to any animal protein source or even beans, and that those who consume a little of these items, probably do so at the most 2 or 3 times per week. Therefore, the nutrient intake for most of the children is probably quite poor, and the true protein quality of such an intake of foods difficult to evaluate. Of the total intake of 325 g, 32% come from corn, food that is ingested in the largest amount, followed on an item basis by beans (Murillo, Cabezas & Bressani, 1974).

Chemical analyses of a diet composite indicated that from the total intake of 325 g, 210 g are water -equivalent to 64.7% - and 115 g dry matter -equivalent to 35% of the total intake. The dry matter provides 14 g protein, 2.9 g fat, 2.6 g minerals and 455 kcal. Protein content of the diet as consumed is 4.3%, with 0.9% fat and 140 kcal/100 g. On the basis of the protein and calorie content of corn and beans as consumed, calculations indicate that lime-treated corn provides 31% of the total protein, and 45% of the

Table 1. Food intake of preschool children
in rural Guatemala.

Food	Food intake as consumed	
	g/day	%
Tortillas*	103.5	31.9
Bread	19.5	6.0
Rice	16.1	4.9
Beans	47.9	14.7
Sugar	28.9	8.9
Meat broth	26.4	8.2
Beef	4.8	1.5
Egg	7.8	2.4
Vegetables	21.2	6.5
Fruits	29.4	9.1
Potato	4.3	1.3
Bean broth	12.5	3.8
Coffee	2.6	0.8
Total	324.9	100.0

*   Lime-treated corn.
    Data taken from Murillo, Cabezas
    & Bressani (1974).

energy intake, while beans supply 24% of the protein
and 12% of the energy. Therefore, in terms of protein
and calorie contribution to the whole diet, corn
constitutes the main food item.

BASIC NUTRITIONAL STUDIES ON THE IMPROVEMENT OF THE PROTEIN QUALITY OF CORN

There are many studies published on the subject
of improving the protein quality of corn proteins, and
it is already well known that these are deficient in
the essential amino acids lysine and tryptophan.

a. Amino Acid Supplementation

Table 2 presents a summary of various studies
carried out in experimental animals with lime-treated
corn. As the evidence indicates, a limited improvement
from lysine addition alone was obtained, but no effect
resulted from the addition of only tryptophan. However,
when both amino acids were added together, a significant
increase in weight gain and protein quality was observed.
The addition of other amino acids together with lysine
and tryptophan did not improve further animal performance (Elías & Bressani, 1972), as has been reported by
other investigators (Sure, 1953; Sauberlich, Chang &
Salmon, 1953). Data of the same nature have also been
obtained in children (Bressani, 1971). The nitrogen
balance results shown in Table 3 summarize the effects
of the addition of amino acids from various studies
when protein intake exclusively from corn was given to
groups of children. As the data indicate, positive
nitrogen balance is obtained when intake of corn
protein was approximately 3.0 g/kg/day. Furthermore,
the single effects of lysine and tryptophan, which
are similar in magnitude are more evident at the higher
nitrogen intake level. The largest improvement in
quality is observed when both amino acids are added
together, improved further by the addition of isoleucine (Bressani,1969). These results indicate, therefore,
the importance of increasing the quality of corn
proteins as a means of improving its utilization and
provide better nutrition to the consumer, particularly
to those who require a higher quantity and better
protein.

Table 2.   Supplementation of lime-treated corn
with amino acids.

Amino Acids added, % *	Average weight gain, g	PER
None	32	1.21
Lysine (0.31%)	41	1.51
Tryptophan (0.10%)	22	1.15
Lysine (0.31%) + Tryptophan (0.05%)	100	2.66
Lysine (0.31%) + Tryptophan (0.05%) + Threonine (0.20%) + Isoleucine (0.20%) + Methionine (0.10%)	112	2.69

*   L-Lysine Hcl, DL-Tryptophan, DL-Isoleucine,
    DL-Threonine, DL-Methionine.

Data taken from Elías & Bressani (1972).

Table 3. Effect of the addition of amino acids to lime-treated corn at various levels of nitrogen intake measured by nitrogen balance in children.

Diet	NI mg/kg/day	NR mg/kg/day	Nitrogen Balance NI mg/kg/day	NR mg/kg/day	NI mg/kg/day	NR mg/kg/day
Lime-treated corn alone (B)	469	14	326	-5	238	-10
B + Tryptophan	465	33	327	-17	-	-
B + Lysine	482	38	335	24	239	-4
B + Try + Lys	461	83	328	36	239	30
B + Try + Lys + Ileu	475	108	335	40	240	46
B + Try + Lys + Ileu + Met	469	90	314	13	240	23
Milk	458	70	364	73	-	-

b.   Protein Supplementation

     Since previous results (Murillo, Cabezas & Bressani,
1974) have shown that the diet consumed by children
is low in total protein, a more adequate improvement
of the protein quality of corn would be one which would
include in a single intervention increased protein
content and higher protein quality. Therefore, studies
were carried out to learn which were the optimum levels,
in terms of protein quality, of various protein supplements to be added to corn. Some of these results measured in experimental animals are shown in Table 4. All
proteins added increased the protein quality of corn,
particularly those which are good sources of the two
limiting amino acids in this cereal grain protein (Bressani & Marenco, 1963). Furthermore, protein content
was also increased in the mixture from about 2 to 4 g.
Other workers have also reported similar improvement
in corn protein quality by protein supplementation
(Del Valle, F. R.; Perez Villaseñor, 1974; Green et
al, 1976; Green et al., 1977 McPherson & Suh Yun L. Ou,
1976).

     Through this approach, it was felt that the basic
corn-bean diet consumed by the child population would
be improved in terms of total protein quality and
quantity. Because of the higher availability of soybeans, its possible local production and relatively
low cost studies with this legume were carried out and
the results are presented in Figure 1. The Figure shows
the effect on weight gain of rats and on protein efficiency as soybean protein is added to a fixed level of
corn. These results suggest that 4-6 g of soybean
protein are probably optimum amounts to add in terms
of protein quality improvement, which are close to the
levels found to interfere less with the physical and
organoleptic characteristics associated with tortillas
(Elías & Bressani, 1972; Bressani & Marenco, 1963).

     More recent considerations suggest that besides
higher protein content and quality, it would also be

Table 4. Recommended levels of protein concentrates to supplement lime-treated corn.

Protein concentrate	Level %	PER
None	–	1.00
Casein	4.0	2.24
Fish protein concentrate	2.5	2.44
Soybean protein isolate	5.0	2.30
Soybean flour	8.0	2.25
Torula yeast	2.5	1.97

Data taken from Bressani & Marenco (1963).

desirable to increase energy content. This was accomplished by the addition of whole soybeans to corn, which increase protein content, improve protein quality and provide energy as well because of the oil they contain (Bressani, Murillo & Elías, 1974). The results of various studies in this regard have indicated that soybeans could be cooked together with corn in the traditional way it is processed in some Latin American

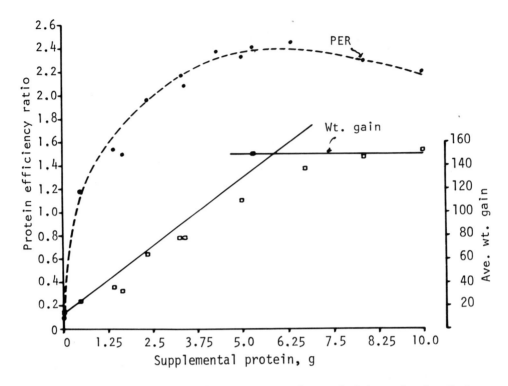

Figure 1. Response to soy supplementation (animals)

countries (Bressani, Murillo, Elías, 1974; Del Valle,
Montemayor, Bourges, 1976; Franz, 1975).

      Some results are shown in Figure 2. In this case
corn and soybeans were cooked together following the
process commonly used by native populations, that is
a cooking treatment with lime, followed by washing,
grinding, dehydration and final grinding to produce a
tortilla flour. These preparations were then fed to
rats at variable protein concentration but with total
dietary fat constant. The results shown in the Figure
indicate optimum protein quality as NPR from the addition of 12-16% soybeans equivalent to 4.6 - 6.1 g of
supplementary protein. These values are not different
from those found when using soybean meal, presented
above or reported in other studies (Bressani, Murillo,
Elías, 1974; Del Valle, Montemayor & Bourges, 1976;
Franz, 1975).

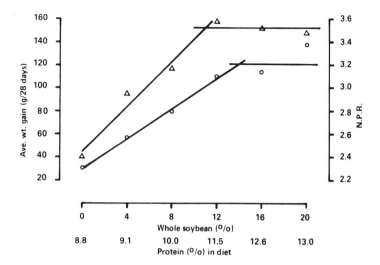

Figure 2.   Response to whole soybean supplementation (animals)

Further studies have been carried out to compare in one experiment the effect of soybean flour and full fat soybeans. Representative nutritional results of this approach are shown in Table 5, where one may observe that a 15% addition of whole soybeans is equal in its effects to 8% soybean flour, both of them inducing an equal or similar increase in protein content and quality. The data shown in the Table also indicate that the additional energy provided by soybeans is of nutritional benefit, as proven by the results in the fourth line of the Table. Therefore, by using 15% whole soybeans, with 85% corn, a food equal to the traditional tortilla but of much better nutritional value, is produced (Bressani, Murillo & Elías, 1974).

Other sources of soybean protein have also been tested. Representative results are presented in Table 6. The values shown are the result of various studies performed with four different soybean products, which include a 50% soybean flour, a soybean protein isolate with 90% protein, texturized soybean protein and whole soybeans. The levels of soybean products shown were chosen on the basis of maximum protein quality improvement, conditioned by technological properties of the

Table 5. Protein quality of lime-treated corn
supplemented with lime-cooked whole soybeans.

	PER	Utilizable protein, %
Lime-treated corn [1,2]	0.95	2.1
85% lime-treated corn + 15% lime-treated whole soybeans [1]	1.98	7.1
92% lime-treated corn + 8% soybean flour [1]	1.98	6.6
85% lime-treated corn + 15% lime-treated whole soybeans [3]	1.98	7.1
Casein [1]	2.60	9.4

[1]   5% refined soybean oil added.
[2]   Diet contained: 9.0% protein. All other diets
       had 12.5% protein.
[3]   No oil added.

Data taken from Bressani, Murillo & Elías (1974).

Table 6. Protein quality improvement of maize from
the addition of various soybean products.

Type of soy product supplement used	Amount added %	Protein efficiency	
		without	with
		supplement	
Flour	8	1.00	2.25
Flour	8	1.26	2.43
Flour	8	1.65	2.50
Flour	8	1.75	2.50
Protein isolate	5	1.00	2.30
TVP	8	1.65	2.31
Beans	15	0.95	1.98
Beans	15	1.17	2.53

final product. The improvement in protein quality is
observed when the PER values of corn with and without
the supplement are compared. The data suggest that
maximum improvement obtained does not go above a PER
value of 2.50. This is considered high enough and it
does not interfere with the technological properties
of the final product. A second aspect of interest is
that all soybean products are capable of increasing the
protein quality of corn to about the same extent. However, it appears to be conditioned by the quality of
the particular sample of lime-treated corn used, when
the supplement provides from 4 to 6 g of additional
protein.

A batch of lime-treated corn supplemented with
soybean and lysine was also tested in children using
the nitrogen balance methodology (Viteri, Martínez
& Bressani, 1972). The results of its nutritional
evaluation are shown in Table 7. At equal nitrogen
intake, the soybean-supplemented corn gave nitrogen
retention values, expressed as percentage of the intake,
similar to those obtained with milk protein, and both
protein sources twice as high as the retention value
from feeding lime-treated corn alone. Of interest is
also the results of feeding corn and common beans,
which resulted in only a small increase in nitrogen
retention.

THE NEED FOR OTHER NUTRIENTS

Research in nutrition, particularly in developing
countries, has concentrated up to recent times in
providing systems to deliver protein quantity and
quality to the human population. More recently the
emphasis has shifted to one of calories, which is
considered to be more limiting than protein. The fact
is that both are really needed, with protein quality
being slightly more important if populations must depend
in future years primarily on cereal grains. As important,
and receiving little attention are other nutrients, such
as vitamins and some minerals. These are needed as
catalysts for the efficient use of energy and protein
by the organism and they may be deficient in the cooked
food consumed. To show their importance some results

Table 7. Protein quality of soybean flour-supplemented tortilla in children.

	Nitr. Balance			Nitrogen	
	Int.	Abs.	Ret.	Absorbed	Retained
	mg/kg/day			%	
Lime-treated corn	192	144	30	75	16
Lime-treated corn + 8% soybean flour + 0.1% Lys	197	154	63	78	32
Milk	195	157	75	80	38
Lime-treated corn (87%) + beans (13%)	207	150	36	72	17

are presented in Table 8 (Elías & Bressani, 1972). In
this case a diet based on corn and beans was supplemented with vitamins and a mineral mixture when the diet
was with and without amino acid supplements. The
results clearly show an improvement in the utilization
of the protein when either a vitamin or mineral mixture
was added. This effect was not observed upon increasing
the energy content of the diet. Furthermore, the
addition of vitamins, minerals, lysine and tryptophan
together resulted in a highly significant improvement
in weight gain and protein efficiency ratio, demonstrating the role they can play to improve the quality of
simple diets of corn and beans. Other studies suggested
thiamine, riboflavin, niacin and Vitamin A to be useful
(Bressani & Marenco, 1963).

Based on the above observations, as well as on
other results, a protein, vitamin and mineral supplement
was formulated to supplement lime-treated corn. The
protein source utilized was soybean flour. The formula
of this supplement is shown in Table 9, and its effectiveness has been tested in animal experiments in the
laboratory (Elías & Bressani, 1972).

PHYSICAL AND BIOLOGICAL CHARACTERISTICS OF TORTILLA WITH AND WITHOUT SUPPLEMENTS

Nutritional improvement of the supplemented corn
is only one of the aspects involved in the solution
of the protein problem. From the chemical and biological point of view, the supplement increases protein
content and that of the limiting amino acids, thus
improving the protein quality. If whole soybeans are
used, oil content also increases. Other added nutrients
such as vitamins, increase the overall nutritive value
of the food. From the industrial and the consumer point
of view, physical and organoleptic characteristics of
the supplemented food are also very important points
to be taken into consideration. The addition of synthetic amino acids is not expected to change those characteristics; however, the use of a protein supplement
may have an effect on the rheological and organoleptic
properties of the corn dough used in the preparation
of tortillas made by the process described in Figure 3.

Table 8. Limiting nutritional factors in basic corn-bean preschool children's diet. [1]

Nutrients added	Average diet intake, g/28 days	Average weight gain, g/28 days	Protein Efficiency Ratio
None	271 ± 8.8 [2]	26 ± 2.3 [2]	1.09 ± 0.072 [2]
Vitamins	367 ± 18.7	49 ± 4.0	1.52 ± 0.06
Minerals	308 ± 15.8	65 ± 4.3	1.91 ± 0.06
Lysine + Tryptophan	266 ± 14.4	26 ± 2.5	1.10 ± 0.08
Vit + Min Lys + Tryp	484 ± 14.7	107 ± 4.9	2.55 ± 0.06

[1] Basic diet: 72.4% corn + 8.1% beans.
[2] Standard error.
Data taken from Elías & Bressani (1972).

Table 9. Formulation of lime-treated corn supplement.

Ingredient	Consumption of the supplement	Content of 8% added to maize, g
Soya flour	97.5000	7.800000
L-Lysine HCl	1.5000	0.120000
Thiamine	0.0268	0.002196
Riboflavin	0.0162	0.001296
Niacinamide	0.1930	0.015440
Ferric Orthophosphate	0.6000	0.048000
Vitamin A 250 SD	0.0313	0.002504
Corn starch	0.1327	0.010616
Total	100.0000	8.000000

Data taken from Elías & Bressani (1972).

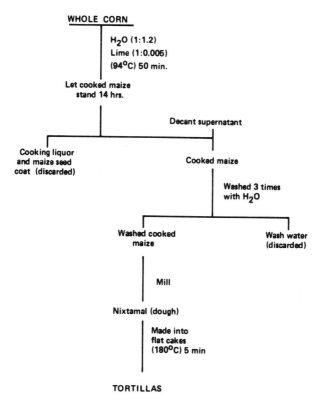

Figure 3.   Tortilla preparation.

Unfortunately, only limited research has been carried out on the rheological characteristics of the corn dough itself, mainly because —at least in some countries— tortilla preparation is a homemade process with only a very small contribution from the industry. Nevertheless, it is expected that as industrialization progresses, convenient corn-based products will have their place in the market of corn-eating countries, and those properties have to be studied. Table 10   summarizes the effect of adding soybean flour,with different nitrogen solubility, to lime-treated corn. The results show the improvement achieved on the protein quality of corn masa and a tendency to obtain better responses with the soybean flour of lesser nitrogen solubility.

Table 10. Improvement of the protein quality of lime-treated corn supplement-ed with soybean flours of different nitrogen solubility.

Supplement	Nitrogen solubility of soybean flour, % 1/	% Protein in the diet	Weight gain g/28 days	PER
None	-	6.8	31	1.65
8% soybean flour - 1	99.7	9.6	78	2.20
8% soybean flour - 3 2/	82.3	9.3	89	2.50
15% whole soybeans	-	11.7	106	2.46

1/ Nitrogen solubility in NaOH 0.02 N.
2/ Lime-treated with 85% corn.

It is also of interest to note that the best
preparation, in terms of weight gain, was that resulting
from the addition of whole soybeans.

Acceptability trials using "The Rank Method" at
laboratory level were carried out on various food
preparations using the type of corn normally consumed
in the Central American countries. Although no significant differences were found among the tortillas,
those prepared from corn and whole soybeans consistently ranked first. Furthermore, differences were found
between the unsupplemented and soybean flour-supplemented corn. However, this did not affect acceptability.

Water retention capacity tests of the supplemented
and unsupplemented tortillas were also carried out,
by weighing the different preparations over a period of
3 days (Elías & Bressani, 1972; Molina et al., 1972).
The results, shown in Figure 4, indicate that over a
72-hour period at room temperature, water retention
was somewhat higher for the different preparations
containing soybean flour. This is an important aspect
from the consumer point of view, since the tortillas
eaten at breakfast are those prepared the previous day;
in a sense, the water-holding characteristics are a
measure of the texture stability of the product through
a definite period ot time.

Other physical measurements were determined in the
corn dough as well as in the corn dough supplemented
with types of soy flour and whole soybeans. Table 11
shows the farinogram values obtained with the different
preparations.

As observed, water absorption by the various preparations during mixing is very similar, although there
is a small tendency to decrease with the addition of
soy flour. This effect is more pronounced in the case of
soybeans.

Since water absorption is related to dough consistency,
the time required for the development of maximum dough
stiffness is longer for the supplemented corn dough

Table 11. Farinographic characteristics of corn dough containing 8% soybean flour.

Supplement	Water absorption ml	Time required for the development of maximum dough stiffness (B), min.	Resistance of the dough to break down (CD), min.	pH
Control	136.0	14.0	8.5	7.05
8% soybean flour - 1	135.0	16.0	4.5	6.95
8% soybean flour - 3	134.0	22.5	7.5	6.95
15% whole soybeans	131.0	23.5	stable	8.70

as compared to the corn dough alone. Again, the corn-whole soybean sample took a longer time to reach maximum stiffness. In summary, these findings show that the addition of soybean flour tends to decrease the break-down resistance of the corn dough, probably due to the reduction of starch contained in these mixtures that was replaced by soy proteins. It is known that soy globulins do not possess the same rheological properties as cereal proteins. Furthermore, the soybean flour added did not received the long cooking time given to corn. The different behavior of the sample with whole soybeans was probably due to the wet heat treatment given to it during preparation of the dough, in comparison to the heat treatment generally applied in the preparation of some soy flours, which have been shown to have an adverse effect on the bread-making potential.

As Table 12 reveals, these observations were confirmed by the amylogram values obtained on those same samples. It can be seen that maximum viscosities were attained with the unsupplemented corn dough and the corn-whole soybeans dough at around 44 minutes and 90 °C. In the case of the latter sample, it is possible that its more alkaline pH influenced the higher viscosity, since it has been demonstrated that there is an effect of pH on the gelatilization and breakdown of corn starch.

From the results obtained it can be said that the use of whole soybeans as a supplement of corn starch. has not only nutritional advantages over soybean flour, but also maintains the physical characteristics of the dough used in the preparation of tortillas.

Although the results obtained with the amylograph and farinograph showed some differences in the physical characteristics of the supplemented dough, they do not appear to be significant from the practical point of view, since the taste panel test carried out with the tortillas prepared with the supplemented corn showed no statistical significant differences, as compared to the tortilla made with normal corn. However, it is

Table 12. Amilographic characteristics of corn dough containing 8% soybean flour.

Supplement	Time maximum viscosity, min.	Temperature for maximum viscosity B. U., °C	Maximum viscosity B.U.	Viscosity at 94°C	Temperature for 500 B.U.
Control	44.0	91.0	1030	996	81.2
8% soybean flour - 1	43.0	89.5	760	708	82.0
8% soybean flour - 3	44.0	91.0	880	840	83.5
15% whole soybeans 1/	43.3	89.9	1130	1150	82.0

1/ Were subjected to an additional tension of 125g.

important to emphasize the fact that the data obtained
suggest that the addition of higher levels of soy
flour to corn flour could affect more drastically the
consistency of the corn dough used to prepare the tortillas. With the present level of soy flour addition,
it seems that the only possible practical problem is
a small increase in the time required to reach the
"normal consistency" usually obtained with normal corn
dough. Furthermore, the addition of soybean flour
does not change the appearance of the tortilla, or its
color, and it can be used to prepare other types of
food.

SYSTEMS FOR ADDITION

From the basic information herein presented, it
is obvious that improvement of the nutritional value
of tortillas can be achieved at laboratory level.
However, the transference of this technology to a
large-scale production is a real problem, partly
because tortilla preparation is almost entirely a
homemade process with a very small but growing participation of industry (Molina et al., 1972). It will
be helpful to introduce at this point the method of
preparing tortillas used in Guatemala in order to
discuss the possibilities of incorporating the supplement at industrial and village level. The traditional
method (Elías & Bressani, 1972; Bressani & Marenco,
1963; Molina et al., 1972) is shown in Figure 3. It
consists in cooking the corn for one hour, using a
calcium hydroxide solution. After cooking and cooling,
the corn is washed with water, operation which removes
the seed coat and eliminates the excess calcium hydroxide.
The cooked maize is calle "nixtamal". It is then ground,
operation which originally was done by hand, using a
grinding stone. Today, however, this is no longer the
case, as the grinding stone has been replaced by wet
corn mills (Figure 4) which operate in many places,
both in the urban and rural areas. The dough is then
made into flat cakes which are cooked over a hot flat
surface. Some conditions of this last cooking step
are summarized in Table 13. These conditions do not
destroy the protein quality of the final product, as

Table 13.   Characteristics of the cooking process of
corn masa for the preparation of tortillas.

Measures

Temperature of the surface	150 – 200 °C
Average time of cooking	3 – 4 min.
Average weight of tortilla before thermic treatment	55
Average weight of tortilla after thermic treatment	44
Moisture content of tortilla before thermic treatment	54.6%
Moisture content of tortilla after thermic treatment	34.6%
Water loss during thermic treatment	20%

Data taken from Elías & Bressani (1972).

judged by chemical analysis or biological assays, as demonstrated in Table 14. In these experiments, synthetic amino acids were used as well as intact proteins. However, for present purposes only the case of amino acids is shown. As it can be seen, the process does not decrease the amounts of added amino acids, lysine and tryptophan, and protein quality remains the same (Elías & Bressani, 1972). This process has been adapted to an industrial scale, however, supplementation can also be performed at home if proper nutrition education measures are taken.

1. Industrial level

The sequency of steps for the industrial preparation of precooked corn flours is basically the same as that used at home level when the alkaline treatment is included in the process. The main differences consist in the cooking time, which is around 1.5 hours, and in the omission of the soaking step after cooking. After grinding, the "nixtamal" (dough) is dehydrated to obtain a precooked flour as the final product.

According to this processing method, the best stage at which to add the supplement is after grinding, the cooked dehydrated grain method which would require a mixing operation before packaging. Experimental data have shown that to attain an efficient homogenous distribution, addition of the supplement as powder is better than in any other form. On the other hand, if the supplement is added as whole soybeans, this can be incorporated from the initiation of the cooking process and preliminary results show this to be adequate (Bressani et al., 1977).

2. Village level

In the rural areas, two are the alternatives of adding the supplement to the corn: at home, or at the mill used to grind the cooked corn (Molina et al., 1972). Evidently, the first procedure is very difficult since from the practical point of view, this mechanism would create numerous problems. The second alternative is more feasible when carried out under controlled conditions,

Table 14. Stability of added amino acids during the conversion of corn dough to tortilla measured by amino acid content and protein efficiency ratio.

	Lysine g/g N		Tryptophan g/g N		PER	
	Before	After[1]/ cooking	Before	After[1]/ cooking	Before	After[1]/ cooking
Corn dough	0.198	–	0.053	–	1.28	–
Tortilla	–	0.199	–	0.055	–	1.25
Corn dough + 0.30% L-Lys HCl + 0.10% DL-Try	0.370	–	0.080	–	2.42	–
Tortilla + 0.30% L-Lys HCl + 0.10% DL-Try	–	0.344	–	0.099	–	2.53

1/ Cooking time applied to make the tortilla: 6 minutes.

but still quite difficult of applying as a general
procedure due to the low education level of the rural
population. At the present time, the addition of
15% whole soybean is being recommended. This amount
is equivalent in nutritive quality to 8% soybean flour.
As indicated before, this may be accomplished by cooking
both grains together following the process described.
Education programs would help the introduction of such
a measure.

Advantages and Disadvantages

The addition of the supplement either at the
industrial or village level, presents both advantages
and drawbacks. From the industrial point of view,
the main advantage is the uniformity of the product
and its availability at all times in different convenient forms. However, the main problem lies in the
fact that in the developing countries food industries
are generally located in the urban areas, and the
supplemented food does not reach the rural areas where
undernutrition is more prevalent. These problems,
of course, can be solved either by locating the food
industries in the rural areas or by recommending
adequate transportation methods. Nevertheless, the
last alternative implies economic factors which are
also important from the consumer's point of view.

EVALUATION OF THE SUPPLEMENTED CORN IN DIETS BASED
ON CEREAL GRAIN AND LEGUME FOODS

Results demonstrating the improvement of protein
quality of lime-treated corn have already been presented
in this paper. We will now discuss selected results
which indicate that the superior quality of supplemented corn and of Opaque-2 corn in comparison with common
corn, is also evident in mixed diets. Some biological
results obtained are shown in Table 15. The data clearly indicate that the protein quality of the diet in
terms of both efficiency and utilization, is increased
by the addition of various supplements such as milk
or yeast, as well as soybean flour. In all cases, small
amounts of lysine were incorporated together with the
protein supplement added because the latter was not able

Table 15. Improvement of the protein quality of a corn-bean diet through amino acid or protein supplementation.

Supplement	Average weight gain, g	PER	Utilizable protein, %
None	52 ± 4.4	1.75 ± 0.12	4.4
Corn + Lys + Try	80 ± 3.6	2.46 ± 0.06	6.3
Corn + 8% soy flour + 0.15% Lys	120 ± 5.4	2.50 ± 0.06	8.2
Corn + 8% skim milk + 0.10% Lys	111 ± 6.1	2.63 ± 0.07	7.7
Corn + 3% Torula + 0.10% Lys	85 ± 5.2	2.24 ± 0.08	6.2

Data taken from Elías & Bressani (1972).

to meet all of the lysine required by corn as previous
results have demonstrated (Elías & Bressani, 1972). A
second example is shown in Table 16. In this case, the
evaluation was done by nitrogen balance, which showed
that the replacement of common corn by Opaque-2 corn
induces a significant increase in nitrogen retention.
This information demonstrates therefore, that either
Opaque-2 corn or protein-supplemented corn, improve
the quality of simple diets based on cereal and beans.

PROSPECTS

The evidence presented proves that a nutritional
intervention such as the one described, is of great
value to improve the nutritional standards of people
consuming poor protein quality diets of low protein
content. The problem, however, is how to make people
accept permanently this type of measure since it has
economic implications which might not be possible for
people to meet. If the lime-treated corn were indus-
trially produced and consumed by all and not only by
the urban sectors, the solution to the problem would
be simple. But as it was indicated, this is not the
case. There are no easy solutions to it. Nevertheless,
one which is very attractive is the use of whole soybeans
together with corn. In this scheme, 85 parts of corn
and 15 parts of whole soybeans are processed together
as indicated (Bressani, Murillo, Elías,1974). Material
balance of this process averaged 85% accounted for, by
the losses of seed coats and poor quality kernels.
Since soybeans are not normally grown in some of these
countries, the success of this possibility would involve
agricultural extension programs designed to teach soybean cultivation, as well as home economics type of
education to show how to use this material together
with corn. A small industry could be developed following a flow diagram, as shown in Figure 5, which would
permit not only the production of soybean-fortified
tortillas, but other food products of higher protein
and energy content, with good protein quality as well.
Obviously, this approach to the problem is not a simple
matter since it requires sustained activity and control
for a prolonged period of time. It has an advantage,
however, and this is the fact that some evidence is

Table 16. Nitrogen retention of young dogs fed a maize-bean diet with and without supplements[1].

Basal diet	Intake	Fecal	Nitrogen balance Urinary	Absorbed	Retained
			mg/kg/day		
Common maize	399	152	206	247	41
Common maize + Lys + Try	347	156	143	218	75
Common maize	357	157	165	200	35
Opaque-2 maize	407	165	127	242	115

[1] Average of 6 dogs and of three nitrogen balances of 4 days each one, by treatment.
Protein intake: 2.5 g/kg/day.

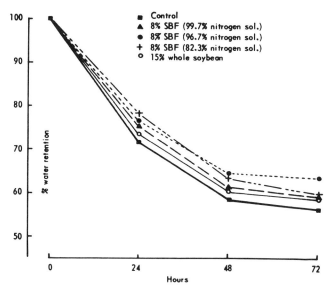

Figure 4. Water retention of tortillas with and without soybean supplement.

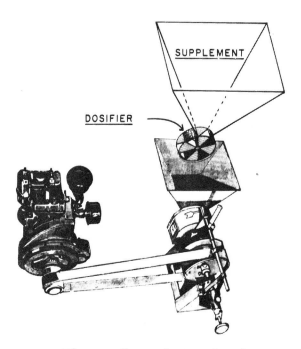

Figure 5. Nixtamal mill.

already available which demonstrates that people consuming such improved foods, derive from them the desired
beneficial effects (Urrutia et al.,1975).

Needs for Research

     Independent of the technology used to supplement
corn, it is important to realize that one of the most
important drawbacks in its implementation from the
industrial point of view is the lack of prestige
of this basic food for people in the high and medium
socio-economic strata. Because bread and other wheat-
based products are imported from Europe and other
developed countries, they have more "prestige" than the
products made from corn. Therefore, although foods
made from corn are consumed by the whole population
they are generally associated with the low income group.
Hence, efforts should be made to correct this situation through an adequate nutritional education and
advertising means. If the industrial intervention is
to be successful it is necessary to estimulate other
research areas as well. Among these it is important to
characterize the technological properties of the corn
dough to be able to establish an adequate quality control for the industry. Furthermore, studies on the
effect of corn varieties on these physical and organo -
leptic characteristics must be established. Very few
studies have been carried out in this area which would
have tremendous advantages as suggested by the impact
wheat technology has had on wheat-derived foods. The
research in this area should be directed not only to
"tortilla" preparation, but also to other forms of
maize-food systems, such as "tacos","atoles" (gruels),
"arepas" and the like. In other words, diversification
of use of the lime-treated corn flour will insure more
success to the industry, because their product will
have greater commercial applications.

     On the other hand, from the engineering point of
view, very little information is found in the literature
in regard to the precooked corn flour or tortilla-indus-
trial preparation. This information has been resctric-
ted by the industries involved in this endeavor, because
they have developed the technology by themselves. From

the nutritional point of view, more research should be
carried out on the significance of urease and trypsin
inhibitors levels in cereal products supplemented with
soybeans. The effect and mechanisms by which the heat
treatment applied during different corn-soybean preparation still is not clear. The results suggest that
the extent of heat penetration is more important than
time of heat exposure, but it is necessary to confirm
and clarify completely those results. Furthermore,
safe levels of those antiphysiological factors should
be established for the benefit of the industry as well
as the consumer.

Finally, it is important to indicate that such
kind of studies should be undertaken by the industry
and research institution in the maize-consuming countries,
if the use of this technology is to become a reality.

REFERENCES

Bressani, R. (1971). Amino acid supplementation of
    cereal grain flours tested in children. In,'Amino
    acid fortification of Protein Foods' , N. S.
    Scrimshaw and A. M. Altschul (Editors). Report
    of an International Conference Massachusetts
    Institute of Technology (MIT), Cambridge, Mass.,
    1969. The MIT Press. p 184-204.
Bressani, R., Elías, L. G., Molina, M. R. & Rubio, M.
    (1977). Further studies on the enrichment of
    lime-treated corn with soybean protein. 37th
    Annual Meeting of the Institute of Food Technolo-
    gists. Philadelphia, Pensylvania, June 6-9.
Bressani, R., Marenco, E. (1963). The enrichment of
    lime-treated corn flour with proteins, lysine and
    tryptophan, and vitamins. J. Ag. Food Chem. 6,
    517-522.
Bressani, R. , Murillo, B. & Elías, L. G. (1974).
    Whole soybeans as a means of increasing protein
    and calories in maize-based diets. J. Food Sci.
    39, 577-580.
Del Valle, F. R., Montemayor, E. & Bourges, H. (1976).
    Industrial production of soy-enriched tortilla flour
    by lime cooking of whole raw corn-soybean mixtures.
    J. Food Sci. 41,349-357.

Elías, L. G. & Bressani, R. (1972). Nutritional value
    of the protein of tortilla flour and its improvement
    by fortification in Central America. In, 'Nutrition
    al Improvement of Maize' , R. Bressani, J. E. Braham
    and M. Béhar (Editors). Proceedings of an Interna-
    tional Conference held at the Institute of Nutrition
    of Central America and Panama (INCAP), G uatemala
    City, March 6-8, 1972. Talleres Gráficos del INCAP.
    p. 168-190.
Franz, K. (1975). Tortillas fortified with whole soy-
    beans prepared by different methods. J. Food Sci.
    40, 1275-1277.
Green, J. R., Lawhon, J. T., Cater, C. M. & Mattil, K.
    F. (1976). Protein fortification of corn torti-
    llas with oilseed flour cottonseed, soybean.
    J. Food Sci. 41, 656-660.
Green, J. R.; Lawhon, J. T., Cater, C. M. and Mattil,
    K. F. (1977). Utilization of whole undefatted
    glandless cottonseed kernels and soybeans to
    protein-fortify corn tortilla. J. Food Sci. 42,
    790-794.
Molina, M. R., Elías, L. G., Gómez Brenes, R. A., Lachan
    ce, P. A. (1972). The technology of maize forti-
    fication in Latin America. In, 'Nutritional
    Improvement of Maize', R. Bressani, J. E. Braham
    and M. Béhar (Editors). Proceedings of an Inter-
    national Conference held at the Institute of Nutri-
    tion of Central America and Panama (INCAP), Guate-
    mala City, March 6-8, 1972. Talleres Gráficos del
    INCAP. p 235-255.
Murillo, B., Cabezas, M. T. & Bressani, R. (1974).
    Influencia de la densidad calórica sobre la utili-
    zación de la proteína en dietas elaboradas a base
    de maíz y frijol. Arch. Latinoamer. Nutr. 24,
    223-241.
McPherson, C. M. & O. Suh Yun L. (1976). Evaluation of
    corn tortillas supplemented with cottonseed flour.
    J. Food Sci. 41, 1301-1304.
Sauberlich, H. E., Chang, W. Y. & Salmon, W. D. (1953).
    The comparative nutritive value of corn of high and
    low protein content for growth in the rat and chick.
    J. Nutr. 51, 623-635.

Sure, B. (1953). Protein efficiency: Improvement in whole yellow corn with lysine, tryptophan and threonine. J. Ag. Food Chem. 1, 626-629.

Urrutia, J. J., García, B., Mata, L. J. & Bressani, R. (1975). Reporte preliminar del efecto biológico de la fortificación del maíz con harina de soya y lisina. En, 'Memorias - Primera Conferencia Latinoamericana sobre la Proteína de Soya' . Asociación Americana de Soya. México, D. F. Nov. 9-12. p. 134-145.

Valle, F. R. del & Pérez-Villaseñor, J. (1974). Enrichment of tortillas with soy proteins by lime cooking of whole raw corn-soybean mixtures. J. Food Sci. 39, 244-247.

Viteri, F. E., Martínez, C. & Bressani, R. (1972). Evaluation of the protein quality of common maize, Opaque-2 maize and common maize supplemented with amino acids and other sources of protein. In, 'Nutritional Improvement of Maize'. R. Bressani, J. E. Braham & M. Béhar (Editors). Proceedings of an International Conference held at the Institute of Nutrition of Central America and Panama (INCAP), Guatemala City, March 6-8, 1972. Talleres Gráficos del INCAP. p. 191-204.

4

ANIMAL AND HUMAN FEEDING STUDIES ON THE BIOLOGICAL AVAILABILITY OF PROTEIN IN SUPPLEMENTS

Rajammal P. Devadas

Sri Avinashilingham Home Science College for Women

Coimbatore 641011, India

INTRODUCTION

The quality of protein from food depends essentially on its ability to meet the body's requirements for amino acids. Although the chemical composition or amino acid analysis of dietary protein may give an elegant representation of the value of a protein, it is necessary to verify its value by actual biological experiments. Hence in the ultimate analysis, protein quality has to be measured in the animal or human system directly with respect to growth, tissue repair or maintenance, and other biological criteria.

AMINO ACID REQUIREMENTS AND PROTEIN QUALITY

The essential amino acid requirements for man per kilogram of body weight decreases with age faster than do nitrogen requirements. Consequently, the quality of proteins for human nutrition differs depending on the age of the subjects consuming them (F.A.O. 1973). Based on the above principle, the potential of cereal-legume based diets to insure adequate protein and amino acid nutrition of preschool children is very significant and practical.

Protein intake of an animal or man can be regarded as nutritionally adequate when it satisfies nitrogen and essential amino acid requirements of that individual. Nitrogen and amino acid requirements are therefore the logical yardsticks of protein quality. Precise knowledge of these requirements is essential. Data regarding amino acid requirements of preschool children are still incomplete. When these gaps are filled, a rational approach to the problem of predicting protein nutritional quality and to the more complex problems of combating protein malnutrition will be possible (Arroyave, 1975).

One important finding is that the requirement of total essential amino acid nitrogen as a per cent of total nitrogen is much lower in the adult than in the infant (Arroyave, 1975). The use of amino acid patterns specific for different age groups is a more logical approach in judging proteins for their nutritional quality than the use of a single pattern. Thus, when proteins are properly scored against age-specific amino acid requirements, their nutritional value is age-dependent, that is, for example, a particular protein may prove very inadequate for the infant and still be very adequate for the adult (NRC, 1976).

PRACTICAL APPLICATIONS

The concept of protein quality evaluation as discussed above has practical applications in overcoming the problem of protein-calorie malnutrition among children. Dietary surveys indicate that calories are also limiting, some times more limiting than protein per se. Evidence is presented in this paper through animal and human studies to show that increasing the intake of the cereal-legume based diets that are presently consumed by rural children in India results in marked nutritional improvement.

EVALUATION OF PROTEIN QUALITY OF INDIGENOUS MIXTURES

A series of cereal-legume mixtures based on suitable local foods were formulated for feeding preschool and school children. These food mixtures were evaluated through animal assays using protein efficiency ratio (PER), net protein utilization (NPU), and net protein calorie per cent (NDP Cal %) as criteria. Out of hundreds of various combinations of cereals, legumes, and oil seeds, six formulations with the most promising amino acid profiles were selected for rat assay. The results are presented in Table 1.

The PER and NPU values of all the various food mixtures were higher than those of the basal diet mixtures. The protein quality of all six food mixtures was satisfactory as judged by Protein Advisory Group (PAG) requirements (PAG, 1971). Girija Bai and Devadas (1972) and Devadas (1973) reported similar PER values for vegetable protein mixtures. The present formulations made from maize together with legumes and oil seeds have been successfully tested by feeding trials with preschool and school children. These findings are discussed later in this paper.

TABLE 1

QUALITY INDEXES OF PROTEIN MIXTURES

Source of protein and their proportions in the mixtures	PER $\pm$ std. error	NPU	NDP Cal %
Skim milk	3.01 $\pm$ 0.07	70	11.41
Maize basal diet	0.87 $\pm$ 0.06	--	--
Maize-cow gram (Vigna Catjang)-green gram (Phaseolus radiatus) (6:1:1:2)-sunflower seed (Helianthus annuus)	2.34 $\pm$	66	6.95
Maize-horse gram-green gram (Biflorus) (6:2:2)	2.24 $\pm$ 0.02	65	9.23
Maize-cow gram-green gram (6:2:2)	2.59 $\pm$ 0.04	65	5.06
Maize-green gram-sunflower seed (6:2:2)	2.44 $\pm$ 0.72	62	6.27
Maize-cow gram-horse gram-groundnut (6:1:1:2)	2.64 $\pm$ 0.05	61	7.15

PROTEIN EVALUATIONS OF SORGHUM-GREEN GRAM DIETS

Another series of experiments was designed to find what proportion of green gram used to supplement sorghum, which is a staple cereal in Coimbatore, Tamil Nadu State of India, would result in the maximum PER value (Nimrala, 1975). The PER values and lysine and methionine contents of the various formulations are given in Table 2.

The diets contained equal amounts of protein derived from different proportions of sorghum and green grams. The maximum protein value was obtained when 60 per cent of the protein in the diet was derived from sorghum and 40 per cent from green gram. These figures correspond to 75 grams of sorghum and 25 grams of green grams in 100 grams of the mixture.

Lysine appears to be the main limiting amino acid when sorghum provides 50 to 100 per cent of the dietary protein. On the other hand, methionine becomes the limiting amino acid when more than half of the protein is provided by green gram. In this series of experiments the optimum proportion of sorghum to green gram was in the ratio 3:1. The results of the various nutritional surveys carried out in Coimbatore, Tamil Nadu State, are shown in Table 3.

TABLE 2

PER VALUES AND LYSINE AND METHIONINE CONTENTS OF FORMULATIONS WITH
VARIED PROPORTIONS OF SORGHUM AND GREEN GRAMS

Protein Ratio:		PER	Amino Acid Content: g/100g	
Sorghum	Green Gram		Lysine	Methionine
100	0	0.87	0.21	0.141
80	20	1.38	0.34	0.157
60	40	2.10	0.43	0.149
50	50	2.04	0.50	0.148
40	60	1.52	0.54	0.143
20	80	0.76	0.63	0.135
0	100	0.77	0.74	0.129

TABLE 3

AMOUNT AND RATIO OF CEREAL (SORGHUM) AND LEGUME (GREEN GRAM) CONSUMED
PER DAY, PER HEAD, IN COIMBATORE (Devadas and Murthy, 1974)

	Sorghum, g/day or other cereals	Green gram, g/day or other legumes	Cereal: legume
Adults	423	50	8.5:1
Children	281	24	11.7:1
	295	26	11.3:1
	277	15	18.5:1
Optimum ratio in this study	75	25	3:1

TABLE 4

MEAN INCREASES IN HEIGHTS AND WEIGHTS OF INFANTS
RECEIVING KUZHANDAI AMUDHU

Groups	Mean height (cm)		Diffe- rence	Mean weight (Kg)		Difference
	Initial	Final		Initial	Final	
Experimental	80.15 ±4.52	86.17 ±3.71	6.02 ±0.81	8.58 ±1.04	10.72 ±1.51	2.14±0.61
Control	79.97 ±3.21	82.60 ±4.51	2.63 ±0.71	8.37 ±1.12	9.56 ±1.61	1.19±0.32
	t value for height: 21.6*			t value for weight: 4.56*		

*Significant at one per cent level

The ratio is ranged from 8 to 18.5. In all cases consumption of sorghum (or cereal) dominates. Thus the quantity and quality of dietary proteins were low. The best ratio for the foods consumed was 75:25 grams or 3:1. This fact is of particular interest in developing mixtures of low-cost indigenous foods to replace imported food mixtures such as corn-soy-milk (CSM) for child feeding programs. Based on these considerations, Devadas and coworkers (1974) have developed an infant food 'Kuzhandai Amudhu', which has been released to the public after standardization and evaluation.

FEEDING TRIALS WITH THE MAIZE-GREEN GRAM KUZHANDAI AMUDHU

One hundred infants in the age range of 6 months to 3 years from two rural communities in Perianaickenpalayam Community Development Block (A Community Development Block is the Unit of Development Work, comprising approximately 100 villages and 66,000 population), Coimbatore District, were selected for the trial. A group of 50 children from the same area with comparable socio-economic background was also selected as controls.

Eighty grams per child per day of the maize-green gram Kuzhandai Amudhu, supplying 305 calories and 11 grams protein, were given to the selected children for a period of 12 months. The mixture was made into balls with boiled cooled water and designated as 'laddus', a prestigious sweet preparation (snack). Two laddus could be prepared with 80 grams of Kuzhandai Amudhu. The laddus were packed in polythene bags for hygienic handling and served to each child daily. The mothers had been persuaded to give the supplement of laddus to their children in the feeding center itself, to ensure consumption.

The data on the heights and weights of the 100 infants who received the Kuzhandai Amudhu, in comparison with those of the 50 children in the control group who did not receive the supplement, are presented in Table 4 (Devadas et al., 1974).

Towards the end of the experiment, children in the experimental group were heavier and taller than their counterparts. The mean differences in the increases in heights and weights between the two groups were significant at the 1% level.

FEEDING TRIAL WITH SORGHUM-BENGAL GRAM KUZHANDAI AMUDHU

Another infant feeding trial was carried out by Devadas et al. (1974) with Kuzhandai Amudhu based on roasted sorghum, Bengal gram, and groundnuts for a period of six months. Twenty five children in the 6 to 30 months age range were given the weaning mixture. Another comparable group of 25 children were given a corn-soy-milk (CSM) mixture with jaggery donated by CARE. A third group of 25 children who did not receive any supplement formed the control. Fifty grams the sorghum-Bengal gram Kuzhandai Amudhu were given per child for those weighing below 7 kg and 100 g per day per child for

those weighing above 7 kg. These amounts were given in four ser-
vings per day for a period of six months. The mixes were distributed to the mothers in quantities adequate for a month. The mothers were instructed to feed each child the day's ration as
porridge, made by adding boiling water, or in any other palatable
and acceptable form. Table 5 gives the results of this trial.

There was a significant increase in body heights and body
weights of the children receiving the weaning mixture and CSM when
compared to the control group. The differences in increase in body
weight gains and heights between the groups on Kuzhandai Amudhu and
CSM were not signficant. The low-cost weaning mixture tried was
geared to the economic reach of the rural families. It can be prepared by mothers in their own homes. Children accepted the weaning
mixture made out of the local foods better than CSM because of the
flavor.

Devadas and Murthy (1974) conducted a study to ascertain the
effect of feeding children, 18 to 30 months of age, diets with high
lysine maize (opaque-2 maize) on their growth and to serve as an
educational program in the popularization of the new maize variety.
The selected 200 children were divided into 4 groups, 50 in the
opaque-2 maize diet, 50 in the ordinary maize diet, 50 in skim milk
group, and 50 receiving no food supplement, serving as control.
The supplement provided 450 calories and 10 grams protein per
child per day. The duration of the feeding was six months. Table
6 shows the changes in weights and heights of the children who participated in the study.

The differences between the increment in body length and weight
of the groups of children receiving the supplements were found to
be significantly higher than those registered by the control group.
However, the differences between the increments among the children
on the opaque-2 maize and skim milk diets were not significant.
The opaque-2 maize was found to be better than ordinary maize in
promoting growth of preschool children. This finding is of great
significance in the Indian context, since opaque-2 maize plays an
important role as a rich and low-cost source of good quality
protein and calories.

Devadas et al. (1973) conducted a study to find the efficacy
of soybean-cereal mixture, in the form of laddu with and without
supplementation with vitamin A and C in feeding selected preschool
children in a slum community (low socio-economic group) in
Coimbatore city. The selected 30 children were assigned groups
A, B, and C with ten children each. Group A received laddu with
beta-carotene and vitamin C; group B received laddu alone; and
group C served as control without any supplement. Seventy grams
of the supplement per child per day supplying 392 calories and
5 grams of protein were given for a period of six months. A comparison of the mean monthly weights of children in the three groups
is given in Table 7.

TABLE 5

MEAN HEIGHTS AND WEIGHTS OF CHILDREN ON SORGHUM-BENGAL GRAM
KUZHANDAI AMUDHU AND CORN-SOY-MILK IN COMPARISON WITH CONTROLS

Group Mean height (cm)	Initial	Final	Difference
A Sorghum-Bengal gram Kuzhandai Amudhu	80.7±3.03	84.3±3.20	3.6±0.67*
B Corn-Soy-Milk	77.8±4.16	82.1±3.57	4.3±0.93*
C Control	81.1±4.38	83.4±3.62	2.3±0.56
Mean weight (Kg)			
A Sorghum-Bengal gram Kuzhandai Amudhu	9.49±1.48	11.15±0.92	1.66±0.59*
B Corn-Soy-Milk	8.86±1.17	10.44±1.21	1.58±0.28*
C Control	9.61±0.57	10.28±0.88	0.67±0.43

*Significant at one per cent level

TABLE 6

MEAN CHANGES IN WEIGHT AND HEIGHT OF THE
TARGET CHILDREN AFTER SIX MONTHS

Diet	Weight, Kg Initial	Final	Difference	Height, cm Initial	Final	Difference
Ordinary maize	11.25	12.11	0.86±0.01	86.20	88.70	2.50±0.0001
Opaque-2 maize	10.90	12.09	1.19±0.01	87.60	90.50	2.90±0.66
Skim milk	11.10	12.27	1.17±0.14	83.36	86.50	3.14±0.19
Control	10.83	11.59	0.76±0.01	80.20	82.30	2.10±0.08

TABLE 7   MEAN MONTHLY WEIGHTS OF THE CHILDREN
Number of children: 10 in each group
Duration of the experiment: 6 months

Group	Initial weight, Kg	1 month	2 months	3 months	4 months	5 months	6 months	Mean increase for 6 months
A	11.45	11.95	12.50	12.80	13.10	13.55	13.90	2.45
B	11.60	12.25	12.55	12.65	13.10	13.50	13.80	2.20
C	11.30	11.30	11.35	11.50	11.85	12.10	12.25	0.95

TABLE 8   MEAN MONTHLY HEIGHTS OF CHILDREN

Group	Initial height, cm	1 month	2 months	3 months	4 months	5 months	6 months	Mean increase for 6 months
A	89.12	90.90	92.16	93.29	94.75	96.73	98.65	9.53
B	87.25	88.74	90.06	91.47	92.97	95.04	96.38	9.13
C	86.60	87.34	88.15	88.89	89.66	90.65	91.34	4.74

TABLE 9   MEAN INCREASE IN WEIGHT AND HEIGHT OF CHILDREN IN THE
CONTROL AND EXPERIMENTAL[+] GROUPS

(Experimental Period: Six months)

Group	Age range, years	Number of children	Initial	Final	Difference	't' value Initial
			Mean weight, Kg			
Control	2.9-4.9	15	9.80	11.03	1.23	1.3000
Experimental	2.9-4.9	15	10.40	12.68	2.28	3.578*
			Mean height, cm			
Control	2.9-4.9	15	87.63	89.68	2.05	0.674
Experimental	2.9-4.9	15	86.26	88.94	2.68	1.020

't' value for weight control vs. experimental 3.995*
't' value for height control vs. experimental 5.314*

*Significant at one per cent level
[+]Given high-protein food: sesame, groundnut, and horse gram mixture

At the end of the experimental period, children in the control group weighed less than those in the two experimental groups. Group A showed greater increases in weight. Although group B had a slightly higher initial weight than that of group A, the final mean weight of group B was lower than that of group A. However, the difference in the mean increases in weight between groups A and B was not significant statistically. The rate of increase of the Control group was lower than that of the experimental group. Thus, supplementation with beta-carotene and vitamin C did not have any additional benefit with respect to weight. The mean monthly height of the three groups of children is presented in Table 7. Group A exhibited a higher mean height than group B at the end of the study. The addition of carotene and vitamin C did not have any further benefit.

Kamalanathan et al. (1970) observed the effects of high-protein food (HPF) blend of groundnut meal, sesame meal, and horsegram on the nutritional status of selected preschool children in the rural area. Groundnut meal and horsegram were selected for their low cost and availability, and sesame meal for its sulfur-containing amino acids. Twenty five children in the age range 2½-5 years admitted to the preschool were included in the experimental group to receive the supplement; 15 children who were identical in all respects, but not receiving the supplement, formed the control group.

The menu was planned to meet two thirds of the allowances recommended by the Indian Council of Medical Research (ICMR) through two meals, namely breakfast and lunch, and an evening snack. A mixture of sesame meal, groundnut meal, and horse gram that provided protein in the ratio 2:1:1 was formulated. This was mixed with jaggery (brown sugar) and made into laddus. One hundred grams of HPF laddus were given per child per day, 50 grams during lunch and 25 grams each for breakfast and evening snack. The target children consumed these supplements in addition to their home diets. The feeding program was evaluated after a period of 6 months. The mean increases in the heights and weights of the two groups of preschool children are presented in Table 9.

The differences between the initial and final weights were significant in the experimental group as were the differences between the weight gains of the control and experimental groups. The differences in the height gains between the experimental and control groups were also significant.

NITROGEN RETENTION IN PRESCHOOL CHILDREN RECEIVING VEGETABLE
PROTEIN SUPPLEMENTS

Devadas et al. (1973) conducted a study to find the nitrogen retention in preschool children on a vegetable protein mixture supplement, through a balance study of 14 days' duration. Five

preschool children of the age range 3 to 4 years, belonging to a
similar socio-economic group and weighing between 8 and 13 kg,
were selected as subjects. The calorie intake was adequate for
all the children during the basal and supplemented periods. The
intake of protein was maintained at a low level (11 to 13.6 g per
child per day) during the basal period and made adequate during
the supplementary period (20.5 to 22.9 g per child per day).
The findings were: (1) The retention of nitrogen from the supplemented diet was 1.945 g. (2) The apparent digestibilities of the
basal and supplemented diets were 75% and 83%, respectively.
(3) The apparent biological value of the supplemented diet (66)
was significantly higher than that of the basal diet (35).

CONCLUSIONS

These results throw doubt on the validity of programs that
supplement cereal-legume diets with concentrated protein sources
alone. Increased consumption of diets based on foods already in
use may be the preferred solution to nutritional problems (Devadas
and Murthy, 1977). This concept does not apply to all situations,
for example, to low-protein cassava-plantain diets. Yet there are
millions of children who at preschool age depend on cereal-legume-
based diets for who proof of this hypothesis may be very valuable.

REFERENCES

Arroyave, G. (1975). Amino acid requirements and age. In "Protein-
    Calorie Malnutrition", R. E. Olson (Ed.), Academic Press,
    New York, 1-18.

Devadas, R. P. and Murthy, N. K. (1977). Nutrition of the preschool
    child in India. World Rev. Nutr. and Diets, 39, 4-5.

Devadas, R. P. and Murthy, N. K. (1974).   Studies on the nutritive
    value of high lysine maize. A report submitted to the Ministry
    of Agriculture, Department of Food, Government of India.

Devadas, R. P., Chandrasekar, U. and Lalitha, M. (1973). Nitrogen
    retention in preschool children on a vegetable protein mixture
    supplement. Am. J. Clin. Nutr., 26, 415-419.

Devadas, R. P., Bhalerao, V. and Vaijayanthi, S. (1973). Use of
    soybean cereal mixture in feeding preschool children: M. Sc.
    Thesis, Madras University, India.

Devadas, R. P., Jamala, S., Chandrasekar, U. and Murthy, N. K. (1974).
    Nutritional evaluation of maize based indigenous infant food
    Kuzhandai Amudhu   Ind. J. Nutr. Diet., 11, 257-263.

Devadas, R. P., Roshan Bibi, A. and Murthy, N. K. (1974). Evaluation
    of weaning mixture based on local foods. Ind. J. Nutr. Diet.,
    11, 209-211.

F. A. O. (1973). Energy and Protein Requirements. Report of a Joint FAO/WHO Expert Group, WHO Tech. Rep. Ser. No 552, p. 121.

Girija, Bai and Devadas, R. P. (1973). Ability of two rice diets to support reproductive and lactation performance in rats. Ind. J. Nutr. Diet., 10, 275.

Kamalanathan, G., Nalinakshi, G. and Devadas, R. P. (1970). Effect of a blend of protein foods on the nutritional status of pre-school children in a rural Balwadi. Ind. J. Nutr. Diet., 7, 288-292.

N. R. C. (1976). Evaluation of Protein Nutrition. 2nd Edition, National Academy of Sciences, National Research Council, Washington, D. C.

Nirmala, P. S. (1975). Nutritive evaluation of the supplementary value of low cost and locally available food namely horsegram, field beans, sesame and amaranthus to poor rice diet. Unpublished.

P. A. G. (1971). Mannual on Feeding Infants and Young Children. Protein Advisory Group of the United Nations System. PAG Document 1, 141/26, pp. 17-18.

5

EFFECT ON NITROGEN RETENTION BY ADULTS OF DIFFERENT PROPORTIONS OF INDISPENSABLE AMINO ACIDS IN ISONITROGENOUS CEREAL-BASED DIETS

Helen E. Clark, Marie F. Brewer and Lynn B. Bailey

Department of Foods and Nutrition and Purdue University

Agricultural Experiment Station, West Lafayette, IN 47907

ABSTRACT

Nitrogen retention of adults who consumed diets in which cereals furnished 6.0 g N and 0.9 g of lysine was improved by increasing lysine to 1.8 g without altering other amino acids. In a second experiment, 70% of the 6.0 g of dietary N was supplied by rice + wheat and 30% by mixtures of amino acids so designed that the total intakes of amino acids were equivalent to those in diets containing 6.0 g N from whole egg (E), egg + potato (EP), rice + wheat (RW), rice + soy (RS), wheat + milk (WM) or corn + beans (CB). Mean N balances of young men in descending order were, g/day: E 0.69 $\pm$ 0.23, RS 0.44 $\pm$ 0.15, EP 0.43 $\pm$ 0.09, WM 0.24 $\pm$ 0.16, CB 0.16 $\pm$ 0.13 and RW -0.02 $\pm$ 0.10. In the same order, these diets provided, g/day: lysine 2.6, 1.9, 2.3, 1.6, 1.4 and 1.0; S-acids 2.2, 1.7, 1.6, 2.2, 1.9 and 2.3; and tryptophan 0.7, 0.4, 0.6, 0.5, 0.3 and 0.4. N balances resulting from diets E, RS and EP did not differ significantly from each other but E was superior to CB and RW (P<0.01). Relative amounts and proportions of the essential amino acids could be varied without altering nitrogen retention until at least one amino acid became limiting. Several patterns of indispensable amino acids therefore may be equally effective in meeting needs of adults, but both amounts and relative proportions should be considered.

INTRODUCTION

Adverse effects of disproportionate amounts of amino acids can be produced readily in growing animals by feeding mixtures of crystalline amino acids. Harper (1974) has suggested that these should be classified as imbalance, antagonism or toxicity. It is difficult to study effects of different proportions of amino acids when foods are incorporated in human diets, but such information is needed to plan experiments, interpret data, develop feeding programs and utilize food resources efficiently. Also, in considering human populations, it is necessary to recognize that disproportionately small amounts of certain amino acids are present in some foods and that deficiencies and excesses may coexist in individual foods or combinations thereof. Deficits in cereal-containing diets of the infant or preschool child can be overcome by supplementation (Graham, 1971), judicious combination of complementary protein sources (Bressani and Elias, 1973) or genetic modification (Pradilla, Harpstead, Sarria, Linares and Francis, 1975).

Several reference patterns of amino acids have been proposed, but none has proven satisfactory. Because amino acid requirements of the infant (Holt and Snyderman, 1965) differ from those of the adult (Rose, 1957) in amount, proportion and relation to body weight, the same scoring pattern (WHO, 1973) should not be applied to both groups. In fact, it may not be possible to develop a single useful pattern for the adult because of variations in requirements of individuals (Rose, 1957) and in zone of tolerance for different amino acids (Kolski, Shannon, Howe and Clark, 1969).

VARIABLE PROPORTIONS OF CERTAIN AMINO ACIDS

The effects of modifying amounts and proportions of certain indispensable amino acids have been investigated in a series of experiments in which diets were isonitrogenous at 6.0 g of nitrogen per day, an amount that clearly reveals deficits or excesses of amino acids when energy needs of individuals are met and other nutrients are adequate. An intake of 6.0 g of nitrogen was equivalent to approximately 0.5 g of protein per kilogram of body weight of the subjects.

A basic mixture of amino acids was developed (Table 1) that approximated minimal requirements of men (Rose, 1957) except that leucine, phenylalanine and valine were slightly higher (Clark, Fugate and Allen, 1967). Amino acids were supplied in part by wheat flour, which was constant, and the mixture of L-isomers of indispensable amino acids replaced the nonspecific nitrogen source in a stepwise manner. There was a significant linear regression of nitrogen retention on intake of indispensable amino acids ($Y = 550X - 585$, when Y is milligrams of nitrogen retained and X is grams of amino acids). This response was consistent not only with the report of Romo and Linkswiler (1969) who administered crystalline amino acids but also with data obtained when one combination of foods provided from 5 to 8 g of nitrogen (Clark, Howe, Magee and

TABLE 1

Basic mixture of amino acids

(Clark, Fugate and Allen, 1967)

Amino acid	Multiple of basic mix			
	1.0	1.5	2.0	2.5
Isoleucine	0.98	1.38	1.78	2.18
Leucine	1.30	1.95	2.60	3.26
Lysine	0.85	1.29	1.74	2.19
Met + cys	0.96	1.60	2.23	2.87
Phe + tyr	1.51	2.23	2.95	3.67
Threonine	0.61	0.91	1.21	1.51
Tryptophan	0.31	0.47	0.62	0.78
Valine	1.03	1.51	1.98	2.46
Total	7.55	11.34	15.11	18.91
N balance, g	−0.07	0.22	0.56	0.72

Malzer, 1972). Each increment of indispensable amino acids present
in the same proportions therefore causes a predictable improvement
in nitrogen retention.

Lysine, tryptophan and sulfur amino acids are most likely to
be inadequate in human diets (WHO, 1973), whereas leucine may be
in excess. Therefore, these amino acids were modified over a
range relevant to human diets while other indispensable amino acids
were constant at one of the multiples designated in Table 1. When
twice the basic mixture of amino acids was consumed, nitrogen
retention improved significantly as lysine increased from 0.9 to
1.8 g (Figure 1), and larger increments also were beneficial
(Clark, Boyd, Kolski and Shannon, 1968). For efficient utilization
of other amino acids in the mixture, it was necessary to provide
at least twice the minimal lysine requirement established earlier
with a mixture of amino acids in which other amino acids were in
excess (Rose, 1957) or when cereals provided part of the amino

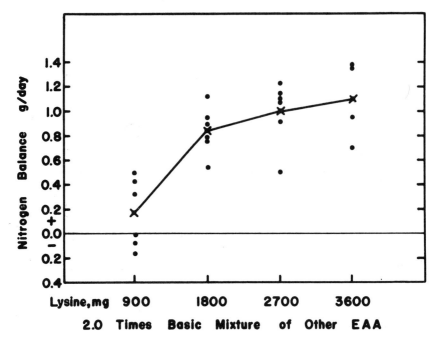

Figure 1. Nitrogen balances of adults who consumed variable amounts of lysine when other amino acids were constant.

acids which were fed in the egg pattern (Clark, Yang, Walton and Mertz, 1960).

In contrast, nitrogen retention was not altered significantly by leucine between 1.3 and 6.6 g in conjunction with 1.5 times the basic mixture which contained 1.4 g of isoleucine (Kolski, Shannon, Howe and Clark, 1969), although there was a trend toward less satisfactory utilization near the lowest intake, which approximated the minimal requirement, and at the highest level. A hypoglycemic response to high doses of leucine has been reported in a few individuals (McArthur, Kirtley and Waife, 1963). The zone of tolerance for valine extended from 1.1 to 4.4 g.

Five levels of tryptophan between 260 and 750 mg fed with 2.5 times the basic mixture did not significantly alter nitrogen retention (Clark, Moon, Malzer, Birt and Pang, 1974). However, because both lysine and tryptophan are low in many foods, it was important to determine whether there was an interaction between them. For this purpose, 75% of the 6.0 g of nitrogen was supplied by cereals and 25% by a mixture of amino acids in the same proportions as in the cereals except that lysine and tryptophan were modified (Clark, Bailey and Brewer, 1977). To reduce tryptophan to 260 mg, it was necessary to limit cereals to 4.5 g of nitrogen and to include cornmeal. The pronounced effect of increasing lysine from 0.9 to 1.8 g and the absence of a significant response to tryptophan was confirmed (Figure 2). In another experiment, plasma amino acids and nitrogen retention showed that lysine was more effective when added to cereals than to the same amounts of crystalline amino acids (Bailey and Clark, 1976). Thus, it is not always appropriate to use interchangeably data obtained with foods and with amino acid mixtures.

Relations between sulfur-containing amino acids and other indispensable amino acids are difficult to quantitate. Most men attained nitrogen equilibrium when they consumed, in conjunction with 1.5 times the basic mixture, 460 mg of methionine plus 340 mg of cystine, although individual requirements ranged from as little as 260 mg of methionine plus 280 mg of cystine to 700 mg of methionine plus 400 mg of cystine (Clark, Howe, Shannon, Carlson and Kolski, 1970). The latter total approximates the requirement for methionine in the absence of cystine (Rose, 1957). When 340 mg of

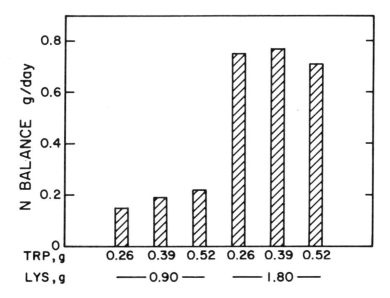

Figure 2. Nitrogen balances of men who consumed variable amounts of lysine and tryptophan when other amino acids were constant

cystine were present, nitrogen retention was not improved significantly by raising methionine from 300 to 900 mg. The sparing action
of cystine, which is present in all foods, presumably changes as
methionine increases. These data suggest that sulfur amino acids
are unlikely to be limiting for adults if cereals are present,
unless the protein sources are poorly digested or total protein
is so low that other amino acids also are deficient.

AMINO ACID PATTERNS

After measuring the effect of variable proportions of individual amino acids, six patterns of indispensable amino acids that
represented major components of human diets were compared (Brewer,
Halvorson and Clark). Rice and wheat together furnished 70% of
the nitrogen and a mixture of indispensable and dispensable amino
acids 30% (Table 2). Each mixture was formulated so that the total
intake of each amino acid was equivalent to the designated source
when fed at 6.0 g of nitrogen. The percentage of nitrogen from
each source that was used to develop the amino acid mixture is
indicated for each diet (Table 2). The basic diet combined with
variable amino acid mixtures permitted investigation of only the
relative proportions of amino acids, apart from differences in
digestibility, availability of amino acids or other characteristics
of individual foods.

TABLE 2

Sources of nitrogen in experimental diets (g)

Source	E	EP	RS	WM	CB	RW
	Egg	Egg + Potato	Rice + Soy	Wheat + Milk	Corn + Beans	Rice + Wheat
	100	60:40	50:50	67:33	67:33	50:50
Rice (146 g)	2.0	2.0	2.0	2.0	2.0	2.0
Wheat (126 g)	2.2	2.2	2.2	2.2	2.2	2.2
L-amino acids	1.8	1.4	1.7	1.5	1.3	1.6
Nonspecific N	0.0	0.4	0.1	0.3	0.5	0.2
Total, g	6.0	6.0	6.0	6.0	6.0	6.0

Hen egg is used frequently to study protein metabolism (Calloway, 1975; Young, Taylor, Rand and Scrimshaw, 1973), and as a basis of comparison. Nitrogen retention of men (Figure 3) was not significantly higher in response to the egg pattern alone than to the equivalent of 60% of nitrogen from egg and 40% from potato (EP). This is not surprising in light of an earlier report that egg + potato was more efficient than egg alone for men (Kofrányi, Jekat and Müller-Wecker, 1970; Kofranyi, 1973). The 50:50 combination of rice and soy (RS) was as satisfactory as egg or egg and potato (EP); and these three caused greater retention than rice and wheat (RW 50:50). Egg alone was superior to wheat plus milk (WM) and corn plus beans (CB) when the cereal provided 67% of the nitrogen. All or most men retained nitrogen when they consumed both diets containing egg or rice plus soy, but only half of them when consuming other diets.

Diets EP and RS provided 16% less total indispensable amino acids than diet E (Table 3). Both contained 25% less sulfur amino acids than egg; and diet RS also supplied 25% less isoleucine,

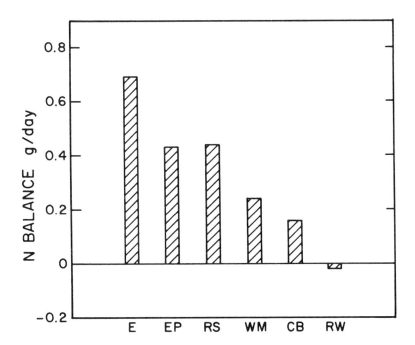

Figure 3. Nitrogen balances of men who consumed different patterns of indispensable amino acids.

TABLE 3

Amino acids in six patterns (g)

Amino acid	E	EP	RS	WM	CB	RW
Ile	2.4	2.0	1.7	1.6	1.5	1.6
Leu	3.3	2.9	3.3	3.1	4.9	3.3
Lys	2.6	2.3	1.9	1.6	1.4	1.0
M + C	2.2	1.6	1.7	2.2	1.9	2.3
P + T	3.7	3.2	3.5	3.6	3.6	3.8
Thr	1.9	1.7	1.4	1.2	1.4	1.2
Trp	0.7	0.6	0.4	0.5	0.3	0.4
Val	2.6	2.2	2.3	2.0	1.9	2.2
Total	19.4	16.5	16.2	15.8	16.9	15.8

lysine and threonine and 40% less tryptophan. Hence, comparison
with egg may seriously underestimate the protein quality of other
dietary sources, whereas a range of amounts represented by rice
plus soy, egg plus potato or other efficient combinations might be
used in preliminary evaluation of foods.

Reductions in nitrogen retention resulting from other diets
were associated with downward trends in intake of some amino acids.
When diet CB was consumed, lysine and total sulfur amino acids
should have been adequate, but the ratio of leucine to isoleucine
was exceptionally high and leucine may have depressed utilization
of tryptophan which was lower than in any other diet. A deficit
of lysine was the obvious cause of inefficient utilization of
diet RW; tryptophan was as high as in diet RS and sulfur amino
acids were equivalent to egg.

These data indicate that both total amounts of essential
amino acids and relative proportions among them can be varied within certain limits without affecting nitrogen retention of adults.
Either several patterns or a range for certain indispensable amino
acids therefore might serve as useful guidelines and be more

useful than any single pattern. Lysine, leucine, sulfur amino
acids and tryptophan need special consideration. Phenylalanine,
threonine and valine are influenced to a lesser extent by dietary
protein source than are the others, and isoleucine requirement is
influenced by leucine. Total amounts of indispensable amino acids
as a group or total nitrogen derived from them are not definitive,
unless total protein is reduced drastically.

FOODS AS SOURCES OF AMINO ACIDS

The concept of improving protein quality of foods implies
that a modification which will facilitate protein synthesis can be
achieved by increasing the amounts of one or more indispensable
amino acids, altering the proportions of certain amino acids or
changing both amounts and proportions. Although neither a serious
deficit nor excess of an amino acid is likely to occur when large
quantities of protein are consumed from many sources, as in the
United States (Phipard, 1974), diets in many areas of the world are
restricted in both source and amount. Furthermore, data obtained
by altering the proportions of individual amino acids or by investi-
gating representative patterns are relevant to the question of
protein and amino acid requirements of man and the fulfillment of
these requirements by various types of diets.

Experiments in which foods have been combined in different
proportions (Howe, Clark, Tewell and Senchak, 1972; Lee, Howe,
Carlson and Clark, 1971) support the data obtained when proportions
of amino acids have been manipulated as described here. That total
amount of protein also is important is shown by the fact that a
combination of rice, milk and wheat was inadequate at 32 g of
protein/day, met minimal requirements at 38 g, and also covered
integumental losses at 44 or 50 g of protein/day, equivalent to
0.6 or 0.7 g per kilogram of body weight (Clark, Howe, Magee and
Malzer, 1972).

Statements concerning protein requirements should specify the
source or sources; differences in amino acid composition (FAO, 1970)
should be recognized. For example, adults would need to consume a
larger amount of the diet containing rice and wheat than rice and
soy to reach the same level of nitrogen retention. Young, Murray,
Rand and Scrimshaw (1975) estimated that to attain nitrogen equilibrium, men not only required a larger amount of protein from
wheat than from beef or egg but the requirement was considerably
higher than that estimated from the data on nitrogen and amino acid
content of the wheat.

In summary, both amounts and proportions of certain indispensable amino acids are of particular significance in determining the ability of dietary proteins to meet requirements of

adult humans, whereas the intakes of others may vary widely provided
that minimal requirements are met. Improvement of protein quality
therefore may require adjustment of both amount and proportions of
amino acids. Several patterns of indispensable amino acids may be
useful for comparative purposes or preliminary screening.

REFERENCES

Bailey, L.B. and Clark, H.E. (1976). Plasma amino acids and nitro-
    gen retention of human subjects who consumed isonitrogenous
    diets containing rice and wheat or their constituent amino
    acids with and without additional lysine. Am. J. Clin.
    Nutr., 29, 1353-1358.
Bressani, R. and Elias, L.G. (1973). Development of highly nutri-
    tious products. In, Man, Food and Nutrition, M. Rechcigl
    (Editor). CRC Press, Cleveland.
Brewer, M.F., Halvorson, J.D. and Clark, H.E. Nitrogen retention
    of young men who consumed selected patterns of essential amino
    acids at a constant nitrogen intake. Am. J. Clin. Nutr.
    In Press.
Calloway, D.H. (1975). Nitrogen balance of men with marginal
    intakes of protein and energy. J. Nutr., 105, 914-923.
Clark, H.E., Bailey, L.B. and Brewer, M.F. (1977). Lysine and
    tryptophan in cereal-based diets for adult human subjects.
    Am. J. Clin. Nutr., 30, 674-680.
Clark, H.E., Boyd, J.N., Kolski, S.M. and Shannon, B. (1968).
    Nitrogen retention of adults given variable quantities and
    proportions of lysine. Am. J. Clin. Nutr., 21, 217-222.
Clark, H.E., Fugate, K. and Allen, P.E. (1967). Effect of four
    multiples of a basic mixture of essential amino acids on
    nitrogen retention of adult human subjects. Am. J. Clin.
    Nutr., 20, 233-242.
Clark, H.E., Howe, J.M., Magee, J.L. and Malzer, J. (1972). Nitro-
    gen balances of adult human subjects who consumed four levels
    of nitrogen from a combination of rice, milk and wheat.
    J. Nutr., 102, 1647-1654.
Clark, H.E., Howe, J.M., Shannon, B.M., Carlson, K. and Kolski, S.M.
    (1970). Requirements of adult human subjects for methionine
    and cystine. Am. J. Clin. Nutr., 23, 731-738.
Clark, H.E., Moon, W.H., Malzer, J.L., Birt, D.F. and Pang, R.L.
    (1974). Nitrogen retention of adult human subjects fed vary-
    ing quantities of tryptophan. J. Nutr., 104, 1121-1126.
Clark, H.E., Yang, S.P., Walton, W. and Mertz, E.T. (1960). Amino
    acid requirements of men and women. II. Relation of lysine
    requirement to sex, body size, basal caloric expenditure and
    creatinine excretion. J. Nutr., 71, 229-234.
FAO. Amino Acid Content of Foods and Biologic Data on Proteins.
    (1970). FAO Nutritional Studies No. 24, Food and Agriculture
    Organization of United Nations. Rome.

Graham, G.G. (1971). Methionine or lysine fortification of dietary protein for infants and small children. In, 'Amino Acid Fortification of Protein Foods', N.S. Scrimshaw and A.M. Altschul (Editors). M.I.T. Press, Cambridge.

Harper, A.E. (1974). Effects of disproportionate amounts of amino acids. In, 'Improvement of Protein Nutriture', Nat'l. Acad. of Sciences, Washington, D.C.

Holt, L.E. and Snyderman, S.E. (1965). Protein and amino acid requirements of infants and children. Nutr. Abst. and Rev., 35, 1-13.

Howe, J.M., Clark, H.E., Tewell, J.E. and Senchak, M.M. (1972). Nitrogen retention of adults fed six grams of nitrogen from combinations of rice, milk, and wheat. Am. J. Clin. Nutr., 25, 559-563.

Kofrányi, E. (1973). Evaluation of traditional hypotheses on the biological value of proteins. Nutr. Repts. Intnl., 7, 45-50.

Kofrányi, E., Jekat, F. and Müller-Wecker, H. (1970). The minimum protein requirement of humans, tested with mixtures of whole egg plus potato and maize plus beans. Hoppe Seyler's Z. Physiol. Chem., 351, 1485-1493.

Kolski, S.M., Shannon, B., Howe, J.M. and Clark, H.E. (1969). Nitrogen balances of adults given leucine and valine. Am. J. Clin. Nutr., 22, 21-26.

Lee, C., Howe, J.M., Carlson, C. and Clark, H.E. (1971). Nitrogen retention of young men fed rice with or without supplementary chicken. Am. J. Clin. Nutr., 24, 318-323.

McArthur, L.G., Kirtley, W.R. and Waife, S.O. (1963). Effect of large doses of L-leucine in animals and man. Am. J. Clin. Nutr., 13, 285-290.

Phipard, E.F. (1974). Protein and amino acids in diets. In, 'Improvement of Protein Nutriture'. Nat'l. Acad. of Sciences, Washington.

Pradilla, A.G., Harpstead, D.D., Sarria, D., Linares, F.A. and Francis, C.A. (1975). Quality protein maize in human nutrition. In, 'High-Quality Protein Maize'. Dowden, Hutchinson and Ross, Stroudsburg, Pa.

Romo, G.E. and Linkswiler, H. (1969). Effect of level and pattern of essential amino acids on nitrogen retention of adult man. J. Nutr., 97, 147-153.

Rose, W.C. (1957). The amino acid requirements of adult man. Nutr. Abst. Rev., 27, 631-647.

WHO. Energy and Protein Requirements. (1973). Report of a Joint FAO/WHO Ad Hoc Expert Committee. WHO Tech. Rept. Series No. 522, World Health Organization, Geneva.

Young, V.R., Murray, E., Rand, W.M. and Scrimshaw, N.S. (1975). Protein requirements of man: comparative nitrogen balance response within the submaintenance-to-maintenance range of intakes of wheat and beef proteins. J. Nutr., 105, 534-542.

Young, V.R., Taylor, Y.S.M., Rand, W.M. and Scrimshaw, N.S. (1973).
    Protein requirements of man: efficiency of egg protein
    utilization at maintenance and submaintenance levels in young
    men. J. Nutr., 103, 1164-1174.

Journal paper 6762, of Purdue University Agricultural Experiment
Station, West Lafayette, Indiana, 47907.

This research was supported in part by U.S.P.H.S., Research
Grant AM 08533 from the National Institute of Arthritis, Metabolism
and Digestive Diseases.

6

COMPARATIVE PROTEIN QUALITY AS MEASURED BY HUMAN AND SMALL ANIMAL

BIOASSAYS OF THREE LINES OF WINTER WHEAT[1]

C.Kies,H.M.Fox,P.J.Mattern,V.A.Johnson and J.W.Schmidt

Dept. of Food and Nutrition and Dept. of Agronony

University of Nebraska, Lincoln, NE 68583

ABSTRACT

Incomplete information on factors contributing to apparent protein quality and to value of food products as sources of protein and how these factors interact necessitate the use of bioassay procedures. Ideally bioassay procedures should be done using the animal species for which the protein is intended. Practical considerations dictate the use of small animal bioassay rather than human bioassays for routine use in protein product evaluation. To be of real value for assays of food products designed for human use, animal bioassays must accurately predict human performance. Surprisingly little information is available on this topic.

In the current project three Nebraska winter wheats of similar genetic backgrounds were evaluated for protein value and for value of the wheats as sources of proteins. Chemical, weanling mouse, adult human and growing human bioassay techniques were employed. Rankings of the grains were similar regardless of species used for protein quality evaluations. Similar rankings were found regardless of species used for protein quality/quantity evaluations. However, ranking varied between methods designed to evaluate protein quality and those designed to measure protein quality/

[1]The research was supported in part by funds from the Agency for International Development, U.S. Dept. of State, Washington, D.C. Contract No. AID/csd-1208 and by Nebraska Agricultural Experiment Station Project 91-007. Published as Paper No. 3633, Journal Series, Nebraska Agricultural Experiment Station.

quantity interrelationships. The results stress the importance of
matching appropriate methodology with information desired. In a
latter project, wheats of dissimilar genetic background were not
as uniformily evaluated. This suggests that other factors known
to affect protein quality and value were more variable in these
wheats.

INTRODUCTION

Because of greater ease, lower expense, and ethical considerations, small animals such as rats and mice are more frequently
used to assess the protein quality of food products destined for
human consumption than are human subjects. Value of results small
animal assays are limited to the extent that they accurately reflect
human performance on similar assays and to the extent that the
parameters in either assay either directly or indirectly measure
factors of concern in human nutrition. Ideal amino acid proportionality patterns vary among various small animal and human
beings. Hence, protein quality of a food product for humans may
be estimated falsely high or low with small animal bioassays.
Futhermore, errors in qualitive/quantitive estimations of first
limiting amino acids may lead to undesirable amino acid supplementation. Protein value of food products for humans is also
influenced by digestibility and by non-specific nitrogen content.
Human and small animal responses to these are not identical.

PROTEIN QUALITY VS. PROTEIN VALUE

In looking at relationships between characteristics of a
food or feed and its protein nutritional value for animal species
consuming it, several questions may be asked. Two of the most
basic of these are:

> What is the nutritional value of the protein contained
> in a test product?
> What is the nutritional value of a test product as a
> source of protein?

These questions are not synonymous since the former involves
measurement of protein quality and the latter implies in the
limited sense measurement of both protein quantity and quality
contained in the product. (Kies, C.,1970) In the broader sense,
this later question also might include all factors influencing the
amount of food product consumed or likely to be consumed by any
human population group or segment thereof. Thus, cultural values,
economic conditions, palatability characteristics could reasonably

be covered. However, this discussion will be limited to the
narrower definitions. Methodologies for evaluations of protein were
developed, tested, and perfected using either relatively purified
proteins or mixtures of purified amino acids. Different problems
in the bioassay of mixtures of purified amino acid proportioned as
in corn protein, purified corn proteins such as zein and corn
protein as contained in corn exist. Reduction in variables make
results with relatively purified materials more predictable in
both human and small animal bioassays. Proteins as contained in
products are far more important as practical sources of dietary
proteins for most human populations at the present time. Hence,
accuracy of methods for these applications is necessary.

METHODOLOGY VARIATIONS: SMALL ANIMAL VS HUMAN BIOASSAYS

     Unfortunately, comparison of data and conclusions drawn from
data obtained from human bioassay studies and small animal bioassay studies are not merely a problem of species differences but
also of methodology difference.   There are a variety of measurements useful in protein bioassays (Friedman, 1975, Bodwell, 1977,
LaChance et al, 1977) using human beings and small animals but in
practice relatively few of these currently receive wide usage.
Growth measurements or derivations of growth measurements are
usually used in small animal studies with protein efficiency ratios
(PER) or feed efficiency ratios (FER) involving weanling rats or
mice being most popular. The nitrogen balance technique is the
most commonly used approach in human bioassay protein studies.

     Because of smaller amounts of test rations required, weanling
mice rather than weanling rats are most commonly used in this
laboratory. Both mouse and human bioassays are employed in the
Department of Food and Nutrition, University of Nebraska. As
interpreted in our laboratory, classical methodology for mouse
bioassay procedures and human bioassay procedures are summarized
in Table 1.

     Rations of small animals are formulated to contain equal
quantities by weight of test product or of test protein and
calculations are accomplished on the amount voluntarily eaten by
the animal. Usually evaluations are done on relatively unprocessed test materials. In human evaluations, a predetermined
amount of test product or protein is determined by the investigator
for subjects to consume. (If they're not willing to eat it,
they're eliminated as subjects.) Test foods are fed in a more
highly processed, cooked form, and are fed as part of a more
liberal diet.

TABLE 1

Protein Bioassay Methodology at

Department of Food and Nutrition

University of Nebraska

Mouse Bioassay	Human Bioassay
Rations formulated to contain quantities of grain or protein on a % of ration basis.	Diets formulated to contain quantities of grain or protein on a 24-hour intake basis.
Growth (weight gain) is indirectly method of assay.	Nitrogen balance is method of assay.
Comparisons made among groups of animals having same genetic background, different test rations.	Subjects have different genetic backgrounds; hence, all experimental variables plus controls must be applied to all subjects during different periods.
Test feeding period per each test grain = 28 days.	Test feeding period per each test grain = 4-7 days.

As previously discussed, growth (weight gain) is the basis of the most popular assays using small animals while the nitrogen balance technique is the method of choice usually in human bioassay approaches. While it is possible to do growth-type evaluations on humans or nitrogen balance-type studies on mice, questions of morality limit the application of the former and questions of practicality in mass screening reduce the usefulness of the latter.

In small animal bioassays, comparisons are made among groups of animals having the same genetic background but fed different test rations. Because of the impossibility in obtaining inbred humans for testing purposes of this type, in human bioassay evaluations all experimental diets plus control diets are usually fed to all subjects during different, short term periods. Experimental feeding periods in classical animal bioassay methods are relatively long--28 days in terms of the life span of the animals. The 4-7 day periods used in human bioassay procedures are obviously short by any standard of evaluation.

Under many circumstances, simply to determine whether or not one product is superior in protein quality to another or to rank products is the type of information wanted. Theoretically nitrogen balance studies or PER studies should give similar answers. Several studies have been conducted in this laboratory using wheat grain flours as the test materials to evaluate this approach.

METHODOLOGY: WHEAT STUDY

Chemical Assay

The 3 wheat grain materials used in this study were Gage, Scout 66 and Scoutland grains ground into a whole wheat flour. These were analyzed for total protein content (nitrogen content by the Kjeldahl method x 5.83) (2). Amino acid profiles were determined by autoanalyzer column chromatography techniques.

Small Animal Bioassay

Male weanling mice (Swiss Webster strain) were randomly assigned to groups of 6 mice each. Groups were equalized for initial weight. Mice were caged individually in wire cages and allowed feed and water ad libitum for the course of the study--26 days.

In one series PER (protein efficiency ratio) evaluations were performed on the test grains. This evaluation measures weight gain per gram of protein consumed by the mice. An increase in PER value is assumed to be indicative of an improvement in protein quality. In this evaluation, rations were formulated to contain either 10% protein or 7% protein from each of the test grains. Rations were fortified with a vitamin mix (2.0%) and a mineral mix (4.2%). They also contained corn oil (10%), sucrose (8.8%), and variable amounts of wheat starch (used to equalize the various wheat flours in amounts necessary to give 7 or 10% protein). Mice were weighed weekly. Feed consumption was determined over the full 26-day feeding period. Details regarding methodology in mouse bioassays used in this laboratory have been given in an earlier study (Kies, 1972b)

In a second series, FER (feed efficiency ratio) evaluations were done. As applied in our laboratory, FER measures the amount of ration required for each gram of weight gained; hence, the lower

the FER number value the better nutritional value of the ration is
assumed to be. This method is used to answer questions on comparative value of test grains quantitatively and qualitatively as
sources of protein. As applied in the evaluation described here,
rations were formulated to contain equal quantities of test grain
(75% by weight). Other constituents of the rations were wheat
starch, sucrose, corn oil, vitamin mix, and mineral mix. Because
rations were formulated to contain equal quantities of grain and
the grains varied in protein content, the rations also varied in
protein content proportional to that found in the original grain.
Other aspects were as described for the first series.

A casein diet (10% protein) and dry skim milk (10% and 7%
protein) were used as positive controls with separate groups of
mice.

Human Bioassay

Several human biological assays of the test grains were
carried out using the nitrogen balance technique. The nitrogen
balance technique measures nitrogen intake minus urinary and fecal
nitrogen. A decrease in body nitrogen loss or an increase in
body nitrogen retention (real or apparent) is assumed to be
indicative or an improvement in protein nutritional value of the
diet qualitatively and/or quantitatively, depending upon the
experimental design.

In the first study, 12 adult subjects were fed 4.0 g N per
day from each of the test grains, an evaluation of protein quality.
The 32-day study was divided into a nitrogen depletion period
(2 days), a nitrogen adjustment period (6 days), and 4 experimental
periods of 6 days each. Purposes and procedures of the nitrogen
depletion and nitrogen adjustment periods have been discussed in
an earlier paper. (Kies, 1972a)

During the experimental periods, nitrogen intake of the 12
adult human subjects was maintained constant at 4.8 g N per day.
(-4.0 g N from the test wheat flours or the dry skim milk control
and 0.8 g N from the basal diet). Diets were supplemented with
vitamins and minerals. The wheat flour was incorporated into a
yeast-raised bread. The experimental periods were randomly
arranged for each individual subject. Other general details
pertaining to human bioassay determinations were described more
fully in an earlier paper (Kies, 1972a).

The 12 young men and women who participated as subjects were
all students of the University of Nebraska-Lincoln. All were in
good health and received approval for subject participation by the

Student Health Division of the University of Nebraska. All maintained their usual class/work/daily life schedules, but ate most of their meals in the Human Metabolism Laboratory.

A second study was essentially a replication of the study just described except 12 - 16 year old boys in the rapid growth stage were used as subjects. Experimental periods were shortened to 4 days each. The 12 boys' personal physicians rather than the University Student Health Division were used as medical consultants.

In a third adult human bioassay study, the 3 test grains were evaluated at equal intakes of grain (150 grams per day), a method designed to compare both quantitative and qualitative aspects of grain. Except for the variation in use of equal levels of grain rather than equal levels of protein, experimental procedures were similar to those described in the first study of the series. (Ten adult men and women were subjects.)

In all 3 studies, nitrogen balance data were based on urinary excretion of nitrogen on 24 hour collections and on stool excretion of nitrogen on full period lots. The Kjeldahl nitrogen procedure (Scales and Harrison, 1920) was used for analysis of urine, stools, and food for nitrogen content. Statistical analysis of variance and Duncan's Multiple Range Test.

RESULTS - WHEAT STUDY

Chemical characteristics of the test grains are given in Table 2.

Protein contents of Gage, Scout 66, and Scoutland were 16.8, 15.8, and 14.8%, respectively. Lysine contents on a percent protein basis were 2.8, 3.1, and 3.1, respectively, and on a percent grain basis were 0.48, 0.48, and 0.46, respectively.

Ranks were assigned from a 1 (best) to 3 (poorest) basis for whatever characteristic or type of data being evaluated. Using this approach, as shown in Table 2, on the characteristic of protein content Gage was ranked 1, Scout 66 ranked 2, and Scoutland ranked 3; on the basis of lysine as a percent protein basis Scoutland and Scout 66 ranked about the same and Gage was ranked 3; on the basis of lysine content on a percent grain basis, there was little difference among the grains. The small variation in lysine content among the grains tested might limit the usefulness of comparison.

PER and FER values of the wheat materials are shown in Table 3. Using the ranking system of evaluation for PER at both the

TABLE 2

Chemical evaluations of Test Grains

Characteristics	Test Grain		
	Gage	Scout 66	Scoutland
Chemical Evaluations			
Protein content			
% Grain	16.8	15.8	14.8
Rank	1	2	3
Lysine content			
% Protein	2.8	3.1	3.1
Rank	3	1.5	1.5
% Grain	0.48	0.48	0.46

10% and the 7% protein intake levels, Scoutland was ranked first, followed by Scout 66 with Gage ranking third. These differences in PER value were small and not statistically significant, reflecting probably the relatively small differences in lysine content among the grains. Ranking according to the FER data gave Gage top value followed by Scout 66 with Scoutland being third.

Human bioassay study results are given in Table 4. In the first study, adult subjects were fed 4.0 g N per day from each of the tests grains, an evaluation of protein quality. Mean nitrogen balances of the 11 adult subjects fed 4.0 g N/day from Gage, Scout 66 and Scoutland were -1.15, -1.15 and -0.93 g N/day, respectively, giving a rank of 1 to Scoutland but failing to differentiate between Gage and Scout 66 for second and third place.

In a similar study, 12 adolescent boys (rapid growth state) were fed 4.0 g N per day from the test grains. Mean nitrogen balances for the 12 boys fed Gage, Scout 66 and Scoutland were

TABLE 3

Mouse Bioassays of Test Grains

Characteristics	Test Grain[1]		
	Gage	Scout 66	Scoutland
Mouse PER values			
10% protein			
PER value	0.86^a	1.26^{ab}	1.42^b
Rank	3	2	1
7% protein			
PER value	1.09^a	1.16^a	1.28^a
Rank	3	2	1
Mouse FER values			
FER value	6.47^a	6.90^{ab}	7.46^b
Rank	1	2	3

[1]Figures with different letter superscripts statistically different from one another, 5% level

-0.08, +0.13 and +0.47 g N/day, respectively, giving rank values of 3 to Gage, 2 to Scout 66 and 1 to Scoutland. (Values for Gage and Scout 66 were not significantly different.)

In a third adult human bioassay study, the 3 test grains were evaluated at equal intakes of grain (150 grams per day), a method designed to compare both quantitative and qualitative nutritional aspects of grain. Mean nitrogen balances of the 10 subjects fed Gage, Scout 66, and Scoutland were -0.12, -0.44 and -1.02 g N/day, respectively. Using the ranking system, Gage ranked 1, Scout 66 ranked 2, and Scoutland ranked 3.

TABLE 4

Human Bioassays of Test Grains

Characteristics	Test Grain[1]		
	Gage	Scout 66	Scoutland
Human N balance values			
N balance - adults 4.0 g N intake/day			
g N/day	-1.15[a]	-1.15[a]	-0.93[b]
Rank	2.5	2.5	1
(milk control = -0.53)			
N balance - adolescent boys 4.0 g N intake/day			
g N/day	-0.08[a]	+0.13[a]	+0.47[b]
(milk control = +1.07)			
N balance - adults 150 g grain intake/day			
g N/day	-0.12[a]	-0.44[b]	-1.02[c]
Rank	1	2	3
(milk control = +0.04)			

[1]Figures designated by different letters in each group are statistically different from one another at the 5% level.

At first, the results seem to be so mixed that no conclusions can be drawn. However, if one remembers that answers to two separate questions were being sought, the data become clearer.

The first question was "What is the rank order of the protein value provided by the 3 test grains?" This is a question of protein quality and relates primarily to comparative amino acid proportionality patterns. The best tests for measuring this characteristic in this series were as follows:

1) Chemical evaluations - lysine content as a percent of protein. The ranks for the 3 test grains were 3 for Gage, 1.5 for Scout 66 and 1.5 for Scoutland.

2) Mouse bioassay evaluation - PER assay. At both 7 and 10% protein intakes, ranks for the test grains were 3 for Gage, 2 for Scout 66, and 1 for Scoutland.

3) Human bioassay evaluations - measurement at equal intake of nitrogen (protein). Rank values for adults were 2.5 for Gage and Scout 66 and 1 for Scoutland; rank values for children were 3 for Gage, 2 for Scout 66 and 1 for Scoutland.

The second question that was asked was "What is the rank order value of the 3 test grains as sources of protein?" This question involves both characteristics of quality and quantity. Best measures of finding the answer to this question are as follows:

1) Chemical evaluations - protein content. Rank values were: Gage - 1, Scout 66 - 2, Scoutland - 3.

2) Mouse bioassay evaluations FER measurements. Rank values were: Gage - 1, Scout 66 - 2, Scoutland - 3.

3) Human bioassay evaluations - equal intake of grain evaluations. Rank values were: Gage - 1, Scout 66 - 2, and Scoutland - 3.

Therefore, the various methods were in fairly close agreement in giving similar answers to the specific questions asked. If one is interested in the comparative value of the protein of the 3 test grains, Scoutland is best followed by Scout 66 with Gage being poorest. However, if one is interested in comparative value of the 3 grains as sources of protein, Gage is best, followed by Scout 66 with Scoutland being poorest. Chemical, animal and human evaluations in general gave fairly comparable rank order.

Since completion of this study another project has been completed using different lines of wheat of different genetic backgrounds. (Kies et al, 1975) Theoretically ranking of these materials
by chemical, small animal, and human bioassays should have been
easier since protein and lysine content differences were greater.
This proved not to be the case. Correlation between chemical and
mouse bioassay results were better than between human and small
animal bioassay results. Results suggested difference in apparent
digestibility of these products among mice and humans might account
for these variations.

These projects do demonstrate the importance of appropriate
matching of methodology to particular knowledge that is wanted and
the danger of over-reliance on any one method of protein quality
assay.

REFERENCES

Bodwell, C.E. (1977). Problems in the development and application
of rapid methods of assessing protein quality. Food
Technology 31, 73-77

Friedman, M. ed. (1975). Protein nutritional quality of Foods and
Feeds. Part I Assay Methods - Biological, Biochemical and
Chemical. New York: Marcel Dekker Inc. c 1975 626 pages

Kies, C. (1972a). Evaluation of the protein value of cereal/plant/
oilseed products by human biological assay techniques in Seed
Proteins. ed by G.E. Inglett, Westport Conn: AVI,
pages 253-264

Kies, C. (1972b). Nutritional evaluation in Proceedings of
International Wheat Conference, Ankara, Turkey, June 5 - 9,
1972, pages 134-139.

Kies, C., Fox, H.M., Mattern, P. and Johnson, V. (1975). Comparative protein nutritive values of whole ground and white flours
from five wheat varieties for humans. Paper presented Spring
Conference, Milling and Baking Division, American Assoc. of
Cereal Chemists, April 24, 1975, Fort Worth, Texas

LaChance, P.A., Bressani, R., and Elias, L.G. (1977). Shorter
protein bioassays. Food Technology 31, pages 82-84

Scales, F.M. and Harrison, A.P. (1920). Boric acid modification
of the Kjeldahl method for crop and soil analysis.
J. Ind. Eng. Chem. 12, pages 350-359

7

UREA AS A DIETARY SUPPLEMENT FOR HUMANS[1]

Constance Kies and Hazel Metz Fox

Dept. of Food and Nutrition, University of Nebraska

Lincoln, NE 68583

ABSTRACT

Use of urea as a nonprotein supplement in the feeding of beef cattle and other ruminant animals is a technique of practical application. Urea, has also been used in human feeding studies. Its early employment was that of an added source of amino nitrogen in studies designed to determine minimum requirements of the essential amino acid. Later studies suggested that it's inclusion in diet containing sub-optimal amounts of protein supplied by various food product could result in the establishment of apparent improvement in protein nutriture. Other studies indicate that urea is not unique in this ability but is only one of many possible sources of amino nitrogen and is actually one of the least effective. Known and potential hazzards definitely prohibit the use of urea supplements to food products other than in research or clinical laboratories at the present time.

INTRODUCTION

Use of urea as a nonprotein nitrogen source in the extending or total replacing of protein in ruminant animal feeds has been widely studied to the extent that it is now currently part of animal nutrition practical practice (Chalupa, 1972, Briggs, 1967). Since explanations for ruminant animal utilization of non-protein

[1]Paper N. 5416, Journal Series, Nebraska Agricultural Research Station Project 91-007.

nitrogen sources including urea have stressed the role of microbial activity in the rumen it is not surprising that possibilities
of nonprotein nitrogen useage in nonruminant animals including
human beings have received comparatively little attention. Studies
on urea and other nonprotein nitrogen sources utilization by swine
and chickens have been reviewed by Hoefer, 1967, Featherston, 1967,
Lewis, D., 1972. This paper will be limited to a discussion of
some of the research involving investigation of nonprotein nitrogen
utilization by human beings in which urea was employed as the non-
protein nitrogen source.

UREA AND MINIMUM ESSENTIAL AMINO ACID REQUIREMENTS

In studies to establish quantitive requirements of the
essential amino acids of humans, it was early recognized that
additional sources of nitrogen to that supplied by the essential
amino acids must be supplied for synthesis of nonessential amino
acids if determined requirements figures were to be truly minimal
(Rose, 1957). This additional nitrogen has been variously termed
nonessential, unessential, or nonspecific nitrogen. Included
under such general headings would be nitrogen from excess essential
amino acids, nitrogen from nonessential amino acids, and amino
nitrogen from such nonprotein sources as glycine and diammonium
citrate and glycine. While it was recognized that such nitrogen
resources should be incorporated into the semi-purfied diets used
in these studies, little consistency existed among researchers on
what kind or how much should be used. Urea was utilized in some
of the studies designed to establish minimal essential amino acid
requirements of adult men and of infants (Rose, 1957, Holt et al,
1960). However, various mixtures of glycine, diammonium and
glutamic acid were usually used in those studies seeking to determine minimal essential amino acid requirements of women(Leverton,
1959).

Level of nonspecific nitrogen supplementation may actually or
apparently affect minimal essential amino acid requirements in
several ways. If omitted or fed at less than optimal levels,
essential amino acids would be needed to fill not only essential
amino acid functions but also for synthesis of nonessential amino
acids; thus, requirements for essential amino acids would be increased. Studies for establishment of minimal essential amino
acids specified a quantitative level of nitrogen balance for
designation of adequacy of intake of a particular amino acid.
Errors inherent to nitrogen balance studies favor more positive
nitrogen balances with increases in total dietary nitrogen (which
does occur with nonspecific nitrogen supplementation) which makes

true improvement somewhat difficult to establish. Nevertheless both of these factors would tend to make essential amino acid requirements established at higher total nitrogen intake levels of less than those established at lower levels of total nitrogen intake.

More recently, several investigations on effects of total nitrogen intake on quantitive requirements of essential amino acid have been reported. Lysine, tryptophan and phenyalanine requirements are apparently lower at higher total nitrogen intake levels than at lower intake levels (Fisher et al, 1968, Fisher et al, 1963, Tolbert and Watt, 1963, Kies et al, 1965, Kies and Fox, 1970).

In a recent study completed in this laboratory, the effects of two levels of urea supplementation of diets containing graded levels of methionine was investigated in an attempt to investigate the effect of total nitrogen intake on methionine requirements of human adults (Kies and Fox, 1975).

In the controlled-feeding study, 14 adult men and women were maintained on diets low in total sulfur-containing amino acids. The basal diet used in the adjustment and experimental periods provided 4.3 g nitrogen per day and 0.40 g of S-containing amino acids from potatoes, soy-meat analog, and a few low protein fruits and vegetables. In each of the 2 parts of the study, crystalline L-form methionine was added as a dietary supplement to provide 0.00, 0.30, 0.60 and 0.90 g of methionine per day, respectively, during each of the 4 experimental periods making up each half. Thus, total sulfur containing amino acid intake varied from 0.40, to 0.70, to 1.00, to 1.30 g per day, respectively. Within each half, order of presentation of the experimental periods was randomized for each subject in order to minimize carry-over and ordering effects. Urea was used to adjust total dietary nitrogen to 4.5 g nitrogen per day in Part A and to 8.5 g in Part B. Order of Parts A and B was reversed for one-half of the subjects. Vitamin and mineral intakes were maintained at adequate levels through use of supplements. Caloric intake was adjusted for each individual at a level for maintenance of weight through alterations in intake of sucrose, butter oil, starch bread and hard candy. The experimental plan is shown on Table 1.

Standard nitrogen balance methodology was used as the criteria of evaluation. As employed in this laboratory, detailed description of this procedure has been described in an earlier paper (Kies, 1977). Analysis of variance and Duncan's Multiple Range Tests were used in statistical analysis of data.

TABLE I

Effect of Urea Supplementation of Diets Containing Graded Levels of Sulfur
Containing Amino Acids (S-cont. AA) on Nitrogen Balances of Adult Men

Period	No. of days	S-cont. A.A. intake		N intake			N balance[1]
		Supplement	Total	Diet	Urea	Total	
		g	g	g	g	g	g
Part A							
Depletion	2	0.00	0.07	0.8	0	0.5	
Adjustment	6	0.00	0.40	4.3	0.2	4.5	
Expt. 1	4	0.00	0.40	4.3	0.2	4.5	-0.91
Expt. 2	4	0.30	0.70	4.3	0.15	4.5	-0.66
Expt. 3	4	0.60	1.00	4.3	0.10	4.5	-0.41
Expt. 4	4	0.90	1.30	4.3	0.05	4.5	-0.36
Part B							
Depletion	2	0.00	0.07	0.8	0.0	0.5	
Adjustment	6	0.00	0.40	4.3	4.2	8.5	
Expt. 5	4	0.00	0.40	4.3	4.2	8.5	-0.50
Expt. 6	4	0.30	0.70	4.3	4.15	8.5	-0.25
Expt. 7	4	0.60	1.00	4.3	4.10	8.5	-0.31
Expt. 8	4	0.90	1.30	4.3	4.05	8.5	-0.27

[1]Mean values of 14 adult men.

As shown in Table 1, mean nitrogen balances while receiving 0.40, 0.70, 1.00 and 1.30 g of total sulfur containing amino acids were -0.91, -0.66, -0.41 and -0.36 g nitrogen, per day, at the 4.5 g nitrogen intake respectively, and -0.50, -0.25, -0.31 and -0.27 g N per day, respectively at the 8.5 g level. Nitrogen equilibrium was not achieved at either level of total nitrogen intake which might have been the result of failure to have a completely adjusted pattern of essential amino acids other than the total sulfur containing amino acids. Statistical improvement in nitrogen retention was found in increasing total sulfur-containing amino acids from 0.4 to 0.7 to 1.0 g per day but not to increasing intake to 1.3 g per day. Thus, one interpretation of data could be that requirement of methionine was between 0.7 and 1.0 g per day at this level of total nitrogen intake. At the 8.5 g nitrogen intake level no improvement in nitrogen retention was achieved by raising total sulfur containing amino acid intake to above 0.70 g per day. Thus, the requirement level would be reduced to between 0.40 and 0.70 g per day at this level of nitrogen intake.

UREA SUPPLEMENTATION OF FOOD PROTEIN RESOURCES

While the need for inclusion of nonspecific nitrogen sources such as urea in purified essential amino acid mixtures for research or therapeutic purposes is generally accepted, the idea that nonspecific nitrogen supplementation of food protein might be demonstrated to have some apparent positive effects is less well recognized and, in fact, is subject to some controversy.

Several authors have observed that feeding foods to provide minimum but adequate amounts of the essential amino acids fail to maintain human subjects in positive nitrogen balance or in nitrogen equalibrium. Bricker, et al(1945) observed that although 0.20 g/kg of cow's milk protein contains adequate quantities of all essential amino acids, 0.45 g protein/kg are needed to maintain nitrogen balance. Snyderman (1967) reported that 0.40-0.50 g/kg of cow's milk are needed. In our own laboratory, 20 g protein from egg has been found to be inadequate to maintain nitrogen equilibrium in human adults although essential amino acids are all provided in amounts equal to or greater than the Rose Minimum Requirement Pattern (1957). Food proteins contain appreciable amounts of nonessential amino acids as well as essential amino acids. Although sources of high quality protein such as egg, milk and beef generally contain proportionally lower amounts of nonessential to essential amino acid than do cereal/plant products, the nonessential amino acids provided more closely match the general patterns found in the protein constituents of the human body. Thus, it would seem surprising that additional sources of nonspecific nitrogen for their synthesis would be needed when the food proteins were fed in amounts to just meet essential amino acid requirements. However, the earlier discussed studies in which the essential amino acid requirements were established involved the feeding of nonspecific nitrogen to essential amino acid nitrogen in proportionately much greater amounts than that found in food.

This seeming inconsistency was studied by Snyderman (Snyderman, 1967, Snyderman et al, 1962). Using human infants for study, milk intake was reduced in a stepwise fashion while keeping energy intake constant until weight gain was arrested or until subnormal nitrogen retention was observed. Addition of either urea or glycine reestablished nitrogen balances at levels indicating adequacy of protein intake and also reestablished the normal pattern of weight gain. Thus, the authors concluded that established "unessential" nitrogen rather than an essential amino acid as being the first limiting factor in milk for human infants. The same authors also reported data from studies involving feeding of labeled "unessential nitrogen" (^{15}N urea and ^{15}N ammonium chloride). Incorporation of these materials into both plasma protein and hemoglobin was found.

In a series of studies from this laboratory involving nonspecific nitrogen supplementation of corn, nonspecific nitrogen was found to be the first limiting nitrogenous factor in ordinary corn protein (Kies et al, 1965a, 1965b, 1967a, 1967b). These studies used various combinations of glycine, diammonium citrate and glutamic acid as nitrogen sources. More recently studies involving urea supplementation of opaque-2 corn have been conducted (Kies and Fox, 1972, Ranum et al 1977, Korslund et al, 1977).

In the first study a low protein opaque-2 corn diet was supplemented with a nonspecific nitrogen source (urea) to provide three different levels of nitrogen intake. A 3-day nitrogen depletion period and three experimental periods of 10 days each were used. The order of the three experimental periods was randomly arranged for each of the 9 adult subjects.

During the three experimental periods the opaque-2 corn provided 4.0 g N/day. Either 0.0, 4.0 or 8.0 g N/day was added to each subject's diet by urea supplementation. Together with the 0.8 g N/day supplied by the basal diet the final nitrogen intakes for the three experimental diets were either 4.8, 8.8 or 12.8 g N/day. Standard nitrogen balance techniques as applied in our laboratory were carried out. In addition venous fasting blood samples were drawn prior to the feeding phase of the study and at the end of each experimental period. Serum's total iron binding capacity (TIBC) was measured as an indication of total amount of serum transferrin. Transferrin levels have been found to be severely depressed in children with kwashiorkor.

Nitrogen balances of subjects receiving urea supplementation of the opaque-2 corn was improved at both levels of supplementation in comparison to values when opaque-2 corn was fed alone as shown in Table 2. It is important to remember that if more opaque-2 corn protein had been fed, positive nitrogen balance could have been achieved by that approach.

TABLE 2

Affect of Urea N Supplementation of Opaque-2 Corn Diets (4.0 g N/day) on Nitrogen Balances of Human Adult Subjects

Subject No.	N balance at following levels of urea N supplementation (g N/day)[1]		
	0	4.0	8.0
	g N/day	g N/day	g N/day
280	-0.17	-0.59	0.38
281	-0.60	0.37	1.86
282	-0.22	0.99	3.60
283	0.14	0.45	1.95
284	-0.58	0.06	0.09
285	0.77	1.09	2.40
286	0.10	0.17	1.12
287	-2.46	-0.35	0.42
288	-0.22	0.27	1.59
Mean	-0.36	0.27	1.49

[1]Mean balances for each subject for the last five days of each 10 day period.

Mean blood serum TIBC of subjects while receiving 0, 4.0, and 8.0 g N/day from urea as a supplement to the corn protein were 328, 343, and 360 μg/100ml, respectively. Values for individual subjects are shown on Table 3. Although not statistically significant, the results do indicate a patterned response of possible biological significance. It would appear that subject's transferrin levels were most   closely similar to pre-experimental values (when it is assumed that subjects were receiving ample protein supplies) when the highest level of urea supplementation was employed.

Several other parameters of protein nutritional status were also measured including blood serum total protein, blood serum albumin/globulin ratios, blood hemoglobin, and blood hematocrit. No consistent changes were seen which could be attributed to urea supplementation of the opaque-2 corn diets.

TABLE 3

Affect of Urea N Supplementations of
Opaque-2 Corn Diets (4.0 g N/day)
on Blood Serum Total Iron Binding
Capacity (TIBC) of Human Subjects

Subject No.	TIBC (ug/100ml) after 10 days on following levels of Urea N Supplementation (g N/day)			
	Pre-study	0	4.0	8.0
280	318	320	292	310
281	312	307	316	339
282	352	273	326	301
283	349	316	323	378
284	376	331	364	400
285	421	387	410	420
286	475	356	387	380
287	332	355	381	386
288	360	303	289	325
Mean	366	328	343	360

In the second study of this series on urea supplementation of opaque-2 corn diets, 7 adolescent doys aged 12 - 16 years were subjects (Korslund et al, 1977). The experimental period was 23 days in length and consisted of a 3-day adjustment period and two 10-day experimental periods. During all experimental periods, opaque-2 corn supplied 6.0 g day/subject/day. During one of the experimental periods a urea supplement supplying 4.0 g N/day was employed while during the other no nonspecific nitrogen supplement was given. Nitrogen balances of subjects were determined for subjects for the last 5 days of each experimental period using techniques customarily employed in this laboratory. In addition fasting blood samples were drawn at the end of each experimental period for additional analyses.

Mean individual and group nitrogen balances for the experimental periods in which 6 g of nitrogen from opaque-2 corn alone or in combination with 4 g nitrogen from urea were fed are shown in Table 4. The mean nitrogen balance of 7 boys when opaque-2 corn was fed alone was +0.63 g/day. When 4 g of nitrogen from urea was added, the mean nitrogen balance was +1.37 g/day. Individual mean balances increased when urea was added for all subjects except subject 402 whose nitrogen balance decreased slightly when urea was added suggesting a true improvement in response to the supplement. Statistical analysis of variance showed that mean nitrogen balances for the 2 treatments were significantly different (P>0.05).

TABLE 4

Nitrogen Balances of Adolescent Boys fed Opaque-2
Corn With or Without Urea Supplementation[1]

Subject No.	Nitrogen Balance	
	Without Supplement	With Supplement
	(g/day)	
390	+1.92	+2.81
392	+0.89	+2.39
393	-0.26	+1.17
397	-0.74	-0.16
398	+1.30	+2.11
399	+1.18	+1.24
402	+0.14	+0.04
Mean N Balance	+0.63	+1.37

[1]Opaque-2 corn fed to supply 6.0 g N/subject/day during all periods. The urea supplement supplied 4.0 g N/subject/day.

Apparent digestibility values for opaque-2 corn measured with and without urea supplementation for individual subjects and mean digestibilities were determined. Mean fecal nitrogen excretion was almost the same (1.79 and 1.83 g/subject/day) for the 2 treatments. The apparent digestibility was higher (83%) when urea was added than when corn was fed alone (73%). This observation indicated that urea was nearly 100 percent digestible. Thus, apparent digestibility increased when urea was fed.

Treatments which resulted in greater nitrogen retention (more positive, or conversely less negative balances) were considered superior to those in which less nitrogen was retained. The results of this study were similar to those observed in adults by Kies and Fox (1972). The addition of urea to the diet resulted in increased nitrogen retention in both studies. If an increase in nitrogen retained is used as the criterion, apparently urea can be used as a source of nitrogen for the synthesis of nonessential amino acids in both growing boys and adults. The possibility that urea may go directly to blood urea nitrogen must be considered since BUN values increased in all cases when urea was added to the diet (Table 5). While the fate of urea in metabolism was not tested in this study, it has previously been observed the BUN values increase in response to any increase in total dietary nitrogen, whether from intact protein, synthetic amino acids or any source of nonspecific nitrogen (Kies et al, 1967b; Kies and Fox, 1970b; Kies and Fox, 1971). The levels of blood urea nitrogen observed in this study were within normal range when high levels of urea supplements were used.

The results of these two studies suggest that nonspecific nitrogen may be the first limiting nitrogenous factor in opaque-2 corn. This does not eliminate all considerations of protein quality. Other studies indicate that feeding of lysine supplements also are effective in improvement in nitrogen balance when opaque-2 corn is feed in less than optimal amounts (Kies and Fox, 1972).

COMPARATIVE EFFECTIVENESS OF UREA AS A NONSPECIFIC NITROGEN SOURCE

Urea may have certain advantages economically as a nonspecific nitrogen source but few studies have been conducted to compare its biological effectiveness with other laboratory-used sources of nonspecific nitrogen. Several studies have been conducted using a wide variety of nonspecific nitrogen resources including essential amino acid mixtures, nonessential amino acid mixtures, diammonium citrate, glycine, glutamic acid, and various combinations of these and others but from which urea was omitted. These studies have been reviewed in an earlier article (Kies, 1974).

TABLE 5

Blood Urea Nitrogen Levels of Adolescent
Boys Fed Opaque-2 Corn With or
Without Urea Supplementation[1]

Subject No.	Blood Urea Nitrogen	
	Without Supplement	With Supplement
	(mg/100 ml)	
390	4	10
392	6	10
393	4	7
397	6	8
398	4	6
399	5	8
402	4	7
Mean	4.7	8.0

[1]Opaque-2 corn fed to supply 6.0 g N/subject/day during all periods. The urea supplement supplied 4.0 g N/subject/day.

Two studies have been conducted in this laboratory to compare the effectiveness of urea and diammonium citrate as sources of nonspecific nitrogen for human adults (Kies and Fox, 1973).

The first study consisted of four experimental parts, each composed of a 5-day nitrogen adjustment period and two experimental periods of 5 days each. During one experimental period an isonitrogenous mixture of glycine and diammonium citrate was the source of nonspecific nitrogen and,during the other, the source of nonspecific nitrogen was an isonitrogenous mixture of urea and diammonium citrate. During the four parts, these nitrogen sources were added to the diets to supply 1.77, 4.77, 7.77, and 10.77 g of N/day. The essential amino acids were fed as defined by the Rose Minimum Requirement Pattern. Accounting for all sources of nitrogen, nitrogen intake ranged from 3 to 6 to 9 to 12 g of N/day.

Mean nitrogen balance of subjects as shown in Table 6 receiving urea and glycine at the 3.0 g of N level was -1.65, a value significantly lower ($p < 0.05$) than the mean value of -1.12 g of N, while receiving diammonium citrate and glycine. At the 6.0 g of N level the comparable values were -0.85 and -0.52 ($p < 0.05$), at the 9.0 g of N level, the values were +0.12 and +0.28 (no significant difference), and at the 12 g of N intake level, the values were +0.74 and +0.72 g of N/day (no significant difference), respectively. Thus as the level of nonspecific nitrogen supplementation was increased, the nitrogen retention of subjects also increased and the difference in effectiveness between the two test sources of nonspecific nitrogen was decreased.

The second study of this series was composed as a 2-day depletion period, a 3-day adjustment period, and two experimental periods of 5 days each. During the two experimental periods, diammonium citrate or urea was fed as a single source of nonspecific nitrogen at a 4.3 g of nonspecific N intake level (6.0 g total N intake). Other aspects of the study were essentially the same as in the one just described. Mean nitrogen balance of subjects as shown in Table 7 receiving the urea supplement was -0.42 g of N and, while receiving diammonium citrate, was -0.24 g of N (p<0.05%). These results clearly suggest that urea is a less efficient source of nonspecific nitrogen than diammonium citrate.

TABLE 6

Nitrogen Balances of Human Adult Subjects
Fed Supplements of Diammonium Citrate
(DAC) + Glycine or Urea + Glycine

Level of Supplementary N[1]	Mean N balance while receiving	
	DAC + Glycine	Urea + Glycine
(g N/day)	(g N/day)	
1.77	-1.12	-1.65
4.77	-0.52	-0.85
7.77	+0.28	+0.12
10.77	+0.72	+0.74

[1]Essential amino acids supplied by a mixture of purified L amino acids as defined by the Rose Minimum Requirement Patterns.

TABLE 7

Nitrogen Balances of Human Adult Subjects
Fed Supplements of Diammonium Citrate
(DAC) or Glycine (4.3 g N/subject/day)

Source of Supplementary N	Mean N Balance
DAC	-0.24
Urea	-0.42

CLINICAL STUDIES INVOLVING UREA UTILIZATION BY HUMANS

Discussion of urea supplementation of human diets must at least mention the use of Giordano - Giovannetti (Gio-Gio) diets in treatment of uremic patients (Giordano, 1963, Giodano et al, 1968, Giovannette and Maggiore, 1964). This work suggests that the high levels of blood urea nitrogen in uremia can be reduced if small amounts of idealized patterns of essential amino acids as purified amino acids or as high quality protein are included in otherwise protein-free diets. In addition to reducing blood urea nitrogen, nitrogen balances of patients are improved with this therapeutic approach. Using both normal and uremic patients, ^{15}N from urea was found in nonessential amino acids of blood albumin. Administration of an antibiotic to reduce intestinal microorganism populations and urease activity resulted in an apparent inhibition of urea utilization.

Currently, some modifications of the Gio-Gio approach have been initiated and others are being recommended. These have been reviewed by Gofferje (1976).

Gallina and Dominquez (1971a) recently investigated the role of calorie intake when nonprotein nitrogen replaced part of a high biological value protein. In 5 obese women fed low calorie milk diets, negative nitrogen balance was induced either by decreasing milk intake or by decreasing carbohydrate intake. In the latter case fat replaced carbohydrate isocalorically. The addition of urea to the diet improved nitrogen retention when milk was the limiting factor but not when carbohydrate was restricted. Carbohydrate precursors are apparently necessary for the synthesis of nonessential amino acids. These authors studied this concept in another way when they induced negative nitrogen balance by removing

valine from the diet of one young woman. The diet contained 10.3
g nitrogen from glycine, diammonium citrate and 8 essential L-amino
acids in the proportion present in egg protein. The ingestion of
the keto analogue, α-ketoisvaleric acid, returned nitrogen balance
to equilibrium when the amount fed was three times that of the
valine removed (Gallina et al, 1971b). The authors speculated
that the amount of the keto analogue needed to maintain nitrogen
equilibrium would be expected to decrease as the subject adjusted
to this metabolic system. A source of nitrogen for ammonia
formation would obviously be necessary for the keto analogue to
be utilized for amino acid synthesis.

CONCLUSION

The topic of urea supplementation of diets must be approached
with greatest caution. Experience with ruminant animal feeding
indicate dangers of ammonia toxicity when care is not employed
in use of urea supplements. Vizek (1972, 1974) has reviewed a
large number of real and potential hazzards as the result of
nonspecific nitrogen supplementation of human diets in general
which may be applied to urea supplementation in particular.
Certainly for the present this is an approach for the research or
clinical laboratory and is not one to be even considered for
practical application. However, it does suggest that protein
quality is not the only factor to consider when determining
adequacy of dietary protein for humans.

REFERENCES

Bricker, M., Mitchell, H.H., and Kinsman, C.H. (1945). The
    protein requirements of adult human subjects in terms of
    various foods and food combination, J. Nutr., 30, 269
Briggs, M.H. (1967). Urea as a Protein Supplement, Pergamon
    Press, 466 pages   c 1967.
Chalupa, W. (1972). Metabolic aspects of nonprotein nitrogen
    utilization in ruminant animals. Fed. Proceedings 31,
    1152-1164.
Featherston, (1967). Utilization of urea and other sources of
    of nonprotein nitrogen by the chicken in Urea as a Protein
    Supplement ed by M.H. Briggs, Pergamon Press, pages 445-454
Fisher, H., Brush, M.K., Griminger, P., and Sostman, E.R., 1968.
    Amino acid balance and the lysine requirement of young
    women. Fed. Proc. 27, 251.
Fisher, H., Brush, M.K., Shapiro, R., Wessels, J.P.H., Berdanier,
C.D., Griminger, P. and Sostman, E.R. (1963). Amino acid balance
in the adult: high nitrogen-low tryptophan diets. J. Nutr. 81,230.

Gallina, D.L. and Dominquez, J.M. (1971). Human utilization of
    urea nitrogen in low calorie diets. J. Nutr. 101, 1029.
Gallina, D.L., Dominquez, J.M., Hoschoian, J.C. and Barrio, J.R.
    (1971). Maintenance of nitrogen balance in a young woman by
    substitution of α-ketoisovaleric acid for valine. J. Nutr.
    101, 1165.
Gofferye, H. (1976). Use of essential amino acids in uremic
    patients. Nutr. Metab. 20, 35-48.
Giordano, C., (1963). Use of exogenous and endogenous urea for
    protein synthesis in normal and uremic subjects. J. Labr.
    and Clin. Med. 62, 231.
Giodano, G., Depascale, C., Balestrieri, C., Cittadini, D., and
    Crescenzi, A., (1968). Incorporation of urea ^{15}N in amino
    acids of patients with chronic renal failure on low nitrogen
    diet. Am. J. Clin. Nutr. 21, 394.
Giovannetti, S. and Maggiore, Q., (1964). A low-protein diet with
    proteins of high biological calue for severe chronic uraemia.
    Lancet I, 1000.
Hoefer, J.A., (1967). The effects of dietary urea on the pig in
    urea as a protein supplement ed. by M.H. Briggs, Pergamon Press,
    pages 431-440.
Holt, L.E. Jr., György, P., Pratt, E.L., Synderman, S.E. and
    Wallace, W.M., (1960). Protein and Amino Acid Requirements
    in Early Life. New York: University Press.
Kies, C., (1974) Comparative value of various sources of nonspecific
    nitrogen for the human. J. Ag. Fd. Chem. 22, 190-193
Kies, C. (1972). Nonspecific nitrogen in the nutrition of human
    beings. Fed. Proc. 31,1172-1177.
Kies, C.,(1977). Techniques in human nitrogen balance studies in
    Evaluation of Proteins for Humans ed. by C.E. Bodwell,
    Westport, Conn.: Avi, c 1977, pp. 162-176.
Kies, C. and Fox, H.M., (1970). Effect of level of total nitrogen
    intake on second limiting amino acid in corn for humans.
    J. Nutr. 100, 1275-1285.
Kies, C. and Fox, H.M., (1973). Comparison of urea and diammonium
    citrate as sources of nonspecific nitrogen for human adults.
    J. Nutr. 103, 664-669.
Kies, C. and Fox, H.M., (1972). Protein nutritional value of
    opaque-2 corn grain for human adults. J. Nutr. 102, 757-765.
Kies, C. and Fox, H.M., (1975). Tryptophan and total sulfur-
    containing amino acid requirements of human adults at two
    levels of total nitrogen intake. Paper presented at FASEB
    annual meeting, Atlantic City, N.J., April 13-18.
Kies, C., Williams, E. and Fox, H.M., (1965a). Determination of
    first limiting nitrogenous factor in corn protein for nitrogen
    retention in human adults. J. Nutr. 85: 350.
Kies, C., Williams, E., and Fox, H.M., (1965b). Effect of "non-
    specific" nitrogen intake on adequacy of cereal proteins for
    nitrogen retention in human adults. J. Nutr. 86: 357.

Kies, C., Fox, H.M., and Williams, E.R., (1967). Effect of non-specific nitrogen intake on minimum corn protein requirement and first limiting amino acid in corn for humans. J. Nutr. 92, 377-383.

Kies, C., Fox, H.M., and Williams, E.R., (1967b). Time, stress, quality and quantity as factors in the nonspecific nitrogen supplementation of corn protein for adult men. J. Nutr. 93: 377-385.

Korslund, M.K., Kies, C, and Fox, H.M., (1977). Protein nutrition value of opaque-2 corn for adolescent boys. Am. J. Clin. Nutr. 30: 371-374.

Lewis, D., (1972). Nonamino and amino nitrogen in nonruminant nutrition. Fed. Proc. 31: 1165-1171.

Leverton, R.M., (1959). Amino acid requirements of young adults in protein and amino acid nutrition. ed by A.A. Albanese, New York: Academic Press, p. 477.

Ranum, P.M., Kies, C., and Fox, H.M., (1977). Effect of low nitrogen intake on serum transferrin of healthy human adults. Nutr. Reports Int. accepted for publications

Rose, W.C., (1957). Amino acid requirements of adult man. Nutr. Abst. Rev. 27: 631-646.

Snyderman, S.E., (1967). Urea as a source of unessential nitrogen for the human in Urea as a Protein Supplement. ed. by M.H. Briggs, New York: Pergamon Press, pages 441-444.

Snyderman, S.E., Holt, L.E. Jr., Dancis, J., Rortman, E., Boyer, A., and Balis, M.E., (1962). "Unessential nitrogen: a limiting factor in human growth. J. Nutr. 78: 57.

Tolbert B. and Watts, J.H., (1963). Phenylalanine requirement of women consuming a minimum tyrosine diet and the sparing effect of tyrosine on phenylalanine requirement. J. Nutr. 80: 111.

Visek, W.J., (1972). Effects of urea hydrolysis on cell life-span and metabolism. Fed. Proc. 31: 1178-1193.

Visek, W.J., (1974). Some biochemical considerations in utilization of nonspecific nitrogen. J. Agric. Fd. Chem. 22: 174-184.

8

NUTRITIONAL CONSEQUENCES OF EXCESS AMINO ACID INTAKE

Hamish N. Munro

Department of Nutrition and Food Science, Massachusetts

Institute of Technology, Cambridge, Mass. 02139

ABSTRACT

Various mechanisms respond to intakes of amino acids in excess of those required for normal tissue function. When excessive amounts of amino acids are taken, catabolism by enzymes in the liver and elsewhere is accelerated when intake exceeds requirements. In addition, changes in the free amino acid levels in the brain signal the nervous system centers regulating food consumption, and eating patterns are affected. This central nervous system mechanism may even determine the proportions of protein and of energy-yielding nutrients chosen in the diet through a mechanism regulated by the entry of tryptophan and other neurotransmitter precursors into the brain. These observations on protective mechanisms are considered in relation to effects obtained by feeding disproportionate amounts of amino acids. Intakes of large amounts of amino acids can produce toxicities, in which plasma concentrations of the administered amino acid rise to very high levels. Antagonisms arise from feeding excess of one amino acid that can be relieved by feeding a structurally related amino acid. Finally, amino acid imbalances are produced by adding surpluses of essential amino acids other than the essential amino acid most limiting for growth; the growth depression caused by this addition can be relieved by adding more of the most limiting amino acid to the diet. In all circumstances involving feeding with disproportionate amounts of amino acids, there is evidence of changes in brain amino acid levels. It is suggested that these changes play an important role in initiating protective responses against abnormal amino acid intakes.

INTRODUCTION

Most dietary proteins do not provide concentrations of amino acids similar to those needed by the body. Furthermore, the supplementation of human diets with amino acids can run the risk of distorting dietary amino acid patterns. In evaluating the hazards of such procedures, the question of nutritional consequences of amino acid excesses should be considered. This chapter outlines mechanisms in the body which permit excesses to be tolerated within certain limits, and describes how various types of disproportion in amino acid intake can induce these mechanisms to respond.

PHYSIOLOGICAL MECHANISMS FOR PROTECTING THE BODY AGAINST EXCESS AMINO ACID INTAKE

The free amino acid levels in the plasma and tissues are low. The sum of the free essential amino acids in the body of a 100 gm rat amounts to about 150 mg, while each gram of protein consumed by such a rat brings in about 500 mg of essential amino acids (Munro, 1970). Thus, if the levels of free amino acids are to be kept reasonably constant, there have to be sensitive mechanisms to protect the tissue against the impact of even normal intakes of amino acids. Such mechanisms are also available to deal with excess intakes of single amino acids.

The protective mechanisms begin with absorption of free amino acids and peptides liberated as end-products of proteolytic digestion of dietary proteins. Several authors (see Fauconneau and Michel, 1970, for review) have demonstrated that glutamic and aspartic acids are extensively transaminated by the mucosal cells after these amino acids are absorbed for the gut lumen. However, the main site of regulation of amino acid catabolism is the liver. The absorbed amino acids pass via the portal vein to the liver, which is the main or exclusive site of catabolism of seven of the essential amino acids (Miller, 1962), the three exceptions being the branched-chain amino acids which are degraded primarily in muscle and kidney (Ichihara and Koyama, 1966). Using dogs fed a large meat meal, Elwyn (1970) has shown that more than half of the incoming amino acids are degraded to urea. Only about a quarter of the incoming load passes into the general circulation as free amino acids, with the branched-chain amino acids predominating. Such a study represents protection against a large excess of incoming amino acids. Nevertheless, at less extreme intakes, this mechanism appears to be sensitive and discriminating in its modulation of degradation of many of the essential amino acids in relation to the needs of the body. When rats are given quantities of an essential amino acid beyond requirements, the enzymes of the corresponding degradative pathway are often induced. In the

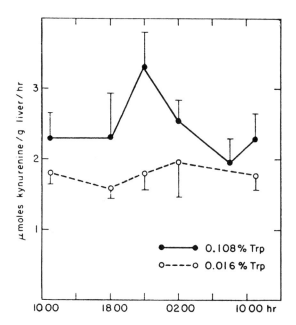

Figure 1. Tryptophan oxygenase activity of the livers of adult rats at various times of day while receiving either an adequate intake of tryptophan (0.108%) or an inadequate level (0.016%). (Young and Munro, 1973)

case of tryptophan oxygenase the enzyme is induced by excessive intakes of substrate at the time of absorption of the meal, the elevated levels lasting for only a few hours (Young and Munro, 1973). Figure 1 shows the levels of this enzyme is the livers of mature rats measured at various times of day when the rats were receiving either a diet low in tryptophan (0.016%) or one more than adequate in tryptophan content (0.108%). The transient elevation of enzyme activity at the higher intake coincides with the absorptive period. In other cases, it appears to take a longer time of adaptation to high levels of amino acid intake, as in the instance of lysine (Brookes, Owens and Garrigus, 1972). This latter study illustrates very clearly the sensitivity of the hepatic degradative process of amino acid intakes beyond the needs of the body. Increasing amounts of lysine were fed to young rats, optimal gain in body-weight being achieved at an intake of 100 mg lysine/day. When ^{14}C-lysine was injected into the rats receiving these various levels of lysine, production of $^{14}CO_2$ was slight at low intakes of lysine, but showed a clear break point with a rapid increase at intakes above 100 mg lysine/day. This indicates that the intake which gave maximal growth corresponded to the point at which the liver began to destroy excess lysine coming from the diet.

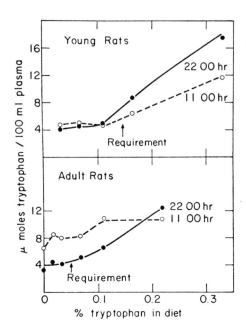

Figure 2. Response of plasma tree tryptophan concentrations in young and adult rats to different levels of dietary tryptophan. Animals were killed at either 1100 or 2200 hours. Each point is the mean value for five animals. The arrows indicate the tryptophan requirements for young and adult rats. (Young and Munro, 1973)

This protective mechanism does not, however, prevent some elevation in the free amino acid content of the peripheral blood. Thus the pattern of rise of lysine level in the blood gives a similar curve to that seen with CO_2 production (Pawlak and Pion, 1968) and this has been used to study requirements for individual amino acids in animals and man, the point of inflection when the plasma level starts to rise being used as an index of requirements. For example, in the course of the studies described in the preceding paragraph, we (Young and Munro, 1973) fed rats on a synthetic diet providing various levels of tryptophan. Plasma concentrations of tryptophan were measured during absorption (22.00 hr) and in the post-absorptive state (11.00 hr) on animals fed these various dietary levels of tryptophan. It was found that the point of inflection varied with age, occurring at lower dietary concentrations for older rats, especially for plasma obtained at 22.00 hr. (Figure 2). Other methods of assessing the tryptophan requirements of growing rats and mature rats showed reasonable concordance with the point of inflection in the plasma levels, thus strengthening the case for such a point.

RESPONSES OF THE CENTRAL NERVOUS
SYSTEM TO AMINO ACID SUPPLY

There is accumulating evidence that the central nervous system, and in particular the region of the basal ganglia, is sensitive to the pattern of amino acids in the plasma. The mechanism of amino acid transport into brain cells is discussed in detail by Pardridge (1977). The usual separate transport systems for basic, acidic and neutral amino acids have been identified. A major point of interest is the competition between neutral amino acids for entry into the brain. This competition is especially effective between branched-chain amino acids and other amino acids (Neame, 1966) and in consequence the levels of these branched-chain amino acids in the plasma can modulate availability to the brain of other amino acids such as tryptophan and phenylalanine. As a result, the amounts of amino acids available for neurotransmitter synthesis can be affected. The level of tryptophan in the brain is known to be rate-limiting for serotonin synthesis, and in consequence a change in the plasma concentrations of branched-chain and other large neutral amino acids will result in the opposite change in brain serotonin levels (Fernstrom, Madras, Munro and Wurtman, 1974). Thus a reduction in neutral amino acid levels will raise brain serotonin synthesis. This mechanism is seen in extreme form in cases of cirrhosis of the liver, in which the levels of phenylalanine and of tryptophan in the plasma tend to be elevated because of lack of regulation of their catabolism by the damaged liver, while the branched-chain amino acid levels are low due to the excessive passage of insulin through the liver into the plasma causing these amino acids to be deposited in muscle. As a result of the elevated level of plasma tryptophan and the depressed levels of other large neutral amino acids (high TRP/NAA ratio), excessive uptake of tryptophan by the brain results and unusually large amounts of serotonin are synthesized and contribute to the coma of liver failure (Munro, Fernstrom and Wurtman, 1975).

Anderson has recently proposed that the regulation of protein intake by animals (Anderson, 1977) and by man (Anderson, Blendis, Shillabeer and Krulewitz, 1978) is related to entry of tryptophan into the brain. He finds that the ratio of plasma tryptophan concentration to the concentrations of the large neutral amino acids in the plasma (TRP/NAA ratio) is inversely correlated with the amount of protein consumed in the diet. Using an experimental design in which rats were allowed to choose the proportion of protein in their diets, he showed that they selected protein intakes that tended to minimize changes in this plasma amino acid ratio. He proposes that changes in the TRP/NAA ratio trigger a feeding mechanism that is used to regulate protein intake. This mechanism may involve serotonin

synthesis from tryptophan, a hypothesis which was strengthened
by showing that injection of 5,6-dihydroxytryptamine (which
destroys the serotonin neurones) causes a decrease in protein
consumption occurring in parallel with the decrease in brain
serotonin level.

As will emerge later, and as appreciated also by Anderson
(1977), this mechanism does not explain some of the changes in
food intake caused by diets containing grossly abnormal proportions of amino acids. Under these latter circumstances,
there is good evidence of involvement of a central nervous system
response mechanism different from the serotonin pathway. This
evidence is considered in the next section.

EFFECTS OF DISPROPORTIONATE AMOUNTS
OF AMINO ACIDS IN THE DIET

Excess amounts or severe disproportions of one or more amino
acids in the diet leads to adverse effects on the growth and
sometimes tissue functions of experimental animals (Harper,
1964). These effects are usually most marked at low intakes of
protein. There is, however, little evidence from human studies
that disproportionate amino acid intakes produce more than mild
effects (Harper, 1973). Harper (1964) recognizes three types of
effect: toxicities, antagonisms and imbalances. Amino acid
toxicity results from intake of large quantities of individual
amino acids, such as tyrosine. Antagonisms are recognized by
growth depression caused by excessive intake of one amino that
can be alleviated by adding a structurally related amino acid to
the diet, such as leucine and isoleucine. Finally, amino acid
imbalances are created by adding surpluses of essential amino
acids other than the essential amino acid in the diet that is
limiting growth; growth is depressed, but can be restored by
adding more of the most limiting amino acid to the diet. These
three types of response to disproportionate amounts of amino
acids will now be considered in more detail.

Studies of the effects of toxic doses of amino acids have
been made with many amino acids. Most attention has been paid
to the effects of feeding large amounts of phenylalanine because
of its relevance to the congenital metabolic disease phenylketonuria, in which lack of phenylalanine hydroxylase in the liver
results in the inability to remove excess phenylalanine as
tyrosine. In order to depress growth of the rats, more than 4
percent of the amino acid must be added to the diet, the effect
being less when the diet is rich in protein (Harper, 1973).
Feeding of excessive amounts of tyrosine causes growth failure
associated with more specific signs, which include redness of the
paws. The most toxic of the naturally occurring amino acids is

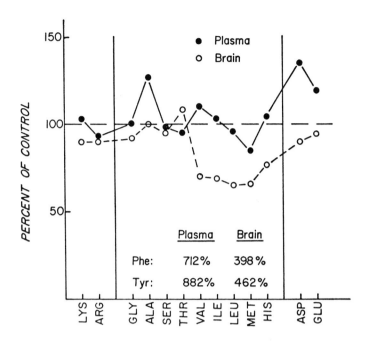

Figure 3. Brain and plasma amino acid changes in rats force-fed a low-protein diet with 5% phenylalanine added. Amino acid concentrations for animals force-fed the basal low-protein diet (---) were assigned values of 100, and rats receiving the high-phenylalanine meal are shown relative to these values for plasma (●—●) and brain (o---o). (Peng et al., 1973)

methionine, which produces growth retardation at 2 percent levels in the diet (Benevenga and Harper, 1967), whereas the least toxic essential amino acid is threonine (Sauberlich, 1961). In general, animals tolerate large doses of non-essential amino acids.

Excessive levels of one branched-chain amino acid in the diet of the rat cause a depression of growth rate that can be relieved by giving additional amounts of another branched-chain amino acid (Benton, Harper, Spivey, and Elvehjem, 1956). Since these three amino acids (leucine, isoleucine and valine) have structural similarities, this special form of toxicity due to amino acid excess is termed by Harper (1964) an antagonism. Another example is the antagonism been lysine and arginine (Jones, 1964).

An interesting finding in all these toxicities is the considerable change in free amino acid concentrations in the brain. In an extensive series of studies, Peng, Gubin, Harper, Vavich and Kemmerer (1973) added large amounts of amino acids (methionine, tryptophan, histidine, leucine, phenylalanine, threonine, lysine, or glutamic acid) singly to a low-protein meal which they fed to rats. Control rats received the low protein meal without added amino acids. In all cases except glutamic acid, there were grossly elevated levels in the plasma and the brain of the amino acid added to the diet. In contrast, the brain levels of many amino acids were depressed, consistent with competition for entry across the blood-brain barrier between the administered amino acid and other free amino acids in the plasma. Figure 3 shows that, following administration of excess phenylalanine, the levels of phenylalanine and tyrosine were much elevated in the plasma and brain. The levels of other amino acids in the plasma were little affected, whereas the levels in the brain of the branched-chain amino acids and of histidine and methionine were severely reduced. This suggests that amino acid-mediated signals to the appetite centers of the brain may well occur and account for the general reduction in food intake of animals on diets with excesses of amino acids.

Amino acid imbalance is a more subtle phenomenon. A typical example is to feed young rats on a diet in which the protein source is provided by 6 percent fibrin in the diet (Kumta and Harper, 1960). On such a diet, rats will gain about 2 gm. daily, a slow rate of growth. If a mixture of essential amino acids lacking histidine is added to this diet, growth is further depressed, but is restored by adding histidine to the mixture. Histidine is the most limiting amino acid in fibrin, and the imbalance created by adding a mixture lacking histidine further impairs the capacity of the rat to grow. This impairment is accompanied by a rapid reduction in food intake. The mechanism underlying such a response to imbalanced amino acid mixtures has been explored by Kumta and Harper (1962), who fed rats a single meal with 6 percent fibrin or the same meal to which had been added a mixture of essential amino acids lacking histidine. Within 6.5 hr., the concentration of histidine in the plasma of the second group of rats had fallen five-fold. In addition, it is known from other studies by Harper and his colleagues that the appetite of such rats becomes rapidly impaired and they consume less of the imbalanced diet within the same short period. We may conclude that the rapid distaste for the imbalanced diet is in some way related to the reduction in the level of histidine in the plasma. It has further been shown that the concentration of the limiting amino acid is reduced in brain in parallel with the change in the plasma (Peng, Tews and Harper, 1972). Rogers and Leung (1973) have explored the possibility when such changes in availability of an essential amino acid to the brain can be responsible for the rapidly impaired appetite of animals fed an imbalanced diet. Rogers and Leung (1973) produced a threonine imbalance in rats by feeding a diet low in threonine and supplemented with other essential amino acids. Injection of threonine into the carotid artery going to the brain restored the drive for food in this group of animals, whereas injection into the jugular vein leaving the head did not elicit this response. This suggests that low levels of single essential amino acids in the blood supply to the brain can inhibit the appetite center. This is presumably a protective mechanism against consuming a diet that will put a strain on amino acid metabolism. The site of action of amino acids within the brain is uncertain. Destruction of the ventromedial hypothalamus, the usual site associated with appetite control, does not abolish the response to imbalanced diets, which appears to depend on other brain locations, notably the prepyriform cortex and the amygdala (Rogers and Leung, 1973). However, high intakes of protein still depress the food intake of rats with lesions in these latter two areas.

CONCLUSION

The capacity of the body to respond to amino acid excess or disproportion is dependent on a series of safety mechanisms, beginning with the gut wall, then the catabolic enzyme pathways of the liver, and finally, the capacity of the brain to monitor plasma levels of amino acids. This last mechanism is responsible for appetite control and is an area of considerable promise for future understanding of homeostatic control of amino acid metabolism in relation to supply in the diet.

REFERENCES

Anderson, G.H. (1977) Regulation of protein intake by plasma amino acids. In, 'Advances in Nutritional Research', H.N. Draper (Editor). Vol. 1, Plenum Publishing Corp.

Anderson, G.H., Blendis, L.M., Shillabeer, G. and Krulewitz, J. (1978) Correlation between the plasma tryptophan to neutral amino acid ratio and dietary protein-energy selection in man. Fed. Proc., 37, 360.

Benevenga, N.J. and Harper, A.E. (1967) Alleviation of methionine and homocystine toxicity in the rat. J. Nutr., 93, 44-52.

Benton, D.A., Harper, A.E., Spivey, H.E. and Elvehjem, C.A. (1956b) Leucine, isoleucine and valine relationships in the rat. Arch. Biochem. Biophys., 60, 147-155.

Brookes, I.M., Owen, F.N. and Garrigus, U.S. (1972) Influence
    of amino acid level in the diet upon amino acid oxidation
    by the rat. J. Nutr. 102, 27-34.

Elwyn, D. (1970) The role of the liver in regulation of amino
    acid and protein metabolism. In, Mammalian Protein Metabolism
    H.N. Munro (Editor) Vol. 4, pp. 523-571, Academic Press, New
    York.

Fauconneau, G. and Michel, M.C. (1970) The role of the gastro-
    intestinal tract in the regulation of protein metabolism.
    In, Mammalian Protein Metabolism, H.N. Munro (Editor), Vol.
    4, pp. 481-522, Academic Press, New York.

Fernstrom, J.D., Madras, B.K., Munro, H.N. and Wurtman, R.J.
    (1974) Nutritional control of the synthesis of 5-hydroxy-
    tryptamine in the brain. In, Aromatic Amino Acids in the
    Brain , Ciba Foundation Symposium. pp. 153-173, Elsevier,
    New York.

Harper, A.E. (1964) Amino acid toxicities and imbalances. In,
    Mammalian Protein Metabolism, H.N. Munro and J.B. Allison
    (Editors), Vol. 2, pp. 87-134, Academic Press, New York.

Harper, A.E. (1973) Effects of disproportionate amounts of amino
    acids. In, Improvement of Protein Nutriture. pp. 138-166,
    National Academy of Sciences, Washington, D.C.

Ichihara, A. and Koyama, E. (1966) Transaminase of branched
    chain amino acids. J. Biochem., Tokyo, 59, 160-169.

Jones, J.D. 1964. Lysine-arginine antagonism in the chick. J.
    Nutr. 84, 313-321.

Kumta, U.S. and Harper, A.E. (1960) Amino acid balance and
    imbalance. III. Quantitative studies of imbalances in
    diets containing fibrin. J. Nutr. 70, 141-146.

Kumta, U.S. and Harper, A.E. (1962) Amino acid balance and
    imbalance. IX. Effect of amino acid imbalance on blood
    amino acid pattern. Proc. Soc. Exp. Biol. Med., 110, 512-
    517.

Miller, L.L. (1962) The role of the liver and the non-hepatic
    tissues in the regulation of free amino acid levels in the
    blood. In, Amino Acid Pools, J.T. Holden, Editor. pp. 708-21.
    Elsevier, Amsterdam.

Munro, H.N. (1970) Free amino acid pools and their role in regulation. In, Mammalian Protein Metabolism, H.N. Munro, Editor. Vol. 4, pp. 299-386, Academic Press, N.Y.

Munro, H.N., Fernstrom, J.D. and Wurtman, R.J. (1975) Insulin, plasma amino acid imbalance, and hepatic coma. Lancet, I, 722.

Neame, K.D. (1966) Effect of neutral and amino acids and basic amino acids on uptake of L-histidine by intestinal mucosa, testis, spleen, and kidney in vitro: a comparison with effect in brain. J. Physiol. 185, 627-645.

Pardridge, W.M. (1977) Regulation of amino acid availability to the brain. In, Nutrition and the Brain. R.J. Wurtman and J.J. Wurtman, Editors. Vol. 1, pp. 141-204, Raven Press, New York.

Pawlak, M. and Pion, R. (1968) Influence de la supplementation des proteines de ble par des doses croissantes de lysine sur la teneur en acides amines libres du sang et du muscle du rat en croissance. Annls Biol. anim. Biochim. Biophys. 8, 517-30.

Peng, Y., Tews, J.K. and Harper, A.E. (1972) Amino acid imbalance, protein intake, and changes in rat brain and plasma amino acids. Am. J. Physiol. 222, 314-321.

Peng, Y., Gubin, J., Harper, A.E., Vavich, M.G. and Kemmerer, A. R. (1973) Food intake regulation: Amino acid toxicity and changes in rat brain and plasma amino acids. J. Nutr., 103, 608-617.

Rogers, Q.R. and Leung, P.M.B. (1973) The influence of amino acids on the neuroregulation of food intake. Fed. Proc., 32, 1709.

Sauberlich, H.E. (1961) Studies on the toxicity and antagonism of amino acids for weanling rats. J. Nutr., 75, 61-72.

Young, V.R. and Munro, H.N. (1973) Plasma and tissue tryptophan levels in relation to tryptophan requirements of weanling and adult rats. J. Nutr., 103, 1756-1763.

9

HAIR AS AN INDEX OF PROTEIN MALNUTRITION

Mendel Friedman* and R. Orraca-Tetteh**

*Western Regional Research Laboratory, U.S. Department
of Agriculture, Berkeley, CA 94710
**Department of Nutrition and Food Science, University
of Ghana, Legon, Ghana

ABSTRACT

Hair samples from seven sick Ghanaian children were analyzed
for amino acids. Cystine was determined by a procedure of
Friedman using tributylphosphine and 2-vinylpyridine to change
residues of cystine (and cysteine, if present) to S-β-
(2-pyridylethyl)-L-cysteine (2-PEC). This acid-stable derivative
is released by normal acid hydrolysis and is eluted as a well-
resolved peak before lysine in conventional ion-exchange amino
acid analysis. The average cystine content of six children suffering from kwashiorkor or marasmic kwashiorkor was found to be about
20% less than that of the one remaining child, whose protein
nutrition was judged adequate. In view of conflicting evidence of
the relation of hair cystine content and nutrition, we believe
further definitive studies of this subject are urgent. No other
substantial difference in amino acid composition was noted.

INTRODUCTION

More than five hundred million people are estimated to be
malnourished, with about fifteen thousand daily deaths attributed
to malnutrition (NRC, 1975). At the same time, no accepted simple
technique is currently available that permits rapid, large-scale
assessment of protein nutritional status (Hartman et al., 1966).
An attractive possibility is that the nutritional status of individuals can be established by analysis of hair because it is
synthesized at a rate about four times as fast as any other tissue
proteins (Sims, 1968; 1970). Since hair is all protein, intake of
dietary protein that is quantititively insufficient or lacking in

specific essential amino acids would be expected to affect its
growth, composition and physical properties. Various studies of
composition changes have not always given conclusive results
(Bigwood and Robazza, 1965; Hartman et al., 1966; Lightbody and
Lewis, 1929; Koyanagi and Takanohshi, 1961; Koyanagi et al., 1965;
Menkart et al., 1966; Morel et al., 1966; Ogura et al., 1962;
Platt and Nagchaudhuri, 1954; Pollitt and Stoner, 1971; Narasinga,
and Gopalan, 1957; Robbins and Kelly, 1970; Sanda, 1966; Sanda and
Bradfield, 1967; Sims, 1970; Sinclair, 1957; Smuts et al., 1932;
Wysocki et al., 1954). Extensive efforts have been made to devise
simple and convenient methods to diagnose malnutrition from other
hair properties (Bradfield, 1968, 1973a, 1973b, 1974; Burley, 1960;
Burley and Horden, 1960; Crounse and Fraser, 1969a, 1969, Fraser
et al., 1972; Gillespie, 1967; Gillespie et al., 1969; Johnson
et al., 1976; Latham, 1966; Kutner et al., 1973; Hartman et al.,
1966; Lee and Luttrell, 1965; Malcolm et al., 1973; Menkart et al.,
1966; MacDonald and Warren, 1961; Sims, 1967; 1968; Tanphaichitr
et al., 1977; Vandiviere et al., 1971; Whitley et al., 1970;
Wilson et al., 1971; Wolfram et al., 1970; Zain et al., 1977) and
other biochemical criteria (Bodwell, 1975; Gopalan et al., 1963;
Gopalan and Srikantia, 1973; Gurson, 1966; Ingenbleek et al.,
1975; Kahawati and McLaren, 1970; Nammacher et al., 1972; Nwuga,
1977; Olson, 1975; Waterlow, 1972; Waterlow and Alleyne, 1971).

None of the proposed methods seems adequate. Thus, Hartman
et al. (1966) point out that estimating nutritional status of
large population groups is difficult in the absence of a single
direct indicator of protein nutriture. They note that although
protein nutritional status may be inferred from several nonspecific indices such as total serum protein, serum albumin, hemoglobin,
stature, weight, hair pigmentation etc., such multiple observations may be uncertain because they are influenced by many
unrelated factors. For further evidence, we have evaluated hair
samples from children suffering from kwashiorkor and related
diseases associated with malnutrition. Several publications (see
below) suggest that the content of the amino acid cystine of
hair may respond to the nutritional status of the child, although
the evidence is by no means consistent. Discrepancies in the
reported relationships of cystine levels in hair of normal and
malnourished subjects could be due, in part, to problems and
inaccuracies in cystine analysis. Direct assay of cystine in protein hydrolysates by ion-exchange chromatography normally gives
low and varying values, because L-cystine is partly destroyed
during acid hydrolysis. Consequently, many attempts have been
made to change cystine residues quantitatively to acid-stable
derivatives that are resolvable in standard amino acid analysis
(Friedman, 1973). Derivatives tried for this purpose include,
among others, cysteic acid, S-sulfocysteine, S-carboxymethylcysteine, and S-carboxyethylcysteine. Most of these, however, are

not formed quantitatively or do not completely escape destruction
during acid hydrolysis, and some are hard to resolve in an amino
acid analyzer. To find a suitable solution to this problem, we
developed new techniques based on alkylating SH groups (generated
by reducing protein disulfide bonds) with vinylpyridines and
2-vinylquinoline (Friedman, 1973, 1972; Friedman and Krull, 1969;
Friedman et al., 1970, 1973; Friedman and Noma, 1970; 1975;
Friedman and Tillin, 1974; Krull et al., 1971; Wu et al., 1971).
We showed that the vinylpyridine derivatives selectively modify
SH groups under mild conditions, are stable to acid as used for
protein hydrolysis, and are eluted conveniently as well-resolved
peaks in standard amino acid analysis. In addition, since both
the pyridine and quinoline derivatives contain ultraviolet absorbing chromophores, they can be determined independently by
ultraviolet spectroscopy. Since these procedures have been found
useful for estimating the cystine content of both soluble proteins
and wool keratin, (Friedman and Noma, 1970; Friedman and Tillin,
1974) it appeared that they would be applicable to human hair, even
though it has a higher cystine content and is, thus, more crosslinked than wool (Cf. Menefee, 1977).

     In this paper we explore the simultaneous reduction and
alkylation of hair from malnourished children by tributylphosphine
and 2-vinylpyridine. The results show that this is a convenient
procedure for determining cystine levels in human hair and that the
cystine content of hair from malnourished Ghanian children may be
lower than in hair from an adequately nourished child.

EXPERIMENTAL

Reductive alkylation

     The following is a typical procedure for simultaneous small-
scale reduction of hair disulfide bonds and alkylation of the
liberated SH groups by 2-vinylpyridine. The hair (about seven mg)
was suspended in a solution consisting of 6 cc of normal propyl
alcohol and 6 cc of pH 7.6 (0.1M) Tris (Tris hydroxylmethyl amino-
methane) buffer containing 8M urea. Nitrogen was bubbled in for
about one minute and 0.1 cc of n-tributyl phosphine (Aldrich) and
0.1 cc redistilled 2-vinylpyridine (Aldrich) were added. The
flask was stoppered and shaken for 48 hours. An additional 0.05
cc, each, of tributylphosphine and 2-vinylpyridine were then added,
nitrogen bubbled in for about one minute, and the flask shaken for
another 48 hours. The hair was then filtered off, washed with
water and propyl alcohol, air-dried, and hydrolyzed for amino acid
analysis.

Amino Acid Analyses

A weighed sample, about 5 mg, of hair was added to about 15 cc of 6N HCl in a commercial hydrolysis tube. The tube was evacuated, placed in an acetone–dry ice bath, and evacuated and refilled with nitrogen twice before being placed in an oven at 110°C for 24 hrs. The cooled hydrolysate was filtered through a sintered–disc funnel, evaporated to dryness in vacuo with the aid of an aspirator at 40°C, and the residue was twice suspended in water and evaporated to dryness. Amino acid analysis was carried out on an aliquot of the residue with a Durrum Amino Acid Analyzer, Model D–500, under the following conditions: single–column Moore–Stein ion–exchange method; resin: Durrum DC–4A; buffer pH: 3.25, and 7.90; photometer: 440 nm and 590 nm; column: 1.75 mm X 48 cm; analysis time: 105 min. Norleucine was used as an internal standard. The 2–PEC appears as a well resolved peak before lysine, as confirmed and standardized with synthetic material (Friedman and Noma, 1970; Friedman et al., 1973).

Calculation of Results

The following equation may be used to calculate the half–cystine content of unmodified hair from chromatographically (or spectrophotometrically) determined 2–PEC content of chemically modified hair:

$$\frac{1 \times 10^5}{[C]} = \frac{1 \times 10^5}{[2\text{-PEC}]} - (M+1) \qquad (1)$$

where $C_{1/2}$ is the calculated number of half–cystine residues in mmoles per 100 g of dry native hair; 2–PEC is the determined concentration of 2–PEC (mmoles per 100 g of dry modified hair); M + 1 is the gram-formula weight of added pyridylethyl group (106) per half–cystine residue, M being the molecular weight of 2–vinylpyridine, equal to 105 and 1 being the molecular weight of hydrogen introduced during the reduction step shown in Figure 1.

Equation 2 is an analogous formula for the number of cystine residues (gram-moles of -S-S- bonds) present in native hair

$$\frac{1 \times 10^5}{[C]} = \frac{2 \times 10^5}{[2\text{-PEC}]} - (2M + 2) \qquad (2)$$

where C is the cystine content of the native hair in mmoles per 100 g.

The half–cystine content of native proteins may be calcualted from chromatographically determined 2–PEC content of S–pyridylethyl proteins by means of equation 1 and 3

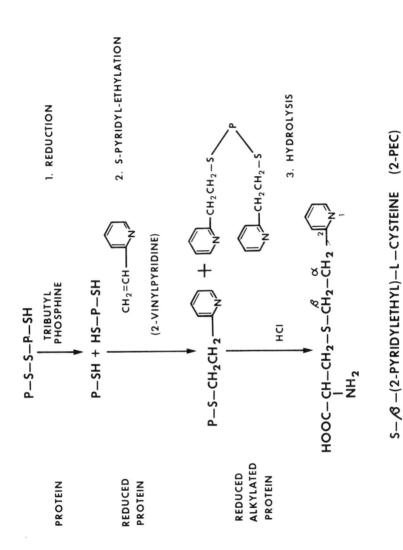

Figure 1. Reduction-alkylation of a protein

$$[C] = [2\text{-PEC}] \times \frac{[\text{Any AA}] \text{ in original hair (HSSH)}}{[\text{Any AA}] \text{ in modified hair (PEH)}} \qquad (3)$$

where AA refers to any amino acid in the hydrolyzate, the content of which is not changed by the treatment chosen as a reference, HSSH designates native hair, and PEH, S-pyridylethyl hair.

Equation 1 is applicable only for those proteins in which the weight increase per half-cystine residue is exactly M + 1. This is probably rarely the case with hair proteins because of high sensitivity to changes during chemical modification.

Equation 3 corrects for all weight changes during chemical modification except loss of soluble protein experienced during the reductive-alkylation. Generally, we prefer to report results in mole-ratios or mole per cent rather than in terms of weight of each amino acid per unit weight of hair. Alanine (or any other amino acid that is unaffected by the treatment) can be chosen as an internal standard. The mole percent or ratio methods are better measures of relative amino acid composition of modified hair because they avoid errors due to weight, moisture content, protein content, molecular weight, and other changes occurring during amino acid analysis (Cf. Cavins and Friedman, 1968; Friedman and Noma, 1970; Friedman, 1978). Note, also, that the use of eq. 3 (which gives the results in weight per cent) requires carrying out amino acid analyses on both untreated and treated hair.

RESULTS AND DISCUSSION

Previous Studies

Previous attempts to relate protein nutritional status to the amino acid composition of hair, and especially with cystine content, will be briefly summarized in chronological order before the new method for assaying the cystine content is discussed.

First, it should be noted that Caucasian hair appears not to differ significantly in amino acid composition and physico-chemical properties from Negro hair (Menkart et al., 1966; Robbins and Kelly, 1970; Wolfram et al., 1970). They do differ, however, in fiber geometry. Menkart et al., (1966) note that Caucasian hair approximates a cylinder and Negro hair a twisted oval rod.

Lightbody and Lewis (1929) found that the cystine requirement for growth of the body takes precedence over the cystine requirement for hair production in the white rat. In a related study, Smuts et al., (1932) reported that supplementing a cystine-deficient diet by either cystine or meat protein resulted in 25%

increase in the cystine content of rat hair. The authors suggest that the lower cystine content of hair produced during a cystine-deficient diet results from defective keratinization of the hair, which contained more of the sulfur-poor medullary substance and less of the sulfur-rich cortex than normal rat hair.

Wysocki et al. (1954) did not observe significant differences in the cystine and methionine contents of hair from normal and malnourished (kwashiorkor) Indonesian children. Hair samples were hydrolyzed in 1:1 mixture of 20% hydrochloric and 88% formic acid for 12 hours at 120–125°C. Cystine content was determined by the Block and Bolling (1945) adaptation of the Winterstein-Folin procedure.

Platt and Nagchaudhuri (1954) extracted two pigments (B and R) from normal (black) and malnourished (red) hair. Pigment B was readily converted into one with chromatographic and spectrophotometric characteristics of R by oxidation with hydrogen peroxide. They also found that the cystine content of hydrolysates of hair yielding R, determined by the method of McFarren and Mills (1952), was less (amount not given) than that of hair yielding pigment B.

Sinclair (1957) reported hair analysis of samples collected before and after a famine in the Netherlands in May 1945. Since food was being dropped from the air to help alleviate the famine, Dr. Sinclair reasoned that analysis for amino acids along the length of the hair might reflect the gradual improvement of protein nutriture after the period of severe protein depletion two weeks or more before. Examination of three different parts of the hair from root to tip, however, showed no meaningful variation of sulfur amino acids.

Narasinga Rao and Gopalan (1957) examined the cystine, methionine, tyrosine, phenylalanine, histidine, arginine, and nitrogen content of Indian and African children suffering from kwashiorkor. Cystine was measured by the Sullivan procedure (Brown and Lewis, 1941) after hydrolysis of the hair samples in 6 N HCl for 12 hours. Although the time of hydrolysis appears insufficient to liberate all the amino acid residues, including cystine, from the keratin protein, the data suggest that cystine but not nitrogen or any of the other amino acids increased after nutritional improvement of the malnourished children. An unsuccessful attempt was made to correlate cystine levels in hair from malnourished patients with hair color changes (dyschromotricia and hypochromotricia) that often accompany malnutrition. The authors speculate, however, that a low concentration of sulfhydryl groups in melanogenic cells, as reflected in a low cystine content in hair, may accelerate conversion of tyrosine to melanin, and favor further oxidation of melanin to brown or colorless pigments. Other nutritional factors, presumably, also regulate this process since malnourishment, with or without decreased hair cystine, is not always accompanied by dyschromotricia.

Close (1958) noted a significantly lower cystine content of hair from malnourished African children compared to that from a normal child (12.54 vs. 14.7%) but not in hair from Guatamalan Indians suffering from the same disease. Cystine was determined as cysteic acid (Bigwood et al., (1954). None of the other amino acids showed significant differences in either case.

Koyanagi and Takanohashi (1961) and Koyanagi et al. (1965) observed a 20-30% increase in cystine content of hair of Japanese children previously suffering from protein malnutrition, after their diets had been supplemented with minerals (phosphorus, iron, iodine, and calcium), vitamins, methionine, and skim milk. Cystine content was determined by the phosphotungstic acid method (Kolb and Toennies, 1952) on one-gram samples hydrolyzed in 3 N HCl at 120°C for 4 hours.

Bigwood and Robazza (1965) examined the amino acid composition and sulfur content of hair from normal and malnourished African patients. Using the cysteic acid procedure (1954), they found that the cystine content of hair from malnourished infants was about 25% less than in hair of a normal child of the same age, brought up in the same environment. The sulfur to nitrogen ratio (S/N) was less by about 10%.

Hartman et al., (1966) examined the influence of nutritional status on changes in diameter, composition, cystine content, and pigmentation of hair from Negro children in Haiti. Multiple regression analysis showed no significant differences among three health groups: normal, kwashiorkor, and marasmus. Nevertheless, cystine contents of pigmented hair were found to be lower than in dyspigmented hair. Amino acid analyses were carried out on 1.0 to 2.5 mg samples of anterior hair hydrolyzed at 121°C in 6 N HCl under nitrogen for 24, 48 and 72 hours. Losses during hydrolysis were taken into account to get zero-time values.

Morel et al., (1966) examined the amino acid composition of hair from normal and malnourished children and normal Europeans. They ascribed the observed lower, and widely varying, cystine and serine levels in hair from the malnourished group to a biochemical abnormality that affects cystine biosynthesis from serine and homocystine via cystathionine, and to possible genetic factors. Cystine was determined by the colorimetric method of Kurzawa (1961).

In addition to diet, genetic disease also seems likely to affect the cystine and sulfur content of hair. Thus, on the basis of a study of the amino acid composition of whole hair, hair extracts, and hair residues from normal and mentally retarded siblings, Pollitt and Stonier (1971) reported that the cystine content (determined as S-carboxymethylcysteine) of a mentally retarded sibling was less than half that of normal hair (6.7. vs. 14.4%).Most other amino acids also differed. The authors accounted for these observations in terms of factors that influence keratin (hair and wool) biosynthesis. (Cf. also Burley, 1960; Burley and Horden, 1960; Fraser et al., 1969).

Not only may changed amino acid patterns be associated with mental retardation of genetic origin but, conversely, protein-calorie malnutrition seems to retard intellectual development (Nwuga, 1977).

Finally, Kutner et al., (1973) have reported statistically meaningful differences in the sulfur content of normal hair compared to that from patients suffering certain diseases that affect hair. They suggest that hair sulfur analysis is a useful diagnostic screen for evaluating such disorders.

Cystine Analysis Applied to Hair

Hair samples were obtained from children admitted for treatment at the Princess Marie Louise Hospital, Accra, Ghana. Histories for six malnourished children and one child (No. 4) admitted to the hospital for illness not related to protein nutrition are summarized in Table 1. Since child No. 4 did not show advanced clinical signs of protein malnutrition the hair of this child is used as a control. Amino acid analyses for these samples are given in Tables 2-5 and Figures 1-9.

The reductive alkylation of the hair was carried out in a mixture of 50 parts by volume of normal propanol and 50 parts of 8 M urea in pH 7.6 Tris – HCl buffer. The procedure was essentially as described for wool (Friedman and Noma, 1970; Friedman and Tillin, 1974) except that the reaction time was increased to four days. Rate studies with normal human hair revealed that complete reductive alkylation of disulfide bonds takes place in about 24 hours. How ever, the longer time period was used to assure complete reaction with the small samples of hair available for this study. The·stoichiometry of reduction is given in eq. 4 and the chemistry of the reductive alkylation of both free and generated SH groups in Figure 1.

$$\text{Protein-S-S-Protein} + n\text{-Bu}_3\text{P} + \text{H}_2\text{O} \xrightarrow{} 2\ \text{Protein-SH} + n\text{-Bu}_3\text{P=O} \quad (4)$$

Protein-S-S-Protein + n–Bu₃P + H₂O → 2 Protein-SH + n–Bu₃P=O (4)
(hair)   (normal tributyl-phosphine)   (reduced hair)   (normal tributyl phosphine oxide)

Table 1. MEDICAL HISTORIES

SAMPLE 1	PATIENT A	Age: 5 years	SAMPLE 2	PATIENT B	AGE: 5 years

Male   Age: 5 years
KWASHIORKOR
Haemoglobin   12.7g or 87%
Edema of feet
Depigmented hair, with greyish and golden strands.
Child was under care of paternal aunt, since his
mother left child with the father. Has a rather
small head and is retarded.

Male   AGE: 5 years
KWASHIORKOR
Haemoglobin   11.2g or 77%
Edema of whole body
Dermatosis, very extensive
Depigmented hair, greyish.
Breast fed for 1 year
Weaning diet was maize porridge.
Fell ill with vomiting and loss of appetite.

SAMPLE 3	PATIENT C	Age: 2 years	SAMPLE 4	PATIENT D	Age: 1 year

Male   Age: 2 years
MARASMIC KWASHIORKOR
Haemoglobin   14.6g or 100%
Wasting of the body
Depigmented hair, long, silky and golden.
Dietary history could not be elicited.

NO PROTEIN MALNUTRITION - TO BE USED AS STANDARD
Haemoglobin   10.5g or 72%
Fever
Vomiting
Watery stool with mucus
Angular stomatitis
Hair normal pitch black and curly.

Table 1   (continued)

SAMPLE 5	PATIENT E	Age: 1-1/2 years

Female
KWASHIORKOR
Haemoglobin   10.65g or 73%
Edema of the legs
Depigmented hair – brownish
Angular stomatitis
Loss of appetite
Castroenteritis
Brochopneumonia
Fed mainly starch food, maize.

SAMPLE 6	PATIENT F	Age: 2-1/2 years

Male
KWASHIORKOR
Haemoglobin   132g or 89%
Edema
Depigmented hair, brownish
Dietary history could not be elicited. (Fed
    mainly on starchy foods.)
Child was under care of grandmother.
Child had measles sometime ago.

SAMPLE 7	PATIENT G	Age: 1-1/2 years

Male
KWASHIORKOR
Haemoglobin   12.7g or 87%
Edema of feet
Depigmented hair – golden brown
Loss of appetite
Loose stools
Brochopneumonia
Breast fed and weaned on to maize porridge.

Table 2. AMINO ACID COMPOSITION OF REDUCED-ALKYLATED HAIR

Numbers are mole or residue per cent (moles of each amino
acid recovered from the ion/exchange column divided by the
sum for all 18 amino acids listed times 100).

Amino Acid	SAMPLE NUMBER						
	1	2	3	4	5	6	7
			control				
$CYSO_3H$	0.301	0.529	0.440	0.236	0.457	0.120	0.491
ASP	6.38	6.18	5.90	5.94	6.15	5.74	5.93
THR	7.01	7.76	8.53	7.90	8.08	7.64	7.94
SER	11.78	12.66	12.68	11.85	11.84	12.50	11.81
GLU	11.32	10.88	10.90	10.41	12.28	10.14	12.82
PRO	6.86	7.47	7.81	7.00	7.40	7.06	7.71
GLY	6.97	6.62	6.31	5.87	5.92	6.27	6.13
ALA	5.35	5.23	4.81	4.83	4.81	4.95	4.78
VAL	5.80	5.75	5.70	5.62	5.37	5.77	5.37
MET	0.687	0.744	0.590	0.606	0.547	0.623	0.560
ILEU	3.07	3.00	2.94	2.90	2.83	2.92	2.78
LEU	7.73	7.43	7.04	7.16	7.24	7.21	7.00
TYR	2.47	2.22	1.99	2.03	1.84	2.16	2.17
PHE	2.12	2.10	1.99	1.87	1.80	1.83	1.78
HIS	0.832	0.740	0.406	0.912	0.601	0.650	0.741
2-PEC	11.82	11.07	12.56	15.53	13.48	15.23	12.54
LYS	2.89	2.90	2.45	2.57	2.47	2.75	2.43
ARG	6.61	6.68	6.93	6.74	6.87	6.42	6.99

Tables 2-4 show that the 2-PEC contents of the samples from
the malnourished children are lower than that for the single control value. The decrease ranges from about 66 percent for sample
No. 2 to 88% for sample 6 compared to sample No. 4 (the control
sample). However, when the values for the six hair samples from
malnourished children are averaged, the difference from sample 4
is about 20% when alanine, valine, isoleucine, and leucine are
used as internal standards and about 25 percent when the ratios
of 2-PEC to glycine are compared. These values correspond to a
cystine content of 12.57% for sample 4 and 8.92 ± 1.20 weight %
for the others (Table 5).

The variation in the cystine level among the six samples may
partly reflect differing nutritional status. If this were the
case, measurement of cystine levels as 2-PEC could be a sensitive
index of nutritional status and could perhaps allow detection and
assessment of marginal or moderate malnutrition not yet clinically
evident. The statistical verification of this possibility remains
to be shown with a larger number of hair samples from persons with
defined nutritional status and of representative genetic and geo-

Table 3. AMINO ACID COMPOSITION (MOLE RATIOS TO ALANINE) OF REDUCED-ALKYLATED MALNOURISHED HAIR

	1	2	3	4 ("Control")	5 ("Control")	6	7	AV ±S.D. (Nos 1-3,5-7)
CYSO$_3$H	0.0563	0.101	0.188	0.152	0.095	0.178	0.103	0.120+0.052
ASP	1.19	1.18	1.23	1.23	1.28	1.16	1.24	1.21+0.045
THR	1.31	1.48	1.77	1.63	1.68	1.54	1.66	1.57+0.17
SER	2.20	2.43	2.63	2.45	2.46	2.52	2.47	2.45+0.14
GLU	2.11	2.08	2.26	2.15	2.55	2.04	2.68	2.29+0.27
PRO	1.28	1.43	1.62	1.45	1.54	1.42	1.65	1.49+0.14
GLY	1.30	1.27	1.31	1.21	1.23	1.27	1.28	1.28+0.03
ALA	1.00	1.00	1.00	1.00	1.00	1.00	1.00	
VAL	1.08	1.10	1.19	1.16	1.12	1.16	1.12	1.13+0.04
MET	0.128	0.142	0.122	0.126	0.114	0.126	0.117	0.125+0.01
ILEU	0.573	0.575	0.611	0.600	0.589	0.580	0.582	0.585+0.014
LEU	1.44	1.42	1.46	1.48	1.50	1.45	1.56	1.47+0.05
TYR	0.462	0.425	0.413	0.420	0.382	0.437	0.453	0.429+0.029
PHE	0.395	0.403	0.414	0.387	0.373	0.369	0.371	0.388+0.019
HIS	0.155	0.142	0.084	0.189	0.125	0.131	0.154	0.132+0.026
2-PEC	2.20	2.12	2.61	3.21	2.80	2.85	2.62	2.53+0.31
LYS	0.540	0.554	0.509	0.533	0.514	0.554	0.508	0.530+0.022
NH$_4$	1.88	2.63	2.43	2.78	2.91	2.15	2.85	2.47+0.40
ARG	1.24	1.28	1.44	1.40	1.43	1.29	1.56	1.37+0.12

Table 4. 2-PEC CONTENT OF HAIR SAMPLES IN TERMS
OF MOLE RATIOS

Sample Number	$\dfrac{\text{2-PEC}}{\text{GLY}}$	$\dfrac{\text{2-PEC}}{\text{ALA}}$	$\dfrac{\text{2-PEC}}{\text{VAL}}$	$\dfrac{\text{2-PEC}}{\text{ILEU}}$	$\dfrac{\text{2-PEC}}{\text{LEU}}$
1	1.69	2.20	2.03	3.85	1.53
2	1.67	2.12	1.92	3.68	1.49
3	1.99	2.65	2.20	4.27	1.78
4 ("Control")	2.64	3.21	2.77	5.35	2.17
5	2.27	2.80	2.50	4.76	1.86
6	2.25	2.85	2.45	4.85	1.96
7	2.04	2.62	2.33	4.50	1.79

Average + S.D.=1.99+0.6 2.54+0.31 2.24+0.23   4.32+0.48 1.74+0.19
(No's 1-3,5-7)

Average
(No's 1-3,5-7)=0.754   0.791   0.809   0.807   0.802
Control   =75.4%   79.1%   80.9%   80.7%   80.25
(No 4)

Table 5. CYSTINE CONTENT OF HAIR DETERMINED AS S-β-
(2-PYRIDYLETHYL-L-CYSTEINE (2-PEC) VIA AMINO ACID
ANALYSIS

Sample No	Cystine content [a] wt. %
1	8.99
2	7.57
3	7.58
4 ("control")	12.80
	12.34 [b]
5	10.68
6	9.13
7	9.54

Average + Std. Dev. (samples 1-3; 5-7) = 8.92 + 1.20

[a] Calculated by means of equation 3 in mmoles per 100 gram of
hair (2 PEC concentration times ratio of alanine concentration in untreated, native hair divided by alanine concentration
in reduced-alkylated hair) and changed to grams per 100 grams
of hair (weight per cent) by multiplying by 120, the molecular
weight of a half-cystine residue. Not corrected for moisture
content.

[b] Hydrolysed for 48 hours.

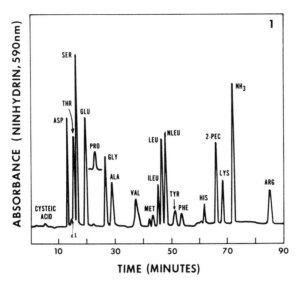

Figure 2.   Amino acid analysis of a hydrolysate of reduced-alkylated
malnourished hair sample 1. Note absence of cystine peak
and presence of 2-PEC peak. Norleucine (NLEU) was added
to the amino acid hydrolysate as an standard.

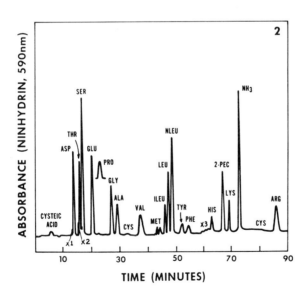

Figure 3.   Amino acid analysis of a hydrolysate of reduced-alkylated
malnourished hair sample 2.

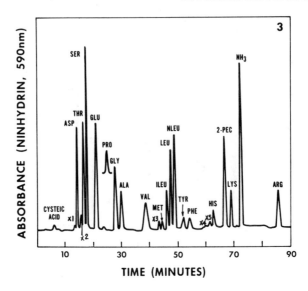

Figure 4.   Amino acid analysis of a hydrolysate of reduced-alkylated
malnourished hair sample 3.

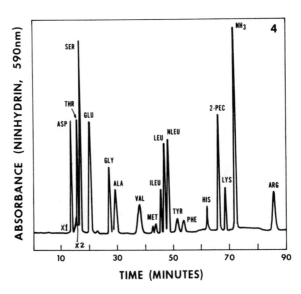

Figure 5.   Amino acid analysis of a hydrolysate of reduced-alkylated
normal hair sample 4.

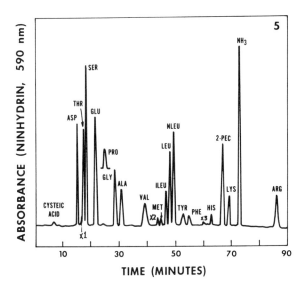

Figure 6.   Amino acid analysis of a hydrolysate of reduced-alkylated malnourished hair sample 5.

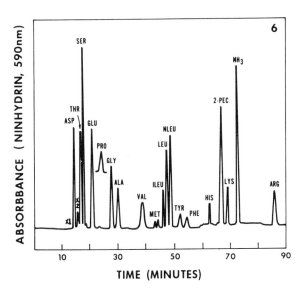

Figure 7.   Amino acid analysis of a hydrolysate of reduced-alkylated malnourished hair sample 6.

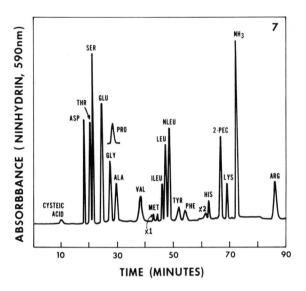

Figure 8.   Amino acid analysis of a hydrolysate of reduced-alkylated hair sample 7.

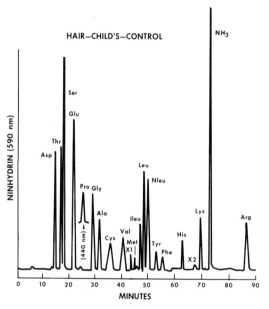

Figure 9.   Amino acid composition of a hydrolysate of untreated normal hair. Sample No. 4. Note cystine peak.

graphical origin. If the correlation between 2-PEC content of hair and nutritional status can be shown to be valid, then the 2-PEC procedure could be simplified and adapted to field conditions since the pyridine chromophore in 2-PEC can also be estimated by relatively inexpensive ultraviolet spectroscopy when an amino acid analyzer is not available.

Direct analysis of protein hydrolysates for cystine is known to be an unreliable measure of cystine content of proteins. In our case, just as in the case for wool (Friedman and Noma, 1970), the direct method gives values which are 10 to 15% lower than the 2-PEC method, although the difference between sample 4 and the average for the others is of the same order for the two methods. Previous studies with wheat gluten (Friedman et al., 1970) and wool (Friedman and Noma, 1970) showed that analysis through PEC is more accurate and more reproducible than direct cystine analysis or determination of cystine as cysteic acid (Schramm et al., 1954).

Note also that the numbers used to express apparent differences in composition among hair samples from normal and (protein) malnourished children vary somewhat depending on the units used to present the results, namely, weight per cent, mole (residue) per cent, mole ratio, etc.

In summary, this study shows that: (a) disulfide bonds in human hair, as in wool, can be quantitatively reduced by tributylphosphine and simultaneously alkylated by 2-vinylpyridine to form $S-\beta-(2-pyridylethyl)-L-cysteine$. The cysteine derivative is eluted in a convenient position in amino acid analysis, permitting quantitative assay; (b) application of this technique to hair from malnourished children reveals that its average cystine content, measured as 2-PEC, is about 20 percent less than that of a hair sample from a child who did not show clinical symptoms of protein malnutrition; however, more work needs to be done to establish the scope and reliability of this observation; and, finally, (c) none of the other amino acids in these samples, with the possible exception of histidine, seems to be systematically affected by protein malnutrition.

ACKNOWLEDGMENTS

It is a pleasure to thank Amy T. Noma for her help with the amino acid analyses and E. Menefee and W. H. Ward for constructive contributions.

REFERENCES

Bigwood, E. J. and Robazza, F. (1965). Amino acid and sulphur
    content of hair in normal African natives and in kwashiorkor.
    Voeding, 16, 251-256.
Bodwell, C. E. (1975). Biochemical parameters as indices of pro-
    tein nutritional value. In "Protein Nutritional Quality of
    Food and Feeds," Part 1, edited by M. Friedman, Marcel Dekker,
    New York, pp. 261-310.
Bogaty, H. (1969). Differences between adult and children's hair.
    J. Soc. Cosmet. Chem., 20, 159-171.
Bolling, D., and Block, R. J. (1945). "The Amino Acid Composition
    of Proteins and Foods." Charles C. Thomas, Springfield, p. 152.
Bradfield, R. B. (1973a). Protein-calorie malnutrition diagnosis
    by hair tissue: a review. Environ. Child Health, 370-375.
Bradfield, R. B. (1973b). Hair tissue in the diagnosis of marasmus
    and kwashiorkor. J. Amer. Med. Women's Ass., 28, 393-394.
Bradfield, R. B. (1974). Hair tissue as a medium for the differen-
    tial diagnosis of protein-calorie malnutrition: A commentary.
    J. Pediatrics, 84, 294-296 and references cited here.
Bradfield, R. B. (1968). Changes in hair associated with protein-
    calorie malnutrition. In "Calorie Deficiencies and Protein
    Deficiencies", edited by R. A. McChance and E. M. Widdowson,
    Churchill, London, 213-220.
Brown, B. H., and Lewis, H. B. (1941). The metabolism of sulfur.
    XXVII. The distribution of sulfur in the ultrafiltrates of blood
    plasma. J. Biol. Chem., 138, 705-716.
Burley, R. W. (1960). Experiments on wool from copper-deficient
    sheep. I. Some physical measurements on intact fibers and
    experiments on the dissolution and fractionation of oxidized
    wool. Text. Res. J., 30, 473-484.
Burley, R. W. and Horden, F. W. A. (1960). The amino acid compo-
    sition of oxidized normal and copper-deficient wool fractions
    and further attempts at fractionation. Text. Res. J., 30,
    484-489.
Cavins, J. F., and Friedman, M. Preparation and evaluation of
    S-β-(4 pyridylethyl)-L-cysteine as an internal standard for
    amino acid analyses. Analyt. Biochem. 35, 489-493. 1970.
Crounse, R. G., Bollet, A. J., and Owens, S. (1970). Quantitative
    tissue of human malnutrition using scalp hair roots. Nature,
    228, 465-466.
Close, J. (1958). Les modifications chimiques et morphologiques
    de cheveux, accompagnant le kwashiorkor. Ann Soc. Belg. Med
    Trop., 38, 95-104.
Fraser, I. E. B. (1969a). Proteins of keratin and their synthesis.
    I. Proteins of prekeratin and keratin. Aust. J. Biol. Sci., 22,
    213-229.
Fraser, I. E. B. (1969b). Proteins of keratin and their synthesis.
    II. Incorporation of (^{35}S) cysteine in prekeratin and keratin
    proteins. Aust. J. Biol. Chem., 22, 231-238.

Fraser, R. D. B., MacRae, T. P., and Rogers, G. E. (1972). "Keratins, Their Composition, Structure, and Synthesis", Charles, C. Thomas, Springfield, Illinois.

Friedman, M. (1978). Inhibition of lysinoalanine synthesis by protein acylation. This volume.

Friedman, M. (1973). "The Chemistry and Biochemistry of the Sulfhydryl Group in Amino Acids, Peptides, and Proteins." Permagon Press, Oxford, England and Elmsford, New York, 485 + viii pages. Chapter 11.

Friedman, M. (1972). Selective chemical modification of protein sulfhydryl groups. Intra-Science Chem. Reports 6, No. 4, 16-34. 1972.

Friedman, M., and Krull, L. H. (1969). A novel spectrophotometric procedure for the determination of half-cystine residues in proteins. Biochem. Biophys. Res. Commun., 37, 630-633.

Friedman, M., Krull, L. H., and Cavins, J. F. (1970). The chromatographic determination of cysteine and half-cystine residues in proteins as S-β-(4-pyridylethyl)-L-cysteine. J. Biol. Chem. 245, 3868-3871.

Friedman, M., and Noma, A. T. (1975). Methods and problems in chromatographic analysis of sulfur amino acids. In "Proteins Nutritional Quality of Foods and Feeds," Part I, edited by M. Friedman, Marcel Dekker, New York, pp. 521-548.

Friedman M., and Noma, A. T. (1970). Cystine content of wool. Text Res. J. 40, 1073-1078.

Friedman, M., Noma, A. T., and Masri, M. S. (1973). New internal standards for basic amino acid analyses. Analyt. Biochem. 51, 280-287.

Friedman, M., and Tillin, S. (1974). Partly-reduced-alkylated wool. Text. Res. J. 44, 578-580.

Gillespie, J. M. (1967). The dietary regulation of the synthesis of hair keratin. In "Fibrous Proteins", W. G. Crewther, Ed., Plenum Press, New York and Sydney, pp. 362-363.

Gillespie, J., M. Broad, A., and Reis, P. J. (1969). A further study on the dietary-regulated biosynthesis of high-sulphur wool proteins. Biochem. J., 112, 41 (1969).

Goodwin, K. O. (1962). Skin, hair, and nail in protein malnutrition. In World Review of Nutrition and Dietetics, 3, 105-128.

Gopalan, C., Reddy, V., and Mohan, V. S. (1963). Some aspects of copper metabolism in protein-calorie malnutrition. J. Pediatrics, 63, 646-649.

Gopalan, C., and Srikantia, S. G. (1973). Nutrition and diseases. World Rev. Nutrition and Dietetics, 16, 98-113.

Gurson, C. T., Neyzi, O., Uzman, Y., and Saner G. (1966). An evaluation of the plasma amino acid ratio in marasmus. Proc. Seventh Int. Congress Nutr. Hamburg, Vol. 1, 112-122.

Hartman, D. R., Fougere, W., and King, K. W. (1966). Diameter and amino acid changes in hair of Negro children with protein-calorie malnutrition. Proc. Soc. Exp. Biol. Med., 123, 542-544.

Ingenbleek, Y., Van Den Schriek, H. G., De Nayer, P., and De Visscher, M. (1975). The role of retinol-binding protein in protein-calorie malnutrition. Metabolism, 24, 633–641.

Horn, M. J., Jones, D. B., and Blum, A. E. (1946). Colorimetric determination of methionine in proteins and foods. J. Biol. Chem., 166, 313, 320.

Johnson, A. A., Latham, M. C., and Roe, D. A. (1976). An evaluation of the use of changes in hair root morphology in the assessment of protein-calorie malnutrition. Am. J. Clin. Nutr., 29, 502–511.

Kahawati, A. A., and McLaren, D. S. (1970). Assessment of marginal malnutrition. Nature, 228, 573–575.

Kolb, J. J., and Toennies, G. (1952). Microdetermination of sulfhydryl and disulfide protein hydrolyzates by phosphotung-state, (1971). Anal. Chem., 241, 1164–1169.

Krull, L. H., Gibbs, D. E., and Friedman, M. (1971). 2-Vinylquino-line, a reagent to determine protein sulfhydryl groups spectrophotometrically. Anal. Biochem., 40, 80–85.

Kurzawa, Z. (1961). Chemia Analityczna (Polish), 6, 1013.

Latham, M. C. (1966). The tensile strength of hair in protein-calorie malnutrition. Proc. Seventh Int. Congress Nutr., Hamburg, Vol. 1, pp. 87–91.

Koyanagi, T. and Takanohashi, T. (1961). Cystine content of hair of children as influenced by vitamin A and animal protein in the diet. Nature 192, 457–458.

Koyanagi, T., Hareyama, S., and Takanohashi, T. (1965). Effect of supplementation of B vitamin, phosphorus, methionine or skim milk on the cystine content of hair, dark adaptation, creatine-creatinine excretion and growth of undernourished children. Tohoku J. Exp. Med., 85, 108–114.

Kutner, M., Miller, K., and Brown, A. C. (1973). A critique: hair sulfur analysis for evaluation of normal and abnormal hair. In "The First Human Hair Symposium", edited by A. C. Brown, Medicom Press, pp. 363–376.

Lea, C. M., and Luttrell, V. A. S. (1965). Copper content of hair in kwashiorkor. Nature, 206, 413.

Lee, L. D. and Baden, H. P. (1975). Chemistry and composition of the keratins. Intern. J. Dermatol., 14, 161–171.

Lightbody, H. D., and Lewis, H. B. (1929). The metabolism of sulfur. XVI. Dietary factors in relation to the chemical composition of the hair of the young white rat. J. Biol. Chem., 82, 663–671.

MacDonald, I., Warren, P. J. The copper content of the liver and hair of African children with kwashiorkor, Brit. J. Nutr. 15, 593–595.

McFarren, E. F., and Mills, J. A. (1952). Quantitative determination of amino acids on filter paper chromatograms by direct photometry. Anal. Chem., 241, 650–653.

Malcolm, L. A., Balasubramanian, E., and Edwards, G. (1973). Effect of protein supplementation on the hair of chronically malnourished New Guinean school children. Am. J. Clin. Nutr., 26, 479-481.

Menefee, E. (1977). Physical and chemical consequences of keratin crosslinking, with application to crosslink density. In "Protein Crosslinking: Biochemical and Molecular Aspects", edited by M. Friedman, Plenum Press, New York, 307-327.

Menkart, J., Wolfram, L. J., and Mao, I. (1966). Caucasian hair, Negro hair, and wool: similarities and differences. J. Soc. Cosmet. Chem. 17, 769-787.

Morel, E., Mentzer, C., and Gessain, R. (1966). Modifications biochimiques des cheveux de jeunes africaines atteints de kwashiorkor. Comptes Rendus Soc. de Biologique, 160, 20-24.

N. R. C. (1975). National Research Council, "Study on World Food and Nutrition". National Academy of Sciences, Washington, D.

Nammacher, M. A., Bradfield, R. B., and Arroyave, G. (1972). Comparing nutritional status methods in a Guatemalan survey. Am. J. Clin. Nutr. 25, 871-874.

Narasinga, Rao, B. S., and Gopalan, C. (1957), Some aspects of the hair changes in kwashiorkor. Ind. J. Med. Res., 45, 85-93.

Nwagua, V. C. B. (1977). Effect of severe kwashiorkor on intellectual development among Nigerian children. Am J. Clin Nutr., 30, 1423-1430.

Ogura, R., Knox, J. M., Griffin, C., and Kusuhara, M. (1962). The concentration of sulfhydryl and disulfide in human epidermis, hair, and nail. J. Invest Dermatol., 38, 69-75.

Olson, R. E. (1975). The effect of variations in protein and calorie intake on the rate of recovery and selected physiological responses in Thai children with protein-calorie malnutrition. In "Protein-Calorie Malnutrition", edited by R. E. Olson, Academic Press, New York, pp. 277-297.

Platt, B. S., and Nagohaudhuri, J. (1954). Nutrition and hair pigmentation. Proc. Nutr. Soc., 13, ix-x.

Pollitt, R. J. and Stoner, P. D. (1971). Proteins of normal hair and of cystine-deficient hair from mentally retarded sibling. Biochem. J., 122, 433-444.

Porter, J. and Fouweather, C. (1975). An appraisal of human head hair as forensic evidence. J. Soc. Cosmet. Chem., 26, 299-313.

Robbins, C. R. and Kelly, C. H. (1970). Amino acid composition of human hair. Text. Res. J., 40, 891-896.

Sanda, M. A. (1966). Hair changes associated with protein-calorie malnutrition. M. S. Thesis, University of California, Berkeley, 68p.

Sanda, M. A. and Bradfield, R. B. (1967). Hair cystine changes in protein-calorie malnutrition. Fed. Proc., 25, 630.

Schramm, E., Moore, S., and Bigwood, E. J. (1954). Chromatographic determination of cystine as cysteic acid. Biochemical J., 57, 33-37.

Sims, R. T. (1970). Hair as an indicator of incipient and
    developed malnutrition and response to therapy-principles and
    practice. In "An Introduction to the Biology of the Skin",
    edited by R. H. Chapman, T. Gillman, A. J. Rook, and R. T. Sims,
    Blackwell, Oxford, England, 387-407.
Sims, R. T. (1968). The measurement of hair growth as an index of
    protein synthesis in malnutrition. Br. J. Nutr., 22, 229-236.
Sims, R. T. (1967). Hair growth in kwashiorkor. Arch. Dis.
    Childhood, 42, 397-400.
Sinclair, H. M. (1957). Nutrition and the skin in man. IVth
    Internation Congress on Nutrition, Proceedings p. A 147-A176.
Smuts, D. B., Mitchell, H. H., and Hamilton, T. S. (1932). The
    relation between dietary cystine and the growth and cystine
    content of hair in the rat. J. Biol. Chem., 95, 283-295.
Tanphaichitr, P., Chasingh, S., Dhanamitta, S., and Tontisirin, K.
    (1977). Differences in hair roots among children with
    differing nutritional status and of different ethnic origins.
    Clin. Pediatrics, 16, 599-600.
Vandiviere, H. M., Dale, Th. A., Driess, R. B., and Watson, K. A.
    (1971). Hair shaft diameter as an index of protein-calorie
    malnutrition. Arch. Environ. Health, 23, 61-66.
Walker, H. G., Jr., Kohler, G. O,. Kuzmicky, D. D., and Witt, S. C.
    (1975). Problems in analysis for sulfur amino acids in feeds
    and foods. In "Protein Nutritional Quality of Foods and Feeds",
    Part I, edited by M. Friedman, Marcel Dekker, New York, pp.
    549-567.
Waterlow, J. C. (1972). Classification and definition of protein-
    calorie malnutrition. Medical Practice, 566-569.
Waterlow, J. C., and Alleyne, G. A. (1971). Protein malnutrition
    in children, Adv. Protein Chemistry, 2, 117-241.
Whiteley, K. J. and Balasubramanian, E., and Armstrong, L. (1970).
    The swelling and supercontraction of sulfur-enriched wool
    fibers. Text Res. J., 40, 1047-1048.
Wilson, P. A., Henrikson, R. C. and Downes, A. M. (1971).
    Incorporation of (Me-^{3}H) methionine into wool follicle proteins:
    a biochemical and ultrastructural study, J. Cell. Sci., 8, 489-
    512.
Wilson, R. H., and Lewis, H. B., (1927). The cystine content of
    hair and other epidermal tissues. J. Biol. Chem., 73, 543-553.
Wolfram, L. J., Hall, K., and Hui, I. (1970). The mechanism of
    hair bleaching. J. Soc. Cosmet. Chem. 21, 875-900.
Wu, Y. V., Cluskey, J. E., Krull, L. H., Friedman, M. (1971).
    Some optical properties of S-β-(4-pyridylethyl)-L-cysteine
    and its wheat gluten and serum albumin derivatives.
    Canad. J. Biochem. 49, 1042-1049.
Wysocki, A. P., Mann, G. V., and Stare, F. J. (1954). The
    cystine and methionine content of the hair of malnourished
    children. Am J. Clin. Nutr., 2(4), 243-245.
Zain, B., Haquani, A. H., Qureshi, N., and el Nisa, I. (1977). Stud-
    ies on the significance of hair root protein and DNA in protein-
    calorie malnutrition. Am. J. Clin. Nutri., 30, 1094-1097.

10

THE PROBLEM OF CURVATURE IN SLOPE ASSAYS FOR PROTEIN QUALITY

J. Murray McLaughlan

Department of National Health and Welfare

Ottawa, Canada   K1A 0L2

ABSTRACT

The dose-response curves in a valid slope-ratio assay must be
linear and meet at the zero protein dose. However in rat bioassays
at least 3 types of curvature are found when the method is applied
to a wide range of samples; the types of curvature result from: 1)
excessive protein 2) lysine deficiency and 3) threonine deficiency.
Whole wheat flour which was limiting in lysine and threonine showed
marked downward curvature after supplementation with threonine.
It can be argued from these results that the slope ratio and
relative protein value method underestimated the protein quality
of lysine-deficient foods.

INTRODUCTION

The protein efficiency ratio (PER) is the official method in
the United States and Canada. Its shortcomings are well-known.
In 1965 Hegsted and Chang proposed a multi-dose rat growth assay
for protein quality (Hegsted and Chang, 1965). The method was
patterned after the bacteriological slope ratio (Finney, 1964) for
vitamin assays; consequently the method was called slope ratio
(SR).

The ideal SR assay is illustrated in Figure 1 (left side).
The dose-response lines of the reference protein and test sample
are linear and meet at a common point on the vertical axis. The
vertical axis is change in body weight and the horizontal axis is
protein consumed. Figure 1 (right side) shows the relationship
between slope ratio and net protein ratio (Bender and Doell, 1957).

155

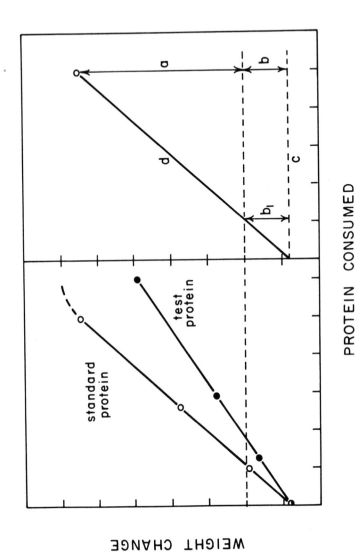

PROTEIN CONSUMED

WEIGHT CHANGE

Figure 1. Idealized growth response curves for multiple doses of protein. (Left side) Response curves for standard and test protein in the slope ratio assay. (Right side) Diagram showing interrelationships among PER, NPR and SR assays. "a" is weight gain. "b" (and "bl") is the weight loss of the non-protein group. "c" is the protein consumed.

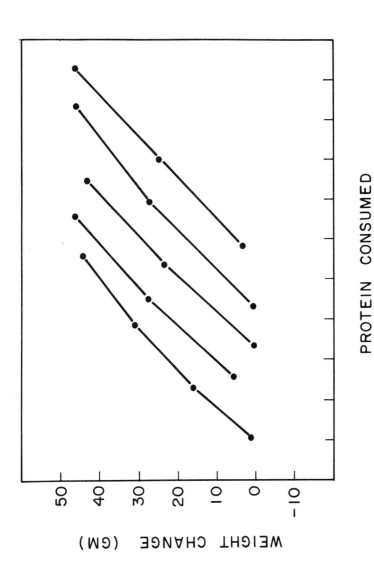

Figure 2. Five consecutive dose-response curves for the standard (lactalbumin).

The slope of the response "d" is a + b/c. Net protein ratio (NPR) is the weight gain of the test group (a) plus the weight loss of the non-protein group (b1) divided by the protein consumed (c). However, b1 is equal to b and therefore SR and NPR are identical providing the SR assay is ideal. PER is weight gain over protein consumed or a/c.

EXPERIMENTAL

In practice few things are ideal. Figure 2 gives standard (lactalbumin) curves for 5 consecutive assays. The highest dosage level is approximately 8% protein. Four of 5 curves show downward curvature. Although curvature for individual assays might not be significant, examination of a series of responses leaves little doubt that we are dealing with curves and not straight lines.

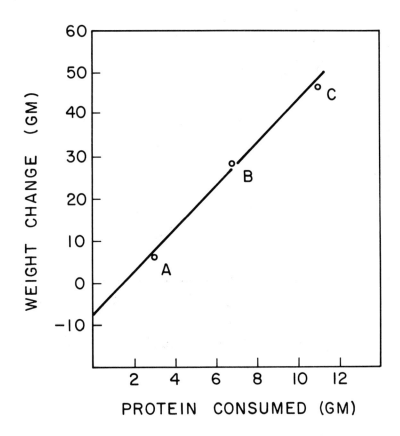

Figure 3.   Dose-response curve for lactalbumin.

Data for one response line with moderate curvature is illustrated in Figure 3. Using the data for protein levels A, B and C the slope is 5.04 and the intercept on the vertical axis is -9.648. If just the data at levels A and C are used the slope is also 5.04. Inclusion of the middle dose is necessary in the SR assay to test for excessive curvature but the data is wasted as far as determination of protein quality is concerned. The slope for AB portion of the line is 5.515 whereas the slope for the BC part is only 4.739.

The dose response data for lactalbumin in 10 consecutive assays were plotted; protein levels ranged from 2 to 8.5% of the diet. The data indicated that the customary response is a smooth curve as shown in Figure 4. This curve is slightly exaggerated but it is useful in illustrating how selection of the dosage levels

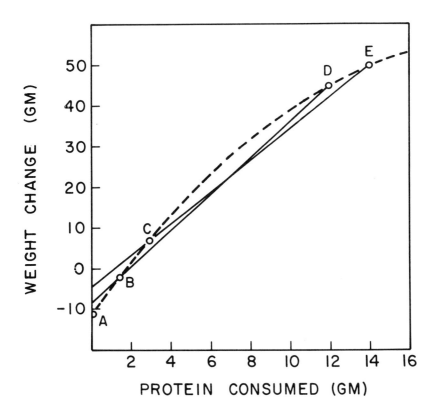

Figure 4. Dose response curve for lactalbumin showing curvature (dashed line).

affects the apparent slope. Selecting the dosage levels of 2%
protein (B) and 8% protein (D) yields a slope of 4.54. Choosing
protein levels of 3% (C) and 8.5% (E) gives a slope of 3.86. (It
was shown in Figure 3 that the middle dose has little or no effect
on the slope). It is obvious that judicious selection of dosage
levels of reference protein and sample could produce considerable
variation in estimates of protein quality.

Downward curvature must occur at high protein intakes. In
our laboratory curvature in the lactalbumin standard curve usually
becomes excessive above 8.5-9.0% protein. Recent studies also
suggest that the level of lipid in the diet can alter the range of

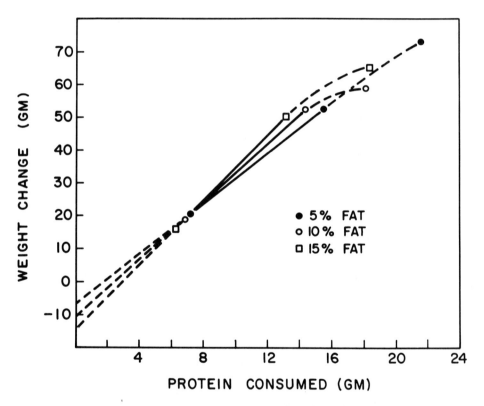

Figure 5. Dose response with three levels of lipid. Protein
levels were 7, 10 and 13%.

"linearity". Figure 5 gives response curves for soy isolate with added methionine and 3 concentrations of lipid 5, 10 and 15%; the protein levels were 7, 10 and 13%. The dose-response curve with 5% lipid had the lowest slope and the greatest range of linearity.

Finally there are the more serious types of curvature associated with specific amino acid deficiencies - the best known being the lysine-deficiency type (Yáñez and McLaughlan, 1970; McLaughlan, 1972). Certain proteins such as wheat gluten yield "horizontal type" curves and show marked downward curvature in the SR assay. To get around this problem the data for the zero-protein group was omitted in the RPV method (Samonds and Hegsted), the true slopes of the response curves being used.

It was reported from our laboratory (McLaughlan and Keith, 1975) that threonine-deficient proteins tended to have slopes which paralleled that of the reference protein (the response curve cut the vertical axis at a point more negative than that of the standard). These curves may show upward curvature in the SR assay. The effects of lysine and threonine deficiencies are illustrated in Figure 6. The protein was provided by whole wheat flour; the limiting amino acids were lysine first limiting and threonine 2nd limiting (McLaughlan, 1977). Addition of lysine made threonine the limiting amino acid.

The curve with closed circles is for the unsupplemented flour. The curve with open circles is with added threonine; this is the typical lysine-deficient response showing marked downward curvature in the SR assay (Fig. 6 left side). The curve for the basal diet with added lysine (threonine deficient) shows upward curvature. Curvature due to deficiencies of lysine and threonine are not obtained in the RPV assay (Fig. 6 right side). However, I think that these data point out a serious flaw in the RPV procedure. Actually threonine was the limiting amino acid in whole wheat flour at the low protein level whereas lysine was deficient at protein levels supporting growth. Addition of threonine markedly increased growth at the low concentration of protein; addition of lysine had no effect at the low protein level. These effects of supplementation were reversed with high protein. Threonine added to whole wheat flour made lysine the limiting amino acid at all protein levels. A similar lowering of the slope of mixtures of foods after addition of threonine has been reported for rice-casein, peanut-sesame-fish and for soya protein with added methionine (McLaughlan and Keith, 1977); the mixtures were limiting in lysine and threonine. Surely the protein quality was not poorer after the addition of threonine but the RPV assay indicated this to be so. These studies indicate that the RPV assay underestimates the quality of lysine-deficient proteins.

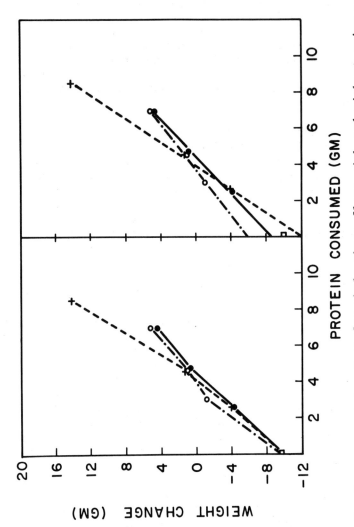

PROTEIN CONSUMED (GM)

WEIGHT CHANGE (GM)

Figure 6. Dose-responses curves for whole wheat flour with and without amino acid supplements. (Left side). Response lines drawn to zero protein dose. (Right side). Response lines extended to vertical axis –zero protein group not included in RPV assay. The response lines with filled circles are for the unsupplemented flour. The lines and unfilled circles are the response with added threonine. The curves with the crosses are the responses with added lysine. The open square represents the non-protein group.

Hackler observed marked differences in apparent protein quality of peanut meal, soy isolate and tuna fish depending on whether or not the protein-free group of rats was used in calculation of the slope (Hackler, 1977). It has become increasingly apparent that a multidose assay should include that the data for the non-protein group (McLaughlan and Keith, 1977; Hackler, 1977; PAG, 1975) yet the SR assay is subject to at least 3 different forms of curvature: 1) the slight (least serious) downward curve of the response shown for lactalbumin 2) lysine-deficient type and 3) threonine-deficient form. Nevertheless the slope ratio is preferable to the RPV assay which does not utilize the non-protein group. The real question however is whether or not any multidose slope assay with its own set of problems is that much superior to NPR to justify the extra cost.

REFERENCES

1. Bender, A.E. and Doell, B.H. 1957 Biological evaluation of proteins. A new aspect. Brit. J. Nutr. 11: 140-148.

2. Finney, D.J. 1964 Statistical methods in Biological assay 2nd Ed. Hafner Publishing Co., New York.

3. Hackler, L.R. 1977 Methods of measuring protein quality: A review of bioassay procedures. Cer. Chem. 54: 803-812.

4. Hegsted, D.M. and Chang, Y. 1975 Protein utilization in growing rats. I Relative growth index as a bioassay procedure. J. Nutr. 85: 159-168.

5. MacLaughlan, J.M. 1972 Effect of protein quality and quantity in protein utilization. In Newer Methods of Nutritional Biochemistry (Albanese ed.). Academic Press, New York, 1972, p 33-64.

6. MacLaughlan, J.M. Multi-dose slope assays and protein quality of cereals. Nutr. Rep. Int. (in press).

7. McLaughlan, J.M. and Keith, M.O. 1975 Bioassays for protein quality. In Protein Nutritional Quality of Foods and Feeds (M. Friedman, ed.). Marcel Dekker, Inc. New York, p. 79-85.

8. MacLaughlan, J.M. and Keith, M.O. 1977 Effect of threonine supplementation in the slope assay for protein quality. J. Ass. Official Analytical Chemists, 60: 1291-1295.

9. Protein Advisory Group (PAG) statement no. 28. volume 5, no. 2, June 1975, published by Protein Calory Advisory Group of the United Nations system.

10. Samonds, K.W. and Hegsted, D.M. (personal communication).

11. Yáñez, E. and McLaughlan, J.M. 1970 The effect of level of protein on protein quality of lysine-deficient foods. Can. J. Physiol. Pharmacol. 48: 188-192.

11

DEFINING DIETARY PLANT FIBERS IN HUMAN NUTRITION[1]

Gene A. Spiller and Joan E. Gates

Department of Nutritional Science
Syntex Research
Palo Alto, California   94304

ABSTRACT

Research on the nutritional aspects of dietary plant fibers in human nutrition has been plagued by many problems of definition, terminology, analytical procedures, as well as insufficient consideration of the interactions of other dietary components with the dietary fiber polymers. The use of the term non-nutritive has also led to some confusion, as many polymers of dietary fiber are digested by intestinal bacteria in humans.

It appears extremely important for the orderly progress of this field that comprehensive terms be used cautiously and that perhaps a new umbrella term (such as plantix) should be introduced. The physiological effects of various polymers have been shown to differ considerably; thus the effect of dietary fiber should not be generalized. Analytical procedure should include both water-insoluble and water-soluble fractions and some consideration should be given to the non-polymeric, enzyme-indigestible compounds such as certain seed and leaf waxes.

Various suggestions have been made by Sandstead, Schaller, Southgate, Spiller and Van Soest at the American Chemical Society Symposium on the definition of fiber (Chicago, August 1977). These suggestions are condensed in this chapter.

INTRODUCTION

Research on the nutritional effects of plant fiber has been plagued by many problems that can be grouped as follows:

A) *DEFINITION AND TERMINOLOGY:*   1) Lack of consensus about which
polymers should be included in the general category of fiber.   2)
Incorrectness of the term *fiber*:   many components are not fibrous.
3) Use of the word *fiber* by many other fields (e.g. textiles).   4)
Use of crude fiber to represent fiber in food tables.   5) Failure
to standardize terminology of fiber-related nutrition papers.   6)
Lack of identification of the physico-chemical conditions of the
fiber (i.e. cooked versus uncooked; purified versus unpurified).
B) *ANALYSES:*   1) Insufficient laboratories performing proper plant
fiber analyses of common foods.   2) Lack of uniformity in present-
ing plant fiber values.   C) *NUTRITIONAL ASPECTS:*   1) Failure to
take into account other dietary components that might interact with
fiber (e.g. fat).   2) Tendency to generalize the nutritional effects
of one fiber polymer, or a specific fiber pattern (e.g. grains) to
fiber in general.   3) Tendency to consider plant fibers as non-
nutritive, although many of them are digested by intestinal bacteria.

PROBLEMS WITH COMPREHENSIVE TERMS

Table 1 lists some of the terms used for plant fibers in
human nutrition.   There seems to be a consensus that all the substances listed in Table 2 should be included in a comprehensive
term.   Some of these compounds are water-soluble; some are not.
Many of them, such as gums, are not fibrous, fiber being defined
by the American Heritage Dictionary (1973) as: "Any slender,
elongated structure; a filament or strand."

TABLE 1

DIETARY PLANT FIBER

COMPREHENSIVE (UMBRELLA) TERMS[a] (Spiller & Gates)

Dietary fiber (DF)
Plant fiber (PF)
Fiber
Non-purified plant fiber (NPPF)
Purified plant fiber (PPF)
Non-nutritive natural fiber
Undigestible carbohydrate (UC)
Unavailable carbohydrate (UC)
Plantix (PX)
Complantix (PX)
Partially digestible plant polymers (PDPP)
Partially digestible biopolymers (PDB)

---

[a]Crude fiber is not listed here as it is <u>not</u> a comprehensive term.

TABLE 2

PLANT POLYMERS THAT SHOULD BE INCLUDED
IN A COMPREHENSIVE TERM (Spiller & Gates)

> Cellulose
> Water-Insoluble Hemicelluloses
> Lignin
> Pectins
> Gums (Seed Gums, Exudates, Etc.)
> Mucilages

Very confusing is the fact that the term is shared with so many other fields. It is typical that in computer searches for fiber-related publications, titles related to non-nutrition papers appear with greater frequency than dietary fiber papers. For instance, listings such as: "Glass fibers as a reinforcement for elastomeric compounds", "Microscopical analysis of graphite fiber reinforced epoxy matrix laminates", "Density profile and fiber alignment in fiberboard from southern hardwoods", "Introduction to optical fiber communication systems", "Extracellular organization of collagen-fibers", and "Differentiation of electrical and contractile properties of slow and fast muscle-fibers" appear quite frequently.

It has been suggested by Godding (1976) that indigestible animal fibers should be included in an all-embracing fiber definition. No action has been taken in this direction, but the suggestion certainly deserves consideration.

Some investigators have recently recommended that the term fiber be entirely dropped or retained only for that fraction of the plant cell wall that is more properly fibrous, namely cellulose and lignin. Spiller and co-workers (Spiller, Fassett-Cornelius, Briggs, 1976; Spiller and Shipley, 1976; Spiller, 1977) would include all the polymers listed in Table 2 under the comprehensive term "plantix". They state (Spiller, Fassett-Cornelius, Briggs, 1976): "We propose a new word, *plantix*, derived from two Latin words: *planta* and *matrix* (plant and matrix). We are obviously dealing with *plant* materials, the undigested compounds form a *matrix* in the digestive system of humans (up to the ileocecal valve), and the action of colonic bacteria on this *matrix* is responsible for many physiological effects. . ." Such adjectives as purified, non-nutritive, and dietary could further particularize the basic plantix.

Trowell (1977) has objected to this change and prefers "dietary fiber" despite the impropriety of the term fiber. Fiber will probably survive as a popular term, while some new scientific

umbrella term will be agreed upon. <u>Plantix</u> appears the only one
concise term that has been suggested so far. Figure 1 illustrates
various umbrella terms, the polymers included, and methods of
analysis.

DIETARY FIBER (PLANTIX) VERSUS CRUDE FIBER

Southgate feels that it is important to have a clear definition of what is meant by the term dietary fiber or whatever term
may be selected, because incorrect or inexact terms lead to confusion that can create problems when one attempts to examine epidemiological data or tries to interpret many clinical or nutritional experiments.

According to Schaller, an immediate problem that has to be
faced is the misinformation that is being perpetuated by using
the antiquated term <u>crude fiber</u>. The problem is illustrated in
Table 3. The table shows a comparison of crude fiber versus
water-insoluble dietary fiber of three sources of fiber: cellulose,
rice bran, and corn bran.   These sources are compared in some
mythical food product on the basis of equal crude fiber content
per serving. The fiber values on a per serving basis are quite
different. The under-estimation of dietary fiber varies according
to the particular ingredient. Presently, crude fiber values are
the only ones available, and can not be used to estimate dietary
fiber; since, as can be seen in Table 3, even among cereal grains
there is no consistent relationship between crude fiber and dietary fiber. The crude fiber analysis results bear no relationship and serve no useful purpose in measuring dietary fiber intake.
Southgate agrees that crude fiber is a difficult and unreliable
method and these values have no place in human nutrition.

This is the reason why it is important to have a clear definition of what is meant by the term dietary fiber.

TABLE 3

COMPARISON OF CRUDE FIBER TO DIETARY
FIBER FOR SOME FOOD INGREDIENTS (Schaller)

	Crude Fiber Per Serving	Crude Fiber	Dietary Fiber Per Serving	Dietary Fiber
	(grams)	(%)	(grams)	(%)
α-Cellulose	1	73	1.3	94
Rice Bran	1	8	2.7	22
Corn Bran	1	19	4.7	89

DEFINITION OF DIETARY FIBER (PLANTIX)

Southgate defines dietary fiber as the sum of the polysaccharides and lignin that are not digested by the endogenous secretions of the human digestive tract. These are the components that are imagined to pass through the small intestine and into the large intestine substantially unchanged by the intestinal secretions.

Southgate emphasizes the following points concerning dietary fiber: 1) dietary fiber is a mixture whose composition will vary according to the types and amounts of food being consumed, 2) it is not equivalent to any specific analytical fraction nor to material that can be recovered in the feces, and 3) it is made up of components derived from the plant cell walls in the diet together with other polysaccharides.

It may well be that other components of the plant cell wall, proteins, lipids, and inorganic constituents, contribute to some of the properties of dietary fiber and that some of the effects of dietary fiber are due to the fact that it is consumed in the physical form of the plant cell wall.

Similarly, Schaller describes the term dietary fiber as those components of plants that are not hydrolyzed by human digestive enzymes. Schaller states that this functional definition allows other components that fit the physiological definition to be added to the group of plant materials known as dietary fiber as our knowledge increases. It allows extremely dissimilar classes of plant components to be grouped under a single term, and it classes materials according to a physiological property important and common to all humans.

Schaller correlates the term dietary fiber to the term vitamin as literal descriptions for the groups of compounds they are to classify. Both are inaccurate; both are now based on functional, physiological properties rather than chemical ones; both are fixed in the literature and in common usage. He feels that it would be futile at this late date to try to change either term. Education as to what is meant by dietary fiber and examination of the importance in the diet are much more valuable ways to spend efforts at this time, according to Schaller.

SOME PROPERTIES OF DIETARY FIBER (PLANTIX)

Summarized in Table 4 are the properties of the dietary fiber complex and the relationship of those properties to nutritional and physiological effects in humans. From this table one can understand the necessity to define the specific components of plant fiber under investigation.

TABLE 4

PROPERTIES OF DIETARY FIBER AND THEIR RELATION TO PHYSIOLOGICALLY
IMPORTANT EFFECTS

Major Properties	Known Effects	Substances Involved	Possible Nutritional/ Physiological Effects
Physical Properties			
Cell wall structures	Texture of foods	Components of plant cell wall	Voluntary food intake
Capacity to bind water		Many polysaccharides including starch	
Formation of gels and viscous solutions	Consistency of contents of stomach and small intestine	Starch, pectin, gums and many other polysaccharides	Physico-chemical effects Gastric emptying Flow through tract Accessibility to enzymes
Chemical Properties			
Functional Groups	Binding of ions and other substances	Uronic acid containing polysaccharides?	Absorption of cholesterol Bile salt excretion
Structural Groups	Indigestible (not hydrolized by intestinal secretions)	Lignin?	Bulk in large intestine Increased excretion of bound components
	Degraded by intestinal flora	Pectins; partial for others	Substrate for microflora
	Not degradable by microflora	Lignin; partial for others	Bulk - increased fecal excretion - water retention

Many polysaccharides (cell wall components plus other poly-saccharides such as starch) have an important role in determining the texture of foods. Texture of a food affects its palatability and it may also influence voluntary food intake. Southgate suggests that the texture of a diet could certainly influence the rate at which it can be eaten.

Many polysaccharides also have the properties of absorbing water, swelling and forming gels or viscous solutions. These properties will affect the consistency of the contents of the stomach and small intestine and may also affect gastric emptying and flow through the gastrointestinal tract. The absorption of other constituents in the gut will be affected by the presence of these polysaccharides because they alter the physico-chemical environment of the intestines.

Various polysaccharides and lignin which are not degraded will contribute to the mass and its consistency in the large intestine. The most consistent effects of gel forming properties of dietary fiber are the production of bulky, moist stools which are easily expelled and a more rapid transit with the stimulus of the volume of the contents.

Southgate emphasizes that to concentrate on one property in defining dietary fiber is to restrict one's view of this highly diverse dietary component.

IMPROPER TITLES AND CONCLUSIONS IN PUBLISHED PAPERS

The tendency to generalize the effects of fiber in both scientific papers and popular articles has unfortunately led to improper conclusions. These two titles were typical of those early articles or papers: "Dietary fiber does not lower serum cholesterol" (this article referred only to wheat fiber; it is known that pectins and gums do lower serum cholesterol); "Low fiber intake of diets in population X" (all the analyses reported were for crude fiber, thus the diet could have been high in pectin, from fruits and vegetables, since no pectin appears in a crude fiber determination).

Fortunately, because of the many publications warning about such improprieties, this tendency is now disappearing and it is hoped it will be only a memory of the early, stormy days of dietary fiber research before too long!

Kay and Truswell's recent paper (1977), "Effect of citrus pectin on blood lipids and fecal steroid excretion in man", is a good example of proper terminology.

TABLE 5

STRUCTURAL FEATURES OF THE COMPONENTS OF DIETARY FIBER (Southgate)

Major Groupings	Principal Structural Types	Main Variations
Structural		
Non-Cellulosic Polysaccharides	Galacturonans	Methoxy groups; side chains
	Xylans, arabino-glucurono-	Branched and linear xylan chain; number and distribution of side chains.
	Mannans, gluco-galacto-	Number and distribution of side chains.
	Galactans, arabino	Branching and side chains.
Cellulose	β-D-Glucan	Degree of polymerization.
Lignins	Aromatic polymer	Type of polymer; functional groups.
Non-Structural		
Pectin	Galacturonans	Methoxy group; side chains.
Gums Mucilages	Great variety including arabino-xylans and gluco- and galacto-mannans	
Algal Polysaccharides	Sulphated Galactans Gulurono-mannuronans	
Modified Celluloses	Ethers, etc. Esters, ethers	Cross-linking.

ANALYSIS AND CHARACTERIZATION OF DIETARY PLANT FIBERS (PLANTIX)

There are a number of methods available for the measurement and characterization of dietary fiber (plantix). The Southgate method and modifications of the Van Soest NDF and ADF methods have found an important place in plant fiber research. But there are still too few laboratories performing proper plant fiber analyses and there is a lack of published analytical data on both total plant fiber and individual components. This latter problem makes epidemiological and applied clinical research rather diffi-cult at times.

The mixture of substances making up dietary fiber in a typi-cal mixed diet contains a wide range of structures, as illustrated in Table 5, and the analysis of this mixture presents some for-midable problems to the analyst (Southgate, 1976c).

The Southgate methods of analysis include both water-soluble and insoluble polysaccharides and those that are susceptible to degradation by the intestinal microflora in addition to those that escape degradation and appear in the feces. This concept of the distinction between water-soluble and water-insoluble frac-tions is an important one and it is quite often overlooked.

It is desirable that the methods characterize the dietary fiber so that the results of the analysis provide a basis for the interpretation of the properties of the mixture being eaten.

Southgate is convinced that the interpretation of experi-mental studies with dietary fibers and of epidemiological data depends on the measurement and characterization of the dietary fiber being consumed, and that analytical methods must attempt to provide this type of information. The research analyst work-ing in this area must have methods that give a measure of total dietary fiber present and of the amounts and types of the various components making up the total. Rapid quality control or screen-ing methods may be useful at times, and must be relatable to the ideal reference type of method, but cannot be used to define dietary fiber.

THE SOUTHGATE METHOD OF ANALYSIS

Dietary fiber must be considered in the general context of the analysis of food carbohydrates (Southgate, 1974, 1976 b,c). The proper preparation of the sample is an often neglected area of food fiber analysis and the sample taken must be representa-tive. The plant cell wall material in many foods is present as large discrete particles which are unevenly distributed in the food and which have a different density to the remainder of the food.

It is known that air-drying at elevated temperatures (100°C) produces artifacts which interfere with the analysis of lignin and it is best to avoid this form of drying (Van Soest and McQueen, 1973). Nevertheless, most human diets include cooked foods which have been taken to much higher temperatures and the normal diet will include these artifacts and our analyses must include them if we are to analyze what is being eaten.

Freeze-drying is probably the best approach, but extraction with aqueous alcohol can be used on fresh foodstuffs if one adjusts the strength of the alcohol to the water content of the sample. The residue is a polysaccharide which is eminently suitable for subsequent analyses.

A crucial aspect of measuring dietary fiber is the definition of the boundary between the available carbohydrates (McCance and Lawrence, 1929; Southgate, 1969 a,b, 1976 b) - those that are digested and absorbed as carbohydrate and which form the major part of the total carbohydrate in most diets - and dietary fiber.

The free sugars and oligosaccharides are conveniently extracted with aqueous alcohol; removal of a lipid, which is essential as some starch granules are resistant to extraction and enzymatic attack if their lipid coats are intact, can be incorporated at this stage (Schoch, 1942).

The selective hydrolysis of starch and dextrins marks the effective boundary between the characteristically α-glucans of the available carbohydrate and the β-glycans of the dietary fiber. The boundary is determined by digestive capacity of the small intestinal secretions and can only be rigorously determined by biological experiment; it is therefore important to seek to mimic the in vivo digestion in an in vitro analytical situation.

Chemical hydrolysis or selective extraction of starch and dextrins are not likely to be sufficiently specific as some components of dietary fiber are very readily hydrolyzed or possess similar solubilities to starch.

Enzymatic hydrolysis seems to offer the most specific approach and the choice of enzyme preparation thus becomes the critical factor in defining the division between available carbohydrate and dietary fiber.

Takadiastase preparations have been widely used for enzymatic hydrolysis (Widdowson and McCance, 1935; Bolton, 1960; Southgate, 1969 a,b) and also other α-amyloglucosidase mixtures such as pancreatin (Williams and Olmstead, 1935; Hellendoorn et al, 1975). Recently the more specific 1→4 and 1→6 α-glucoamylases which are now available have been used. These are highly active and attractive as analytical reagents because of their high specificity and uniformity. However, they do require very careful preparation of the sample. In Southgate's view, the acid pretreatment used in some methods is not acceptable as it will hydrolyze some non-starch polysaccharides (Southgate, 1974, 1976 b).

After enzymatic hydrolysis, some polysaccharides will dissolve in the buffer system used and these must be reprecipitated with alcohol before the next stages.

The extraction of the water-soluble components is a difficult stage to standardize in practice. It may be desirable to add EDTA to the extracting medium to ensure that all pectin complexed with calcium is extracted.

The non-water soluble material includes cellulose, lignin, (plus cutin, etc.) and a range of non-cellulosic polysaccharides. The latter can be extracted with dilute alkali, but it is a difficult technical operation with many diets and it is preferable to hydrolyze them directly with dilute acid ($1\underline{N}$ H_2SO_4 or $2\underline{N}$ CF_3CO_2H) and measure the component sugars. The analyses can be made using relatively non-specific colorimetric methods for the major classes present (i.e. anthrone for hexose, ferric chloride/orcinol/HCl for pentoses and carbazole for uronic acids) but gas-liquid or high performance liquid chromatography provide a better and more specific approach. Uronic acid-containing polysaccharides are difficult to hydrolyze completely and the carbazole method remains the most practicable at present.

The cellulose in the residue after acid hydrolysis can be measured after extraction into 72% w/w H_2SO_4 leaving the residual lignin. This procedure has been applied to a wide range of foodstuffs (Southgate et al, 1976) and the values obtained are compatible with the limited but more detailed studies of the plant cell wall in some of these foods and with other types of procedures developed for specific foods (Fraser et al, 1956).

It is important to know how these values from the Southgate method compare with other procedures, mainly with the detergent fiber method of Van Soest. Acid detergent fiber (ADF) values appear to provide the same type of values for cellulose and lignin as the method outlined for a number of foodstuffs. The lignin values in some foods by both methods are rather higher than one would expect but undoubtedly include heat-induced artifacts.

Neutral detergent fiber (NDF) values should agree with the non-water soluble fractions of dietary fiber and give values that are lower than what Southgate thinks should be called total dietary fiber. In wheat products the difference is rather small because they contain only small amounts of water-soluble components, but in many other foods the NDF values are much lower.

Schaller emphasizes that a major difficulty appears in translating the definition (of dietary fiber) into actual values for applied nutritional use. A method or methods of analysis have to be accepted; these methods of analyzing for dietary fiber have to be accurate and suitable for the use intended. The Food Fiber Committee of the American Association of Cereal Chemists is currently evaluating different methods of analyzing for dietary fiber. Recently, during a collaborative study, Southgate's unavailable carbohydrate analysis, Van Soest's neutral detergent fiber method (for water-insoluble fiber) modified for use with foods, and an enzyme digestion method from Saunders[2] were compared for their ability to measure water-insoluble fiber.

The results of the study for wheat bran are shown in Table 6. As one can see, essentially the same results were obtained with all methods. Southgate's detailed method of analysis was compared to a general gravimetric method and a general enzyme digestion. More information was available from the detailed method including the water-soluble fiber components. Southgate's method and other similar methods of analysis are able to give exact amounts of the components of dietary fiber in addition to the total amount, but in monitoring total amounts, these methods were comparable in this study.

Schaller states that the depth of information that is supplied by each of these analyses is not the same and the choice of methods will be dictated by the end use of the results. The method that gives detailed results may be necessary for testing a scientific hypothesis. The day-to-day monitoring of ingredients of products generally requires a different approach.

There are methods of analysis suitable for the quick, accurate estimation of dietary fiber, such as the modified Van Soest analysis as well as more detailed methods for in-depth research such as Southgate's method. According to Schaller, they all need to be accepted and used for estimating dietary fiber or portions of it.

TABLE 6

DIETARY FIBER ANALYSES ON

WHITE WHEAT BRAN (Schaller)

(%)

Southgate (Unavailable Carbohydrate)	37
NDF (Modified for use with foods)	36
Enzymatic Analysis (+ regression equation)	35

According to Southgate, values for total dietary fiber <u>must</u> include any water-soluble components and ideally the analytical method should characterize the polysaccharides present - by giving the component sugars for example. Van Soest's methods are more rapid and have been partially automated. For many foods, however, the water-soluble fraction is substantial and is important in determining some of the properties of the dietary fiber in the food.

Figure 1 shows a schematic comparison of various methods of analysis.

All this has led Southgate to state that it would be unfortunate if the term dietary fiber was defined as a function of any one standard method. The cell wall in many plants has a different composition and the selection of one method that is completely applicable to all foods and diets is probably an unattainable aim. Southgate expresses the viewpoint that dietary fiber should be left as a philosophical ideal and that analytical procedures remain what they are, approximations to the measurement of the ideal.

THE ROLE OF DIETARY PLANT FIBER IN GUT FERMENTATION

An important concern in discussing the term dietary fiber is the presumption made by various authors that fiber is non-nutritive or indigestible. This is far from correct. Solid evidence demonstrates that plant fiber can represent a significant source of nutrition by means of fermentative digestion in the lower G.I. tract of humans. The fermentative digestion by intestinal bacteria produces certain metabolites (volatile fatty acids) which may be absorbed into the systemic circulation or the lymph. Plant fibers such as pectin, hemicellulose and cellulose may be extensively fermented in the lower digestive tract, yielding low recoveries of these substances in feces.

The topic of fiber and its role in gut fermentation is, according to Van Soest, essentially a story of symbiotic bacteria in normal gut fermentation. Gut microflora are capable of degrading a wide variety of substances. Generally, the lower tract fermentation will metabolize most residue escaping from or secretions arising from digestion in the upper digestive tract. Substances that are degraded by gut microflora can be classified in two groups: those resistant to animal digestive enzymes and those escaping or arising from animal digestion. Resistant water-insoluble substances include those in the fiber matrix of plant foods such as cellulose, hemicellulose, lignin and a group of relatively soluble gum-like carbohydrates including pectin and galactins, mucilages and gums. Substances escaping from the upper tract include starches, mucoid secretions and lactose (in lactose intolerance). Van Soest emphasizes that these adventitious substances should be considered

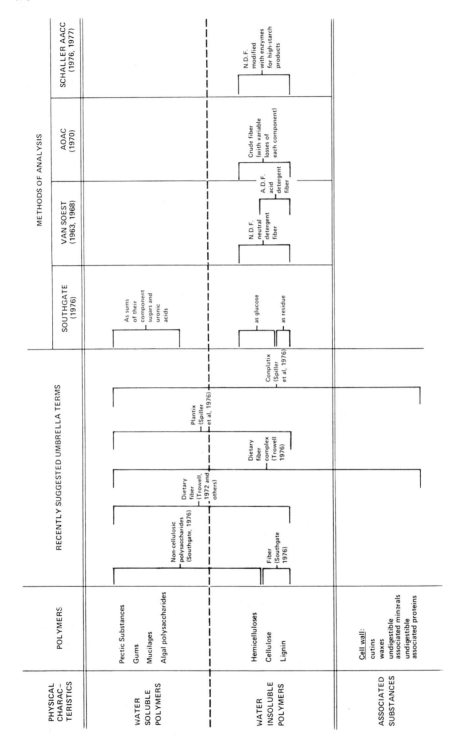

Fig. 1. Suggested umbrella terms and analytical procedures for dietary fiber or its fraction.

by those who wish to define fiber as the fraction in plants resistant to animal digestive enzymes.

There are also substances which escape microbial degradation
to become voided in the feces. These include matter which is
obligately resistant to microbial degradation and that which is
potentially degradable.

Obligately undegradable matter includes condensed structures
such as lignin, cutin, or Maillard polymers and compounds of high
carbon and hydrogen density (saturated long chain fatty acids or
resistant proteins such as skin and hair). G.I. fermentation is
obligately anaerobic and it is unable to derive free energy from
substrates low in oxygen content.

Lignin is the most resistant of plant cell wall components
by virtue of its condensed phenolic structure and relatively low
oxygen content as compared with carbohydrates. Phenols are metabolized with difficulty in most anaerobic systems. The lignin
also protects a portion of the associated cell wall carbohydrates
(cellulose and hemicellulose) from fermentative degradation.
According to Van Soest, the resistance of this carbohydrate to
degradation is apparently dependent on ester linkages to lignin,
since treatment of cereal straws with sodium hydroxide can render
the whole available without the removal of any lignin (Hartley
and Jones, 1976; Rexen et al, 1975).

One of the dietary significances of the undegraded fiber is
its bulking effect in the lower bowel and in the stool. Highly
fermentable fiber sources provide less of this effect, as for
example, cabbage which has a digestibility of greater that 90%
in the human (unpublished observations).

The extent of degradation of potential degradable carbohydrates is dependent upon a number of factors among which are included the potential fermentation rate, the residence time of the
substrate at the fermentation site, and ecological conditions of
pH, Eh osmotic pressure (Hungate, 1967). Degradation is also
dependent on a requisite microflora, the development of which is
influenced by the relative rates of passage and microbial generation time. Fast rates of passage tend to cause loss of slowly
fermenting substrates such as crystalline cellulose (Van Soest,
1975).

Purified celluloses are relatively unfermented vegetable
fibers, while pectin may be largely catabolized by bacteria to
volatile fatty acids and gaseous products.

The potential fermentation rate is an intrinsic characteristic of each substrate. Fiber substances vary both in the extent

TABLE 7

FERMENTABILITY OF VEGETABLE FIBERS (Van Soest)

Fiber Source	Fermentation		Maximum Extent	L/C[a]	15 hour Digestion Coeff.
	Lag (hour)	(rate/hr)	(%)		(%)
Cauliflower	4	.42	.94	.05	.93
Cabbage	3	.40	.93	.04	.90
Onions	5	.23	.91	.09	.57
Corn Bran	5	.10	.94	.12	.54
Wheat Bran	3	.06	.43	.47	.33
Bagasse	4	.04	.45	.31	.23
Cellulose	9	.06	.94	.03	.26
Cotton	17	.04	.98	.00	.18

[a]L/C = ratio of lignin to cellulose.

of degradability and in the potential rate at which the degradable part can be fermented (Table 7). Van Soest writes that the factor of fermentability is an important property of plant fibers since it reflects the amount of microbial products in the bowel.

The organisms producing fermentation in the cecum, large intestine and colon are an exceedingly diverse group comprising as many as 500 species, the majority of which are obligate anaerobes (Holdeman et al, 1976). Organisms possessing the ability to ferment cellulose and hemicellulose are a relatively fastidious group with special nutrient requirements. Requirements for various species may include carbon dioxide, ammonia, acetate, isobutyrate, isovalerate, heme and various vitamins (Bryant, 1974).

The whole culture fermentation of any substrate gives rise to the production of microbial cells, short chain fatty acids (VFA), carbon dioxide and methane. The distribution of fermentation products is presented in Table 8. The principal fatty acids are acetic, propionic and butyric.

The portion of the fermented substrate converted to microbial cells is a major factor influencing loss of nutrients in feces. Microbial matter forms the largest single organic fraction in the feces of most animals, comprising in man 60-80% of the dry weight of feces. This microbial mass which consists mainly of dead cells is formed from undigested food residues reaching the lower tract in addition to endogenous secretions and sloughings from the host.

TABLE 8

DISTRIBUTION OF FERMENTATION PRODUCTS
IN COLONIC FUNCTION[a] (Van Soest)

	Dry Weight	Carbon
	(gram)	(moles)
Fiber Carbohydrate	100	3.67
NH_3 Requirement	3.6	
Product		
Acetate	21.9	.73
Propionate	17.8	.72
Butyrate	7.7	.35
CO_2	16.3	.37
CO_4	2.4	.15
Microbial Cells	30	1.35
Total VFA	47.4	1.80

[a]Calculated from the volatile acid ratios reported by Argenzio
and Southworth (1974) for the pig and the estimates of mircrobial
yield according to Baldwin (1970).

This matter includes virtually all of the so-called metabolic fecal
nitrogen (Mason, 1969). The loss of microbial matter can be viewed
both positively and negatively. The loss of nutrients--minerals,
vitamins, protein--is counterbalanced by binding of potentially
toxic matter, and the high water-holding capacity of this matter
is probably a factor in softness of the stool.

The quantity of microbial matter found in gut fermentation is
variable and dependent upon a number of factors:

First, microbial yield is generally proportional to the amount
of substrate fermented. Thus the addition of fermentable fiber
carbohydrate increased fecal microbial loss, which is measured
mainly as metabolic fecal nitrogen.

A secondary factor influencing the distribution of cells and
fermentation products involves the rate of fermentation, generation
time of bacteria and the rate they are washed out through transit
and passage. The addition of unfermentable fiber increases passage
rate and therefore promotes fecal microbial loss.

The third set of factors influencing microbial yield are the
efficiencies of microbial species. The conversion to cell yield
is dependent upon the amount of ATP individual strains can extract

out of the substrate and the efficiency with which ATP can be converted to cell mass. Anaerobic bacteria vary considerably in this respect depending on their ecological strategy for survival.

Bearing on the previous discussion, Van Soest speculates on a unifying hypothesis of bowel cancer as related to fiber and diet. High protein-low fiber diets of meat-eating Western man produce long transits and prolonged microbial refermentation of residues in the bowel into potentially toxic products. As a result of bacterial fermentation in the gut, excess dietary nitrogen from such diets appears in the lumen as ammonia, amines and other nitrogenous bases that can be toxic to the gut wall, increasing cell death and turnover in these tissues (Visek, 1977). The extra ammonia absorbed from the gut during proteolytic fermentation is reconverted to urea by the liver. This extra load is a problem in liver disease and can be relieved by feeding a source of fermentable carbohydrate such as lactulose. The addition of fermentable fibrous carbohydrate increases microbial mass. The increased microbial nitrogen requirement pulls urea from the blood through diffusion, thus diverting urinary nitrogen to the feces where it is excreted in the form of microbial matter. In ruminants fed low-protein, high-carbohydrate diets, it is possible through this mechanism to reduce urinary nitrogen loss to virtually zero. From this viewpoint, bowel cancer etiology from high beef diets may be contrasted with high fiber diets that are systematically lower in protein. It is difficult to decide between high protein or low fiber since they are a part of the same effect.

The composition of the intestinal flora in animals is altered by diet. This point is emphasized by the large differences seen in ruminants of the same species on low and high fiber diets. A major difference between humans and experimental animals is the constancy of diet. Humans follow a free-choice pattern of eating compared to the uniformity of experimental animal diets such as rat chow. The intestinal microflora respond and adapt to the substances they are offered. In humans, they must be continually changing and adapting. For this reason, Van Soest suggests that the only relevant animal models are humans themselves. Alternately, Spiller and co-workers have suggested certain old world monkeys (*Macaca nemestrina*) as one of the better animal models even though they agree that humans are the model of choice.

Humans do not have digestive enzymes capable of hydrolizing the carbohydrates in plant cell walls. They have instead developed a symbiotic relation with gut microflora to obtain energy from plant material such as cellulose and hemicellulose. It has been assumed that fiber is non-nutritive and that the products of fermentation are not utilized. This contrasts with results from animal and human experiments. Tables 9 and 10 illustrate the fact that fiber may be used to obtain energy in a number of different species.

TABLE 9

DIGESTIBILITIES OF FIBERS IN ANIMAL SPECIES (Van Soest)

Animal	Fiber Source	Hemicellulose	Cellulose	Reference
		(% dry matter)	(% dry matter)	
Cow	Alfalfa	49	51	Keys et al, 1969
Sheep	Alfalfa	46	50	Keys et al, 1969
Rat	Alfalfa	47	21	Keys et al, 1969
Pig	Alfalfa	43	40	Keys et al, 1969
Dog	Cereal	47	18	Visek and Robertson, 1973
Man	Mixed	72-98	15-44	Southgate and Durnin, 1970
Man	Bran	68	51	Williams and Olmstead, 1936
Man	Alfalfa	-	14	Williams and Olmstead, 1936

TABLE 10

ENERGY OBTAINED FROM VOLATILE FATTY ACIDS[a] (Parra)

Animal	Fermentation Site	
	Foregut	Hindgut
	$(Kcal/w^{.75})$	$(Kcal/w^{.75})$
Cattle	70-80	0-15
Sheep	57-79	0-?
Goat	37-46	
Deer	25	
Langur monkey	>100	
Rabbit		8-12
Porcupine		6-39
Beaver		19
Rat		9
Pig		5-28
Man		0.7-10

[a]The energy contribution of fiber in the form of VFA is dependent upon the level of fermentable fiber in the diet.

TABLE 11

ESTIMATE OF DIETARY ENERGY SUPPLIED BY FIBER[a] (Van Soest)

	Wheat Bran	Carrots	Corn Germ	Sugar Beet Pulp	Peas	Cabbage
Intake[b] (gm)	243	226	329	164	163	211
Fiber digestion[b] (gm)	42	75	89	61	38	63
Net VFA[c] (meq)	391	521	623	424	263	442
VFA excreted[b] (meq)	101	97	110	98	45	135
VFA absorbed (meq)	190	424	513	326	218	307
VFA absorbed (%)	65	81	82	77	83	69
VFA absorbed[d] (Kcal)	58	129	157	99	67	94
Kcal/gm dig. fiber	1.38	1.72	1.76	1.62	1.76	1.49
Kcal/gm food	.24	.57	.48	.60	.41	.45

[a]Calculated from the data of Williams and Olmstead, 1936.

[b]Original values, average of three subjects.

[c]Calculated assuming a 30% yield of microbial cells from fermented carbohydrate (Baldwin, 1970) with remaining carbon distributed between VFA, CO_2 and CH_4 according to the stoichiometric equations of Wolin, 1960.

[d]Volatile fatty acids (VFA) assumed to have molar ratios similar to that observed in the lower bowel of the pig (Argenzio and Southworth, 1974), of acetic:propionic:butyric of 52:35:13; an average moles carbon per equivalent of 2.61; and 117 Kcal per carbon equivalent.

Data in Table 11 provide an estimate of dietary energy supplied by different plant fiber sources. These results of Williams and Olmstead indicate that up to 80% of the expected volatile fatty acid production is absorbed by human subjects. About 50% of the total carbon in fermentable carbohydrate is converted to volatile fatty acids (Table 12). Volatile fatty acids (VFA) are probably largely absorbed as free acids and may be a significant source of metabolizable energy.

The amount of carbohydrate fermentable in the bowel may be greater than the sum of fermented cellulose and hemicellulose since any starches, pectins or other carbohydrates reaching the lower tract can ferment.

TABLE 12

CARBON-HYDROGEN BALANCE EQUATIONS[a] (Van Soest)

$$Glucose \rightarrow 2 \text{ Acetate} + 2CO_2 + 8H$$
$$Glucose \rightarrow Butyrate + 2CO_2 + 4H$$
$$Glucose + 4H \rightarrow 2 \text{ Propionate}$$
$$CO_2 + 8H \rightarrow CH_4 + 2H_2O$$

Net[b]: 3 Glucose $\rightarrow$ 2 Acetate + Butyrate +
2 Propionate + $3CO_2$ + CH_4 + $2H_2O$

---

[a]Deficiency or excess of oxygen expressed as hydrogen where:
$O = -2H$, (Wolin, 1975).

[b]Actual experimental yields are variable and a decrease in methane output is usually associated with increased propionate production. Hydrogen may also appear as a product.

Conversely, Southgate and Durnin (1970) concluded that dietary fiber is of little importance as an energy source for humans. Disagreeing, Van Soest states that the kind of dietary fiber in the studies of those investigators at higher levels was mainly bran which is a relatively lignified and less available source of energy than other fibers. Data of Williams and Olmstead (1936) agree with Southgate that the energy value of fiber carbohydrate will be less than 10%. However, their conclusion underestimates the value of fruits and vegetables.

Van Soest emphasizes that the assumption that fiber has negligible food value is inaccurate. In the case of low fiber Western diets, he feels that it would be more appropriate to say that the intake of digestible fiber is negligible. He suggests that the intake of fermentable energy from dietary fiber might be significant in a high fiber consuming population.

DIETARY FIBER SHOULD NOT BE CALLED "NON-NUTRITIVE"

The role of fiber in human nutrition and disease, states Van Soest, can not be comprehended merely in terms of its amount and physical properties. Fiber is the substrate for an important gastrointestinal fermentation through which it is involved in a complex way in metabolism. Through the medium of fermentative digestion, fiber can represent a significant food value. In the face of animal studies, there is little justification for the use of the term non-nutritive residue. This term implies inertness, which even indigestible fiber is not, since it has an effect on

transit and on the environment of the digestive tract and is capable of adsorbing minerals (McConnell et al, 1974; Jones, 1977) and
promoting fecal loss of lipids and microbial nitrogen. Fiber is
admittedly a nutrient of relatively low (and variable) caloric
value but with its own distinctive characteristics and effects.

APPLICATIONS OF PROPER DEFINITIONS, ANALYSES
AND EXPERIMENTAL DESIGN TO NUTRITIONAL RESEARCH

It appeared appropriate that the symposium would end with a
report by Sandstead of a study that shows a careful definition of
the dietary fiber used, without attempting sweeping generalizations. Furthermore, fiber analyses are properly presented. In
addition, the background diet was a typical U.S. diet, fairly
high in animal proteins. All in all, this study indicates the
direction we should follow, without preventing further refinements.

The influence of dietary fiber on fecal bivalent ion excretion is incompletely defined and is an area in need of more extensive study. One concern is that an excess of plant fiber in
the diet may result in nutritional deficiencies (such as zinc or
other minerals). To complicate the issue, dietary fiber, since
it is a highly interacting agent, will be expected to affect bivalent metal excretion differently depending on the other components of the diet and the nutritional status of the individual.

Much of the work in this area has been done on persons fed
diets rich in vegetables and cereals, but containing less than
30 g of animal protein per day. It appears from these studies
that consumption of liberal amounts of bread prepared from unre-
fined wheat flour may impair the absorption of zinc and iron.
But it should be pointed out that these studies were done on persons consuming a Middle Eastern diet which is substantially different from the typical American diet and it is unreasonable to
apply these results to persons consuming a Western-type diet.

A study presently in progress at the USDA Human Nutrition
Laboratory in North Dakota by Sandstead and co-workers[3] on the
effect of selected fiber sources on mineral balance in humans is
attempting to take into account all dietary factors and to make
the results applicable to the typical American diet. This study
appears to be a well controlled study of the effects of cereal
brans on bivalent ion metabolism in persons consuming a well defined Western diet.

Sandstead and co-workers are interested in determining
whether increased intakes of sources of dietary fiber could have
adverse effects on the availability of zinc, copper and iron for
intestinal absorption.

TABLE 13

FIBER COMPOSITION[a] (Sandstead)

	SWW	HRS	CB	SH
	(%)	(%)	(%)	(%)
Water-Insoluble Hemicellulose	30.0	35.0	71.0	33.0
Cellulose	9.0	9.3	22.0	53.0
Lignin	2.5	3.5	0.1	0.7
Ash	5.6	7.8	0.6	4.3
Starch	33.0	20.0	1.0	0.0
Protein	15.0	20.0	5.5	8.0
Oil	4.0	3.9	0.6	0.9
Phytate Phosphorus	0.5	0.4		
Percent Dietary Fiber	42.0	48.0	93.0	86.0

[a]Water-soluble dietary fiber not reported.

Human volunteers living in a controlled metabolic environment were fed a constant mixed diet similar to that consumed by many U.S. men. Each study period was 28-30 days in length. Following an initial 16-18 day adaptation period, fecal and duplicate diets were collected for 12 days. Throughout the studies, energy intake and expenditure were maintained constant so that body weight changed very little.

Approximately 26 g/day of American Association of Cereal Chemists soft white wheat bran (SW), hard red spring wheat bran (HR), corn bran (CB), soybean hulls (SH), apple powder (AP), or carrot powder (CP) were incorporated into the daily bread to increase the fiber content of the diet. The composition of the fiber sources is shown in Table 13. Both soft white wheat (SW) and hard red spring wheat bran (HR) contained less than 50% dietary fiber and both corn bran (CB) and soybean hulls (SH) contained more than 80% dietary fiber. The wheat brans contained much more lignin than the other two brans. They were also higher in protein. Soft white wheat and hard red spring wheat bran contained approximately 20% starch.

To date, zinc, iron and copper balance has been determined for SW, CB, SH and HR. The results of copper balance are summarized in Figure 2. These preliminary results suggest that volunteers tended to be in more positive balance when fed SH and HR than when fed SW or CB.

Preliminary observations of the authors suggest that 26 g/day of SW, CB or SH in bread do not appear to impair iron balance. They are unable to draw conclusions about the effects of the dietary fibers on iron balance at this time.

Figure 2 also presents a summary of the results of zinc balance. From this figure, it can be seen that there were no significant differences among the fibers compared to basal. However, the net zinc balance when hard red spring wheat bran was fed was negative. The authors' preliminary interpretation of these results suggests that HR may inhibit zinc absorption in some persons.

It is important to note that the four cereal brans examined did not show the same effects on zinc, copper and iron balance in the volunteer subjects. This study exemplifies the point that it is crucial not to generalize the effects of dietary fiber in human nutrition.

Sandstead and co-workers conclude that the differences in their findings from those reporting the effects of Middle Eastern diets rich in bread might be due to the marked difference in the dietary content of protein in these two quite dissimilar diets. They hope that future studies will clarify the discrepancies between their findings and those reported previously.

The problem of possible effects of increased intakes of plant fibers and deficiencies of bivalent cations might well be correlated to a number of factors including the composition of the remainder of the diet, the nutritional status of the individual, the specific type of plant fiber consumed, and the amount of plant fiber ingested.

The overall impression obtained by examining Figure 2 is that none of the dietary plant fibers meaningfully changed mineral balances when fed with an otherwise typical American diet with sufficient animal proteins present. Notice that some subjects are in negative balance on the diet without any added dietary fiber.

This field needs much more study and it is hoped that investigators will take into account some of the concepts expressed in this symposium.

SUMMARY AND CONCLUSIONS

There seems to have been a consensus among the participants at this symposium that:

1. We need always to define carefully the dietary fiber (plantix) used. This means: a) Presentation of proper

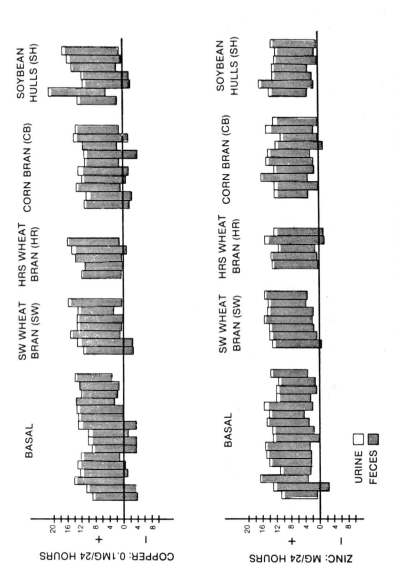

Fig. 2. Copper and zinc balances in healthy human subjects fed various high dietary fiber substances according to Sandstead and co-workers.

analytical data. b) Avoidance of the term crude fiber.
c) Careful description of any natural product used including its source, preparation, region of production,
season of harvesting, etc. d) Careful limitation of
conclusions in papers and popular writings to the materials studied (e.g. cooked, raw, finely ground, purified,
part of a natural food, etc.).

2.   We need to avoid generalizations of the effects of dietary fiber, as the overall diet might affect the action
of the fiber. There are some exceptions such as the
general bulking effect in the colon of certain products,
which might be independent of the remainder of the diet,
except perhaps total caloric intake.

At the round table that followed the symposium, there was no
consensus as to a possible new term for dietary fiber or whether
the word fiber should be totally dropped because of its imprecise-
ness. The term plantix suggested by some of us has not yet found
universal acceptance. It was agreed that various scientific bodies
should take into consideration the various proposals and come up
with some recommendations.

In spite of these problems, research on the medical, epidemiological and nutritional aspects of dietary fiber in humans has
progressed a great deal in the last three to four years, but some
confusion persists. There is a tremendous amount of research to
be done and this research must be done well. Scientific journals
have the responsibility of accepting only properly executed research or review papers and should be extremely strict in allowing
only the proper terminology to be used. As these journals are the
channels that bring dietary fiber (plantix) research to the scientific community, they have the key to insuring that only good
research will be published.

The authors of this chapter have frequently used the term
plantix in parentheses after dietary fiber, as a way to show a
possible way to introduce a new term.

There is no doubt that dietary fiber (plantix) has a much
more important function in human health than previously suspected.
This symposium was an attempt to clarify some confused concepts -
we hope it was a step in the right direction.

ACKNOWLEDGMENT

The authors acknowledge the assistance of Elizabeth A. Shipley
of Syntex Research in the preparation of this symposium.

FOOTNOTES

[1]This chapter was compiled using the typescripts by the various speakers from the presentations made at the American Chemical Society, 1977, Chicago National Meeting, in the Symposium: DEFINING FIBER IN HUMAN NUTRITION. The following symposium speakers are extensively quoted in this chapter: G.A. Spiller, Syntex Research, Palo Alto, CA; D.A.T. Southgate, Medical Research Council, Cambridge, U.K.; P. Van Soest, Cornell University, Ithaca, N.Y.; D. Schaller, The Kellogg Co., Battle Creek, MI; and H. Sandstead, Human Nutrition Laboratory, U.S.D.A., Grand Forks, N.D. Whenever these authors are quoted herein without reference to the bibliography, the reference refers to their symposium presentation and their contributions have been made an integral part of the text.

[2]R. Saunders, Western Regional Laboratories, U.S.D.A., Albany, California.

[3]J. Junoz, L. Klevay, R. Jacob, S. Reck, F. Dintzis, G. Inglett and W. Shuez.

REFERENCES

American Heritage Dictionary. Morris, W., Editor. American Heritage Publishing Co., Houston. 1973.

Argenzio, R.A. and M. Southworth. 1974. Sites of organic acid production and absorption in gastrointestinal tract of the pig. Am. J. Phys., 228, 454-460.

Baldwin, R.L. 1970. Energy metabolism in anaerobes. Am. J. Clin. Nutr., 23, 1508-1513.

Bolton, W. 1960. The determination of digestible carbohydrates in poultry foods. Analyst, 85, 189-192.

Bryant, M.P. 1974. Nutritional features and ecology of predominant anaerobic bacteria of the intestinal tract. Amer. J. Clin. Nutr., 27, 1313-1319.

Cummings, J.H. 1976. What is fiber? In "Fiber in Human Nutrition", G.A. Spiller and R.J. Amen (Eds.), Plenum Press, New York.

Fraser, J.R., M. Brendon-Bravo and D.C. Holmes. 1956. The proximate analysis of wheat flour carbohydrates I methods and scheme of analysis. J. Sci. Food Agric., 7, 577-589.

Fruda, I. 1977. Fractionation and examination of biopolymers from dietary fiber. Cereal Food World, 6, 252-254.

Godding, E.W. 1976. Dietary fiber redefined. Lancet, i, 1129.

Hartley, R.D. and E.C. Jones. 1976. Diferulic acid as a component
    of cell walls of lolium multiflorum. Phytochem, 15, 1157-60.

Hellendoorn, E.W., M.G. Nordhoff and J. Slagman. 1975. Enzymatic
    determination of indigestible residue (dietary fibre) content
    of human foods. J. Sci. Food Agric., 26, 1461-1468.

Holdeman, L.V., I.J. Good and W.E.C. Moore. 1976. Human fecal
    flora: variation in bacterial composition within individuals
    and a possible effect of emotional stress. Applied and En-
    vironmental Microbiology, 31, 359-375.

Hungate, R.E. 1967. "The Rumen and Its Microbes". Academic Press,
    New York.

Jones, L.H.P. 1978. Mineral components of plant cell walls.
    Proc. NIH Symp. on the Role of Dietary Fiber in Health.
    Roth, H., Editor. Am. J. Clin. Nutr. (in press).

Kay, R.M. and Y.S. Truswell. 1977. Effect of citrus pectin on
    blood lipids and fecal steroid excretion in man. Am. J.
    Clin. Nutr., 30, 171-175.

Keys, J.E. Jr., P.J. Van Soest and E.P. Young. 1969. Comparative
    study of digestibility of forage cellulose and hemicellulose
    in ruminants and non-ruminants. J. An. Sci., 29, 11-15.

Mason, V.C. 1969. Some observations on the distribution and
    origin of nitrogen in sheep feces. J. Agric. Sci. Camb.,
    73, 99-111.

McCance, R.A. and R.D. Lawrence. 1929. The carbohydrate content
    of foods. Spec. Rep. Med. Res. Coun. Lond. No. 195 (HMSO
    Lond.).

McConnell, A.A., M.A. Eastwood and W.D. Mitchell. 1974. Physical
    characteristics of vegetable foodstuffs that could influence
    bowel function. J. Sci. Food Agr., 25, 1457-1464.

Parra, R. 1973. Comparative aspects of the digestive physiology
    of ruminants and nonruminants. Paper in Comparative Gastro-
    enterology, NY State Vet. Coll. Library, Ithaca, New York.

Rexen, F.P., P. Stigsen and V.F. Kristensen. 1975. The effect
    of new alkali technique on the nutritive value of straw.
    Proc. Ninth Nutrition Conf. for Feed Manufacturers, Univer-
    sity of Nottingham, England, Jan. 5-7.

Schoch, T.J. 1942. Non-carbohydrate substances in the cereal starches. J. Amer. Chem. Soc., 64, 2954-2956.

Southgate, D.A.T. 1969a. A determination of carbohydrates in foods I available carbohydrates. J. Sci. Food Agric., 20, 326-329.

Southgate, D.A.T. 1969b. Determination of carbohydrates in foods II unavailable carbohydrates. J. Sci. Food Agric., 20, 331-335.

Southgate, D.A.T. 1974. Problems in the analysis of polysaccharides in foodstuffs. J. Assoc. Pub. Analysts, 12, 114-118.

Southgate, D.A.T. 1976a. The chemistry of dietary fiber. In "Fiber in Human Nutrition", G.A. Spiller and R.J. Amen (Eds.), Plenum Press, New York, 31-72.

Southgate, D.A.T. 1976b. "Determination of Food Carbohydrates", Applied Sci. Publishers, London.

Southgate, D.A.T. 1976c. The analysis of dietary fiber. In "Fiber in Human Nutrition", G.A. Spiller and R.J. Amen (Eds.), Plenum Press, New York, 73-107.

Southgate, D.A.T., B. Bailey, E. Collinson and A.F. Walker. 1976. A guide to calculating intakes of dietary fibre. J. Hum. Nutr., 30, 303-313.

Southgate, D.A.T. and J.V.G.A. Durnin. 1970. Caloric conversion factors. An experimental reassessment of the factors used in the calculation of the energy value of human diets. Brit. J. Nutr., 24, 517-535.

Spiller, G.A. 1977. "Fiber" in the vocabulary of nutrition. Lancet, i, 198.

Spiller, G.A., G. Fassett-Cornelius and G.M. Briggs. 1976. A new term for plant fibers in nutrition. Am. J. Clin. Nutr., 29, 934-935.

Spiller, G.A. and E.A. Shipley. 1976. New perspectives on dietary fiber. Food Prods. Dev., 10, (8), 54-57.

Trowell, H.C. 1974. Definition of fiber. Lancet, i, 503.

Trowell, H.C. 1977. A new term for dietary fiber? Am. J. Clin. Nutr., 30, 1003.

Van Soest, P.J.   1975.   Physico-chemical aspects of fibre digestion. Proc. IV. Intr. Ruminant Congress, 351-365.

Van Soest, P.J. and R.W. McQueen.   1973.   The chemistry and estimation of fibre.   Proc. Nutr. Soc., 32, 123-130.

Visek, W.J.   1977.   Diet and cell growth modulation by ammonia. Proceedings of the NIH Symp. on the role of dietary fiber in health.   H. Roth, Editor.   Am. J. Clin. Nutr.

Visek, W.J. and J.B. Robertson.   1973.   Dried brewers grains in dog diets.   Proc. Cornell Nutrition Conf., 40-49.

Widdowson, E.M. and R.A. McCance.   1935.   The available carbohydrate of fruits.   Determination of glucose, fructose, sucrose and starch.   Biochem. J., 29, 151-156.

Williams, R.D. and W.H. Olmstead.   1935.   A biochemical method for determining indigestible residue (crude fiber) in faeces, lignin, cellulose and non-water soluble hemicellulose.   J. Biol. Chem., 108, 653-666.

Williams, R.D. and W.H. Olmstead.   1936.   The effect of cellulose, hemicellulose and lignin on the weight of the stool: A contribution to the study of laxation in man.   J. Nutr., 11, 433-449.

Wolin, M.J.   1975.   Bacterial species of the rumen: Interactions between bacterial species of the rumen.   In "Digestion and Metabolism in the Ruminant".   Proc. IV.   International and ACI.   Warner.   The University of New England Publishing Unit. 134-148.

12

PHOTOSYNTHESIS AND INCREASED PRODUCTION OF PROTEIN

Steven G. Platt* and James A. Bassham**

*Western Regional Research Center, U.S. Department
of Agriculture, Berkeley, California 94710
**Laboratory of Chemical Biodynamics, Lawrence Berkeley
Laboratory, University of California, Berkeley,
California 94720

ABSTRACT

Photosynthesis, the use of light energy in the conversion of CO_2 and inorganic nutrients into plant material, is the ultimate source of the food protein necessary to man's existence. Given certain assumptions, the overall maximal theoretical photosynthetic efficiency of agricultural plants can be calculated. Actual measured maximal growth rates of plants are equivalent to efficiency levels well below that theoretical maximum. In air, C4 plants can come closer to the theoretical value than C3 plants, perhaps because C4 plants avoid the occurrence of measurable photorespiration and oxygen inhibition of photosynthesis.

Alfalfa, a C3 legume, is an extremely productive protein source. Its protein yield per acre can surpass that of commonly grown C4 crops (corn, sorghum) and C3 seed crops (soybean, wheat, rice). Alfalfa leaf protein is of high nutritional quality and can apparently be used directly in the human diet, eliminating the protein loss involved in animal production.

Plant protein productivity can be raised as part of an increase in overall crop yield. The growth of plants in atmospheres with elevated CO_2 levels can result in increased yields. In C3 plants this is due, at least in part, to the suppression of photorespiration and oxygen inhibition of photosynthesis. We have investigated the effect of CO_2 concentration on alfalfa photosynthetic metabolism. Our results support the contention that alfalfa productivity can be increased by an environment of elevated CO_2.

A second approach toward increased plant protein productivity is through regulation of carbon flow during photosynthesis so as to increase protein production relative to that of other plant constituents. In particular, we have investigated whether ammonia (the form in which plants first incorporate nitrogen) can act to regulate leaf carbon metabolism. Our results indicate that NH_4^+, in part through stimulation of pyruvate kinase, brings about increased production of amino acids at the expense of sucrose production in alfalfa. That effect may be of considerable importance in the regulation of green leaf protein synthesis.

INTRODUCTION

Photosynthesis is the process by which carbon dioxide and various inorganic nutrients are converted into plant matter. That conversion requires an energy input, and is driven by sunlight. Man is totally dependent (directly and indirectly) on photosynthesis for the production of protein essential to human life. It is clear that in a time of protein shortage, one approach toward increasing the production of that material for human use must be an attempt to increase the efficiency and hence the productivity of the photosynthetic process. Yet, as recently as 1975 the Committee on Agricultural Production Efficiency of the National Research Council was able to state the following in its report "Agricultural Production Efficiency" (Committee on Agricultural Production Efficiency, 1975): "Of all the basic research on photosynthesis, essentially none has yet found its way into the farmer's field to contribute to agricultural production efficiency, and hence, to fill the food carts in the supermarket". This situation has become intolerable to many photosynthesis researchers, and there is a strong movement toward directing research into areas ultimately beneficial to crop production. Many recent papers on photosynthesis, and the proceedings of meetings between plant physiologists, agricultural scientists, and photosynthesis researchers, (Brown et al., 1975; Burris and Black, 1976; Cooper, 1975; Marcelle, 1975) clearly indicate the desire to obtain basic knowledge about photosynthesis which would allow us to increase agricultural productivity.

In this chapter we will first discuss the process of photosynthesis--the initial incorporation of light energy and the fixation of CO_2 (the source of 90-95% of the dry weight of plants). We will then describe some of our ideas and recent research results regarding both increasing photosynthetic efficiency and controlling the flow of fixed carbon so as to bring about increased protein production.

PHOTOSYNTHETIC CARBON REDUCTION

Photosynthetic carbon reduction in green plants is the use of light energy in the synthesis of organic compounds from carbon dioxide, with the concomitant release of oxygen. Electrons are transferred from water to carbon dioxide. The overall process can be thought of as consisting of two events: (1) the absorption of light energy, and its use to produce oxygen, high-potential reducing agents and energy-storing compounds; (2) the use of the energy storing compounds and reducing agents to carry out carbon dioxide reduction. The reduced carbon compounds produced are used for the synthesis of the diverse macromolecules essential to plant life, including starch, cellulose, proteins, fats, nucleic acids, and pigments. Transformation of the intermediates of photosynthesis into such compounds can be accomplished both with or without the intermediate production of free carbohydrates as carriers of stored carbon, energy, and reducing power.

The Light Event: Photosynthetic Electron Transport

The absorption of light energy and CO_2 reduction both take place in the chloroplast (Fig. 1). That organelle consists of an outer double membrane; internal lamellar layers of membranes forming the grana, visible as stacks of hollow disc-like structures called the thylakoids; and a viscous internal cytoplasmic region, the stroma, surrounding the grana.

The grana contain chlorophyll and carotenoid pigments that are capable of absorbing light energy. The chemical energy produced from light energy in the grana is used to drive electron transport which results in the oxidation of water to produce O_2, the reduction of ferredoxin (a soluble, low-molecular weight non-heme iron protein), and the production of ATP from ADP and inorganic phosphate. A theoretical scheme summarizing electron flow during the light event of the photosynthetic process is shown in Fig.2. Key to the process are the two photochemical steps (shown in Fig. 2 by heavy arrows) in which light energy absorbed by forms of chlorophyll (P680 and P700) is used to transfer electrons from donors to acceptors (Traps II and I). The electron flow in the photochemical steps is against the thermodynamic gradient of reduction potentials, and it is the light energy input that makes possible the transfer of electrons from the weaker reducing agents (P680 and P700) to the stronger reducing agents. The overall path of electron flow and the energy considerations involved are as follows: Water is oxidized by an oxidant produced through the action of light ($h\nu_{II}$) on P680 which results in the transfer of an electron to trap II. The electron then flows down a potential energy gradient (through several electron carriers decreasing in reducing power) to an electron hole brought about by light excitation of P700. The absorption of a second quanta of light

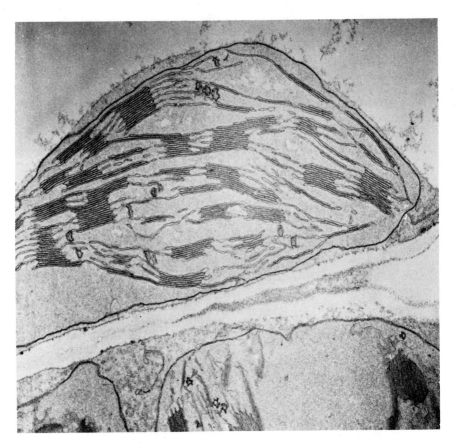

Figure 1. Spinach chloroplast electron micrograph.

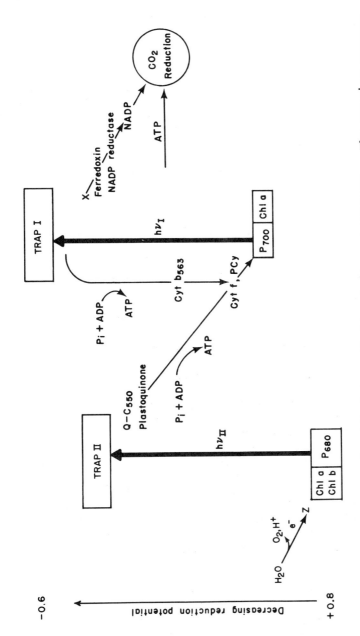

Figure 2. A representation of photosynthetic electron transport. The precise energy-conserving sites are in doubt; however, there appear to be two sites which result in a total of as much as 1 1/2 molecules ATP formed for each pair of electrons flowing from water to ferredoxin (non-cyclic electron flow).

($h\nu_I$) transfers an electron to Trap I and forms a material with low reduction potential. An electron from that trap then flows down an energy gradient to form reduced ferredoxin and then NADPH, which is of sufficiently low potential to be used in the stroma (along with ATP) to bring about the reduction of CO_2.

Accompanying the flow of electrons from water to P680 and from Trap II to P700, energy is stored in the membranes as an electrical potential plus a gradient of H^+ ions across the membrane. This energy is used to drive the conversion of ADP and Pi to ATP in a protein complex attached to the thyalkoid membrane. For each pair of electrons transferred from water to ferredoxin, about 1 1/2 molecules of ATP are formed. Electrons can also be "short-circuited" from Trap I back to P700 in a process of cyclic electron flow, again with energy storage in the membrane. Use of this energy for ATP formation can also occur, and is referred to as cyclic photophosphorylation.

An equation for the light event of photosynthesis is:

$$2\ H_2O + 2\ NADP^+ + 1\ H^+ + 3\ ADP^{-3} + 3\ Pi^{-2} \xrightarrow[\substack{(4\ \text{electrons} \\ \text{transferred})}]{8\ \text{photons}}$$

$$2\ NADPH + 3\ ATP^{-4} + O_2 + 3\ H_2O$$

It should be noted that water is the source of the oxygen released.

The Reductive Pentose Phosphate Cycle

The reductive pentose phosphate (RPP) cycle (Fig. 3) is the basic enzymatic pathway whereby carbon dioxide is converted to reduced metabolites during photosynthesis (Bassham and Calvin, 1957). Apparently, all known green plants and algae capable of oxiding water to O_2 employ the RPP cycle. In some plants that cycle is used for the initial incorporation of CO_2 as well as for CO_2 reduction. Those plants have been labeled "C3" plants, as their primary carboxylation product is the three-carbon acid 3-phosphoglyceric acid (PGA). A second class of higher plants utilizes an additional cycle (to be outlined below) for the initial incorporation of CO_2, but later release it to the RPP cycle for reduction.

The RPP cycle occurs in the stroma. It begins with the carboxylation of ribulose-1,5-diphosphate (RuDP) to form a transient six-carbon intermediate which decomposes to give two molecules of PGA. That reaction is catalyzed by ribulose-1,5-diphosphate carboxylase. CO_2 incorporation through reaction with RuDP is thermodynamically favorable (Bassham and Krause, 1969), but ATP and NADPH, formed by means of the light events (Fig. 2), are

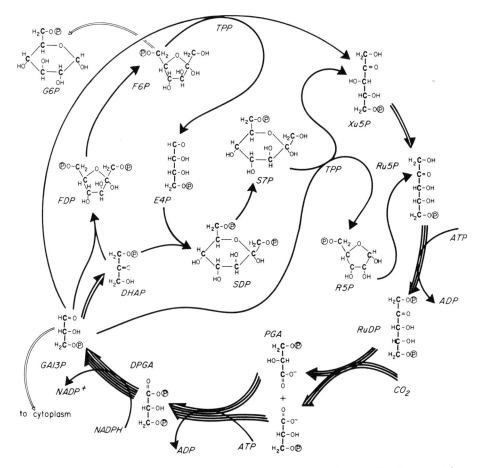

Figure 3. The reductive pentose phosphate cycle. The heavy lines indicate reactions of the RPP cycle; the faint lines indicate removal of intermediate compounds of the cycle for biosynthesis. The number of heavy lines in each arrow equals the number of times that step in the cycle occurs for one complete turn of the cycle, in which three molecules of CO_2 are converted to one molecule of GA13P. Abbreviations: RuDP, ribulose 1,5–diphosphate; PGA, 3-phosphoglycerate; DPGA, 1,3–diphosphoglycerate; NADPH and NADP$^+$, reduced and oxidized nicotinamide-adenine dinucleotide phosphate, respectively; GA13P, 3-phosphoglyceraldehyde; DHAP, dihydroxyacetone phosphate; FDP, fructose 1,6–diphosphate; F6P, fructose 6-phosphate; G6P, glucose 6-phosphate; E4P, erythrose 4-phosphate; SDP, sedoheptulose 1,7–diphosphate; S7P, sedoheptulose 7–phosphate; Xu5P, xylulose 5-phosphate; R5P, ribose 5-phosphate; Ru5P, ribulose 5-phosphate, and TPP, thiamine pyrophosphate.

necessary to continue the RPP cycle. PGA is converted to 1,3
diphosphoglycerate (DPGA) using ATP, and then to 3-phosphogly-
ceraldehyde (GA13P) using the reducing agent NADPH. In the cycle
as shown in Figure 3, three molecules of RuDP are carboxylated
to produce six molecules of PGA and then six molecules of GA13P.
Five molecules of GA13P are converted to three molecules of
ribulose-5-phosphate (Ru5P) by the series of isomerizations, con-
densations and rearrangements shown. The three molecules of Ru5P
are phosphorylated (again using ATP, generated by the light reactions) to regenerate three molecules of RuDP. As only five GA13P
were used to regenerate the three molecules of Ru5P, the cycle's
operation has resulted in a net gain of one molecule of GA13P
for each three CO_2 molecules incorporated. An equation for the
net photosynthetic production of one molecule of GA13P by the
RPP cycle is as follows:

$$3 \ CO_2 + 9 \ ATP^{-4} + 6 \ NADPH + 5H_2O \longrightarrow 1 \ GA13P^{-2} + 8 \ Pi^{-2} + 9 \ ADP^{-3} + 6 \ NADP^+ + 3H^+$$

Formation of sufficient NADPH to carry out the above reaction
required, per mol of CO_2, the transfer of 4 mols of electrons
from H_2O to $NADP^+$ and the liberation of 1 mol of O_2 from the water.
Based upon the scheme shown in Fig. 2, this requires the absorption
of 8 mols of photons per mol of CO_2 (2 steps x 4 e^-) = 8 einsteins
of light.

The extra GA13P molecule produced allows for synthesis of new
plant material. It can be used in the synthesis of starch within
the chloroplast or, following isomerization to dihydroxyacetone
phosphate (DHAP), it can be exported to the cytoplasm. Upon
leaving the chloroplast, the DHAP can be isomerized back to GA13P,
which can then be reoxidized to PGA with concomittant formation
of cytoplasmic reducing power (NADH) and ATP through what is essentially a reversal of the two-step process occurring in the RPP
cycle (Heber, 1974). Transport of GA13P from the chloroplast
therefore can carry reduced carbon, energy in the form of high
energy phosphate bonds, and reducing power, to the rest of the
cell. Other transport mechanisms exist, although carbon seems
to be mainly transported in this way. The exported reduced carbon,
ATP and NADH can be used in the synthesis of energy transport
compounds (such as sucrose) and storage compounds (such as fat),
and also in the synthesis of macromolecular compounds necessary for
plant or cell growth (phospholipids, proteins, cellulose, nucleic
acids, etc.).

Only three reactions of the RPP cycle require cofactors from
the light reactions--the phosphorylation of PGA, the reduction of
DPGA and the phosphorylation of Ru5P. In those steps ATP and NADPH
are used, yielding ADP and $NADP^+$. Continued operation of the RPP
cycle depends on regeneration of ATP and NADPH by the light events

shown in Fig. 2. None of the reactions of the RPP cycle are themselves photochemical steps; but this is not to say that the sole
tie between the light and dark events is the transfer and recycling
of ATP and NADPH. There are numerous regulatory effects of the
light reactions on key enzymes of the RPP cycle including enzymes
which do not directly use ATP or NADPH as cofactors but whose activities are mediated by changes in ion, cofactor, and electron
carrier concentrations (Bassham, 1978). The regulatory interactions essentially provide for levels of operation of the RPP cycle
that are consonant with the level of operation of the light steps
and the withdrawal of reduced carbon compounds for starch and other
macromolecule synthesis inside the chloroplast and export of
reduced carbon to the cytoplasm.

The C4 Cycle

Certain plants growing in areas where sunlight intensity and
temperature are high and water is limited, have evolved an additional carbon dioxide-fixing cycle. That cycle is called the C4
cycle, because the first product of CO_2 incorporation is the four
carbon dicarboxylic acid oxaloacetic acid (OAA).

One version of the C4 cycle of CO_2 incorporation is presented
in Figure 4. The features of this cycle have been recently discussed by Black (1973) and by Chollet and Ogren (1975). In another
version (not shown) OAA is converted into aspartate rather than
malate for transport, but the major features of the cycle remain
unchanged. In the C4 cycle as shown atmospheric CO_2 is first
incorporated into OAA by phosphoenolpyruvate carboxylase in plant
mesophyll cells. These mesophyll cells have little or no RuDP
carboxylase. After transformation into a four-carbon transport
compound, carbon is carried into chloroplasts of the plant bundle
sheath cells (near the leaf vascular system) where CO_2 is released.
The three-carbon material pyruvate, produced upon release of CO_2,
is recycled (Fig. 4). The released CO_2 is fixed by RuDP carboxylase in the bundle sheath cells and reduced by the RPP cycle, which
operates in the chloroplasts of those cells. A key point is that
the C4 cycle results in transport of CO_2 from the atmosphere to
the bundle sheath chloroplasts, and not in CO_2 reduction, which
remains the function of the RPP cycle. The cost of the extra
transport cycle is apparently at least two additional ATP mols per
mol of CO_2 fixed.

The major C4 crop plants are maize, sorghum, and sugar cane.
Most crop plants, including rice, barley, oats, wheat, and soybeans, do not have the C4 pathway, and fall into the C3 class.
The presence of the C4 cycle in a plant seems to increase its
photosynthetic efficiency in air under conditions of high light
intensity and temperature.

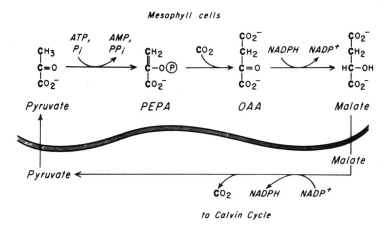

Figure 4.   The C4 cycle of photosynthesis. This is one version
            of the preliminary CO_2 fixing cycle which occurs in
            certain tropical grasses as well as in a scattering of
            other plant species. This cycle by itself does not
            result in any net fixation of CO_2 into organic compounds,
            but rather serves as a vehicle to move CO_2 from cell
            cytoplasm and perhaps outer leaf cells into the chloro-
            plasts of the vascular bundle cells in these plants.
            This CO_2 transport is thought to be responsible for the
            minimization of photorespiration in these cells (see
            text). In some plants, another version (not shown) of
            the C4 cycle is found in which OAA is converted to
            aspartate rather than malate for transport. Abbrevi-
            ations: PEP, phosphoenolpyruvate; OAA, oxaloacetate.

THE EFFICIENCY OF PHOTOSYNTHETIC CARBON REDUCTION

One approach toward increasing plant protein productivity is
to increase photosynthetic efficiency, thereby increasing the
overall yield of plant material. The maximum expected energy efficiency of carbon reduction in green plants is directly predictable
from our knowledge of the detailed mechanism of photosynthesis
(Loomis and Williams, 1963; Loomis et al., 1971; Loomis and Gerakis,
1975; Bassham, 1977). To arrive at a reasonable approximation of
plant photosynthetic efficiency one can consider photosynthesis
to be complete when carbon dioxide has been reduced to the glucose
moiety of starch and cellulose. The formation of 1/6th of a mole
of the glucose moiety (CH_2O) by photosynthesis is represented by
the following net equation:

$$CO_2 + H_2O \rightarrow (CH_2O) + O_2$$

The chemical free energy stored by this reaction is approximately
114 kcal per mol of CO_2 reduced. The corresponding light energy
input is equal to that of 8 einsteins of absorbed light. Light
usable by green plants for photosynthesis (photosynthetically
active radiation, PAR) falls in the range of 400 to 700 nm, making
up only 43% of the total solar radiation reaching the earth's
surface. All the PAR is used as though it were 700-nm light, but
at the earth's surface the energy input in the range 400-700 nm is
equivalent to that of monochromatic light at 575 nm. An einstein
of light of 575 nm wavelength has an energy of 49.74 kcal. The
theoretical maximum energy efficiency for the photosynthetic reduc-
tion of CO_2 using PAR is therefore $\frac{114 \text{ kcal}}{8 \times 49.74} = 0.286$. The
efficiency based on the total available solar radiation is 0.43 x
0.286 = 0.123. That is, if all PAR were absorbed, and used to
reduce CO_2, the efficiency of photosynthesis would be 12.3%. It
has been established that the upper limit of PAR that can actually
be absorbed by the leaf canopy of a land plant when fully developed
(leaf canopy completely covers the ground), is 80% (Loomis and
Williams, 1963; Loomis et al., 1971). Incorporating this factor
we now have a maximum efficiency of 0.123 x 0.8 = 0.0984 for day-
time efficiency in the green cells of leaves. As a final factor,
we must consider that plant cells use up stored energy through
dark respiration. Substantial respiration occurs at night in the
entire plant, and in roots and stems during the day. Mitochondrial
respiration may continue during the day even in green tissue
(Zelitch, 1971; Chapman and Graham, 1974). As a rough estimate,
respiration may reduce agricultural efficiency by a third giving
us an efficiency factor of 0.67. Hence, taking into account all
these factors (0.43 x 0.286 x 0.80 x 0.67 = 0.066) we arrive at
an estimated 6.6% overall maximum daily energy efficiency for
photosynthesis.

We can now calculate the plant growth rate expected, given an energy efficiency of 6.6%, the theoretical maximum. Glucose has a molecular weight of 180, but in cellulose or starch one water molecule (molecular weight 18) is removed per glucose added to the chain. Hence, the molecular weight of carbohydrate added per CO_2 reduced is 162/6 = 27. For each kcal of total solar radiation a maximum of 0.066 kcal of energy can be stored, and this is equivalent to $\frac{0.066}{114}$ = 0.00058 mols of CO_2 reduced to starch or cellulose or 0.00058 x 27 = 0.0157 grams of starch or cellulose.

Table 1 presents data on the incident solar energy in the United States (averaged over 24 hr per day and 365 days per year) and maximum storable energy given optimal conditions of plant growth (including optimal temperature, water, fertilizer, leaf canopy), as calculated on the basis of an efficiency of 6.6%. It also presents data on maximum theoretical dry yields, based on a factor of 0.0157 g cellulose/1 kcal total energy.

Table 1

Incident solar energy, maximum storable energy, and maximum Yields in the U.S.

	Incident Solar Energy kcal/m^2·day	Maximum Storable Solar Energy kcal/m^2·day	Maximum Yield g/m^2·day
Average (annual basis)	3930	259	61
U.S. Southwest (annual basis)	4610	304	72
U.S. Southwest (summer)	6775	447	106

The maximum theoretical yields can be compared to maximum measured plant yields. Table 2 shows the actual measured rates of growth (yields per day) for several selected species, obtained during their time of most rapid growth. Yearly yields are reported as extrapolations of those maximum measured short-term growth rates and are given in parenthesis. (Actual annual yields are reduced from the extrapolated maximum partly because the plants are not grown year round or grow more slowly in the winter).

Table 2

Maximum theoretical photosynthetic productivity and maximum measured
yields of selected plants
(Values given are for total dry matter).[a]

	Growth rates $gm/m^2 \cdot day$	Yields[b] metric tons per hectare·yr	Percent efficiency[c]
Theoretical maxima (Table 1):			
U.S. average, annual basis	61	224	
U.S. Southwest, annual basis	72	263	
U.S. Southwest, summer	106	387	
Maxima measured C4 Plants:			
Sugar Cane	38	(138)	2.4
Sudan Grass (Sorghum)	51	(186)	3.2
Napier Grass	39	(139)	2.4
Corn	52	(190)	3.2
C3 Plants:			
Sugarbeet	31	(113)	1.9
Alfalfa	23	(84)	1.4

[a]Plant data from Alich and Inman, 1973.

[b]Values in parenthesis are calculated from maximum measured daily yields.

[c]Efficiency calculated based on U.S. Southwest, summer light energy conditions.

The extrapolated yearly yields during the maximum growth season for the C4 plants, corn and sorghum, are equivalent to 1/2 the theoretical maximal efficiency of 6.6%, and those for the C3 plants reported are even lower. Clearly, there is room for improvement in the use of available solar energy.

AN ADDITIONAL LIMIT ON PHOTOSYNTHETIC EFFICIENCY: PHOTORESPIRATION

It was noted above that the maximal extrapolated yearly yields and efficiency for the C4 crop species given in Table 2 exceed those for the C3 crop species reported. Several other differences have been noted to exist between C3 and C4 plants, although there are some data suggesting that the separation between C3 and C4 plants may not be as sharp as has been generally believed (Lloyd et al., 1977; Kennedy, 1976; Quebedeaux and Chollet, 1977; Zelitch, 1975c).

1) The CO_2 compensation point is defined as the equilibrium concentration of CO_2 that will be obtained in a closed gas system by a photosynthesizing plant. At the CO_2 compensation point the rate of photosynthetic CO_2 uptake equals the total rate of respiratory CO_2 release and the CO_2 concentration will remain constant. C3 higher plants have CO_2 compensation points (air level oxygen, 25°C) in the range of 30 - 70 ppm CO_2. Under such conditions C4 plants have CO_2 compensation points of from 0-10 ppm (Black, 1973; Moss, 1962; Krenzer et al., 1975). In the absence of oxygen, the CO_2 compensation point of C3 higher plant species drops to approximately that of the C4 species (Zelitch, 1971; Forrester et al., 1966a).

2) Stimulation of the net photosynthetic rate is observed in C3 plants (high illumination, air-level CO_2) when the oxygen level in the surrounding atmosphere is decreased from 21 to 2%, but C4 photosynthesis is essentially unaffected by that change (Zelitch, 1971).

3) An oxygen-stimulated post-illumination CO_2 outburst occurs in C3 plants, but not in C4 plants (Decker, 1955; Forrester et al., 1966ab). The outburst is apparently due to an elevated respiratory rate that is measurable immediately after turning out the light. The rate of respiration soon decays to a lower value.

4) Extrapolation of the curve relating net photosynthesis and CO_2 concentration in C3 plants (air-level oxygen, 25°C) to zero CO_2 results in a large negative value of fixation that is greater than measured dark respiration (Decker, 1957; Jackson and Volk, 1970; Zelitch, 1971). In corn, a C4 plant, the extrapolated value was zero (Hew et al., 1969).

The gas exchange differences, observed between C3 and C4 plants with respect to compensation points, oxygen sensitivity of the net photosynthetic rate, crop growth and photosynthetic rates, CO_2 outburst, and compensation point are attributable at least in part to the existence of a respiration process called photorespiration which occurs rapidly in the light in C3 plants, but not in C4 plants (Zelitch, 1971; Jackson and Volk, 1970). In essence, photorespiration is a process by which some of the carbon dioxide initially fixed by the RPP cycle in C3 plants is lost to the atmosphere through reoxidation to CO_2 (Zelitch, 1975a; Chollet and Ogren, 1975). In that regard, it is the reverse of photosynthesis and to the extent to which it occurs, it reduces the observed photosynthetic rate. Photorespiratory CO_2 losses result from oxidation of substrate produced in the light by photosynthesis; but no photo-steps are involved. Apparently, most of the energy and reducing power liberated by that oxidation are not conserved (unlike the situation of mitchondrial respiration) and the overall process is therefore wasteful. There is substantial evidence that glycolate is the photorespiratory substrate (Jackson and Volk, 1970; Tolbert 1973ab; Zelitch 1975a, 1971; Chollet and Ogren, 1975). Both photorespiration (as measured by gas exchange) and glycolate metabolism (its synthesis and further oxidation) generally appear to be stimulated by O_2 and repressed by very high levels of CO_2. Photosynthesis and plant productivity on the contrary are stimulated by CO_2 and inhibited by oxygen.

There is disagreement in the literature regarding the predominant mechanism of glycolate formation and the predominant mechanism of photorespiratory CO_2 release (Zelitch, 1975ac; Chollet and Ogren, 1975). Evidence has been obtained that glycolate arises from oxidation of the two carbon glycolyl moiety transferred in the trans-ketolase reactions of the RPP cycle (Wilson and Calvin, 1955; Shain and Gibbs, 1971; Bassham and Kirk, 1973) and also by means of the RuDP carboxylase-mediated oxidation of RuDP by O_2 (oxygenase activity) to produce P–glycolate, which is then hydrolyzed to glycolate (Bowes et al., 1971, Chollet and Ogren, 1975). Zelitch (1965) has presented evidence for glycolate synthesis in the light by reactions that are largely separate from those of the RPP cycle. Several contributing mechanisms are of course possible in vivo, although evidence increasingly points to the major role of the RuDP oxgenase mechanism (Krause et al., 1977). After its synthesis, glycolate may be oxidized (at least in part) to photorespiratory CO_2 by two possible pathways. Both involve initial oxidation of glycolate to glyoxylate. One proposed path of CO_2 release is the glycolate pathway sequence glycolate→glyoxylate→glycine→serine + CO_2 (Tolbert, 1973 ab, 1971a). Another proposed path is the direct oxidative decarboxylation of glyoxylate and possibly further oxidation of resultant formate (Zelitch, 1975ac).

Some of the gas exchange differences between C3 and C4 plants may be due in part to competitive inhibition of RuDP carboxylase activity by oxygen (Chollet and Ogren, 1975). A number of authors

(Chollet and Ogren, 1975; Ludwig and Canvin, 1971; Laing et al., 1974; and Ku and Edwards, 1977a) have concluded that about 2/3 of the observed oxygen inhibition of apparent photosynthesis is due to that competitive inhibition and only about 1/3 of it is due to photorespiratory CO_2 release. This is, however, a matter of some controversy (Zelitch, 1975bc; Ogren, 1975).

The absence of significant photorespiratory CO_2 release in C4 species has been attributed to mechanisms which have their origin in the anatomy and metabolism of these plants (Zelitch, 1975ac; Chollet and Ogren, 1975). One proposed mechanism is that the C4 cycle, which operates between the mesophyll and bundle sheath cells, concentrates CO_2 in the bundle sheath cells. The high level of CO_2 at the site of the RuDP carboxylase reaction and the RPP cycle then limits glycolate formation, prevents the occurrence of measurable photorespiration, and reduces the direct inhibition of photosynthesis by O_2. It is also possible that C4 plants can, by means of the C4 cycle, refix any small amounts of photorespiratory CO_2 released in the bundle sheath cells. Refixation would occur in the mesophyll cells before the CO_2 escaped from the leaf.

Data tabulated by Zelitch (1971, 1975abc), obtained by several methods of estimating photorespiration, indicates that photorespiration is equal to a substantial fraction of the net photosynthetic rate in C3 plants and exceeds their rates of dark respiration. Some illustrative data are presented in Table 3.

Table 3

Minimal rates of photorespiration
(Selected values from Zelitch 1971, 1975abc)

Species	Photorespiration (% of net photosynthesis in air)	Ratio of photorespiration to dark respiration
C3: Soybean	42	1.9
Sugar beet	47, 40	8.5, 1.4
Tobacco	25	3.5
C4: Maize	0, 5.7	0 - .15

Lesser values of photorespiration as a percentage of photosynthesis have been estimated by some authors, based upon the characteristics of RuDP carboxylase-oxygenase, and have been confirmed by some photorespiration assays (Chollet and Ogren, 1975; Ogren, 1975; Laing et al., 1974). However, those authors indicate that in the absence of both photorespiration and the associated direct oxygen inhibition of photosynthesis, C3 photosynthesis at air level CO_2 would increase by about 45%-an amount equivalent to what would be expected on the basis of the data in Table 3.

Due to disagreement as to the exact nature of photorespiration and how best to measure it (Chollet and Ogren, 1975; Jackson and Volk, 1970; Ludlow and Jarvis, 1971; Zelitch, 1975b), all estimates of photorespiration seem to be crude indications of the extent to which that process is occurring. Estimates of photorespiration may always be in doubt, because one is attempting to measure it while at least three complex processes are occurring simultaneously: photosynthesis, photorespiration, and perhaps mitochondrial respira ration. However, it does seem reasonable that repression of photorespiration and of any associated direct inhibition of photosynthesis by oxygen, can lead to substantially increased rates of photosynthesis and plant growth for C3 plants. Evidence for such an effect will be presented below.

INCREASING PROTEIN PRODUCTION

Our work on improving the production of protein through photosynthesis consists of two main approaches. One is to examine the possiblity of increasing crop yields through atmospheric manipulation, resulting in a concommitant increase in protein yield. Our experiments have been designed to gain an understanding of the biochemical effects of elevated levels of CO_2 on plant metabolism (Platt et al., 1977a). The second approach is to learn how to regulate the direction of carbon flow during photosynthesis so as to increase protein production relative to the production of other plant constituents. In particular, we have investigated the effects of ammonium ion on amino acid production in leaf tissue (Platt et al., 1977b). Amino acid production is, of course, a necessary prerequisite for increased protein synthesis in plants. While most plant protein currently used directly in human nutrition comes from seeds, we believe that leaf protein may play a major role in human nutrition in the future.

Alfalfa: A Source of Protein for Direct Human Consumption

An effective increase in the efficiency of agricultural protein production occurs when plant protein is directly utilized by human beings instead of first feeding it to animals for meat production. Approximately 40% of the human diet in the United States is presently derived from animals that consume 80% of the feed energy annually harvested from crops. Half of the daily energy intake of beef cattle consists of feed necessary for maintenance without weight gain (Committee on Agricultural Production

Efficiency, 1975). Use of plant material in this way cannot be justified using the argument that animals eat wild grasses (or non-protein nitrogen) not otherwise useful for human consumption. Much of the meat we consume comes, in actuality, from cattle fattened with grain and other concentrates in lieu of roughage (Committee on Agricultural Production Efficiency, 1975). Bowman (1973) has tabulated data (Table 4) showing the efficiency of protein utilization occurring in animal agriculture. The protein lost ranges from 77-97%. Clearly, direct consumption of plant protein by man is preferable on this basis—but which plant and type of plant protein to use?

Leafy plants, such as alfalfa, can be more efficient protein producers than the grain and bean crops, generally thought of as our sources of dietary plant protein. Stahmann (1968) has collected the midwest U.S.D.A. experiment station results presented in Table 5.

Table 4

The efficiency of conversion of feed protein intake
to edible protein in lifetime performance of
farm species
(Bowman, 1973)

Animal	Edible protein/feed protein produced (percent)
Diary herd	23
Diary and beef herd	20
Sheep flock	3
Pig	12
Broiler	20
Egg flock	18
Beef herd	6

Table 5

Crude protein production (Stahmann, 1968)

Crop	Pounds crude protein per acre
Forage:	
Alfalfa	2400
Sorghum-Sudan	2100
Corn	1500
Seed:	
Corn	800
Soybean	700
Wheat	300
Rice	200

Forage crops (crops grown for their total aerial portion) produced 3-10 times more protein per acre than the four major seed crops shown. Alfalfa, an extremely leafy and protein-rich plant, produced more protein per acre than any of the other crops listed, even more than the C4 plant corn. But is that protein nutritionally suitable for direct human consumption? Leaf-protein concentrate (LPC) prepared from many plant species, including alfalfa, contains more lysine than the best high lysine corn, more methionine than soybean protein, and compares well with animal protein with respect to amino acid composition (Stahmann, 1968; Gerloff et al., 1965). The biological value of leaf protein from both enzymatic hydrolysis and rat growth assays (Table 6) is superior to wheat and soy protein, and in fact is superior to beef on this basis (Stahmann, 1968). Limited studies have indicated the value of LPC as a protein-rich supplement in the treatment of human malnutrition (Bickoff et al., 1975; Stahmann, 1968).

Table 6

The biological value of proteins from enzymatic
hydrolysis and rat growth (Stahmann, 1968)

Protein	Enzyme Hydrolysis	Rat Growth
Whole egg	97	96, 97
Whole milk	83	85, 84
Leaf protein concentrate	78 – 89	81 – 86
Beef	75	76
Soybean	65	57, 59 (75, 74)
Wheat flour	50	52

LPC has been advocated as a source of protein for direct
human consumtion for some years; however, major problems seen
in its usage, as generally isolated, have been its poor color
and flavor qualities. Researchers at the Western Regional
Research Center of the United States Department of Agriculture
(G. Kohler and his associates) have therefore directed part
of their research effort toward production of a white and
bland-tasting LPC, useful for blending into customary foods
of people in both developed and developing countries. While
research is still continuing, methods for isolating a white
LPC have been developed through the pilot plant stage (DeFremery
et al., 1973; Edwards et al., 1975). The white LPC contains
approximately 90% protein and should be more acceptable for
human consumption than previous LPCs. The process, as presently
designed, removes a fraction of the total leaf protein, leaving
the residual plant material for use as ruminant feed, an aspect
believed to be necessary at this time to make the process
economically feasible. A major part of the white LPC is ribulose
diphosphate carboxylase (Bickoff et al., 1975). The amino acid
score for human diets of white LPC obtained by the USDA process
is comparable to that of egg, meat, or milk protein and is
much superior to seed proteins. Furthermore, white LPC protein
is 97% digestible (Bickoff et al., 1975). Feeding studies
(mandatory to detect toxic or growth-inhibiting substances) with
rats have shown white LPC to have a protein efficiency ratio that
is equivalent or superior to that of the casein standard (Bickoff,
et al., 1975).

To the extent that alfalfa LPC is utilized for direct consumption by human beings, and the leaf residue used to substitute for grain in animal nutrition, agricultural efficiency will be improved.

Elevated CO_2: A Means of Improving Crop Yield

We noted above that the process of photorespiration appears to limit the photosynthetic rate and productivity of C3 plants, such as alfalfa. In C4 plants, the process of photorespiration (and the associated direct inhibition of photosynthesis by oxygen) may be prevented through biochemical and anatomical provision for concentration of CO_2 at the site of the RPP cycle. With C3 plants a similar physiological end may be attained through use of elevated levels of CO_2 in the plant environment.

Increased levels of CO_2 result in sharply increased photosynthetic rates for C3 plants (Table 7). That these increases are not solely due to repression of photorespiration is shown by the increase in photosynthetic rates observed for C4 species (generally, a smaller percentage than noted for C3 plants).

Table 7

Rate of photosynthesis at ambient and elevated CO_2 levels
(Wittwer, 1974)

Plant	Rate mg dm^{-2} hr^{-1}	
	Ambient CO_2	Elevated CO_2
Corn, sorghum, sugar cane	60 – 75	100
Rice	40 – 75	135
Sunflower	50 – 65	130
Soybean, sugar beet	30 – 40	56
Cotton	40 – 50	100
Tobacco	20 – 25	67
Tomato, lettuce	20 – 25	50

Suppression of photorespiration and glycolate metabolism by high levels of CO_2 has received much support in the literature. Whittingham and Pritchard (1963) reported that glycolate excretion during photosynthesis by Chlorella decreased as the CO_2 level was increased above 0.1%. Wilson and Calvin (1955), working with Scenedesmus, found increased labeled glycolate when the $^{14}CO_2$ level was changed from 1% to 0.003%. Robinson and Gibbs (1974) found that photosynthetic glycolate formation by isolated chloroplasts decreased (albeit not to zero) when bicarbonate concentration was increased. Glycolate synthesis in tobacco tissue was inhibited by 0.5% CO_2 relative to air-level CO_2 (Zelitch and Walker, 1964). Egle and Fock (1967) found that at high levels of CO_2 (0.12%) the CO_2 post-illumination outburst did not occur in liverwort, or in attached bean and sunflower leaves. Inhibition of photosynthesis by oxygen was lessened by increased levels of CO_2 (Jackson and Volk, 1970; Forrester et al., 1966a; Jolliffe and Tregunna, 1968; Ku et al., 1977b). Mahon et al. (1974) found that photorespiration in sunflower leaf discs was high and similar at 115 ppm CO_2 and 400 ppm CO_2, but was inhibited at 967 ppm CO_2.

Increases in photosynthetic rates brought about by elevated CO_2 have generally resulted in substantially increased rates of crop growth and increased yields. For example, the following increases in dry weight yield have been reported at elevated CO_2: lettuce 120%, tomato plants 115%, soybean straw 45%, soybean seed 37% (Zelitch, 1971); total wheat crop 32%, wheat grain 43% (Gifford, 1977), sugar beet, barley and kale about 50% (Ford and Thorne, 1967). Proper environmental conditions must be maintained to allow a crop to take full advantage of elevated levels of CO_2 and grow more rapidly (Hofstra and Hesketh, 1975).

Growth of a legume such as alfalfa with an increased level of CO_2 may have an additional advantage relative to growth of a non-legume crop under this condition. Hardy and Havelka (1975) have found that CO_2 enrichment (to about 0.1% CO_2) during soybean growth results in an approximately 5-fold increase in fixation of nitrogen (nitrogen fixed increased from 75 to 425 kg/hectare) and a significant drop in nitrogen obtained from the soil (decreased from 220 to 85 kg/hectare). Note that the overall nitrogen uptake increased by approximately two-thirds. (Presumably the increase in symbiotic nitrogen fixation occurred because photosynthate supply is a limiting factor in that process.)

What sort of yields and photosynthetic efficiencies could we expect at elevated CO_2? With year-round growth under optimal conditions and CO_2 enrichment a 3- 4% or greater conversion rate might be achievable with alfalfa, equal to the best rates achieved with C4 plants (Table 2). This would be equivalent to a total dry-matter production of 200 or more tons/hectare yr (Table 2). The growth of plants under conditions of elevated CO_2 might be best brought about through the use of protected cultivation (Wittwer, 1974), although enrichment with CO_2 may be feasible with open field conditions (Harper et al., 1973). Protected growth under plastic covers would most easily allow for maintenance of higher-than-normal atmospheric CO_2 concentrations without risking the loss of the additional CO_2. The source for enriching the atmosphere with CO_2 might be the appropriately scrubbed exhaust of fossil fuel power plants. Alternatively, CO_2 available from subterranean gas wells (Wittwer, 1974) could be utilized. Closed-environment growth would allow water recycling and allow farming in regions, such as the American Southwest, which have ample sunlight but little water (Bassham, 1977). Initially, enrichment and "covered" agriculture might be carried out on a small scale, with production of both white alfalfa LPC (for direct human consumption) and residual material (for ruminant consumption) as the goal. Eventually, such a system of plant growth, carried out on a very large scale, could make a contribution to our energy needs through combustion of plant material from which protein has been extracted (Bassham, 1977). Certainly, the engineering and economics of CO_2-enriched, closed-environment systems for increasing alfalfa yield requires additional investigation. Further investigation seems justified in view of the increased overall crop and protein yields, increased nitrogen fixation, potential use of barren areas and energy contribution, made possible by closed system agriculture.

Photosynthesis in Alfalfa at Elevated CO_2

Because of the probable advantages of growing alfalfa at elevated CO_2 (particularly the increased yield and nitrogen fixation) and the potential use of alfalfa leaves as a source of protein for direct human consumption, we have investigated the effect of elevated levels of CO_2 concentration on alfalfa photosynthetic metabolism using $^{14}CO_2$ as a tracer (Platt et al., 1977a). We made use of a recently designed apparatus and set of experimental procedures that allow us to obtain data on the concentrations of numerous labeled metabolites during photosynthesis with $^{14}CO_2$ by whole alfalfa leaflets (Platt et al., 1976; Platt and Bassham, 1977). With this method, the flow of labeled carbon during perturbed steady-state photosynthesis (Bassham, 1973) in whole leaflets can be investigated to a degree that was not previously possible. We have also conducted several experiments in which alfalfa photosynthetic parameters including the CO_2 compensation point and the photosynthetic rate as a function of CO_2 and O_2 concentration were determined.

The basic plan of the steady-state experiment (Bassham, 1971; 1973) is to allow plant material to photosynthesize in the presence of $^{14}CO_2$. The concentration and specific activity of the tracer is held constant throughout the experiment (except in those cases where the substrate concentration is deliberately varied). Samples

of plant material are removed as a function of time and killed.
The plant material is then extracted and labeled compounds analyzed
by two-dimensional paper chromatography. Our procedures have been
described previously (Platt, et al., 1976; Platt and Bassham, 1977).
A typical chromatogram is shown in Fig. 5. The amount of tracer
accumulating in each separated soluble metabolite can be determined
using a Geiger or scintillation counter and is then related to
either chlorophyll content or surface area of the leaflets. The
amount of ^{14}C fixed as insoluble products can be analyzed using
an apparatus that collect the $^{14}CO_2$ produced by combustion of the
tissue residue.

As photosynthesis proceeds, the concentration of labeled
material in some active metabolic pools (such as those of the RPP
cycle) rises until they are saturated with ^{14}C, i.e., until the
^{14}C content of a given metabolite reaches a constant value during
a steady-state photosynthesis experiment. The specific radioactivity of such active metabolic pools is then identical to that of
the incoming $^{14}CO_2$ (neglecting possible contributions from endogenous sources). The amount of radioactivity in those metabolites
is then a direct measure of the amount of material in the pool.
Active pool sizes are calculated by dividing the ^{14}C content of
the metabolite at saturation by the specific radioactivity of the
$^{14}CO_2$. Some metabolites do not reach saturation during a given
experiment, but continue to increase in label content as photosynthesis proceeds. This can occur when a metabolite is an end product
of photosynthetic metabolism or whenever the flow of recently fixed
carbon through a pool is small in relation to the total pool size.
Metabolic pools close to the initial CO_2 fixation step, through
which a rapid flow of recently fixed carbon occurs, tend to reach
saturation before pools more distant from that step. Data prior
to saturation indicate the amount of a metabolite that has arisen
from recently fixed $^{14}CO_2$, rather than the total active pool size.
Such values permit comparison between the overall rate of $^{14}CO_2$
fixation and its flow into individual compounds.

In the perturbed steady-state photosynthesis experiment, once
some early metabolic pools are saturated with label under a given
environmental condition, the system is perturbed by imposing an
environment change which alters the steady state. (An alternative
experimental approach is to study photosynthesis under two conditions, in the presence and absence of some material). Samples are
taken, killed, and analyzed as they were prior to the environmental
change. Changes which are observed in the level of label accumulating in the compounds studied can be used to draw conclusions
about metabolic interrelationships and general plant metabolism
under the two conditions. The data can indicate probable sites of
regulation that allow the leaflet to adjust to the new environmental
condition.

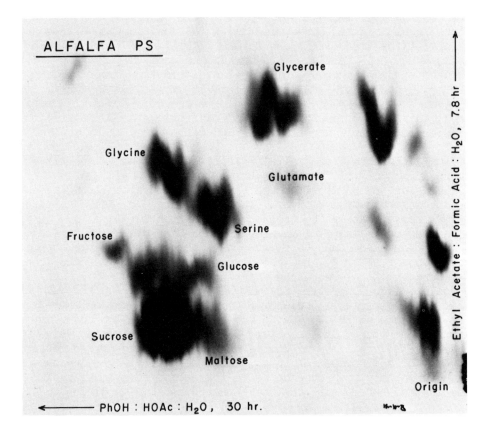

Figure 5.   Radioautograph of two-dimensional paper chromatogram.

In our investigation of alfalfa photosynthesis at an elevated level of carbon dioxide, whole leaflets were exposed to $^{14}CO_2$ using the device shown in Figures 6 and 7 (Platt et al., 1976). The apparatus for the recirculation of gas through the leaflet exposure chamber is visible on the right in Figure 6. The leaflet exposure chamber itself is shown in Figures 6 and 7. The gas flow system has recently been improved by using newly designed push-pull glass valves (Platt et al., 1978). Light of about 40% of the intensity of sunlight is provided by two banks of fluorescent lamps. Instruments continuously measure and record levels of CO_2, O_2, and $^{14}CO_2$. Various regulators and reservoirs allow for manipulation of the contents of the circulating gas stream. Individual samples (each consisting of four leaflets) can be removed from the apparatus without disturbing the remaining leaflets. In the tracer experiments to be presented, leaflets were first exposed to approximately air-level $^{14}CO_2$ followed by a period of elevated $^{14}CO_2$. In Experiment A, this was followed by a period of air-level $^{14}CO_2$ again; the final period of low concentration $^{14}CO_2$ was omitted in Experiment B.

The dependence of the alfalfa leaflet's net photosynthetic rate upon carbon dioxide concentration is presented in Fig. 8. At low levels of carbon dioxide, the rate of photosynthesis increased with increasing carbon dioxide. The photosynthetic rate at saturation was approximately 50% greater than that at air-level CO_2 (0.03% CO_2) and approximately 70% greater than than at 0.026% CO_2. Photosynthesis was also found to be strongly dependent on the atmospheric oxygen content (Fig. 9), the photosynthetic rate increasing as the O_2 concentration was decreased. A photosynthetic rate increase of 50% was obtained upon lowering the oxygen concentration from 21% to 2%. The compensation point (18°C) determined for the leaflets in the presence of 20% O_2 was 49 ppm. The compensation point value was oxygen sensitive and decreased to below 10 ppm in the presence of 5% O_2. The variation of photosynthetic rate with oxygen concentration, the high compensation point of the leaflets at air-level oxygen, and the oxygen dependence of that compensation point are evidence that substantial photorespiration and O_2 inhibition of photosynthesis occur in alfalfa (Chollet and Ogren, 1975; Forrester et al., 1966ab; Zelitch, 1971). This is consistent with the classification of alfalfa as a C3 plant.

The rate of photosynthesis doubled in both tracer experiments when the $^{14}CO_2$ concentration was raised (data shown for Experiment A, Fig. 10). The increase was reflected in the rates of labeling of both soluble and insoluble products with approximately 40% of the total increase accounted for by increased labeling of solubles. The labeled products, separated by paper chromatography were generally similar to those reported in other higher plant species (Tamas & Bidwell, 1970; Jensen and Bassham, 1966; Norris et al., 1955) and included sugar phosphates, sugars, amino acids, and organic acids. Tracer carbon flow from the RPP cycle (Fig. 3) to

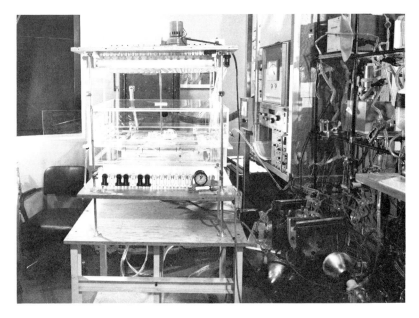

Figure 6. Steady-state leaflet exposure system.

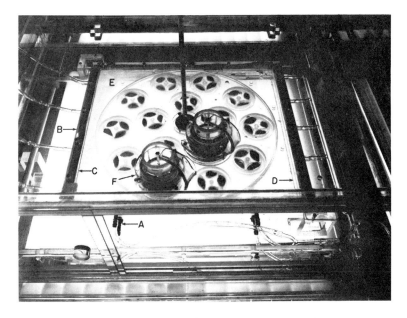

Figure 7. Whole-leaflet exposure device.

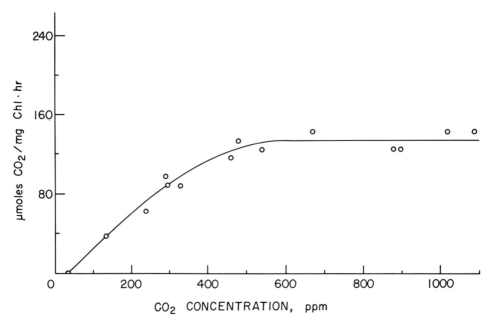

Figure 8.   Photosynthesis in relation to carbon dioxide concen-
             tration. Alfalfa leaflets at 23% O_2 18°C, and 3,600
             ft-c.

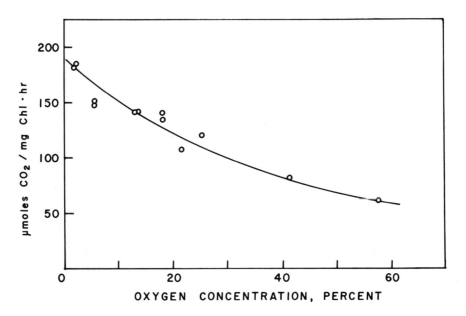

Figure 9.   Alfalfa leaflet photosynthetic rate in relation to O_2
             concentration at 0.035% CO_2, 23°C, and 3,600 ft-c.

other intermediates appeared to be occurring by paths consistent
with the pattern shown in Fig. 11. It must be emphasized that the
paths shown are intended to give only a general picture of major
connections between the RPP cycle and later biosynthetic pathways.
Many details of carbon metabolism are still in doubt.

Sucrose (Fig. 10) was the major soluble product formed. While
its absolute labeling rate increased greatly under elevated $^{14}CO_2$,
there was no major shift in the proportion of carbon flow into
sucrose at elevated $^{14}CO_2$. Sharp increases in relative sucrose
labeling at elevated $^{14}CO_2$ observed in some previous nonkinetic
and shorter term experiments with other plant species (Osmond and
Bjorkman, 1972; Snyder and Tolbert, 1974) may be partly due to
differences in the extent of saturation of sucrose precursors at
high and low CO_2.

Elevated $^{14}CO_2$ concentration brought about an immediate
increase in the rates of labeling of alanine (Fig. 12), malate,
citrate, aspartate, and glutamate (Fig. 13) during experiments A,
and B (data not shown). This suggests that there was an increased
anaplerotic ("filling up") carbon flow into the TCA cycle at
elevated $^{14}CO_2$ available for amino acid production (Fig. 11). This
could be due to stimulation of the carboxylation of phosphoenolpyruvate (PEP) and perhaps also of pyruvate at elevated CO_2. The
increased rate of labeling of alanine suggests an accelerated conversion of PEP to pyruvate, also providing for more rapid acetyl
CoA production.

In experiment A, PGA (Fig. 14) and the sugar mono- and diphosphates (labeling curves similar in shape to that shown for PGA),
reached saturation during the initial period of photosynthesis with
low concentration $^{14}CO_2$, and approximately doubled in steady-state
pool size when the $^{14}CO_2$ concentration was raised. The total
labeling increase observed for the RPP cycle metabolites was 0.9 μg
atoms $^{14}C/mg$ Chl, which is equivalent to less than 1 min of the
additional ^{14}C incorporation occurring with elevated carbon dioxide
(1.3 μg atoms $^{14}C/min \cdot mg$ Chl). During Experiment B, the steady-
state pool sizes of PGA and the other identified RPP cycle
metabolites (sugar mono- and diphosphates) were virtually unchanged
when the $^{14}CO_2$ concentration was raised (data shown only for PGA,
Fig. 15). The RPP metabolite labeling data indicate the precise
regulation of the RPP cycle and of the carbon flow from it.
Absolute steady-state pool sizes of the RPP cycle metabolites PGA
and the sugar mono- and diphosphates were essentially unchanged
during Experiment B, and increased in Experiment A by only a small
amount relative to the additional $^{14}CO_2$ incorporation occurring
at elevated $^{14}CO_2$. This occurred even though $^{14}CO_2$ was clearly
limiting and the photosynthetic rate doubled. Carbon withdrawal
from the RPP cycle for use in leaf metabolism increased almost as
rapidly as did $^{14}CO_2$ influx.

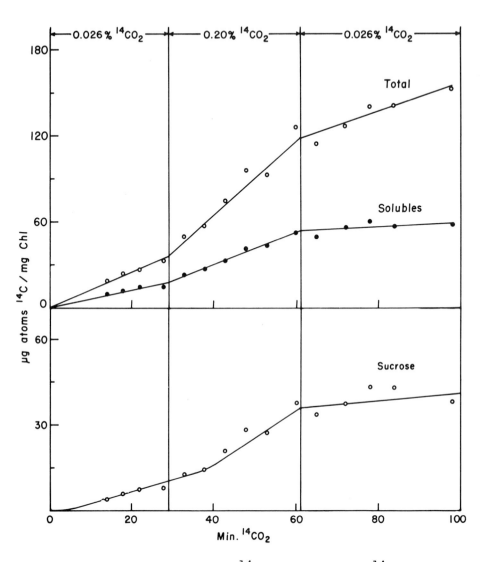

Figure 10.   Total photosynthetic ^{14}C incorporation, ^{14}C incorporation into soluble products, and ^{14}C incorporation into sucrose by alfalfa leaflets exposed to $^{14}CO_2$ in air at 3,600 ft-c. (Experiment A).

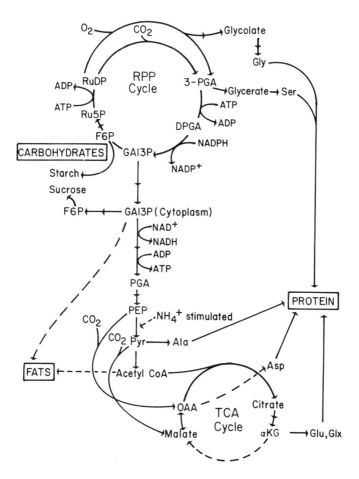

Figure 11. Suggested metabolic paths from the RPP cycle to end
products. Many steps, intermediate compounds, reaction
locations and other details are omitted from this diagram which is intended to give an overall picture of
metabolic connections. Abbreviations: RuDP, ribulose
1,5-diphosphate; 3-PGA, 3-phosphoglycerate; DPGA,
1,3-diphosphoglycerate; $NADP^+$ and NADPH, oxidized and
reduced nicotinamide-adenine dinucleotide phosphate;
GA13P, 3-phosphoglyceraldehyde; F6P, fructose
6-phosphate; Ru5P, ribulose 5-phosphate; Gly, glycine;
Ser, serine; PEP, phosphoenolpyruvate; Pyr, pyruvate;
Ala, alanine; OAA, oxaloacetate; α-KG, alpha-ketogluta-
rate; Asp, aspartate; Glu, glutamate, Glx, glutamine.

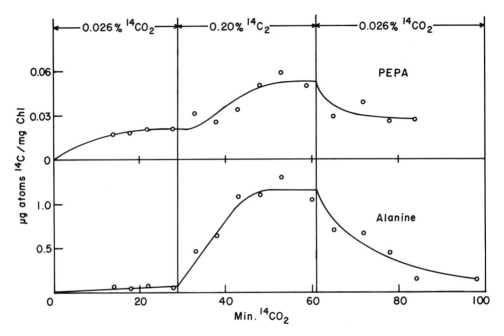

Figure 12.   Labeling of phosphoenolpyruvate (PEPA) and alanine in
             alfalfa leaflets photosynthesizing with $^{14}CO_2$.
             (Experiment A).

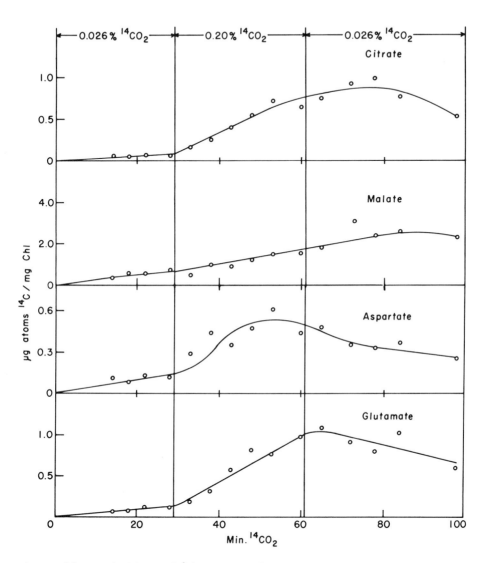

Figure 13.   Labeling of citrate, malate, aspartate, and glutamate in alfalfa leaflets photosynthesizing with $^{14}CO_2$. (Experiment A).

The data obtained in these experiments have led us to draw
some interesting conclusions about glycolate and photorespiratory
metabolism in alfalfa. Formation of glycolate, glycine, and serine
in C3 plants has been often attributed to the glycolate pathway
sequence glycolate→→glycine→serine→glycerate, which is sometimes
equated with the occurrence of photorespiration (Snyder and Tolbert,
1974; Rabson et al., 1962; Tolbert 1971b, 1973ab). However, an
alternative path for synthesis of glycine and serine has been
proposed which does not depend upon glycolate synthesis and any
concomittant photorespiration (Randall et al., 1971). That alternative path consists of the sequence, PGA→glycerate→→serine→glycine
that is initiated by 3-phosphoglycerate phosphatase, an enzyme
present in many plants including alfalfa (Randall et al., 1971).
Evidence has already been obtained for production of glycerate
from PGA during photosynthesis in several species of C3 plants
other than alfalfa (Hess and Tolbert, 1966; Rabson et al., 1962),
although serine in those experiments appeared to be synthesized
predominantly from glycolate. In our experiments, an elevated concentration of $^{14}CO_2$ resulted in decreased levels of label in glycine
and glycolate (Fig. 14 and 15), presumably due to decreased glycolate formation and decreased tracer carbon flow to glycine. In
marked contrast, serine and glycerate steady-state levels during
both experiments reflected the size of the PGA pool (increasing
or remaining constant, as did PGA concentration) and not the label
in glycine and glycolate (Fig. 14 and 15). These results indicate
that glycine is made from glycolate, whereas the predominant production of glycerate and serine is from PGA. Label in serine and
glycerate either increased or remained constant at elevated $^{14}CO_2$
so that ^{14}C flow to those metabolites was apparently not inhibited.

Glycine- and serine- labeling data have often been used in
drawing conclusions about the extent of operation of glycolate
pathway metabolism and photorespiration (Burris et al., 1976;
Snyder and Tolbert 1974; Lee and Whittingham, 1974; Osmond and
Bjorkman, 1972). Aside from the controversy (Zelitch, 1975c)
surrounding identification of the glycine to serine transformation
as the main source of photorespiratory CO_2, conclusions about
photorespiration, drawn on the basis of data on those two amino
acids, can be of only limited value, as shown by our observation
that their labeling may respond quite differently to environmental
perturbation. Information on only the sum of glycine and serine
can be especially misleading, as it may conceal different responses.
Separate data on glycolate, glycine, and serine should be obtained.
Serine labeling should not be taken to be indicative of glycolate
metabolism unless that amino acid has been shown to arise from
glycolate and not from glycerate under all conditions studied.
In fact, our results cast some doubt on the notion that the conversion of glycine to serine is the major source of photorespiratory
CO_2 in alfalfa. The predominant serine production from PGA in
alfalfa, and our evidence for the occurrence of substantial

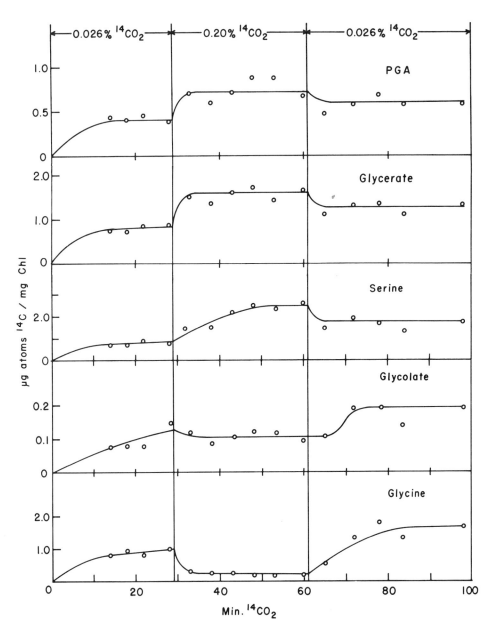

Figure 14.   Labeling of several metabolites in alfalfa leaflets
photosynthesizing with $^{14}CO_2$. (Experiment A).

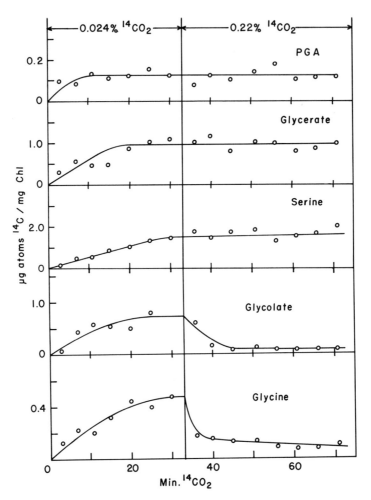

Figure 15.   Labeling of several metabolites in alfalfa leaflets
            photosynthesizing with $^{14}CO_2$ in air at 3,600 ft-c.
            (Experiment B).

photorespiration at least under low $^{14}CO_2$, indicate that alfalfa photorespiratory CO_2 release may occur mainly by mechanisms of glycolate oxidation that do not involve serine formation (Zelitch, 1975c). Alternatively, it is possible that the high compensation point and measured O_2 inhibition of photosynthesis in alfalfa is mainly a result of the competitive inhibition of RuDP carboxylase by oxygen, rather than due to glycolate formation and oxidation.

In summary, increased $^{14}CO_2$ concentration resulted in a doubled rate of photosynthesis. The rate increase was accounted for by increased labeling of both soluble and insoluble products. A large increase in ^{14}C flow through the RPP cycle occurred with only a small absolute increase in the total pool size of RPP cycle intermediates. Sucrose labeling appeared to account for only a slightly larger portion of the overall fixation rate at elevated $^{14}CO_2$. Tracer carbon flow to tricarboxylic acid cycle metabolites and amino acid production increased. In particular, aspartate and glutamate, key precursors of many other amino acids essential for protein synthesis (Miflin and Lea, 1977), were produced at a greater rate at high CO_2. The general conclusion is that alfalfa photosynthetic carbon metabolism is well balanced with increased ^{14}C flow at elevated $^{14}CO_2$ occurring to and through most soluble metabolite pools examined. Only glycolate production and ^{14}C flow along the glycolate pathway to glycine was apparently inhibited at elevated $^{14}CO_2$. Repression of glycolate (and any associated photorespiratory CO_2 release) at elevated $^{14}CO_2$ may have contributed to the observed photosynthetic rate increase. However, much of that increase may be due to decreased O_2 inhibition of photosynthesis at elevated CO_2, and not only repression of photorespiratory CO_2 release. The results of our tracer experiments, and also the experiments with unlabeled CO_2 in which alfalfa photosynthesis was found to be strongly stimulated by high levels of CO_2 and inhibited by O_2, are supportive of the idea that alfalfa protein productivity could be significantly enhanced by an environment of elevated CO_2.

Regulation of Carbon Flow During Photosynthesis: The Ammonia Effect

Products of carbon dioxide fixation by the RPP cycle are ultimately used as precursors for biosynthetic paths leading to the production of carbohydrates, fats, proteins, and other macromolecules (Fig. 11). As the metabolite needs of a green leaf cell change with time, the relative channeling of fixed carbon into those biosynthetic paths must change. For example, in a simplified view, a young expanding cell might channel a large portion of the fixed carbon into production of materials necessary for cell growth; amino acids for use in protein production, fatty acids for use in membrane synthesis, cellulose for cell wall synthesis, and so on. In a green cell in a more mature leaf, the major product may be sucrose for translocation to growing parts of the plant, including new leaf cells, and expanding root and stem systems. Additionally, such

changes could occur on a shorter-term basis due to the diurnal
variation in a plant's environment. Variations in photosynthate
translocation, intermediate-metabolite production, and protein
synthesis have been observed by many researchers (Steer, 1974;
Dickmann and Gordon, 1975; Larson and Gordon, 1969; Loewenberg,
1970). Ultimately, a complete understanding of carbon flow and
its regulation in plants may allow for manipulation of their metabolic processes to cause enhanced production of desired constituents. One might, for example, perhaps increase the production
of hydrocarbon in rubber trees, sugar in sugar beets, or protein
in alfalfa. One way in which increased carbon flow from the photosynthetic cycle to the beginning of a particular biosynthetic
pathway might be accomplished is by allosteric regulation of the
activity of an enzyme at a metabolic crossroad. In vivo, such
a change could be a direct or indirect result of numerous factors,
including nutrient availability, hormonal action, or developmental
state.

   A key element in plant nutrition (particularly with regard to
protein production) is, of course, nitrogen. The initial step of
nitrogen assimilation in higher plants is apparently the incorporation of ammonia into glutamine and then glutamate, with other amino
acids arising by transamination (Lea and Miflin, 1974; Miflin and
Lea, 1976, 1977). The ammonia itself can arise from nitrate reduction or nitrogen fixation. The overall process of nitrate reduction
and ammonia incorporation into amino acids in higher plant leaves
(along with the role of light in that process) has been the subject
of appreciable recent research (Canvin and Atkins, 1974; Lea and
Miflin, 1974; Miflin and Lea, 1976; Beevers and Hageman, 1969;
Magalhaes et al., 1974). Given the production of amino acids as
well as sucrose during photosynthesis (Norris et al., 1955), it
is of interest to determine whether leaf regulatory mechanisms
involve ammonia. The intracellular NH_4^+ level could influence leaf
carbon metabolism during photosynthesis with respect to sucrose
synthesis versus the amino acid synthesis necessary for protein
production and leaf growth. Steer (1974) has noted (in studies of
the diurnal variation of photosynthetic products in Capsicum leaves)
that pyruvate kinase appears to be activated during periods of amino
acid synthesis. Kinetic studies of ^{14}C-labeled compounds formed
in the unicellular green alga Chlorella pyrenoidosa during photosynthesis with $^{14}CO_2$ have indicated that ammonia brings about
increased amino acid synthesis in part due to stimulation of
pyruvate kinase (Kanazawa et al., 1970). In view of our interest
in regulating carbon flow during photosynthesis so as to increase
leaf protein production, we have now investigated the possibility
that a similar regulatory mechanism involving ammonia is active
in leaves of alfalfa (Platt, et al., 1977b). It should be noted
that even nodulated legumes (soybean, field bean, pea, peanuts) in
the field appear to obtain appreciable amounts of nitrogen from the
soil (Hardy and Havelka, 1976, 1975; Cooper et al., 1976). Alfalfa

leaves have the capability of reducing nitrate (Plaut et al., 1976; Eskew et al., 1973) and field-grown, nodulated alfalfa also seems to obtain nitrogen from the soil (Eskew et al., 1973). Hardy and Havelka (1975) have concluded that the major part of the nitrogen in the United States soybean crop may come from fixed nitrogen already in the soil.

In our experiment, techniques of kinetic tracer analysis of steady-state photosynthesis, similar to those described earlier were used. Fixation of labeled carbon dioxide by alfalfa leaf discs in the presence and absence of NH_4Cl was studied. Leaf discs were exposed to carbon dioxide in flasks made from ground-glass joints and having transparent upper and lower surfaces. Each flask was fitted with gas inlet and outlet tubes and a serum stopper (allowing for addition of reagents during experiments). Immediately after being cut, the leaf discs were floated on 4 ml of pH 7.4 phosphate buffer in the disc exposure flasks. The flasks were placed in a temperature-regulated shaking device (previously described for chloroplast experiments (Jensen and Bassham, 1966)) and attached to the closed gas-circulation system (described earlier) through manifolds. After several minutes of preincubation in the dark, the lights were turned on and ammonium chloride in the pH 7.4 buffer was injected into half of the flasks to give a final concentration of 5 mM NH_4Cl. Following photosynthesis with $^{12}CO_2$ for several minutes, the unlabeled carbon dioxide in air was replaced by 0.038% $^{14}CO_2$ in air. Samples of control and ammonium-treated leaf discs were removed and killed at time intervals, and analyzed essentially as described above. Samples were also analyzed for α-ketoacid content as the 2,4-dinitrophenylhydrazone derivatives (Platt et al., 1977b).

The presence of ammonium chloride did not affect the total rate of leaflet photosynthesis, nor the rate of incorporation of ^{14}C into total soluble products, but it did bring about a decrease in sucrose labeling (Fig. 16). Decreased tracer incorporation into sucrose was accompanied by sharply increased labeling of the amino acids glutamate and aspartate (Fig. 17). Glutamine labeling, which was extremely low in the absence of NH_4Cl, was quite high in its presence (Fig. 17). Labeling of other identified amino acids (alanine, glycine, serine) also increased (Fig. 18). Tricarboxylic acid cycle intermediates varied in their response to NH_4^+: Citrate labeling increased, while malate labeling was unchanged (Fig. 19). α-Ketoglutarate (α-KG) labeling decreased, while OAA labeling was unchanged. Neither compound reached saturation with label (Fig. 20). The decline in α-KG labeling (Fig. 20) was substantially less than the increased labeling of glutamate and glutamine (Fig. 17). Uridine diphosphoglucose (UDPG), a precursor of sucrose, increased in labeling in the presence of ammonia (data not shown).

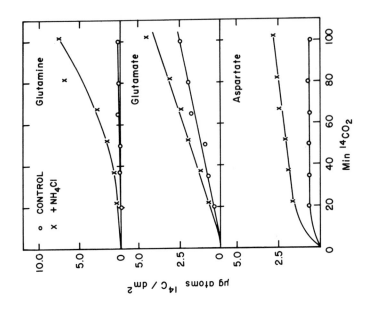

Figure 17. Effect of NH_4^+ on the labeling of glutamine, glutamate, and aspartate in alfalfa leaf discs photosynthesizing with $^{14}CO_2$ under the conditions described in Fig. 16. 0, control; x, 5mM NH_4^+.

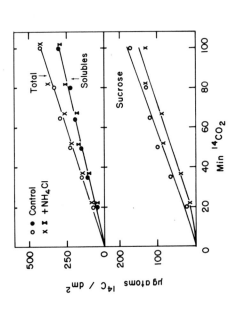

Figure 16. Effect of NH_4^+ on total photosynthetic ^{14}C incorporation, ^{14}C incorporation into solubles, and ^{14}C incorporation into sucrose by alfalfa leaf discs exposed to 0.038% $^{14}CO_2$ in air (20% O_2) at 2400 ft-c. o, ●, control; x, ▮, 5mM NH_4^+.

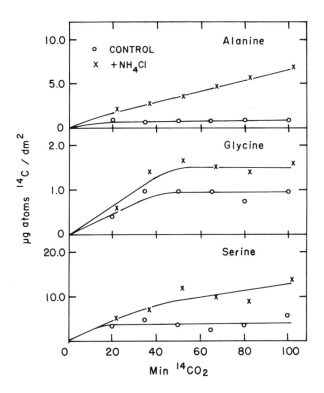

Figure 18. Effect on NH_4^+ on the labeling of alanine, glycine, and
serine in alfalfa leaf discs photosynthesizing with
$^{14}CO_2$ under the conditions described in Fig. 16. o,
control; x, 5mM NH_4^+.

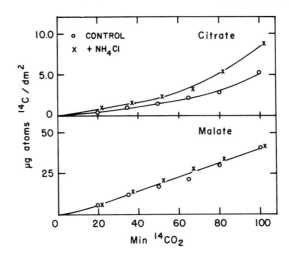

Figure 19.   Effect of NH_4^+ on the labeling of malate and citrate
in alfalfa leaf discs photosynthesizing with $^{14}CO_2$
under the conditions described in Figure 16. o, control;
x, 5 mM NH_4^+.

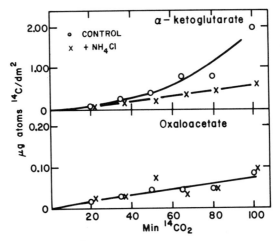

Figure 20.   Effect of NH_4^+ on the labeling of α-ketoglutarate and
oxaloacetate in alfalfa leaf discs photosynthesizing
with $^{14}CO_2$ under the conditions described in Figure 16.
o, control; x, 5mM NH_4^+.

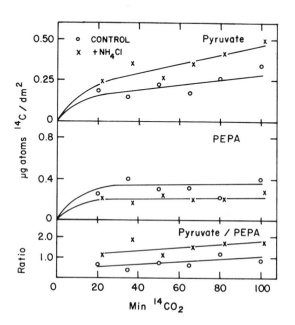

Figure 21. Effect of NH_4^+ on the labeling of pyruvate, phosphoenolpyruvate and the ratio of labeled pyruvate to phosphoenolpyruvate in alfalfa leaf discs photosynthesizing
with $^{14}CO_2$ under the conditions described in Fig. 16. o,
control; x 5mM NH_4^+.

Differences between the two experimental conditions in the levels of pyruvate and phosphoenolpyruvate (PEP) were of particular interest, because of the position of these metabolites between the RPP cycle and probable pathways of carbon utilization, particularly those of amino acid synthesis (Fig. 11). The conversion of PEP (and ADP) to pyruvate (and ATP) is presumably mediated by pyruvate kinase. Pyruvate labeling increased, while the steady-state level of PEP decreased, when the discs were exposed to NH_4Cl (Fig. 21). The ratio of pyruvate to PEP doubled (Fig. 21).

In the presence of NH_4^+, active steady-state pool sizes of several metabolites, including glycolate, phosphoglyceric acid, and the total sugar diphosphates, were unchanged from the control values, while the total steady-state pool size of the sugar monophosphates was slightly lower than the control value (data not shown).

It might be expected that greater intracellular ammonia would result in increased amino acid synthesis for a brief period of time, due to a greater availability of substrate ammonia for incorporation into amino acids. However, for increased amino acid synthesis to proceed for an extended period without a comparable decrease in the level of amino acid precursors (the α-ketoacids), it is necessary that an increase occur in the rate of flow of carbon through rate-limiting steps controlling the production of those ketoacids. Our data show that this happened upon addition of ammonia to the photosynthesizing leaf discs; i.e., ammonia acted not only as a substrate but also as a regulator of carbon flow.

Greatly increased alanine labeling (Fig. 18) in the presence of NH_4^+ required more utilization of pyruvate, the α-ketoacid from which it is presumably synthesized by transamination (Heber, 1974; Kirk and Leech, 1972). α-KG, the carbon skeleton for glutamate and glutamine, is made by anaplerotic reactions of the TCA cycle. Increased synthesis of α-KG requires both increased OAA from C3 carboxylation, and acetyl CoA from pyruvate oxidation (Fig. 11). Increased synthesis of glutamate and glutamine (Fig. 17) in the absence of a comparable decline in α-KG (Fig. 20), as well as increased citrate synthesis (Fig. 19), therefore also required more utilization of pyruvate (Fig. 11). If greater labeling of alanine, glutamate and glutamine was solely due to increased availability of ammonia for incorporation, the level of pyruvate would have decreased. In fact, pyruvate labeling increased, even though the steady-state level of its precursor PEP was lower (Fig. 21). Our observation of increased pyruvate level and decreased PEP pool size in the presence of ammonia is therefore a clear indication of activation of pyruvate kinase.

Alternative pathways from PEP to pyruvate are conceivable: e.g., through reactions meadiated by PEP carboxylase, malic

dehydrogenase, and malic enzyme. The malate labeling curve
(Fig. 19) was differently shaped from those of PEP and pyruvate
(Fig. 21), and the rate of malate labeling was unchanged by the
presence of NH_4^+. Malate thus seems unlikely as an intermediate
between PEP and pyruvate. Activation of pyruvate kinase, an enzyme
widely recognized to be of importance in metabolic regulation
(Duggleby and Dennis, 1973; Seubert and Schoner, 1971), is the
simplest conclusion consistent with our data.

While nitrate reduction occurs in the cytoplasm, nitrite
reduction and concommitant ammonia formation and incorporation
in leaves seemingly occur in the chloroplast (Lea and Miflin, 1974;
Miflin and Lea, 1977; Mitchell and Stocking, 1975). Ammonia
apparently can penetrate the chloroplast membrane to some extent
(Mitchell and Stocking, 1975). Regulation by means of ammonia
requires an interaction with pyruvate kinase and possibly other
enzymes producing amino acid carbon skeletons. Those enzymes are
located mainly outside the chloroplast (Heber, 1974; Kirk and
Leech, 1972; Mitchell and Stocking, 1975). Direct activation of
pyruvate kinase in higher plants by ammonia is supported by work
with the partially purified enzyme. NH_4^+ stimulates pea- and
cotton-seed as well as carrot pyruvate kinase (Tomlinson and Turner,
1973; Miller and Evans, 1957). However, the effect of NH_4^+ may be
indirect. For example, it may affect pyruvate kinase through
changes in ATP and ADP levels (Kanazawa et al., 1972). It is
unlikely that the direct effector is either glutamate or glutamine.
Those two amino acids have been found not to affect the activity
of the partially purified higher plant enzyme (Duggleby and Dennis,
1973; Nakayama et al., 1976). In Chorella, where pyruvate kinase
was also concluded to be activated in the presence of ammonia, more
immediate labeling changes occurred in pyruvate and PEP than in
glutamate and glutamine when ammonia was added (Kanazawa et al.,
1970). In additional alfalfa experiments similar to that just
described (but conducted at low O_2 pressure) our group has found
that exogenously supplied NO_3^- as well as NH_4^+ resulted in activation of pyruvate kinase and increased amino acid formation during
photosynthesis with $^{14}CO_2$ in alfalfa leaf discs (Plaut et al.,
1976). That activation is most simply interpreted as being a result
of an increase in ammonia availability resulting from nitrate reduction followed by nitrite reduction. Future investigations on
isolated green-leaf pyruvate kinase should help to reveal the exact
mechanism of ammonia stimulation of that enzyme.

Increased labeling of glutamate, glutamine, aspartate (Fig.
17), and citrate (Fig. 19) in the presence of NH_4^+ suggests that
oxaloacetate was formed and utilized at an increased rate and that
a stimulation of anaplerotic carbon flow had occurred (Fig. 11).
Malic enzyme may have been simply responding to the increased level
of its substrate pyruvate. It is possible that PEP carboxylase or
malic enzyme was also activated by NH_4^+.

The absence of major change in alfalfa steady-state levels of RPP cycle intermediates, when the discs were supplied with NH_4Cl-containing buffer, indicates that the reactions of the photosynthetic cycle were well regulated. Increased carbon withdrawal to yield amino acids (Figs. 17 and 18) was compensated for by the decreased rate of carbon withdrawal to form sucrose (Fig. 16).

Condensation of fructose-6-phosphate and UDPG is possibly the major path of sucrose synthesis in leaves (Zelitch, 1971). The decrease in sucrose labeling (Fig. 16), in the presence of an increased level of UDPG, suggests an inhibition by NH_4^+ of sucrose phosphate synthetase, the enzyme which catalyzes the rate limiting step in sucrose synthesis. The same reaction was apparently inhibited by ammonia in algae (Kanazawa et al., 1970). However, in alfalfa (in contrast to the situation in algae) the production of sucrose did not completely cease, but only declined when NH_4^+ was supplied. Hence, it appears that in higher plants a balance is maintained between amino acid synthesis and sucrose synthesis, and one process is not completely inhibited to provide for greater operation of the other. Thus, the continuing need for sucrose export from leaves to nonphotosynthetic tissue and developing cells in higher plants is satisfied.

Our data support an in vivo regulatory role for the ammonia effect on amino acid synthesis in leaves. We have observed that increased labeling of amino acids formed by numerous metabolic paths (Figs. 11, 17, 18) occurred in the presence of NH_4^+. Such regulation by ammonia may be an important aspect of the control of leaf protein synthesis.

CONCLUDING REMARKS

We have discussed the nature of the photosynthetic carbon reduction process and its efficiency. We have also discussed two approaches toward increasing protein production: Firstly, increasing photosynthetic efficiency through growth of protein-rich alfalfa at elevated CO_2 is perhaps ready for small-scale field tests now. Secondly, the channeling of photosynthate flow into the most desirable biosynthetic pathways (in particular, the effect of ammonia on amino acid synthesis) is still in an early stage of investigation; more research is necessary in order to understand fully the natural means of regulating carbon metabolism.

ACKNOWLEDGMENTS

We are grateful to B. Platt and L. Rand for assistance in manuscript preparation. We thank E. Heftmann for reviewing our manuscript and M. Friedman for inviting us to contribute to this volume.

REFERENCES

Alich, J. R., Jr. and Inman, R. E. (1973). 'Effective utilization of solar energy to produce clean fuel.' National Science Foundation RANN report under grant GI 38723.

Bassham, J. A. (1971). The control of photosynthetic carbon metabolism. Science, 172, 526-534.

Bassham, J. A. (1973). Control of photosynthetic carbon metabolism. In, 'Symposium of the Society for Experimental Biology 27, Rate Control of Biological Processes'. University Press, Cambridge.

Bassham, J. A. (1977). Increasing crop productivity through more controlled photosynthesis. Science, 197, 630-638.

Bassham, J. A. (1978). The reductive pentose phosphate cycle and its regulation. In, Encyclopedia of Plant Physiology, New Series. Photosynthesis II. Regulation of Photosynthetic Carbon Metabolism and Related processes; M. Gibbs and E. Latzko (Editors). Springer Verlag, Berlin.

Bassham, J. A. and Calvin, M. (1957). 'The Path of Carbon in Photosynthesis.' Prentice-Hall, Englewood Cliffs, N.J.

Bassham, J. A. and Kirk, M. (1973). Sequence of formation of phosphoglycolate and glycolate in photosynthesizing Chlorella pyrenoidosa. Plant Physiol., 52, 407-411.

Bassham, J. A. and Krause, G. H. (1969). Free energy changes and metabolic regulation in steady-state photosynthetic carbon reduction. Biochem. Biophys. Acta., 189, 207-221.

Beevers, L. and Hageman, R. H. (1969). Nitrate reduction in higher plants. Annu. Rev. Plant Physiol., 20, 495-522.

Bickoff, E. M., Booth, A. N., de Fremery, D., Edwards, R. H., Knuckles, B. E., Miller, R. E., Saunders, R. M. and Kohler, G. O. (1975). Nutritional evaluation of alfalfa leaf protein concentrate. In, 'Protein Nutritional Quality of Foods and Feeds', M. Friedman (Editor). Marcel Dekker, New York.

Black, C. C. (1973). Photosynthetic carbon fixation in relation to net CO_2 uptake. Annu. Rev. Plant Physiol., 24, 253-286.

Bowes, G., Ogren, W. L., and Hageman, R. H. (1971). Phosphoglycolate production catalyzed by ribulose diphosphate carboxylase. Biochem. Biophys. Res. Commun., 45, 716-722.

Bowman, J. C. (1973). Possibilities for changing by genetic means the biological efficiency of protein production by whole animals. In, 'The Biological Efficiency of Protein Production,' J. G. W. Jones (Editor). Cambridge University Press, London.

Brown, A. W. A., Byerly, T. C., Gibbs, M. and San Pietro, A. (Editors). (1975). 'Crop Productivity-Research Imperatives.' Michigan Agricultural Experiment Station, East Lansing, MI.

Burris, R. H. and Black, C. C. (Editors). (1976). 'CO_2 Metabolism and Plant Productivity.' University Park Press, Baltimore, MD.

Burris, J. E., Holm-Hansen, O. and Black, C. C. (1976). Glycine and serine production in marine plants as a measure of photorespiration. Aust. J. Plant Physiol., 3, 87-92.

Canvin, D. T. and Atkins, C. A. (1974). Nitrate, nitrite, and ammonia assimilation by leaves: effect of light, carbon dioxide and oxygen. Planta, 116, 207-224.

Chapman, E. A. and Graham, D. (1974). The effect of light on the tricarboxylic acid cycle in green leaves. Plant Physiol., 53, 879-885.

Chollett, R. and Ogren, W. L. (1975). Regulation of photorespiration in C3 and C4 species. Bot. Rev., 41, 137-179.

Committee on Agricultural Production Efficiency. (1975). 'Agricultural Production Efficiency.' Board on Agriculture and Renewable Resources, Commission on Natural Resources, National Research Council. National Academy of Sciences, Washington, D. C.

Cooper, D. R., Hill-Cottingham, D. G. and Lloyd-Jones, C. P. (1976). Absorption and redistribution of nitrogen during growth and development of field bean, Vicia faba. Physiol. Plant, 38, 313-318.

Cooper, J. P. (Editor). (1975). 'Photosynthesis and Productivity in Different Environments.' Cambridge University Press, Cambridge.

Decker, J. P. (1955). A rapid, postillumination deceleration of respiration in green leaves. Plant Physiol., 30, 82-84.

Decker, J. P. (1957). Further evidence of increased carbon dioxide production accompanying photosynthesis. J. Sol. Energy Sci. Eng., 1, 30-33.

deFremery, D., Miller, R. E., Edwards, R. H., Knuckles, B. E., Bickoff, E. M. and Kohler, G. O. (1973). Centrifugal separation of white and green protein fractions from alfalfa juice following controlled heating. J. Agric. Food Chem., 21, 886-889.

Dickmann, D. I. and Gordon, J. C. (1975). Incorporation of ^{14}C - photosynthate into protein during leaf development in young populus plants. Plant Physiol. 56, 23-27.

Duggleby, R. G. and Dennis, D. T. (1973). The characterization and regulatory properties of pyruvate kinase from cotton seeds. Arch. Biochem. Biophys., 155, 270-277.

Edwards, R. H., Miller, R. E., de Fremery, D., Knuckles, B. E., Bickoff, E. M. and Kohler, G. O. (1975). Pilot plant production of an edible white fraction leaf protein concentrate from alfalfa. J. Agric. Food Chem., 23, 620-626.

Egle, K. and Fock, H. (1967). Light respiration - correlations between CO_2 fixation, O_2 pressure and glycolate concentration. In, 'The Biochemistry of Chloroplasts', T. W. Goodwin (Editor). Academic Press, New York.

Eskew, D. L., Schrader, L. E. and Bingham, E. T. (1973). Seasonal patterns of nitrate reductase activity and nitrate concentration of two alfalfa (Medicago sativa L.) cultivars. Crop Science, 13, 594-597.

Ford, M. A. and Thorne, G. N. (1967). Effect of CO_2 concentration on growth of sugar-beet, barley, kale and maize. Annals of Bot., 31. 629-644.

Forrester, M. L., Krotkov, G. and Nelson, C. D. (1966a). Effect of oxygen on photosynthesis, photorespiration and respiration in detached leaves. I. Soybean. Plant Physiol., 41, 422-427.

Forrester, M. L., Krotkov, G. and Nelson, C. D. (1966b). Effect of oxygen on photosynthesis, photorespiration and respiration in detached leaves. II. Corn and other monocotyledons. Plant Physiol., 41, 428-431.

Gerloff, E. D., Lima, I. H. and Stahmann, M. A. (1965). Amino acid composition of leaf protein concentrates. J. Agric. Food Chem., 13, 139-143.

Gifford, R. M. (1977). Growth pattern, carbon dioxide exchange and dry weight distribution in wheat growing under differing photosynthetic environments. Aust. J. Plant Physiol., 4, 99-110.

Hardy, R. W. F. and Havelka, U. D. (1975). Nitrogen fixation research: A key to world food? Science, 188, 633-643.

Hardy, R. W. F. and Havelka, U. D. (1976). Photosynthate as a major factor limiting nitrogen fixation by field-grown legumes with emphasis on soybeans. In, 'Symbiotic Nitrogen Fixation in Plants', P. S. Nutman (Editor). Cambridge University Press, Cambridge.

Harper, L. A., Baker, D. N., Box, J. E. and Hesketh, J. D. (1973). Carbon dioxide and the photosynthesis of field crops. A metered carbon dioxide release in cotton under field conditions. Agron. J., 65, 7-11.

Heber, U. (1974). Metabolite exchange between chloroplasts and cytoplasm. Annu. Rev. Plant Physiol., 25, 393-421.

Hess, J. L. and Tolbert, N. E. (1966). Glycolate, glycine, serine, and glycerate formation during photosynthesis by tobacco leaves. J. Biol. Chem., 241, 5705-5711.

Hew, C. S., Krotkov, G. and Canvin, D. T. (1969). Determination of the CO_2 evolution by green leaves in light. Plant Physiol., 44, 662-670.

Hofstra, G. and Hesketh, J. D. (1975). The effects of temperature and CO_2 enrichment on photosynthesis in soybean. In, Marcelle, R. (1975).

Jackson, W. A. and Volk, R. J. (1970). Photorespiration. Annu. Rev. Plant Physiol., 12, 385-432.

Jensen, R. G., and Bassham, J. A. (1966). Photosynthesis by isolated chloroplasts. Proc. Nat. Acad. Sci. U.S.A., 56, 1095-1101.

Jollife, P. A. and Tregunna, E. B. (1968). Effect of temperature, CO_2 concentration, and light intensity on oxygen inhibition of photosynthesis in wheat leaves. Plant Physiol., 43, 902-906.

Kanazawa, T., Kirk, M. R. and Bassham, J. A. (1970). Regulatory effects of ammonia on carbon metabolism in photosynthesizing Chlorella pyrenoidosa. Biochim. Biophys. Acta., 205, 401-408.

Kanazawa, T., Kanazawa, K., Kirk, M. R., and Bassham, J. A. (1972).
    Regulatory effects of ammonia on carbon metabolism in Chlorella
    pyrenoidosa during photosynthesis and respiration. Biochim.
    Biophys. Acta., 256, 656–669.
Kennedy, R. A. (1976). Photorespiration in C3 and C4 tissue cul-
    tures. Significance of Kranz anatomy to low photorespiration
    in C4 plants. Plant Physiol. 58, 573–578.
Kirk, P. R. and Leech, R. M. (1972). Amino acid biosynthesis by
    isolated chloroplasts during photosynthesis. Plant Physiol.,
    50, 228–234.
Krause, G. H., Thorne, S. W. and Lorimer, G. H. (1977). Glycolate
    synthesis by intact chloroplasts. Studies with inhibitors of
    photophosphorylation. Arch. Biochem. Biophys., 183, 471–479.
Krenzer, E. G., Moss, D. N. and Crookston, R. K. (1975). Carbon
    dioxide compensation points of flowering plants. Plant
    Physiol., 56, 194–206.
Ku, S.-B. and Edwards, G. E. (1977a). Oxygen inhibition of photo-
    synthesis. Plant Physiol., 59, 991–999.
Ku, S.-B. Edwards, G. E. and Tanner, C. B. (1977b). Effects of
    light, carbon dioxide, and temperature on photosynthesis,
    oxygen inhibition of photosynthesis and transpiration in
    Solanum tuberosum. Plant Physiol., 59, 868–872.
Laing, W. A. Ogren, W. L., and Hageman, R. H. (1974). Regulation
    of soybean net photosynthetic CO_2 fixation by the interaction
    of CO_2, O_2, and ribulose 1,5-diphosphate carboxylase. Plant
    Physiol., 54, 678–685.
Larson, P. R. and Gordon, J. C. (1969). Leaf development, photosyn-
    thesis, ^{14}C-distribution in Populus deltoides seedlings.
    Amer. J. Bot., 56, 1058–1066.
Lea, P. J. and Miflin, B. J. (1974). Alternative route for nitrogen
    assimilation in higher plants. Nature, 251, 614–616.
Lee, R. B. and Whittingham, C. P. (1974). The influence of partial
    pressure of carbon dioxide upon carbon metabolism in the tomato
    leaf. J. Exp. Bot., 25, 277–287.
Lloyd, N.D.H., Canvin, D. T. and Culver, D. A. (1977). Photosyn-
    thesis and photorespiration in algae. Plant Physiol., 59,
    936–940.
Loewenberg, J. R. (1970). Protein synthesis in Xanthium leaf
    development. Plant and Cell Physiol., 11, 361–365.
Loomis, R. S. and Gerakis, P. A. (1975). Productivity of agricul-
    tural ecosystems. In, Cooper, J. P. (Editor). (1975).
Loomis, R. S. and Williams, W. A. (1963). Maximum crop producti-
    vity: An estimate. Crop Sci., 3, 67–72.
Loomis, R. S., Williams, W. A. and Hall, A. E. (1971). Agricultural
    productivity. Annu. Rev. Plant Physiol., 22, 431–68.
Ludlow, M. M. and Jarvis, P. G. (1971). Methods for measuring
    photorespiration in leaves. In, 'Plant Photosynthetic Produc-
    tion Manual of Methods,' Z. Sestak, J. Catsky, and P. G. Jarvis
    (Editors). Dr. W. Junk, The Hague.

Ludwig, L. J. and Canvin, D. T. (1971). The rate of photorespiration during photosynthesis and the relationship of the substrate of light respiration to the products of photosynthesis in sunflower leaves. Plant Physiol., 48, 712-719.

Magalhaes, A. C., Neyra, C. A. and Hageman, R. H. (1974). Nitrite assimilation and amino nitrogen synthesis in isolated spinach chloroplasts. Plant Physiol., 53, 411-415.

Mahon, J. D., Fock, H. and Canvin, D. T. (1974). Changes in specific radioactivity of sunflower leaf metabolites during photosynthesis in $^{14}CO_2$ and $^{12}CO_2$ at three concentrations of CO_2. Planta, 120, 245-254.

Marcelle, R. (Editor). (1975). 'Environmental and Biological Control of Photosynthesis'. Dr. W. Junk, The Hague.

Miflin, B. J. and Lea, P. J. (1976). The pathway of nitrogen assimilation in plants. Phytochemistry, 15, 873-885.

Miflin, B. J. and Lea, P. J. (1977). Amino acid metabolism. Annu. Rev. Plant Physiol., 28, 299-329.

Miller, G. and Evans, H. J. (1957). The influence of salts on pyruvate kinase from tissue of higher plants. Plant Physiol., 32, 346-354.

Mitchell, C. A. and Stocking, C. R. (1975). Kinetics and energetics of light-driven chloroplast glutamine synthesis. Plant Physiol., 55, 59-63.

Moss, D. N. (1962). the limiting carbon dioxide concentration for photosynthesis. Nature, 193, 587.

Nakayama, H., Fujii, M. and Miura, K. (1976). Partial purification and some regulatory properties of pyruvate kinase from germinating castor bean endosperm. Plant and Cell Physiol., 17, 653-660.

Norris, L., Norris, R. E. and Calvin, M. (1955). A survey of the rates and products of short-term photosynthesis in plants of nine phyla. J. Exp. Bot., 6, 64-74.

Ogren, W. L. (1975). Control of photorespiration in soybean and maize. In, Marcelle, R. (1975).

Osmond, C. B. and Bjorkman, O. (1972). Simultaneous measurements of oxygen effects on net photosynthesis and glycolate metabolism in C3 and C4 species of Atriplex. Carnegie Inst. Washington Yearbook, 71, 141-148.

Platt, S. G. and Bassham, J. A. (1977). Separation of ^{14}C-labeled glycolate pathway metabolites from higher plant photosynthate. J. Chromatog., 133, 396-401.

Platt, S. G., Plaut, Z. and Bassham, J. A. (1976). Analysis of steady-state photosynthesis in alfalfa leaves. Plant Physiol., 57, 69-73.

Platt, S. G., Plaut,Z. and Bassham, J. A. (1977a). Steady state photosynthesis in alfalfa leaflets: Effects of carbon dioxide concentration. Plant Physiol., 60, 230-234.

Platt, S. G., Plaut, Z. and Bassham, J. A. (1977b). Ammonia regulation of carbon metabolism in photosynthesizing leaf discs. Plant Physiol., 60, 739-742.

Platt, S. G., Erwin, W. and DeGroot, C. W. (1978). Simple push-pull glass valves. J. Chem. Ed., in press.

Plaut, Z., Platt, S. G. and Bassham, J. A. (1976). Nitrate and ammonium regulation of carbon metabolism in photosynthesizing alfalfa leaf discs. Plant Physiol., 57, S-58.

Quebedeaux, B. and Chollet, R. (1977). Comparative growth analyses of Panicum Species with differing rates of photorespiration. Plant Physiol., 59, 42-44.

Rabson, R., Tolbert, N. E. and Kearney, P. C. (1962). Formation of serine and glyceric acid by the glycolate pathway. Arch. Biochem. Biophys., 98, 154-163.

Randall, D. D., Tolbert, N. E. and Gremel, D. (1971). 3-Phospho-glycerate phosphatase in plants. II. Distribution, physiological considerations, and comparison with P-glycolate phosphatase. Plant Physiol., 48, 480-487.

Robinson, J. M. and Gibbs, M. (1974). Photosynthetic intermediates, the Warburg effect, and glycolate synthesis in isolated spinach chloroplasts. Plant Physiol., 53, 790-797.

Seubert, W. and Schoner, W. (1971). The regulation of pyruvate kinase In, 'Current Topics in Cellular Regulation, Volume 3,' B. L. Horecker and E. A. Stadtman (Editors). Academic Press, New York.

Shain, Y. and Gibbs, M. (1971). Formation of glycolate by a reconstituted spinach chloroplast preparation. Plant Physiol., 48, 325-330.

Snyder, F. W. and Tolbert, N. E. (1974). Effect of CO_2 concentration on glycine and serine formation during photorespiration. Plant Physiol., 53, 514-515.

Stahmann, M. A. (1968). The potential for protein production from green plants. Econ. Bot., 22, 73-79.

Steer, B. T. (1974). Control of diurnal variations in photosynthetic products. Plant Physiol., 54, 758-761.

Tamas, I. A. and Bidwell, R. G. S. (1970). $^{14}CO_2$ fixation in leaf discs of Phaseolus vulgaris. Can. J. Bot., 48, 1259-1263.

Tolbert, N. E. (1971a). Leaf peroxisomes and photosynthesis. In, 'Photosynthesis and Photorespiration', M. D. Hatch, C. B. Osmond and R. O. Slayter, (Editors). Wiley-Interscience, New York.

Tolbert, N. E. (1971b). Microbodies-peroxisomes and glyoxysomes. Annu. Rev. Plant Physiol., 22, 45-74.

Tolbert, N. E. (1973a). Compartmentation and control in microbodies. In: 'Symposia of the Society for Experimental Biology 27, Rate Control of Biological Processes'. University Press, Cambridge.

Tolbert, N. E. (1973b). Glycolate biosynthesis. In: 'Current Topics in Cellular Regulation, Volume 7, B. L. Horecker and E. A. Stadtman (Editors). Academic Press, New York.

Tomlinson, J. D. and Turner, J. F. (1973). Pyruvate kinase of higher plants. Biochem. Biophys. Acta, 329, 128-139.

Whittingham, C. P. and Pritchard, G. G. (1963). The production of
    glycolate during photosynthesis in Chlorella. Proc. R. Soc.
    London B, 157, 366-380.
Wilson, A. T. and Calvin, M. (1955). The photosynthetic cycle.
    CO_2 dependent transients. J. Amer. Chem. Soc., 77, 5948-5957.
Wittwer, S. H. (1974). Maximum production capacity of food crops.
    Bioscience, 24, 216-224.
Zelitch, I. (1965). The relation of glycolic acid synthesis to the
    primary photosynthetic carboxylation reaction in leaves. J.
    Biol. Chem., 240, 1869-1876.
Zelitch, I. (1971). Photosynthesis, Photorespiration, and Plant
    Productivity. Academic Press, New York.
Zelitch, I. (1975a). Improving the efficiency of photosynthesis.
    Science, 188, 626-683.
Zelitch, I. (1975b). Environmental and biological control of
    photosynthesis: General assessment. In, Marcelle, R. (1975).
Zelitch, I. (1975c). Pathways of carbon fixation in green plants.
    Annu. Rev. Biochem., 44, 123-145.
Zelitch, I. and Walker, D. A. (1964). The role of glycolic acid
    metabolism in opening of leaf stomata. Plant Physiol., 39,
    856-862.

13

CONTROL THROUGH BREEDING METHODS OF FACTORS AFFECTING

NUTRITIONAL QUALITY OF CEREALS AND GRAIN LEGUMES

Alessandro Bozzini* and Vittorio Silano**

*Crop and Grassland Production Service, Plant Production
and Protection Division, FAO, Rome, Italy

**Laboratory of Toxicology, Istituto Superiore di Sanita,
Rome, Italy

ABSTRACT

The comparison of nutritional quality parameters of proteins
from cultivated cereal and legume species with animal proteins
indicate the poor nutritional value of these plant products.
The nutritive value of different cereal and legume species is very
variable and large differences have also been observed coming from
cultivars belonging to the same species. Many interpreting factors,
such as protein content, essential amino acid composition and
availability, protein digestibility and others are involved in such
a high variability. In addition, cereals as well as legumes may
contain large amounts of antinutritional factors which can have
serious effects under particular circumstances (i. e. tannins in
a low-protein diet or phytates in a metal-deficient diet). Some
legume species also contain chemicals of a different nature
(i. e. lathyrogens, cyanogenetic glycosides, and others) which may
be extremely toxic when ingested in significant amounts. The plant
breeder attempting to develop higher-yielding, disease-resistant
and nutritionally-improved crop varieties should be aware of such
a complex of factors and alert to the possible production or increse
of undesirable products or deleterious changes in chemical composition. Available data, although rather limited, indicate valuable
breeding approaches to the improvement of nutritive value of cereal
and legume grains for humans.

INTRODUCTION

As has also been stated by the Protein Advisory Group (PAG) of the United Nations (1973), the first order of priority of cereal and legume breeders is the improvement of productivity, adaptability, and yield stability, whereas the improvement of acceptability and food nutritional value should be considered of second order. Therefore, changes in chemical composition, recommended as nutritional goals for cereal and legume breeders, are worthwhile only if produced in crops characterized by high yield and good acceptability. Further constraints for breeders attempting to increase the nutritive value of foods may derive from food consumption patterns of specific populations within the context of different levels of social and economic development (IAEA, 1977).

While each one of the 28 cereal and 45 legume edible, cultivated species has specific, useful features of adaptation and nutritional value to deserve local attention, particularly for emergency food supplies, it is evident that only a few species possess the greatest potential for significant contributions to the diet of the world population. Cereals are by far the most important staple foods of mankind and provide the major portion of energy and protein and much of the other nutrients needed. Wheat, rice, and maize account for about three-quarters of the total world cereal production; barley sorghum, oats, and millets for the remaining one-quarter (Cf. Pomeranz, 1975). World production of legumes is about one-tenth that of cereals (Cf. Burr, 1975). However, since pulses have a much higher protein content than cereals, their contribution to the total protein production is of paramount importance. Moreover, legumes are cheap sources of calories and contain vitamins as well as minerals essential for human nutrition. The PAG of the United Nations (1973) recommended urgent research attention to eight major food legumes (common bean, pigeon pea, cowpea, chick pea, broad bean, common pea, soybean, and groundnut), which, as a whole, account for about 93% of the total world legume production.

Some nutritional quality parameters of proteins from the main cultivated cereal and legume species which show the poor nutritive value of these plant products are listed in Tables 1 and 2. As shown by the variation ranges of the three biological indicators reported, the nutritive value of different cereal and legume species is very variable and large differences have also been observed coming from cultivars belonging to the same species (Tables 1 and 2).

PROTEIN CONTENT

It is generally accepted that about 5% of total energy of the human diet is required as high-quality protein and that compensation for inferior digestibility and lower nutritional value of many cereal proteins requires that they must provide more than

TABLE 1

Nutritional Quality of Some Cereal Crops

Cereal species	Indicators of nutritional quality					
	Limiting amino acids		Chemical score (A/T)	Biological value %	Protein efficiency ratio	Net protein Utilization %
	Gross deficiency	Marginal deficiency				
Barley	Lys	Ileu, Thr	54	74	1.6–2.0	59–60
Maize	Lys	Try	41	53–60	0.9–1.3	49–60
Oats	Lys	Meth, Thr, Ileu	57	65–75	1.8–2.5	59–66
Rice	Lys	Meth, Thr, Ileu	57	64–89	1.8–2.3	54–70
Rye	Lys	Phe, Ileu, Try	46	74	1.6–2.3	–
Sorghum	Lys	Meth, Try, Phe	31	51–73	0.2–2.0	48–56
Wheat	Lys	Ileu, Try	44	58–67	0.9–1.7	40–60

Table 2

Nutritional Quality of Some Legume Crops

Legume species	Limiting amino acids		Indicators of nutritional quality			
	Gross deficiency	Marginal deficiency	Chemical score (A/T)	Biological value %	Protein efficiency ratio	Net protein Utilization %
Broad bean	Met, Cys	Try	28	55	–	48
Chick pea	Met, Cys	Try	40	52–78	1.1–2.2	52–64
Common bean	Met, Cys	Try, Val	34	45–73	0.0–1.9	31–47
Common pea	Met, Cys	Try	37	48–66	0.3–2.2	41–50
Cow pea	Met, Cys	Ileu	41	49–66	–	35–51
Groundnut	Met, Cys	Ileu, Thr	43	51–63	1.5–1.8	52–55
Pigeon pea	Met, Cys	Try	27	46–74	0.7–1.8	52
Soybean	Met, Cys	Val	47	68–77	0.7–2.4	58–71

8% and often more than 10% of the energy in those diets in which
they are the nearly exclusive protein source (IAEA, 1977). On average, the the percentage of protein in cereal grains is 7 to 13%
of dry matter and in legume seeds 15 to 35%. It is not surprising,
therefore, that the poor nutritional value of cereals, particularly
when they represent the major part of the diet, also depends upon
protein quantity.

Among all the cereal species, rice has the lowest protein mean
content (7% at 17% moisture in milled rice). Biological studies with
man and rats have shown that the utilization of milled rice protein
is basically related to its protein content (Juliano et al., 1973;
Hegsted and Juliano, 1974; IRRI, 1974 and 1976). Therefore, since
rice protein quality is relatively high, increasing protein content
is the main nutritional goal for this crop. In fact, rice has a balanced amino acid composition, and with an increase in protein content
as high as 40 to 72%, only a slight drop in the first limiting amino
acid lysine was noted (Baldi et al., 1972; Juliano, 1977). Difficulties have been encountered in the breeding programmes intended to
improve the protein content of the rice grain because of the complex
nature of inheritance of protein in triploid tissues and the environmental contribution to variability of protein content within a variety (IRRI, 1974). Grain yield and protein content have a quadratic
relationship so that both characters can be increased simultaneously
only up to a point beyond which an increase in protein content
implies a decrease in yield (Narahari and Bhatia, 1975; Juliano,
1977). Selection on protein per cent as well as on protein per
grain basis can select for low-yielding plants, whereas protein
yield per hill or unit area appears to be a better selection criterion in rice (Narahari and Bhatia, 1975). Physiological studies
indicate that high-protein content in rice grain is due mainly to
the more efficient mobilization of foliar nitrogen into the grain
rather than to an enhanced nitrogen uptake from the soil (Perez
et al., 1973). Rice cultivars with a very high protein content
(as high as 18%) have been obtained through both selection or mutation breeding, but their impact on rice production has been very
poor up to now mainly because of their low yield.

The selection of high-protein cultivars, although desirable,
cannot solve by itself the nutritional inadequacy of the cereal
species, other than rice, and a more balanced amino acid pattern
is needed. For the legume crops, a higher protein concentration is
often emphasized in breeding programmes for their primary importance
in complementing and supplementing the protein-deficient diets generally prevailing among populations in developing countries. In general, the increase of limiting essential amino acids does not parallel
the increase in protein content. Negative relationships have usually
been found in legumes between protein percentage and methionine
content per unit of protein (Bliss and Hall, 1977). A similar
relationship exists in some cereals between lysine and protein con-

tent (Mossé and Baudet, 1969; Johnson and Lay, 1974). A further
inconvenience is that percentage protein has been usually found
negatively related to seed yield in both legumes (Rutgers, 1970;
Porter, 1972; Kelley, 1974; Adams, 1975) and cereals (Johnson
et al., 1967; Swaminathan et al., 1969; Favret et al., 1970;
Narahari and Bhatia, 1975; Narahari et al., 1976).

PROTEIN AMINO ACID COMPOSITION

As shown in Tables 1 and 2, the first limiting amino acid for
all cereal proteins is lysine, whereas the amino acid level requiring
improvement in most legume species is methionine. The non-essential
amino acid cystine, which can partly replace dietary requirements for
methionine, is also found to be at very low concentration levels in
legume proteins. According to Kies et al., (1972), methionine is the
first limiting amino acid in oatmeal and, according to Bressani (1973),
tryptophan may be as limiting as the sulfur-containing amino acids
in pigeon peas. Amino acid supplementation experiments (Table 3)
show that a significant improvement in nutritional value can be expected from an increase of lysine in cereals and of sulfur-amino
acids in legumes. Moreover, such an improvement is not equally
large among all the species and not even among all the cultivars
of the same species. The primary deficiency in lysine is further
intensified by a secondary deficiency, which for most cereal species
is threonine and, for maize, tryptophan. Tryptophan is also the second
limiting amino acid in common bean, cow pea, mung pea, lima beans,
and green pea; valine is the second limiting amino acid in soybeans.

Extensive research, undertaken to provide understanding of the
low nutritional quality of cereal proteins indicates that some cereal
proteins are not only deficient in one or more amino acids, but contain excess of others which can affect protein utilization. Such
effects are classified as amino acid imbalance and amino acid antagonism. Amino acid imbalance is observed, for example, when wheat
gluten is the only source of lysine in the diet. Under such conditions the lysine requirements of the rat for maximum growth is increased. Amino acid imbalance was observed in some studies in which
amino acid supplements were tested for their ability to improve low-
protein diets consisting largely of cereal products. Addition of
mixtures of several amino acids, each in small amounts, decreased
nitrogen retention in adult men consuming a rice diet and in children consuming a protein diet based on maize (Hundley, 1957).
Addition of methionine to the diet depressed nitrogen retention and
the addition of isoleucine was needed to prevent the effect
(Scrimshaw et al., 1958). Amino acid antagonism may be typically
observed with maize and sorghum, where an excess of leucine depresses
utilization of isoleucine. This amino acid imbalance, together with
a deficiency of available nicotinic acid and tryptophan causes
pellagra, a human nutritional disorder (Gopalan, 1968, 1970). In
a study of pellagra in South Africa, Hanke et al., (1971) also

TABLE 3

Effect of Lysine or Methionine Supplementation upon Protein
Efficiency Ratio of some Cereal and Legume Varieties

Species	Protein Efficiency Ratio			
	No. Lys	with 0.2–0.3% Lys	No. Met	with 0.3% Met
Barley	1.6	1.9	–	–
Maize (normal)	1.1	1.5	–	–
Maize (O$_2$)	2.3	2.6	–	–
Oats	1.8	2.5	–	–
Pearl Millet	1.8	2.9	–	–
Sorghum	0.7	1.8	–	–
Wheat	0.9	1.4	–	–
Chick pea	–	–	1.7	2.8
Common bean { black	–	–	0.0–0.9	3.5–3.8
red	–	–	0.0	1.7
white	–	–	1.2	2.7
Cow pea	–	–	1.0	1.7
Pigeon pea	–	–	1.8	1.5
Lentil	–	–	0.0	0.9

concluded that the high leucine content of maize depresses the synthesis of nicotinamide-adenine dinucleotide phosphate in the body.
The excess of arginine in relation to lysine seems to be a contributing factor to the poor utilization of millet protein (Genopathy
and Chitrie, 1970).

As is well known, cereal seed endosperm proteins are usually
divided according to their solubility in different solvent systems
into albumin, globulins, prolamins, and glutelins. Prolamins and
glutelins are exclusively confined to the starchy endosperm, whereas
albumin and globulin proteins are also found in the aleurone layers
of the seed and in the embryo. The proportion of each protein fraction in the endosperm varies according to the cereal species
(Table 4). With the main exception of oats protein, which is mainly
globulin, prolamins and glutelins make up roughly 80 to 90% of the
total grain protein. Albumins and globulins account for the remainder. Prolamins and glutelins are present in approximately equal
amounts in wheat, barley, and rye, whereas in sorghum and corn, prolamins are in excess compared to glutelins. Rice is unique in that
its protein is largely glutelin (Table 4). In spite of possible
varietal and specific signifcant variations, each protein fraction
tends to have a characteristic amino acid composition and the relative proportion of each fraction strongly affects the level of any
amino acid in the total grain protein (Johnson and Lay, 1974).
Since prolamins are most deficient in the essential amino acid lysine (0.1 to 0.8%), followed by glutelins, globulins, and albumins
in increasing order of sufficiency, the general deficiency of lysine
in cereals is essentially the consequence of their low content of
albumins and globulins. It should be stressed that endosperm albumins and globulins (which are also designated as "soluble proteins")
usually not only have a high lysine content, but also exhibit a well-
balanced amino acid composition, similar to that of animal proteins
of superior nutritional value. It appears then that, with the main
exceptions of rice and oats, a consistent enrichment of cereal protein quality can be accomplished by developing new cultivars with
a higher content of endosperm soluble proteins and a lower content
of prolamins (Nelson, 1969; Mertz, 1975). Such cultivars should be
characterized also by an increase in the most essential amino acids.
Moreover, such a breeding approach should prevent the possibility
of spending efforts in selecting cultivars whose high lysine character depends upon an increased embryo/endosperm ponderal ratio or on
an increased number of lysine-rich, undigestible aleurone cell
layers. This conclusion is also consistent with the fact that low
levels of lysine in prolamins make it unlikely that a substantial
improvement of the lysine content of cereals can be achieved by genetic manipulation of these components (Kasarda et al., 1976).
Indeed, even though breeders were not specifically looking for it,
the improvement in biological value associated with high lysine
mutations in maize, barley, and sorghum can be largely attributed
to a reduction in the proportion of prolamins together with a con-

TABLE 4

Relationship between Prolamin and Lysine Content of Some Cereal Cultivars

Sample	Prolamin % of protein	Glutelin % of protein	Lysine % of protein
Barley	35–45	35–45	3.6
Barley (Risø 1508)	10	35	5.3
Barley (Hiproly)	20	51	4.3
Maize	45–55	30–45	2.8
Maize (O_2)	18	43	4.5
Maize (fl_2)	24	41	4.3
Sorghum	55–70	25–30	2.2
Sorghum (hl)	40	34	3.2
Rye	30–40	30–50	4.3
Rice	1–5	85–90	4.4
Wheat	30–40	30–40	3.4

commitant enrichment in the amount of albumins, globulins and glutelins in the endosperm (Table 4) (Axtell, 1976; EEC, 1976). In fact,
the major cause of the increase in lysine content in opaque-2 maize
(Mertz et al., 1964) and in the Risö 1508 barley (Doll et al., 1974)
is a decreased amount of prolamins, as well as increased amount of
soluble proteins and glutelins. These mutants also show an increased
embryo/endosperm ratio and increased levels of free amino acids, including lysine in the endosperm. As pointed out by Munck (1976),
the Hiproly barley is high in lysine mainly because of the increase
in a small, very lysine-rich albumin fraction of the endosperm
(Munck et al., 1970). Similarly, compared to normal sorghums, the
hl mutant in sorghum is characterized by about a 50% reduction of
prolamins and by a 100% increase in soluble proteins and a 30% increase in glutelins (Axtell, 1976). The mutant genes responsible
for the high-lysine character in all these mutants are simply inherited and the protein change is expressed in the endosperm, apparently independently of the rest of the plant (Rabson and Atkins, 1975).
An increasing amount of evidence is accumulating which suggests that
variation in the level of lysine (and of methionine-cystine in legumes) depends more upon regulatory genes that control the proportions
of the various protein fractions in the seed than upon genes controlling the synthesis of these amino acids per se. The possibility of
changing the proportions of the four groups of seed endosperm proteins, without affecting individual amino acid compositions of each
fraction, appears to be a most favorable approach for improving the
nutritional value of cereal proteins, preserving at the same time
their technological quality. In fact, it is questionable whether
cereal varieties (and particularly wheat varieties) with high lysine
prolamins, if they exist, might have desirable technological dough,
baking, and spaghetti-making properties. The insertion of a high
number of lysine residues in the primary structures of gliadins and
glutelins would probably affect conformations of these proteins and,
as a consequence, interfere with the highly specific cooperative
phenomena that determine rheological properties of dough (Kasarda
et al., 1976). It seems, therefore, more convenient to focus breeding efforts toward the selection of cereal (and particularly wheat)
mutants with increased levels of "soluble proteins" at the expense
of prolamins. For a long time it was thought that enzymes make up
the bulk of cereal "soluble proteins". There is still some resistance, therefore, to accept a breeding strategy based on the alteration of levels of "soluble proteins" which are supposed to be biologically active and essential for variability of the seed. However,
it is now well established that the total enzymatic activity
amounts, in terms of concentration, to only a small fraction of the
total endosperm "soluble proteins". Although the bulk of the albumin and globulin fractions from the seed endosperm is still largely
obscure, it is reasonable to suggest on the basis of the present
evidence, that these fractions behave as a peculiar type storage
protein of the seed. The cereal species in which nutritionally

superior types have been discovered (maize, barley, and sorghum).
are all diploid species, whereas large surveys of tetraploid and
hexaploid wheats from the world collection and extensive mutation
experiments in wheat have failed to show any exceptionally high
lysine genotype. This might be due to the polyploid nature of the
cultivated wheats which, because of the presence of duplicate and
triplicate loci, makes the genetic control of protein content and
composition much more complex than in other diploid cereals
(Bathia, 1976).

Protein classes from legume seeds are less heterogenous than
cereal proteins, consisting of only two main fractions (albumins
and globulins). Normally, globulins represent as much as 80% of
the total seed protein. In general, albumins contain a higher
amount of essential amino acids than globulins, particularly of
lysine and sulfur amino acids. Although to-date there have been no
reports of major genes that alter the amino acid composition of legume seeds in a manner similar to those altering lysine content of
cereals, heritable differences for levels of sulfur amino acids have
been reported in several legumes (Porter, 1972; Leleji et al., 1972;
Bliss et al., 1973; Kelley, 1974; Evans, 1975). Hereditability
values in Phaseolus vulgaris for sulfur amino acid content ranged
from 0.1 to 0.85%. Methionine content showed medium level of hereditability in Vigna unguiculata (0.46 to 0.54%), while cystine content showed low hereditability. There is definite evidence that,
at least for some legume species, an increase in methionine-cystine
levels can be obtained by increasing the albumin content at the expense of the globulins (Bajaj et al., 1971a, 1971b; Bajaj, 1973).
By analysing a number of Pisum sativum cultivars with protein
efficiency (PER) ratios ranging from 0.46 to 2.20, these authors
demonstrated a correlation coefficient as high as 0.95 between the
PER value and the albumin content of the pea cultivars tested.
In contrast, the PER and total nitrogen or globulin amount were as
low as 0.42 and 0.32, respectively. Consequently, these authors
suggested that PER values of pea cultivars can be estimated by chemical assay of the albumin content. These findings were attributed
to the fact that pea albumins contain all the essential amino acids,
with the exception of sulfur amino acids, at nutritionally adequate
levels. Moreover, although limited, the sulfur amino acid content
of the albumin fraction is twice as much as that of the globulin
fraction. The lysine level in albumins is also higher than in globulins. In line with these results, an improvement of the protein
quality in Pisum mutants could be achieved by a genetically conditioned alteration of the globulin-albumin ratio (Gottschalk et al.,
1975). A larger quantity of lysine and sulfur amino acids has also
been reported in the albumin fraction of Cicer arietinum (Mathur
et al., 1968). Moreover, protease inhibitors of the albumin-type
that are present in many legume species are well-known for their
high cystine content, which makes them attractive as sulfur-depot
proteins (Pusztai, 1972). The probability of selecting legume

cultivars with an increased albumin content seems to be rather significant because albumins present in legume species and cultivars
could vary from 8 to 40% of the total protein, the remainder being
stored as globulins (Bajaj, 1973; Kelly, 1973). A change of methionine-cystine levels in legume seeds can also result from a shift
in the ratio of high-sulfur globulins to low-sulfur ones. The presence of globulin fractions with different sulfur contents has been
demonstrated in legume seeds after fractionation on the basis of
sedimentation behaviour or electrophoretic mobility. When subjected
to sedimentation in an ultracentrifugal field, legume seed globulins
usually yield two main fractions with sedimentation coefficients
7S (vicilin-like) and 11S (legumin-like) which differ largely in
sulfur-amino acid content (Derbyshire et al., 1976). In several
legume species (Pisum, Vicia, Glycine, and Phaseolus), the 11S
fraction is higher in sulfur amino acids than the 7S one (Boulter
and Evans, 1976), whereas in Arachys, the situation is the opposite.
Moreover, it has been reported (Kelley, 1973) that the electrophoretically characterized α-globulin from navy beans was richer in cystine, methionine, and tryptophan than β-globulin. Wood et al., (1969)
proposed that varieties high in methionine could be developed by
combining into a single genotype the regulatory genes that control
the presence of specific proteins already high in methionine.
After characterization of the Gl globulin (a 7S-related globulin
fraction), it was found that the Gl globulins from modified
Phaseolus vulgaris strains having lower levels of methionine contained only two discernible bands in sodium-dodecylsulfate (SDS)
gel electrophoresis, whereas the Gl globulins from strains richer
in methionine contained three distinct bands (Sun et al., 1974;
Romero et al., 1977). Such a simple inheritance behavior could be
related to the ploidy level of dicotiledons storage organs (2n),
in contrast to the triploidy level present in cereal endosperm.
The association between level of available methionine and polypeptide
subunit structure of the Gl globulin may offer a means for altering
the levels of methionine in Phaseolus vulgaris. Seeds of Lupinus
angustifolius contain three globulins (conglutin α, β, and γ with
methionine contents of 0.2, 0.0, and 1.3%, respectively), which were
resolved and estimated by electrophoresis on cellulose acetate
(Gillespie et al., 1976). This legume species, grown in the virtual
absence of sulphate and visibly sulfur-deficient, produces low sulfur
vaiable seeds with about the normal protein content, but with most
of the usual conglutins α and γ replaced by conglutin β. A significant improvement in sulfur amino acid content of lupin seed may,
obviously, be achieved by selecting varieties rich in conglutin γ.

To summarize, a first nutritional screening for improved
protein quality of both cereals and legumes based on the evaluation
of relative amounts of seed protein fractions should provide more
comprehensive nutritional information than screening based on the
evaluation of certain essential amino acids such as lysine, methionine, or on the analysis of total amino acid profiles. In addition,

the first approach is the only one which relates the protein changes to the genetic mechanism controlling nitrogen accumulation and
which could allow the selection of mutants of high interest for
chromosome engineering, even if it is not characterized by increased
essential amino acid levels. Moreover, such an approach should be
effective in lowering the probability of selecting mutants which,
in spite of higher essential amino acid content, may have a higher
nutritional value because of increases of essential amino acids in
parts of the seed not nutritionally available. The routine evaluation of relative amounts of endosperm protein fractions can be
carried out with limited amounts of seeds utilizing analytical procedures that are comparable, if not preferable, in speed and accuracy to those now available for the complete analysis of amino acid
patterns (Maes, 1962; Nelson, 1969; Mertz, 1975; Laundry and Moureaux,
1970; Bajaj et al., 1971 b; Dalby, 1974; Rhodes, 1975; EEC, 1977).

PROTEIN DIGESTIBILITY

   Low digestibility is a major nutritional problem in high-tannin
sorghum cultivars whose protein digestibility for different animal
species varied from 30 to 80% depending on tannin content (Silano,
1977). High tannin levels have especially been found in brown-
seeded, bird-resistant sorghums (1.3 to 2.0%), compared to a tannin
content of 0.2 to 0.4% for the other cultivars. Over 60% of 472
sorghums from the world collection were classified as low tannin
by Purdue researchers, but 80% of 288 sorghums from Cameron
(Africa), were classified as high tannin lines (Johnson and Lay,
1974). In high-tannin sorghums, an increased lysine content does
not improve the extremely low biological value (Axtell, 1976).
Adverse effects caused by tannins in the nutrition of man and animal species have been recently reviewed by Silano (1977). Although
the important interaction between tannin content and protein quality observed in sorghum is not found in any other cereal species,
tannins are at least in part also responsible for the relatively
low protein digestibility of some barley cultivars (Eggum and
Christensen, 1975). Moreover, a strong correlation was noted
between the digestion coefficients of crude protein in different
cultivars of peas and field beans (Lindgren, 1975). The effect
of tannins on protein digestibility is due to the formation of soluble and insoluble complexes which are poorly digestible and therefore, partially or totally unavailable (Van Buren and Robinson,
1969; Feeney, 1969; Eggum and Christensen, 1975). Furthermore,
tannins inactivate a number of enzymes including trypsin, α-amylase,
and lipase (Tamir and Alumont, 1969; Milic et al., 1972). Because
free tannins also have carcinogenic activity (Singleton and Kratzer,
1973), it appears that protein-tannin complexes present in some
cereal and legume seeds may actually represent partially detoxified
tannins. Tannins are thermo-stable and cannot be inactivated by
heat-treatments.

Some reports (Subramanyan et al., 1955) describe a low deges-
tibility (55%) for Eleusine coracana protein in human adults.
In vitro studies (Swaminathan et al., 1970) showed that mature proteins of several minor millets (Paspalum, Setaria, and Eleusine)
with low Net Protein Utilization (NPU) were extremely resistant
to the action of papain. Protein fractionation studies revealed
(Swaminathan et al., 1970) that most of the minor millets contain
a large portion of unextractable proteins, because of the cellulose
envelope in which proteins are enclosed. The presence of indigestible cellulosic structures reduces protein digestibility, which
averages 80% for major cereal species, with a range of 92% (some
wheat cultivars) to 67% (some barley cultivars), compared to casein
digestibility of 100% (Eggum, 1970, 1973, 1977; Bodwell, 1977;
Hackler, 1977; Juliano, 1977). Although the role of such structures
in preventing the contact of dietary proteins with proteases of the
digestive apparatus has been studied more extensively with wheat
(Munck, 1972; Saunders and Kohler, 1972; Saunders et al., 1972), it
is obvious that they are a more important factor in cereals such as
barley and oats, which have a higher crude fiber content (4.6 and
10.3% of dry matter, respectively), than in maize, rye, wheat, or
triticale (Eggum, 1977). Since the increase in lysine content of
cereals through breeding may occur in the indigestible protein of
the aleurone cells, the role of cellulosic structures in preventing
the utilization of proteins of good nutritional value should not
be disregarded when maximum nutritional quality of cereals is desired.

A further factor to be taken into account, when considering
the reasons for limited digestibility of cereal proteins, is that
these proteins, because of their high proline content, might have
fairly large numbers of lysylprolyl and/or arginylprolyl bonds that
are resistant to trypsin attack (Kakade, 1974). It has been observed that because of its higher content of arginyl and lysyl residues,
rice protein is cleaved by trypsin to smaller peptide fragments to
a greater extent than other cereal proteins (Kakade, 1974; Shukla,
1975). The ratio of arginine plus lysine to proline in rice is 4.0
compared to an average of 1.0 for other cereals, in line with the
higher digestibility and biological value of rice protein.

Some legume proteins are examples of foods whose digestibility
is low. Bressani (1973) has reviewed several reports on the protein
digestibility in human adults and children which show decreased
dietary nitrogen retention when egg is substituted with Pisum
sativum and milk with Phaseolus vulgaris. Low protein digestibility
of legume grains has been observed to vary not only among species
but also among varieties of the same species (Bressani, 1973).
Different cultivars of Cajanus cajan showed protein digestibilities
ranging from 59 to 90% (Jaffé, 1950). Protein digestibilities
that varied from 44 to 84% have also been reported for different
varieties of Phaseolus vulgaris (Jaffe, 1950, 1973 a, 1973 b;
Kakade, 1974; Pusztai et al., 1975). Comprehensive fractionation

studies of seeds of two varieties of kidney beans by Pusztai et al.,
(1975) offer a good understanding of the limited digestibility of
legume protein fractions. True digestibilities by the rat of the
albumin (25.7% of total nitrogen) and globulin (37.3% of total nitrogen) fractions were 82 and 76%, respectively. Furthermore, a large
part of total nitrogen (28.7%) was associated with the water-insoluble residue consisting mainly of protein bound to structural and
cell wall polysaccharides; true digestibility of this fraction was
72%. The low digestibility of the globulin fractions is in line
with the presence in Phaseolus vulgaris of a globulin fraction that
comprises a large part of the bean protein, which is resistant to
in vitro digestion by a number of proteolytic enzymes, even after
thermal and urea treatments (Jaffé and Vega Lette, 1968; Seidel
et al., 1969). Similarly, the limited digesitibility of the albumin
fraction may be related to the presence in this fraction of trypsin
inhibitors from a number of legume species whose cystine is not released by digestive enzymes (Liener, 1975; Liener and Kakade, 1969;
Kakade et al., 1969). Moreover, about 30% of the albumin fraction
and 10% of the globulin fraction consist of lectins whose in vitro
breakdown by trypsin after 24 hours amounted to about 10%, compared
to casein which was completely digested in one hour, (Pusztai et al.,
1975). Lectins from Phaseolus vulgaris also proved to be resistant
to digestion by pepsin and proteolytic bacteria (Jaffé and Hanning,
1965; Jayne-Williams and Burgess, 1974).

   The low digestibilities of some cystine-rich legume proteins
and wheat albumins (Petrucci et al., 1976; Macri et al., 1977) may
depend on their yielding, after treatment with proteases, core
fractions which are resistant to further cleavage and which contain
large amounts of cystine of the original material(Almquist et al.,
1966; Fukushima, 1968; Kakade et al., 1972). Another factor that
depends on protein conformation and which may give a measure of
resistance to proteases of the alimentary canal is the low solubility of certain cereal and legume proteins under physiological conditions. Such a low solubility is an expression of highly organized,
tightly folded, compact structures which prevent hydration of protein
molecules and protect peptidase-susceptible bonds from enzyme attack.
This may be an important factor which explains the low digestibility
of legume globulins and may also be responsible for the low digestibility of zein, thus causing maize to be less utilized in man than
rice (De Muelenaere et al., 1961; Chen et al., 1962; Bressani and
Elias, 1968; De Muelenare et al., 1967). It may also explain the
presence of undigested protein bodies in feces of man on a rice
diet (Juliano, 1977). The presence of crystalline-type protein
bodies has been observed in subaleurone (the outermost cell layers)
layers of rice endosperm (Harris and Juliano, 1977). Finally, the
remarkable stability of many plant lectins against the action of
a great number of proteolytic enzymes may depend, at least in part,
on the glycosidic constituent of the lectins.

In any case, the intrinsic low digestibility of several legume proteins is a significant nutritional problem which can only be partially solved by heat denaturation treatments intended to disrupt internal protein structure and to expose susceptible peptide bonds to proteinases (Jaffe, 1973 a, 1973 b; Kakade, 1974). Several authors have pointed out the very large difference in availability of methionine to the rat from various heat-treated legume proteins containing equal amounts of methionine and/or cystine (Evans and Brandeman, 1962; Kakade, 1974). Rat growth rates became similar in all cases studied following addition of 0.2 to 0.3% methionine to the diet. This observations suggests that certain bean proteins are more resistant to denaturation. According to Kakade (1974), the greater resistance of some legume proteins to heat denaturation may be due to a major role played by   hydrophobic and disulfide bonds, as compared to hydrogen bonds, in stabilizing protein structure.

One interesting point is that reduced protein digestibility is highly undesirable not only because it causes losses of nutritive material, but also because the consequent presence of undigested protein materials in the gut may   elicit an increased secretion of pancreatic enzymes rich in sulfur-containing amino acids, thus accentuating the deficiency of these amino acids typical of plant proteins (Green et al., 1973).   Indeed, Kakade et al., (1973) have shown that soy protein devoid of trypsin-inhibitory activity caused pancreatic enlargement and growth depression in rats.

It appears, therefore, that in order to prevent selection of mutants characterized by poor correspondence between chemically determined levels of amino acids and amounts of these amino acids which are biologically available, protein digestibility must be kept under control. Of course, animal   bioassays would be highly desirable in this respect, but in vivo tests, as is well known, require rather large amounts of material and are, therefore, not suitable for early generation screening. This problem might be partially solved by use of an in vitro method (Hsu et al., 1977) useful for predicting in vivo digestibility (Bodwell, 1977 a). If in vitro digestibility estimates obtained with a multi-enzyme 10-minute assay of Hsu et al., (1977) are shown to correlate with digestibility in humans, such an assay might reflect general changes in amino acid availability (Cf. also, Stahmann and Woldegiorgis, 1975). This method is very simple and could be modified to analyze small samples of cereals and legume grains containing as little as 0.05 to 0.1 grams of protein (Bodwell, 1977 b). It can also be used to test different protein fractions extracted from grains. Eventually the seed and/or protein samples could be submitted to standard thermal treatments to stimulate cooking, thus making it possible to discover more suitable cooking conditions. According to Bodwell (1977 b), assays involving in vitro enzymatic digestion followed by amino acid analysis not only are too time-consuming but also do not appear to have much of an advantage beyond that provided by indices or scores calculated from amino acid composition analyses.

ANTI-NUTRITIONAL FACTORS

It should be clear that in view of the proteinase and α-amylase inhibitory activities associated with albumin fractions from several cereal (Buonocore et al., 1977; Silano, 1977) and legume (Jaffé and Vega Lette,1968; Jaffé et al., 1973; Liener, 1975; Marshall and Lauda, 1975; Richardson, 1977) species, the selection of mutants with a more balanced amino acid composition may lead to the selection of mutants with higher content of protease and amylase inhibitors. Such mutants could offer a higher resistance to insects (Birk et al., 1963; Green and Ryan, 1972; Pressey, 1972; Buonocore et al., 1977). Moreover, in some legume species hemagglutinating activity is associated with both the albumin and globulin fractions (Pusztai et al., 1975). Lectins, also named hemmaglutinins, are widely distributed in legume species and are not necessarily toxic for man or animal species used for testing (Lotan and Sharon, 1977). For example, lectins present in peas, lentils, and peanuts do not affect growth of rats, whereas those from kidney beans, field beans, and soy beans adversely affect rat growth and eventually also cause their death (Liener, 1973; Jaffé, 1973 b; Jayne-Williams and Burges, 1974; Pusztai and Watt, 1974; Pusztai et al., 1975). While their low digestibility is well established, the exact nutritional signficance for man of hydrolase inhibitors and lectins at levels usually found in legume and cereal seeds is difficult to assess. Lectins and trypsin inhibitors are heat-labile. Normal cooking destroys their specific activity. Amylase inhibitors persist in part during bread baking. They are found in the center of bread loaves and a number of wheat-based breakfast cereals consumed by humans also contain α-amylase inhibitory activity; this may also be the case for other wheat foods (i. e. cakes). Although it generally seems likely that the importance of these protein antinutritional factors from legume and cereal grains as toxic agents for man, if any, may be be small, unusually large amounts of these compounds may have an adverse nutritional action if appropriate food cooking or processing is not adopted. Furthermore, since animals are fed raw seeds, unusually large amounts of the anti-nutritional factors may influence animal nutrient utilization.

It is obvious that, to be nutritionally effective, the described desirable changes in relative amounts of endosperm protein fractions should be produced in cereal and legume cultivars devoid of antinutritional factors whose harmful effects have been well-established under conditions of consumption. Therefore, constitutents such as tannins, toxic amino acids(Bell, 1973), flatus-inducing compounds (Patwardhan and White, 1973), cyanogenetic glycosides (Conn, 1973); alkaloids (Keller, 1969), and factors causing favism (Patwardhan and White, 1973) should be, whenever possible, monitored in breeding programs in very early generations. These factors are thermostable, difficult to remove in a household with simple procedures, and their action cannot be counteracted by nutrients. Anti-nutritional factors

such as phytates (Lorenz and Lee, 1977), lectins, hydrolase inhibitors, and lathyrogens (Bell, 1973), and goitrogens (Van Etten and
Wolff, 1973), which can be counteracted by other nutrients or inactivated by special procedures of food preparation, should prefer-
ably be monitored in advanced cereal and legume lines   and
before commercial release. Unfortunately, suitable screening procedures are not available for evaluation of all these anti-nutritional factors. In particular, there are no screening methods for
flatus-inducing and favism-causing compounds and for goitrogens
(Cf. however, Olson et al., 1975). Other anti-nutritional factors
(e.g. estrogenic glycosides, saponins, anti-vitamins, and resorci-
nols) deserve further study to clarify their nutritional significance. At the present time, they do no appear to be of especially
high interest to the breeder. Anti-nutritional factors are not
equally important in different cereal and legume species and need
not be controlled in all species. As previously mentioned in this
paper, tannins are found mainly in sorghum and barley cultivars,
anti-metabolic amino acids in common bean and vetch as well as in
djenkol and jack beans; flatus-forming compounds in soy beans, and
alkaloids in lupin cultivars. Lima bean cultivars are likely to have
a high HCN-producing capacity. Causative factors of favism are
a main concern only in broad beans. Alpha-amylase inhibitors are
present in large amounts in cereals such as wheat, barley, and rye.
Proteinase inhibitors are known to occur mainly in legumes. With
the possible exception of wheat germ agglutinin, lectins pose no
major nutritional problems in cereals. They should be controlled
in legumes such as kidney and field beans and in soy beans.
Lathyrogens are almost limited to Lathyrus species and among
legume and cereal grains, goitrogenic glucosinolates have only been
found in peanut and soy bean. In certain susceptible individuals,
wheat gluten induces a malabsorption syndrome called celiac disease
(Kasarda, 1975).

CONCLUSIONS

     In conclusion, in vitro estimates of protein digestibilities
plus chemical evaluations of relative amounts of seed protein fractions and of the levels of limiting amino acids should all be incorporated in an analysis designed to predict nutritive value for
humans. Such an analysis, integrated with a time-programmed assay
of relevant anti-nutritional factors, should be very useful as
a screening tool in breeding programmes intended to select cereal
and legume cultivars with higher nutritive value.

REFERENCES

Adams, M. W. (1975). On the quest for quality in the field bean. In 'Nutritional Improvement of Food Legumes by Breeding'. M. Milner (Ed.), Wiley and Sons, New York.

Attia, F. and Creek, R. D. (1965). Studies on raw and heated wheat germ for young chicks. Cereal Chem., 42, 494-497.

Almquist, H. J., Christensen, H. L. and Maurer, S. (1966). Sulphide liberation from raw soybean protein. Proc. Soc. Exptl. Med. Biol., 122, 913-914.

Axtell, J. D. (1976). Naturally occurring and induced genotypes of high lysine sorghum. In 'Evaluation of Seed Protein Alteration by Mutation Breeding', IAEA, Vienna, Austria, 45-53.

Bajaj, S., Mickelsen, O., Baker, L. R. and Markarian, D. (1971a). The quality of protein in various lines of peas. Brit. J. Nutr., 25, 207-212.

Bajaj, S., Mickelsen, O., Lillerik, H. A., Baker, L. R., Bergen, W. G. and Gil, J. L. (1971b). Prediction of protein efficiency ratio of peas from their albumin content. Crop Sci., 11, 813-815.

Bajaj, S. (1973). Biological value of legume protein as influenced by genetic variation. In 'Nutritional Improvement of Food Legumes by Breeding', M. Milner (Ed.), Wiley and Sons, New York, 223-232.

Baldi, G., Buiatti, M. and Salamini, F. (1972). Introduzione al miglioramento genetico qualitativo. Edagricole, Bologna, Italy, 25-27.

Bathia, C. R. (1976). Prospects for using aneuploids and their derivatives for wheat protein improvement. In 'Evaluation of Seed Protein Alteration by Mutation Breeding', IAEA, Vienna, Austria, 63-67.

Bell, E. A. (1973). Aminonitriles and amino acids not derived from proteins. In 'Toxicants Occurring Naturally in Foods', Natl. Acad. Sci., Natl. Res. Council, Washington, D.C., 153-169.

Birk, Y., Gertler, A. and Kholz, S. (1963). Separation of a Tribolium proteinase inhibitor from soybeans on a calcium phosphate column. Biochim. Biophys. Acta, 67, 326-328.

Bliss, F. A. and Hall, T. C. (1977). Food Legumes - compositional and nutritional changes induced by breeding. Cereal Foods World, 22, 106-113.

Bliss, F. A., Barker, L. N., Franckowiak, J. D. and Hall, T. C. (1973). Genetic and environmental variation of seed yield, yield components and seed protein quantity and quality of cowpea. Crop Sci., 13, 656.

Bodwell, C. E. (1977a). Application of animal data to human protein nutrition: A review. Cereal Chem., 54, 958-984.

Bodwell, C. E. (1977b). The use of enzymatic assays for the determination of nutritional quality. In 'Evaluating the Nutritional Quality of Mutants with Altered Grain Protein Characteristics'. IAEA, Vienna, Austria.

Boulter, D. and Evans, I. M. (1976). Legume proteins, their nutritio-
    nal improvement and screening techniques. In 'Evaluation of
    Seed Protein Alterations by Mutation Breeding', IAEA, Vienna,
    Austria, 147-150.
Bressani, R. (1973). Legumes in human diets and how they might be
    improved. In 'Nutritional Improvement of Food Legumes by
    Breeding', M. Milner (Ed.), Wiley and Sons, New York, 15-42.
Bressani, R. and Elias, L. G. (1968). Processed vegetable protein
    mixtures for human consumption in developing countries.
    Adv. Food Res., 16, 1-103.
Buonocore, V., Petrucci, T. and Silano, V. (1977). Wheat protein
    inhibitors of α-amylase. Phytochemistry, 16, 811-820.
Burr, H. K. (1975). Pulse proteins. In 'Protein Nutritional Quality
    of Foods and Feeds', Part 2, M. Friedman (Ed.), Marcel Dekker,
    New York, 119-134.
Chen, K. L., Rogers, Q. R. and Harper, A. E. (1962). Observation on
    protein digestion in vivo. Further observation on the gastro-
    intestinal contents of rats fed different dietary proteins.
    J. Nutr., 76, 235-241.
Conn, E. E. (1973). Cyanogenetic glycosides. In 'Toxicants Naturally
    Occurring in Foods', Natl. Acad. Sci., Natl. Res. Council,
    Washington, D. C., 299-308.
Dalby, A. (1974). Rapid method for determining the zein content of
    whole maize seed or isolated endosperm. Cereal Chem., 51,
    586-592.
De Muelenaere, H. J. H., Chen, K. L. and Harper, A. E. (1961). Stu-
    dies on availability of amino acids. Effects of alcohol
    treatment of corn gluten. J. Nutr., 74, 125-130.
De Muelenaere, H. J. H., Chen, K. L. and Harper, A. E. (1967).
    Assessment of factors influencing estimation of availability of
    threonine, isoleucine and valine in cereal products. J. Ag.
    Food Chem., 15, 318-323.
Darbyshire, E., Wright, D. J. and Boulter, D. (1976). Legumin and
    vicilin, storage proteins of legume seeds. Phytochem., 15,3-24.
Doll, H., Køie, B. and Eggum, B. O. (1974). Induced high lysine
    mutants in barley. Radiat. Bot., 14, 73-78.
EEC (Commission of the European Communities) (1977). Techniques for
    the separation of barley and maize proteins. B. J. Miflin and
    P. R. Shewry (Eds.), Coordination of Agricultural Research
    (EUR 5687e), 1-111.
Eggum. B. O. (1970). Current methods of nutritional protein evalu-
    ation. In 'Improving Plant Protein by Nuclear Techniques',
    IAEA, Vienna, Austria, 289-302.
Eggum, B. O. (1973). Biological availability of amino acid consti-
    tuents in grain protein. In 'Nuclear Techniques for Seed Pro-
    tein Improvement' IAEA, Vienna, Austria, 391-408.
Eggum, B. O. (1977). The nutritive quality of cereals. Cereal Res.,
    Commun., 5, 153-157. See also paper by B. O. Eggum, this volume.

Eggum, O. and Christensen, R. D. (1975). Influence of tannin on pro-
    tein utilization in feedstuffs with special reference to barley.
    In 'Breeding for Seed Protein Improvement Using Nuclear
    Techniques', IAEA, Vienna, Austria, 135-143.
Evans, A. M. (1975). Genetic improvement of Phaseolus vulgaris.
    In 'Nutritional Improvement of Food Legumes by Breeding',
    M. Milner (Ed.), Wiley and Sons, New York.
Evans, R. J. and Bandemer, S. L. (1967). Nutritive value of legume
    seed protein. J. Ag. Fd. Chem., 15, 439-443.
Favret, E. A., Manghers, L., Solari, R., Avila, A. and Monesiglio,
    J. C. (1970). Gene control of protein production in cereal
    seeds. In 'Improving Plant Protein by Nuclear Techniques',
    IAEA, Vienna, Austria, 87-96.
Feeney, P. P. (1969). Inhibitory effect of oak leaf tannins on the
    hydrolysis of proteins by trypsin. Phytochem., 8, 2119-2126.
Fukushima, D. (1968). Internal structure of 7S and 11S globulin
    molecules in soybean proteins. Cereal Chem., 45, 203-224.
Gillespie, J. M., Blagrove, R. J. and Randall, P. J. (1976). Regu-
    lation of the globulin of lupin seed. In 'Evaluation of Seed
    Protein Alterations by Mutation Breeding', IAEA, Vienna,
    Austria, 151-156.
Gonopathy, S. N. and Chitrie, R. G. (1970). Simple method for deter-
    mining lysine and tryptophan in high lysine and normal maize.
    Fed. Proc., 29, 761 (Abstract).
Gopalan, C. (1968). Leucine and pellagra. Nutr. Rev., 26, 323-326.
Gopalan, C. (1970). Some recent studies in the nutrition research
    laboratories. Am. J. Clin. Nutr., 23, 35-51.
Green, G. H., Olds, B. A., Mattens, G. and Lyman, R. L. (1973).
    Protein as a regulator of pancreatic enzyme secretion in the
    rat. Proc. Soc. Exptl. Med. Biol., 142, 1162-1167.
Gottschalk, W., Müller, H. P. and Wolff, G. (1975). Relations between
    production protein quality and environmental factors in Pisum
    mutants. In 'Breeding for Seed Protein Improvement Using Nuc-
    lear Techniques', IAEA, Vienna, Austria, 105-123.
Green, T. R. and Ryan, C. A. (1972). Wound-induced proteinase inhi-
    bitor in plant leaves: a possible defense mechanism against
    insects. Science, 175, 776-777.
Hackler, L. R. (1977). Methods of ensuring protein quality: A review
    of bioassay procedures. Cereal Chem., 54, 984-995.
Hankes, L. V. Leklem, J. E., Brown, R. R. and McKel, R.C.P.M. (1971).
    Tryptophan metabolism in patients with pellagra: Problem of
    vitamin B_6 enzyme activity and feedback control of tryptophan
    pyrrolase enzyme. Am. J. Clin. Nutr., 24, 730-739.
Harris, N. and Juliano, B. O. (1977). Ultrastructure of endosperm
    protein bodies in developing rice grains differing in protein
    content. Ann. Bot., 41, 1-12.
Hegsted, D. M. and Juliano, B. O. (1974). Difficulties in assessing
    the nutritional quality of rice protein. J. Nutr., 104, 772-781.

Hsu, H. W., Varak, D. L., Satterlee, L. D. and Miller, G. A. (1977).
A multi-enzyme technique for estimating protein digestibility.
J. Food Sci., 42, 1269-1273.

Hundley, J. M. (1957). Lysine, threonine and other supplements to
rice diets in man: amino acid imbalance. Am J. Clin. Nutr., 5,
316-326.

IAEA (International Atomic Energy Agency) (1977).'Nutritional
Evaluation of Cereal Mutants', Vienna, Austria.

IRRI (International Rice Research Institute) (1974). Annual Report
for 1973. Los Banos, Philippines.

IRRI (International Rice Research Institute) (1976). Annual Report
for 1975. Los Banos, Philippines.

Jaffe', W. G. (1950). Protein digestibility and trypsin inhibitor
activity of legume seeds. Proc. Soc. Exptl. Biol. Med., 75,
219-220.

Jaffe', W. G. (1973a). Toxic proteins and peptides. In 'Toxicants
Occurring Naturally in Foods', Natl. Acad. Sci., Natl. Res.
Council, Washington, D. C., 106-129.

Jaffe', W. G. (1973b). Factors affecting the nutritional value of
beans. In 'Nutritional Improvement of Food Legumes by Breeding',
Wiley and Sons, New York, 43-48.

Jaffe', W. G. and Hanning, K. (1965). Fractionation of proteins from
kidney beans (Phaseolus vulgaris). Arch. Biochem. Biophys., 109,
80-91.

Jaffe', W. G., Moreno, R. and Wallis, V. (1973). Amylase inhibitors
in legume seeds. Nutr. Repts. Int., 7, 169-174.

Jaffe', W. G. and Vega Lette, G. L. (1968). Heat-labile and growth-
inhibiting factors in beans. J. Nutr., 94, 203-210.

Jayne-Williams, D. J. and Burgess, C. D. (1974). Further observation
on the toxicity of navy beans (Phaseolus vulgaris) fo Japanese
quail (Coturnix coturnix Japonica). J. Applied Bact., 37, 149-169.

Johnson, V. A. and Lay, C. L. (1974). Genetic improvement of plant
protein. J. Agr. Food Chem., 22, 558-566.

Johnson, V. A., Mattern, P. J., and Schmidt, J. W. (1967).
Crop Sci., 7, 664-667. See also paper by V.A. Johnson and
P. A. Mattern, this volume.

Juliano, B. O. (1977). Recent developments in rice research.
Cereal Food World, 22, 284-287.

Juliano, B. O., Antonio, A. A. and Esmama, B. V. (1973). Effects of
protein content on the distribution and properties of rice
protein. J. Sci. Food Agr., 24, 295-306.

Kakade, M. L. (1974). Biochemical basis for the differences in plant
protein utilization. J. Agr. Food Chem., 22, 550-555.

Kakade, M. L., Arnold, R. L., Liener, I. E. and Warbel, P. E. (1969).
Unavailability of cystine from trypsin inhibitors as a factor
contributing to the poor nutritive value of navy beans.
J. Nutr., 99, 34-42.

Kakade, M. L., Simons, N., Liener, I. E. and Lambert, J. E. (1972).
Biochemical and nutritional assessment of different varieties
of soybeans. J. Agr. Food Chem., 20, 87-90.

Kakade, M. L., Hoffa, D. D. and Liener, I. E. (1973). Contribution of trypsin inhibitors to the deleterious effects of unheated soybeans fed to rats. J. Nutr., 103, 1772-1778.

Hsu, H. W., Varak, D. L., Satterlee, D. D. and Miller, G. A. (1977). A multi-enzyme technique for estimating protein digestibility. J. Food Sci., 42, 1269-1273.

Kasarda, D. D. (1975). Celiac disease: malabsortion of nutrients in- duced by a toxic factor in gluten. In 'Protein Nutritional Qua- lity of Foods and Feeds, Part 2, M. Friedman (Ed.), Marcel Dekker, New York, 565-593.

Kasarda, D. D., Bernardin, J. E. and Nimmo, C. (1976). Wheat proteins. In 'Advances in Cereal Science and Technology', Y. Pomeranz (Ed.), American Association of Cereal Chemists, St. Paul, MN, 158-236.

Keeler, R. F. (1969). Toxic and teratogenic alkaloids of Western range plants. J. Agr. Food Chem., 17, 473-482.

Kelly, J. F. (1973). Increasing protein quantity and quality. In 'Nutritional Improvement of Food Legumes by Breeding', M. Milner (Ed.), Wiley and Sons, New York, 179-184.

Kelley, J. D. (1974). Genetic modification of protein quantity and quality in beans, Phaseolus vulgaris L., Ph. D. Thesis, University of Wisconsin, Madison, Wisconsin.

Kies, C., Petersen, M. R. and Fox, H. M. (1972). Protein nutritive value of amino acid-supplemented and unsupplmented precooked dehydrated oatmeal. J. Food Sci., 37, 306-309.

Laundry, J. and Moureaux, T. (1977). Hétérogeité des glutelins du grain de mais - Extraction selective et composition des acides amines de trois fractions isolees. Bull. Soc. Chim. Biol., 52, 1021-1037.

Leleji, O. I., Dickson, M. H. and Hackler, L. R. (1972). Effect of genotype on microbiologically available methionine content of bean seeds. Hort. Sci., 7, 277.

Liener, I. E. (1975). Effects of anti-nutritional and toxic factors on the quality and utilization of legume proteins. In 'Protein Nutritional Quality of Foods and Feeds, Part 2: Quality Factors- Plant Breeding, Composition, Processing, and Antinutrients', M. Friedman (Ed.), Marcel Dekker, New York, 523-550.

Liener, I. E. (1973). Antitryptic and other nutritional factors in legumes. In 'Nutritional Improvement of Food Legumes by Breeding', M. Milner (Ed.), Wiley and Sons, New York, 239-258.

Liener, I. E. and Kakade, M. L. (1969). Protease inhibitors. In Toxic Constitutents of Plant Foodstuffs', I. E. Liener(Ed.), Academic Press, New York.

Lindgreen, E. (1975). The nutritive value of peas and field beans for hens. Swed. J. Agr. Res., 5, 159-161.

Lorenz, K. and Lee, V. A. (1977). The nutritional and physiological impact of cereal products in nutrition. CRC Food Science and Nutrition, 8, 383-458.

Lotan, R. and Sharon, N. (1977). Modification of the biological pro- perties of plant lectins by chemical crosslinking. In 'Protein Crosslinking: Biochemical and Molecular Aspects', M. Friedman (Ed.), Plenum Press, New York, 149-169.

Macri, A., Valfre, F., Parlamenti, R., and Silano, V. (1977). Adaptation of the domestic chicken, Gallus domesticus, to continuous feeding of albumin amylase inhibitors from wheat flour as gastroresistant microgranules. Poultry Sci., 56, 434-441.

Maes, E. (1962). Progressive extraction of proteins. Nature, 193, 880.

Marshall, J. J. and Lauda, C. H. (1975). Purification and properties of phaseolomin, an inhibitor of α-amylase from the kidney bean, Phaseolus vulgaris, J. Biol. Chem., 150, 8030-8037.

Mertz, E. T. (1975). Breeding for improved nutritional value in cereals. In 'Protein Nutritional Quality of Foods and Feeds, Part 2: Quality Factors - Plant Breeding, Composition, Processing, and Antinutrients', M. Friedman (Ed.), Marcel Dekker, New York, 1-12. See also paper by E. T. Mertz, this volume.

Mertz, E. T., Bates, L. S. and Nelson, O. E. (1964). Mutant gene that changes protein composition and increases lysine content in maize endosperm. Science, 45, 279-280.

Milic, B. L., Stoyanovic, S. and Vucurecic, N. (1972). Lucerne tannins: Isolation of tannins from lucerne, their nature and influence on the digestive enzymes in vitro. J. Sci. Food Agr., 23, 1157-1162.

Mosse, J. and Baudet, J. (1969). Etude intervarietale de la qualite proteique des orges: taux d'zote, composition en acides amines et richesse en lysine. Ann. Physiol. Veg., 11, 51-66.

Munck, L. (1972). Improvement of nutritional value in cereals. Hereditas, 72, 1-128.

Munck, L., Karlsson, K. E., Hagberg, A. and Eggum, B. O. (1970). Gene for improved nutritional value in barley seed protein. Science, 168, 985-989.

Munck, L. (1976). Aspects of the selection, design and use of high lysine cereals. In 'Evaluation of Seed Protein Alterations by Mutation Breeding', IAEA, Vienna, Austria, 3-17.

Narahari, P. and Bathia, C. R. (1975). Induced mutation for increasing protein content in wheat and rice. In 'Breeding for Seed Protein Improvement Using Nuclear Techniques', IAEA, Vienna, Austria, 23-29.

Narahari, P., Bathia, C. R., Gopalakrishna, T, and Mitra, R. K. (1976). Mutation induction of protein variability in wheat and rice. In 'Evaluation of Seed Protein Alterations by Mutation Breeding', IAEA, Vienna, Austria, 119-127.

Nelson, O. E. (1969). Adv. Agron., 21, 171-194.

Olson, A. C., Becker, R., Miers, J. C., Gumbmann, M. R. and Wagner, J. R. (1975). Problems in the digestibility of dry beans. In 'Protein Nutritional Quality of Foods and Feeds,' Part 2, M. Friedman (Ed.), Marcel Dekker, New York, 551-563.

PAG (Protein Advisory Group) Statement 22 (1973). In 'Nutritional Improvement of Food Legumes by Breeding', M. Milner (Ed.), Wiley and Sons, New York, 349-380.

Patwardhan, V. N. and White, J. W. (1973). Problems associated with
    particular foods. In 'Toxicants Naturally Occurring in Foods',
    Natl. Acad. Sci., Natl. Res. Council, Washington, D. C.,477-507.
Perez, C. M., Cagampang, B., Esmana, V., Monserrate, R. U. and
    Juliano, B. O. (1973). Protein metabolism in leaves and deve-
    loping grains of rice differing in grain protein content.
    Plant Physiol., 51, 537-542.
Petrucci, T., Rab, A., Tomasi, M. and Silano, V. (1976). Further
    characterization studies of the α-amylase protein inhibitor
    of gel electrophoretic mobility 0.19 from wheat kernel.
    Biochem. Biophys. Acta, 420, 288-297.
Pomeranz, Y. (1975). Protein and amino acids of barley, oats,
    and buckwheat. In 'Protein Nutritional Quality of Foods and
    Feeds',Part 2, M. Friedman (Ed.), Marcel Dekker, New York,
    13-78.
Porter, W.M. (1972). Genetic control of protein and sulfur contents
    in dry bean, Phaseolus vulgaris, Ph. D. Thesis, Purdue Univer-
    sity, West Lafayette, Indiana.
Pressey, R. (1972). Natural enzyme inhibitors in plant tissues.
    J. Food Sci., 37, 521-523.
Pusztai, A., Grant, G. and Palmer, R. (1975). Nutritional evalua-
    tion of kidney beans (Phaseolus vulgaris): the isolation and
    and partial characterization of toxic constituents.
    J. Sci. Food Agric., 26, 149-156.
Pusztai, A. and Watt, W. B. (1974). Isolectins of Phaseolus vulgaris.
    A comprehensive study of fractionation. Biochem. Biophys. Acta,
    365, 57-71.
Pusztai, A. (1972). Metabolism of trypsin-inhibitory proteins in
    the germinating seeds of kidney beans. Planta, 107, 121-129.
Rabson, R. and Atkins, C. A. (1975). Workshop report: Genetic and
    physiological basis of seed protein synthesis as related to
    nuclear technology. In 'Breeding for Seed Protein Improvement
    Using Nuclear Techniques', IAEA, Vienna, Austria, 211-216.
Richardson, M. (1977). The proteinase inhibitors of plants and
    microorganisms. Phytochemistry, 16, 159-169.
Rhodes, A. P. (1975). A comparison of two rapid screening methods
    for the selection of high-lysine barleys. J. Sci. Food Agric.,
    26, 1793-1805.
Rutgers, J. N. (1970). Variation in protein content and its relation
    to other characters in beans (Phaseolus vulgaris L.). Report
    Dry Bean Res. Conference, Davis, California, 10, 59-68.
Saunders, R. H. and Kohler, G. O. (1972). In vitro determination of
    protein digestibility in wheat millfeeds and monogastric
    animals. Cereal Chem., 49, 98-103.
Saunders, R. H., Connor, M. A., Edwards, R. N. and Kohler, G. O.
    (1972). Enzymatic processing of wheat bran: effects on nutrient
    availability. Cereal Chem., 49, 436-442.
Scrimshaw, N. S., Bressani, R., Bchar, M. and Viteri, F. (1958).
    Supplementation of cereal proteins with amino acids.
    J. Nutr., 66, 485-514.

Seidl, D., Jaffé, M. and Jaffé, W. G. (1969). Digestibility and
    proteinase inhibitory action of a kidney bean globulin.
    J. Agr. Food Chem., 17, 1318-1321.
Shukla, T. P. (1975). Cereal protein: chemistry and food applica-
    tions. CRC Rev. Food Sci. Nutr., 6, 1-77.
Silano, V. (1977). Factors affecting digestibility and availability
    of protein in cereals. In 'Nutritional Evaluation of Cereal
    Mutants', IAEA, Vienna, Austria.
Singleton, V. L. and Kratzer, F. H. (1973). Plant Phenolics.
    In 'Toxicants Occurring Naturally in Foods', Natl. Acad. Sci.,
    Natl. Res. Council, Washington, D. C., 309-345.
Stahmann, M. A. and Woldegiorgis, G. (1975). Enzymatic methods for
    protein quality determination. In 'Protein Nutritional Quality
    of Foods and Feeds, Part 1: Assay Methods - Biological,
    Biochemical, and Chemical', M. Friedman (Ed.), Marcel Dekker,
    New York, 211-234.
Subramanyan, V., Narayanarao, M., Rannarao, G. and Swaminathan, H.
    (1955). The metabolism of nitrogen, calcium and phosphorus in
    human adults on a poor vegetarian diet containing ragi.
    Brit. J. Nutr., 9, 350-357.
Sun, S. M. McLeester, R. C., Bliss, F. A. and Hall, T. C. (1974).
    Reversible and irreversible dissociation of globulins from
    Phaseolus vulgaris seed. J. Biol. Chem., 249, 118-123.
Swaminathan, M. S., Naik, M. S., Kaul, A. K. and Austin, A. (1970).
    Choice of strategy for the genetic upgrading of proteins in
    cereals, millets and pulses. In 'Improving Plant Protein by
    Nuclear Techniques', IAEA, Vienna, Austria, 165-183.
Swaminathan, M. S., Austin, A., Kaul, A. K. and Naik, M. S. (1969).
    In 'New Approaches to Breeding for Improved Plant Protein',
    IAEA, Vienna, Austria.
Tamir, M. and Alumont, E. (1969). Inhibition of digestive enzyme
    by condensed tannins from green and ripe carobs.
    J. Sci. Food Agric., 20, 199-202.
Van Buren, J. P. and Robinson, W. B. (1969). Formation of complexes
    between protein and tannic acid. J. Agric. Food Chem., 17,
    772-777.
Van Etten, C. H. and Wolff, I. A. (1973). Natural sulfur compounds.
    In 'Toxicants Naturally Occurring in Foods', Natl. Acad. Sci.,
    Natl. Res. Council, Washington, D. C., 210-234.
Wood, P. R., Waide, J. J., Cole, C. V. and Ross, C. (1969).
    Improving bean protein. Report Ninth Dry Bean Research
    Conference, ARS 74-50, U. S. Department of Agriculture,
    Washington, D. C.

14

METHODS FOR IMPROVING CEREAL PROTEIN QUALITY

Edwin T. Mertz

Department of Biochemistry

Purdue University, West Lafayette, Indiana 47907

ABSTRACT

Three methods for improving cereal protein quality are discussed.
Two older methods are supplmentation with limiting essential amino
acids and with protein concentrates high in those amino acids. The
most recent method (since 1964) is the replacement of the normal
cereal grain with its high lysine mutant counterpart. Three high
lysine cereals are now available, corn, barley, and sorghum. In animal feeding, least cost formulas will determine which of the three
improvement methods will be used. In human nutrition, cost, availability, palatability and acceptance are all equally important
factors.

In animals, pounds of gain per pound of feed will be the final
measure of cereal protein quality. In humans, especially preschool
children, the most important criterion will be the ability of the
improved cereal protein to build a strong immune defense system.
Animal studies show that protein quality is more important than
calories when calories are restricted to less than _ad libitum_ consumption. It is therefore essential that children restricted in
their total energy intake have the best cereal protein quality
possible to protect their immune system.

INTRODUCTION

The first limiting amino acid in all cereals is lysine (Jansen
and Howe, 1964). Because of this limitation, cereal proteins have
lower quality than animal proteins. Until 1964, nutritionists had
two methods for raising the protein quality of cereals. One was
to supplement the cereal with pure lysine (corn also needs tryp-

275

tophan). The other was to use a protein source that would supply additional quantities of lysine (and in the case of corn, tryptophan) in the diet.

In 1964, Mertz and coworkers showed that the lysine and tryptophan content of corn endosperm could be doubled by the introduction of the opaque-2 mutant gene (Mertz, Bates, and Nelson, 1964; Misra, Mertz, and Glover, 1975, 1976). After this discovery, plant breeders searched for similar mutations in the economically important cereal grains. Two high lysine types of barley were discovered. The first, a naturally occurring mutation from Ethiopia was discovered in 1968 by Munck and coworker (Munck, 1972). A chemically induced high lysine mutant of barley was also identified by Ingversen and coworkers (Ingversen, Koie, and Dahl, 1973). In addition, a high lysine mutant gene (hl) that improves protein quality and biological value of grain sorghum was found by Axtell and coworkers (Singh and Axtell, 1973). A chemically induced high lysine mutant of sorghum was also identified (Mohan and Axtell, 1974).

The distribution of amino acids in the endosperms of these three high lysine cereals are similar (Misra, Mertz, and Glover, 1976; Munck, 1972; Ingversen, Koie, and Dahl, 1973; Guiragossian, Chibber, Van Scoyoc, Jambunathan, Mertz, and Axtell, 1978). The lysine is almost doubled in the endosperm of all three cereals, and the tryptophan is doubled in the endosperm of corn. Feeding tests in animals show that the relative protein value of each of these mutant cereals is approximately twice that of their normal counterpart. In preschool children, kwashiorkor, a severe protein deficiency disease, has been cured with high lysine corn as the only source of protein (Byrnes, 1969; Reddy and Gupta, 1974).

Lysine in Animal Feeds. The weekly newsmagazine of the American Chemical Society (Anonymous, 1978) reported recently that the demand for feed grade lysine will probably double to about 2,500 metric tons annually in Central and South America by 1982. The lysine is used to supplement cereal grains in the diet of swine, poultry and beef. In the United States and Europe, protein supplements such as fish meal and soybean meal are added to cereals to supply the necessary additional lysine (and tryptophan) in animal diets. The high cost of these two protein supplements in Central and South America (and in parts of the Orient) is the main reason why lysine is able to compete as a supplement. Most of the lysine produced at the present time is made in Japan by fermentation methods, but a competitive process involving chemical synthesis is now on stream in that country. Present world production of pure lysine is estimated at 33,000 tons.

High Lysine Corn in Animal Feed. A study carried out by N. S. Hadley (Hadley, 1966) showed that whenever the price of soybean meal equals or exceeds twice the cost of corn, and the yield of high

lysine corn is at least 95% of normal hybrid corn, the farmer can
make a profit by feeding high lysine corn in place of normal corn
to swine. Since corn is deficient in both lysine and tryptophan,
the addition of pure lysine alone would not be as effective as using
high lysine corn which supplies both lysine and tryptophan. Therefore, in any situation where pure lysine becomes competitive with
soybean meal as a supplement in the rations of poultry, swine and
beef, there is a good probability that high lysine corn would also
be competitive. Animal nutritionists must compare the relative
cost of using high lysine corn versus pure lysine and tryptophan
to normal corn. Synthetic tryptophan is available commercially
but the cost is high. High lysine barley and sorghum would probably also be competitive under these conditions.

Better Quality Protein in Cereal Human Nutrition Taste, palatability and food preferences are extremely important in the nourishment
of humans. In animal production, weight gain per unit of food consumed is the primary measuring stick. Until recently, increase
in weight (and in stature) were the most important criteria for
evaluating nutritive value of foods for the preschool child. However, in a recent study carried out in Guatemala (Urrutia, Garcia,
Bressani, and Mata, 1976),preschool children receiving a diet of
normal maize fortified with soybean meal and lysine showed no significant differences in height and weight when compared with a
control group receiving unfortified normal maize. Nevertheless,
the group receiving the fortified maize showed a greater resistance
to disease and a lower death rate. Therefore, a more sensitive measure of cereal protein quality in the human in this authors opinion,
is its ability to improve the immune system.

Value of Better Quality Cereals in Low Calorie Diets. The question
has been raised as to how much, if any, benefit would be obtained
by fortifying cereal· grains with limiting amino acids, or breeding
cereals for better protein quality, if total food energy is in short
supply and children do not eat enough food. Rat studies carried
out by Jansen and coworkers (Jansen and Verberg, 1977) show that
the net protein ratio and the net protein utilization values obtained with lysine (and threonine) fortified bread fed at 70% of ad
libitum consumption were 1.5 to 2 times those obtained with unfortified bread, in spite of the fact that the latter rats consumed
25% more energy. In additional studies on rats, Jansen and coworkers (Jansen and Monte, 1977) showed that all parameters measured
in the offspring of dams fed lysine and threonine fortified bread
at 70% ad libitum consumption were significantly increased over
the values obtained in the offspring of dams fed unfortified bread
ad libitum even though they had consumed 13% less protein and
dietary energy during pregnancy and lactation periods. The parameters measured were weaning weight, and weight, protein, and DNA
of whole brain and major regions of the brain at weaning. These

studies in rats strongly suggest that nutritionists should make
every effort to improve the protein quality of cereal <u>even</u> <u>under</u>
<u>circumstances</u> <u>where</u> <u>the</u> <u>preschool</u> <u>child</u> <u>or</u> <u>preganant</u> <u>woman</u> <u>is</u> <u>not</u>
<u>consuming</u> <u>adequate</u> <u>amounts</u> <u>of</u> <u>food</u> (i. e., amounts recommended by FAO
to meet "normal" energy requirements). The data strongly suggest
that extra amounts of high quality cereal protein would be retained
in the preschool child and pregnant woman even when inadequate
levels of calories are consumed. Furthermore, the extra protein
retained would increase the immune defense of the child and make
him less susceptible to disease. It would also produce healthier
offspring in pregnant women.

CONCLUSIONS

Scientists and other health workers trained in human and in
animal nutrition now have three methods for improving the protein
quality of cereals. The cereal can be balanced with the first
limiting, and if necessary, the second limiting amino acid produced
in pure form by either fermentation or chemical synthesis. The
second method is to supplement the cereal with protein or proteins
which would supply the deficient amino acid(s). The third method
is to use one of the high lysine cereals available, (maize, barley,
and sorghum). There is also the possibility that combinations of
these three methods could be used effectively.

In animal feeding, the choice of the final diet mixture would
be based on least cost factors. In formulating improved cereal
foods for humans, factors such as palatability, acceptance, and
the ability of the improved cereal to increase the immune defense
mechanisms of the preschool child and the prenatal health of babies
would be of paramount importance.

REFERENCES

Anonymous (1978). Chem. and Eng. News, 56 (2), Jan 9, p. 15

Byrnes, F. C. (1969). A Matter of Life and Death. Rockefeller
    Foundation Quaterly, I, 4-20.

Guiragossian, V., Chibber, B. A. K., Van Scoyoc, S., Jambunathan,
    R., Mertz, E. T. and Axtell, J. D. (1978). Characteristics
    of proteins from normal, high lysine, and high tannin sorghums.
    J. Ag. Food Chem., 26, 219-223.

Hadley, N. S. (1966). Proceedings High Lysine Conference, Corn
    Industries Research Foundation, Corn Refiners Association,
    Washington, D. C., pp. 161-165.

Ingversen, J., Koie, B. and Doll, H. (1973). Induced seed protein
    mutant of barley. Experientia, 29, 1151-1152.

Jansen, G. R. and Howe, E. E. (1964). World problems in protein nutrition. <u>Am</u>. <u>J</u>. <u>Clin</u>. <u>Nutr</u>., <u>15</u>, 262-274.

Jansen, G. R. and Monte, W. C. (1977). Amino acid fortification of bread fed at varying levels during gestation and lactation in rats. <u>J</u>. <u>Nutrition</u>, <u>107</u>, 300-309.

Jansen, G. R. and Verburg, D. T. (1977). Amino acid fortification of wheat diets fed at varying levels of energy intake to rats. <u>J</u>. <u>Nutrition</u>, <u>107</u>, 289-299.

Mertz, E. T., Bates, L. S. and Nelson, O. E. (1964). Mutant gene that changes protein composition and increases lysine content of maize endosperm. <u>Science</u>, <u>145</u>, 279-280.

Misra, P. S., Mertz, E. T. and Glover, D. V. (1975). Studies on corn proteins. VI. Endosperm protein changes in single and double endosperm mutants of maize. <u>Cereal</u> <u>Chem</u>., <u>52</u>, 161-166.

Misra, P. S., Mertz, E. T. and Glover, D. V. (1976). Studies on corn proteins. IX. Comparison of the amino acid composition of Landry-Moreaux and Paulis-Wall endosperm fractions. <u>Cereal</u> <u>Chem</u>., <u>53</u>, 699-704.

Mohan, D. P. and Axtell, J. D. (1974). Chemically induced high lysine mutants in sorghum bicolor (L.) Moench. <u>Agronomy</u> <u>Abstr</u>., p. 66.

Munck, L. (1972). Improvement of nutritional value in cereals. <u>Hereditas</u>, 72, 1-128.

Reddy, V. and Gupta C. P. (1974). Treatment of kwashiorkor with opaque-2 maize. <u>Am</u>. <u>J</u>. <u>Clin</u>. <u>Nutr</u>., <u>27</u>, 122-124.

Singh, R. and Axtell, J. D. (1973). High lysine mutant gene (hl) that improves protein quality and biological value of grain sorghum. <u>Crop</u> <u>Sci</u>., <u>13</u>, 535-539.

Urrutia, J. J., Garcia, B., Bressani, R. and Mata, L. J. (1976). Report of the maize fortification project in Guatemala. <u>In</u> "Improving the Nutrient Quality of Cereals". II. Report of Second Workshop on Breeding and Fortification. Agency for International Development, Washington, D. C. 20523, pp. 26-68.

15

THE CURRENT STATUS OF BREEDING FOR PROTEIN QUALITY IN CORN

David Deutscher

Department of Agronomy, University of Missouri

Columbia, Missouri 65201, USA

ABSTRACT

The current rapid expansion of the human population on earth, particularly in the less developed countries, raises the possibility of widespread, serious malnutrition and starvation for many unless agricultural technology can intervene with appropriate answers to these problems. Plant breeders have been charged with developing varieties that will yield larger quantities of improved quality protein. Since the realization that maize having the opaque-2 gene has markedly improved protein quality, much work has been done in many areas of research to apply this discovery as well as to learn more about alternative methods to attain the same goals. This discussion will be a review of the advances so far attained by plant breeders in their efforts to develop maize with improved protein quantity and quality. Work concerning the utilization of mutant genes that improve protein quality and efforts at exploiting the naturally occurring variation for protein quality and quantity will be examined. Work that has been done in other related fields that has relevance to the protein improvement problem will also be examined. Screening and subsequent regeneration of tissue cultures as well as work concerning the biochemical energetics of yield and protein improvement will be examined in order to bring the problem of breeding for protein improvement into perspective. Finally, the corn industry's experience with improving protein quality and quantity will provide a basis for discussing the economic considerations of such improvement.

The basis for attempting to alter the quantity and quality of cereal proteins is the highly publicized, fashionable "protein problem" of the developing nations. More correctly characterized as the protein-calorie malnutrition problem, a comprehensive evaluation of the situation will show it to be complex and defying rigid numerical assessment. If all of the dietary protein available in the world today were equally distributed, everyone would have an adequate supply and a 70% surplus would remain (Hanson, 1974).

Despite these encouraging statistics, the protein-calorie malnutrition problem is not a myth but a reality to millions, primarily because of distribution inequities. Eighty percent of the world's dietary protein supply is consumed by 20% of the world's population that live in the highly developed industrialized nations. Within the developing countries, the remaining 20% of the world's dietary protein supply is divided among the remaining 80% of the world's population with richer people eating more protein than the poor. Among poor families, the working adults receive the most of the best food available. Individuals suffering from intestinal disease such as diarrhea or recovering from severe fevers like malaria, as well as young children and pregnant and nursing mothers, have an increased requirement for dietary protein. Considering these factors and conditions that have a bearing on protein-calorie malnutrition, it is evident that there exists a vast population of poor people living in the developing countries of the world that have a major malnutrition problem. The problem is enhanced by inadequate marketing and distribution patterns and low levels of sanitation and medical support. These people rely heavily on bulky, cheap, readily available foods that are relatively poor in protein quality and quantity as their major source of nourishment (Hanson, 1974; United Nations, 1973).

The improvement of the protein-calorie malnutrition problem is particularly suited to cereal improvement. Fifty percent of world dietary protein supplies come from cereals (wheat, maize, rice, sorghum, barley, etc.), 20% from legumes (mostly soybeans, dried peas, and dried beans), and about 30% from animal products (meat, milk, eggs, and fish). But in the developing countries of the world, 70% of the dietary protein is supplied by cereals (Glover, 1976; Hanson, 1974). Cereals are the most economical food supply readily available to the poor in the developing countries. The improvement of the protein quality and quantity in cereals probably offers the most economical method of improving dietary protein levels of the vulnerable groups in the developing countries without requiring any changes in dietary patterns or distribution procedures (Hanson, 1974).

Maize accounts for roughly 25% of the world production of protein obtained from all cereals. In the developing countries of Latin America, maize provides 50-60% of the dietary protein. Alterations in the quantity and quality of maize protein could have a significant impact on the protein-calorie malnutrition problem (Vasal, 1974).

Traditional maize varieties are not particularly desirable protein sources as are all other cereals. Cereal protein is low quality
because of the low levels of lysine and tryptophan. These essential
amino acids were shown to be the first and second limiting amino
acids, respectively, for maize fed to growing or finishing pigs
(Eggum, 1977). Other studies have shown the importance of these
essential amino acids in other non-ruminant animal and human nutrition.

The discovery nearly a decade and a half ago by Mertz and his
co-workers (Mertz, Bates, and Nelson, 1964) that the single gene
opaque-2 could drastically improve the quality of maize endosperm
protein, touched off a flurry of research, thought, and speculation
about solving the world's protein-calorie malnutrition problem
through the genetic manipulation of specific seed constituents. The
implicatons of a single, simply inherited, recessive gene that could
improve maize protein by increasing lysine levels 70% and and tryptophan levels 100% and increase the net protein utilization from
about 50% to 90% were great (Hanson, 1974). The distinctive endosperm phenotypic expression of the opaque-2 gene also provided a
rapid, cheap and accurate method of selecting genotypes with improved
protein quality.

Maize protein having nearly the net protein utilization of eggs
was hailed by the popular press as an answer to solving the protein
problems of the developing world and revolutionizing the swine industry in the U.S. But, despite the research and development that
has occurred since 1964, there still exists a vast protein problem
in developing countries and the U.S. swine industry still relies on
soybean meal as a protein source.

The improvement of cereal protein quality is a complex problem
that has generated a great deal of basic knowledge about plant
genetic systems and biochemistry, the economics of new crop development, and the complexities of developing countries; but no significant change has occurred in the world's ability to provide adequate
protein to those people targeted as vulnerable to protein deficiencies.

Although the discovery of the effects of the opaque-2 gene was
for the most part responsible for getting plant breeders interested
in developing crop varieties with improved protein quality and
quantity, other methods have been tried since then to attain the
same goals. The search for alternative methods of improving cereal
protein quality expanded as researchers learned that no single method would be adequate to solve such a complex problem. The areas of
interest that are currently being investigated include:
   (1) utilization of the opaque-2 gene,
   (2) utilization of "modifier" genes the alter the
       phenotypic expression of the opaque-2 gene,

(3) utilization of endosperm double-mutants,
(4) taking advantage of the naturally occurring
    variation in maize for protein and lysine
    levels, and
(5) the development of cell and tissue culture
    techniques and amino acid screening techniques
    that make possible the identification of specific
    amino acid overproducer mutants.

In 1964, Mertz (Mertz, Bates, and Nelson, 1964) reported that
the opaque-2 gene improved the protein quality of the maize endosperm. He associated the increased levels of lysine he observed
with a reduced zein fraction. About 40% of the protein in normal
corn is low quality zein but in opaque-2 maize, the zein fraction
is reduced to about 15%. It is now known that the lysine content
of various protein fractions is altered as well. The lysine in the
alkalai-soluble and residue protein is nearly doubled, as can be
seen in Table 1 (Frey, 1973).

The opaque-2 gene is a simply inherited, single gene that expresses its phenotype in the maize endosperm when it is in the
homozygous recessive condition. Whereas the normal corn kernel has
a hard, vitreous and shiny endosperm, the opaque-2 kernel is soft,
chalky and dull in appearance. This difference allowed the rapid
manipulation of this gene in backcross breeding programs so that

Table 1

Fractional distribution of protein and percents of lysine in

various protein fractions in opaque-2 and normal grain

(Frey, 1973)

Protein fraction	% Fraction of total protein		% Lysine content	
	Opaque-2	Normal	Opaque-2	Normal
Saline solution	21	6	2.1	1.8
Butanol solution	2	7	0.4	0.2
Ethanol solution	16	33	0.4	0.3
Alkali solution	39	27	4.1	1.7
Residue	18	22	6.2	2.8

it was possible to improve the protein quality of corn by a rapid visual screening procedure.

The agronomic effects of the opaque-2 gene were not as favorable as the nutritional aspects. Several serious agronomic problems are associated with opaque-2 varieties of maize. When compared to their normal counterparts, opaque-2 conversions have reduced yields, increased susceptibility to insect and disease pests and higher moisture content at maturity. In addition, the dull, chalky kernel phenotype is unacceptable to many maize-eating people and is not suited to modern processing procedures.

The most important agronomic fault of opaque-2 varieties of corn is their lower yielding ability. Grain yields of opaque-2 varieties are generally 10-15% lower than their normal counterparts and the yield component affected is the kernel test weight which is reduced 10-15% (Dudley, Alexander, and Lambert, 1975; Glover, 1976; Singh and Asnani, 1975). Agronomists believe that the lower test weight of the grain is due to loose packing of the starch particles in the endosperm (Singh and Asnani, 1975).

Maize breeders have put a great deal of effort into improving the serious agronomic shortcomings of opaque-2 varieties. Opaque-2 varieties with yields equivalent to their normal counterparts are sometimes reported, as in Table 2 (CIMMYT, 1976; Dudley, Alexander, and Lambert, 1975; Singh and Asnani, 1975) but, generally, opaque-2 varieties have more or less poorer yields than their normal counterparts. Table 3 gives the results of a uniform test of experimental opaque-2 hybrids conducted in four corn belt states (Iowa, Illinois, Indiana, Missouri) during 1973. This study indicated that the yields of the opaque-2 hybrids ranged from 50 to 94 quintels/ha. and that some of these experimentals gave yields that would be competitive with some of the better normal commercial hybrids. But on the average, the yields of these experimental opaque-2 hybrids range from 80% to 90% or slightly more of the normal hybrids (Glover, 1976).

Although opaque-2 versions of hybrid maize are generally considered to be lower yielding than their normal counterparts, Dudley (Dudley, Alexander, and Lambert, 1975) believes that there is cause for optimism concerning the improvement of yields in opaque-2 hybrids. In tests conducted in 1966, the near-isogenic opaque-2 versions yielded 85% of their normal counterparts on the average, while in 1967 the opaque types yielded 92% of their normal maize counterparts on the average. The eight highest yielding opaque-2 hybrids included in a 1972 test averaged yields that were 99% of that of six commercial dents included in the same test. The best yielding commercial dent exceeded the best opaque-2 by only 7% (Dudley, Alexander, and Lambert, 1975).

Table 2

Some populations having better performance in opaque-2 version

(Singh and Asnani, 1975)

Population	Version	Yield (g/plant)	Ear Length (cm)	Ear Diameter (cm)	Shelling (%)
Cuba 11J	Normal	45.3	14.8	3.5	64
	Opaque-2	50.3	16.1	3.5	66
Cuba V66	Normal	49.1	17.2	3.8	67
	Opaque-2	58.1	13.3	4.0	70
Waimea Dent	Normal	60.7	18.3	3.6	70
	Opaque-2	74.4	18.4	4.0	72
C.D.[1] at 5%		21.5	1.4	0.3	5

[1]C.D., critical difference

    Maize breeders are optimistic about improving the yields of opaque-2 hybrids and varieties. It is known that the opaque-2 gene interacts with different genetic backgrounds. When opaque-2 hybrids are reconstituted some are poor yielders while others compare favorably with their normal counterpart (Glover, 1976). It is believed that adequate variability is available to allow the improvement of quality traits and desirable agronomic characteristics of opaque-2 hybrids and varieties (Singh and Asnani, 1975). The occasional reports of opaque-2 hybrids yielding as well as their normal counterparts tends to support this conclusion, but the concurrent selection of quality traits and agronomic components adds another dimension to the program of a maize breeder attempting to develop improved protein quality maize.

    The dull, chalky appearance of the opaque-2 endosperm has been as serious a drawback as lower yields in getting opaque-2 hybrids into production. It is believed that an improvement of the classical endosperm phenotype of opaque-2 maize to that of normal maize, which is hard and vitreous, will be a significant factor in eliminating or at least improving the problems of consumer acceptance, insect and disease damage, poor milling characteristics and seed damage caused by harvesting and handling (Vasal, 1974).

Table 3

1973 data on opaque-2 hybrid uniform test[1]

(Glover, 1976)

Pedigree	Yield ave. q/ha[2]	L/P
H49^{cm}s x N28^{ht} check	103.5	3.07
Va43 x N28 o_2	94.0	4.49
(B37 x H84) x 00379-A o_2	92.0	4.64
Mo2^{rf} x K55 o_2	90.2	4.32
B37^{cm}s x N28^{ht} check	87.8	3.21
W64 x W117 o_2	50.5	4.74
(A632 x B14A) x C123 o_2	50.0	4.28
Mo2^{rf} x 33-16 o_2	49.5	4.06

[1]Conducted in four states (Illinois, Iowa, Indiana, Missouri)

[2]q = quintel = 100 kilo

When maize breeders started to convert inbred lines of maize to opaque-2 versions by backcross breeding procedures, they noted deviations from the expected phenotypic ratio of 3 normal kernels to 1 opaque-2 kernel in their recoveries. Kernels with varying proportions of vitreous endosperm tissue that could not be phenotypically classed as opaque-2 or normal were observed. This modification of the classical opaque-2 phenotype to a more vitreous endosperm type offered a possible solution to the problems associated with the soft opaque-2 endosperm.

The effects of the so-called "modifier" genes of the opaque-2 gene can be summarized from CIMMYT studies as follows (Vasal, 1974).

(1) Vitreousness in opaque-2 kernels is due to the action of modifying genes,
(2) vitreous kernels in general have a higher percentage of protein in the endosperm, and
(3) hard and soft fractions of modified phenotype opaque-2

kernels differ in protein content and quality. Small
differences are observed in some cases, however,
(4) protein fractions of different materials vary in the
way they are related as a result of modifier selections,
(5) Selection for modifiers can help increase vitreousness and kernel test weight.
(6) Grain size seems to be under the influence of modifiers
and is affected differently in different genotypes,
(7) Modifiers are complexly inherited. Additive gene
effects are more important than dominance in the
expression of kernel vitreousness.
(8) Reciprocal differences have been observed in crosses
between opaque and modified materials, suggesting
some degree of maternal influence in the expression
of this character.

Researchers at Purdue University have concluded that the
modifier genes that act on the expression of the opaque-2 gene are
heritable, tend to be recessive and in most sources probably involve more than one gene. The expression of modifier genes is
variable with different environments. Lower temperatures appear
to enhance the expression of the modified phenotype (Glover, 1976).

Dudley (Dudley, Alexander, and Lambert, 1975) and his co-
workers working with modifiers of opaque-2 have developed several
tentative models of the gene action, but none have been satisfactory
when extensively tested.

Handling the modified materials can be complicated because some
of the modified opaque-2 kernels do not have the level of protein
quality that truly opaque-2 kernels have. Investigators working
with the modified selections all emphasize the necessity of chemical
analysis to screen for modified opaque-2 kernels that have acceptable protein quality (Dudley, Alexander, and Lambert, 1975; Glover,
1976; Vasal, 1974).

Glover (Glover, 1976) at Purdue University has studied the
effects of selection for higher lysine content in modified opaque-
2 synthetics as well as the genetic and environmental stability of
the modified opaque-2 expression. He concluded that selection for
higher lysine content in these modified synthetics was effective
and remained stable through subsequent generations of random mating.
The degree of modification also remained stable indicating that
with the exception of outcrossing to normal maize, modified opaque-
2 varieties would maintain their nutritional quality as well as
their kernel modification when grown by the farmer.

While the genetic manipulation of opaque-2 modifier genes is
generally considered to be complex, two recent reports indicate that
more simply inherited modifiers may be available for maize breeders

to use. Glover (Glover, 1976) reports the discovery of an opaque-2 gene modifier that appears to be simply inherited, with some degree of dominance, that gives a vitreous kernel appearance. The phenotypic expression of the modifier varies in different backgrounds, but the modification does not significantly reduce the lysine levels from those of opaque-2. Illinois researchers report the isolation of a modifier complex (O1716) from an opaque-2 synthetic. The modified kernels have endosperm protein quality comparable to opaque-2 kernels but appear very similar to normal dent kernels (Dudley, Alexander, and Lambert, 1975).

It is probable that other modifiers of the opaque-2 gene will be found as the conversion of varieties, synthetics and inbreds to opaque-2 continues. With the modification of the chalky, dull appearance of opaque-2 kernels to a harder, more vitreous appearance, the problems of consumer acceptance, insect and disease infestation, and handling damage will probably be reduced but there is no evidence to date that modified opaque-2 varieties will have yields comparable to normal maize (Glover, 1976).

Other endosperm mutants of maize are known that alter the nutritional aspects of the grain. One in particular has become increasingly important to the problem of improving the nutritional quality and agronomic performance of opaque-2 maize. The sugary-2 opaque-2 endosperm double-mutant combination results in the improved vitreousness of opaque-2 maize without any loss of protein quality. The kernel density of the su_2o_2 combination is nearly as great as normal maize but the kernel size is considerably reduced. This double-mutant combination suppresses zein synthesis while raising lysine and protein values slightly above those of opaque-2 counterparts. Compared to its normal counterpart, sugary-2 opaque-2 maize has a higher oil content and approximately a 1% increase in germ size. The biological value of su_2o_2 maize is equal to or greater than that of opaque-2 maize (Glover, 1976).

The vitreous endosperm and the good protein quality associated with the su_2o_2 combination make this a desirable method of producing high quality protein maize. But even though the kernel density is improved, the lower yields associated with this double-mutant combination will probably retard its commercial acceptance until yields comparable with normal dent maize are realized.

So far, this discussion has centered around the opaque-2 gene as a method of improving the protein quality of maize. Even though modifier genes of the opaque-2 gene as well as the use of other endosperm mutants are considered, the opaque-2 gene has remained a relatively universal constant in maize protein improvement. Other methods of achieving the same goals in the absence of mutant endosperm genes are being investigated.

Exploiting the naturally occurring variation for lysine and protein content could be a method of improving the nutritional quality of maize without the associated problems of the opaque-2 kernel phenotype. In surveying the normal kernels obtained from 100 segregating families (ears) of the original random mated versions of two populations, Glover (Glover, 1976) found protein content to vary from 7.3 to 14.6%, lysine content to vary from 0.150 to 0.238%, and lysine as a percent of protein to vary from 1.26 to 2.28. He concluded that the variation for these traits is sufficient to insure some limited progress in selecting for protein quality in these normal populations.

Our research at the University of Missouri has attempted to take advantage of the variation for lysine percentage in whole grain from normal populations. Three open pollinated populations, Logan County Composite, Midland Yellow Dent, and Reid Yellow Dent were selected to undergo cyclic selection for increased lysine content. The results are shown in Table 4. Cyclic selection for lysine content of the whole grain was somewhat successful in Logan County Composite and Reids Yellow Dent. No change was observed in the Midland Yellow Dent. These results also show that year-to-year environmental variation can be greater than actual genetic variation for these traits suggesting that the separation of environmental and genetic variation will be difficult and will tend to keep progress by selection slow (Zuber, 1975).

The results also indicate that cyclic selection for lysine content resulted in a gradual increase in protein content, with the exception of Midland, which decreased between the 2nd and 3rd cycles. Correlation coefficients were calculated for each of the three cycles of selection. The results are shown in Table 5. Significant correlations were found between lysine and protein for all three cycles and the three populations. In all three populations, the magnitude of the r values decreased from the 1st to the 3rd cycles (Zuber, 1975).

Zuber (Zuber, 1976; Zuber 1975; Zuber and Helm, 1975) concluded that lysine content can be increased by cyclic selection in some populations of normal dent corn in the absence of endosperm mutants. Further evaluation of this work is needed to assess any changes in yield characteristics or biological value that may have occurred during selection for increased lysine content.

The developing technologies of cell and tissue culture techniques and amino acid screening techniques may provide agricultural scientists with the means to make the next quantum jump in breeding for improved protein quality. The use of these methods could allow the plant breeder to screen large populations of cell or tissue cultures or germinating whole kernels for specific amino acid over-producers.

Table 4

Results of recurrent selection for high lysine in normal-
endosperm corn grown in the same and different years
(Zuber, 1975)

	Percent Lysine		Percent Protein	
	diff. yr.	same yr.	diff. yr.	same yr.
LOGAN COMPOSITE				
original population	0.27	0.34	13.1	11.6
2nd cycle	0.40	0.35	13.7	13.0
3rd cycle	0.44	0.42	14.4	13.2
REID YELLOW DENT				
original population	0.26	0.29	12.3	10.8
2nd cycle	0.34	0.31	12.3	11.7
3rd cycle	0.36	0.34	12.0	12.1
MIDLAND YELLOW DENT				
original population	0.26	0.32	13.4	10.5
2nd cycle	0.35	0.32	13.6	12.9
3rd cycle	0.34	0.32	13.5	11.6

Table 5

Correlation coefficients between lysine and protein for
each of three cycles of recurrent selection for high lysine.
All correlation coefficients are significant at the 1% level
(Zuber, 1975)

	Logan	Reid	Midland
1st cycle	0.70	0.56	0.65
2nd cycle	0.57	0.41	0.49
3rd cycle	0.33	0.38	0.46

Based on biochemical studies of bacteria, it is believed that in higher plants the metabolic pathways for the synthesis of lysine, threonine, and methionine are under the control of end-product feedback inhibition and/or repression of enzyme synthesis. When lysine synthesis reaches its normal level, these control mechanisms come into operation to prevent the overproduction of lysine. If these control points were inactivated or bypassed, there would be an excess amount of the free amino acid in the tissue (Green, 1974; Nelson, 1975). Brock (Brock, Friederich, and Langridge, 1973) suggests that two mutations would be required in higher plants to by-pass the control mechanisms of lysine synthesis.

When maize cell or tissue cultures or germinating whole seeds are allowed to develop in a medium containing inhibitory levels of lysine and threonine, their growth is stopped. The presence of these amino acids in the media activates the metabolic control mechanisms in the developing tissue which then cannot develop further because of the absence of lysine, threonine or methionine synthesis. Tissues that continue to develop in the presence of lysine and threonine in the media would be expected to have mutated so that the control mechanisms are ineffective. The lack of control in the metabolic pathway for lysine should result in plants having the ability to overproduce lysine, threonine, or methionine (Green, 1974; Nelson, 1975).

This work is in the early stages of development. The isolation and subsequent regeneration of viable plants through this screening technique will allow further evaluation of this method. No data exists to date that indicates regenerated overproducer mutants will have improved nutritional characteristics of the grain without adversely affected agronomic traits.

As this discussion concerning methods of improving the nutritional quality of maize through breeding has developed, one issue has been a consistent factor in limiting the commercial acceptance of these nutritionally desirable strains of maize. Although modifier complexes of the opaque-2 gene and the endosperm double-mutant sugary-2 opaque-2 have been utilized to modify the soft, chalky endosperm phenotype of opaque-2 maize and restore many desirable agronomic characteristics, no breeder has had widespread success improving the yield characteristics of these strains of maize. As previously mentioned, some investigations have at times observed opaque-2 conversions that have yields equivalent to their normal counterparts. But these reports are not frequent enough to change the well-used rule of thumb that opaque-2 varieties yield from 10 - 15% less than their normal counterparts.

Mertz (Mertz, 1976) has stated that, "The breeder who attempts to breed for more protein quantity and quality in cereals is faced with an unfavorable interaction between these two variables and yield". Many investigators have found this relationship to exist in their protein quality improvement programs for maize. In the Illinois selection program for protein quality, Dudley (Dudley, 1973; Dudley, Lambert and de la Roche, 1976) reports that the mean protein level has increased 215% of the mean of the original population. However, the kernel size has decreased and a significant negative correlation between yield and percent protein and percent oil was found. Gains in breeding for nutritional improvement in other cereals have been associated with yield reductions (Mertz, 1976).

Recently Bhatia and Rabson (Bhatia and Rabson, 1976) considered the bioenergetics of breeding for protein improvement in cereals. They concluded that in cereals a 1% increase in the seed protein concentration would require about a 1% increase in net overall photosynthetic production. If the additional demand for photosynthate is not met by a photosynthetically more efficient plant, a depression in yield must occur. In modern cereal cultivars having a high level of photosynthetic efficiency as indicated by high grain yield, it may be very difficult to improve the nutritional quality of the grain without reducing yield.

The increased nitrogen requirement for producing more protein in the grain was also calculated. A 1% increase in grain protein concentration required a 6 to 11% nitrogen increase for grain protein stoichiometry alone, depending on the crop variety and the initial protein level. If the increased nitrogen requirement was not supplied by additional nitrogen fertilization, it must come from increased mobilization of nitrogenous materials from the leaves and/or the development of root systems that make more efficient use of available soil nitrogen (Bhatia and Rabson, 1976).

They also concluded that there was a higher energy cost for producing high lysine proteins than normal protein in both maize and barley. When comparing the high lysine mutant barley strain 1508 with the normal barley cultivar 'Eva', a maximum increase of about 2.5% in glucose requirement was needed to just alter the amino acid composition. Any additional protein production would require additional photosynthetic inputs.

Plant breeders intent on improving the protein quality and quantity of cereals must be aware of the costs involved. Reduced yields and increased nitrogen fertilizer requirements may be necessary costs of producing such crops. Until selection schemes that identify plants having the photosynthetic efficiency to produce top yields and improved nutritional quality are successful, it is unlikely that the general association of reduced yields and improved quality will be broken.

For monogastric animals, including man, the nutritional benefits
of improved protein quality cereals have been well documented and
discussed in other places, so there is no need here to do more
than repeat that those benefits have been illustrated. Such benefits
should make the acceptance of high lysine maize desirable for the
swine feeding industry which must rely on protein supplements and
to the maize-eating peoples of the developing world whose diets often
lack adequate protein. However, acceptance of opaque-2 varieties has
been extremely limited despite extensive research to correct undesirable agronomic characteristics.

Although nearly all countries having maize breeding programs
conduct research on opaque-2 maize, only Colombia, Mexico, the U.S.,
Brazil, India, and Nigeria have developed and released opaque-2
varieties for general cultivation. Experimental materials are
available in some other countries (Singh and Asnani, 1975; Vasal,
1974). Research and development of opaque-2 maize for commercial
purposes probably accounts for as little as 1% or less of the world
wide maize breeding efforts. The use of such maize has been limited
to regions where its price is supported at levels profitable to the
grower or to special contract production operations (Brown, 1975).

The negative association between maize yields and protein quality is probably the single most important factor limiting its
acceptance. Generally, there are no price incentives to produce
opaque-2 maize for commercial sale so that any yield reduction
associated with growing such maize would be costly to the farmer
growing it as a cash crop. As long as the yields of high lysine
maize are less than that of normal varieties, farmers will grow the
normal corn unless there is a premium paid for producing the high
lysine maize.

Swine feeders in the U.S. could find the nutritional benefits
of opaque-2 maize profitable despite some yield reduction. For
swine feeders who grow and use their own maize, high-lysine corn
can only be grown profitably as long as the savings in protein
supplement costs offset the yield reduction.

Using computer programming techniques and a variety of swine
ration inputs, as listed in Table 6, Mann (Mann and Scott, 1973)
calculated breakeven points for price premiums and yield reductions.
He proposed a low price set of dietary inputs and a high price set
of the same inputs to account for price fluctuations. He compared
two high lysine varieties. The better quality No. 1 variety had
0.49% lysine and 0.15 % tryptophan be weight and the poorer No. 2
variety had 0.38% lysine and 0.12% tryptophan by weight.

Table 6

Grain and protein supplement prices

(Mann and Scott, 1973)

	Prices	
	Low	High
Feed ingredient	Dollars per bushel or ton	Dollars per bushel or ton
Wheat	$1.06/bu.	$1.48/bu.
Barley	$ .97/bu.	$1.28/bu.
Oats	$ .62/bu.	$ .76/bu.
Sorghum	$ .90/bu.	$1.16/bu.
Corn	$ .95/bu.	$1.35/bu.
Soybean meal	$ 69/ton	$ 107/ton
Cottonseed oil meal	$ 67/ton	$ 97/ton
Menhaden fish meal	$ 137/ton	$ 202/ton
Linseed meal	$ 70/ton	$ 90/ton
Meat and bone scrap	$ 80/ton	$ 130/ton
Tankage	$ 84/ton	$ 112/ton
Blood meal	$ 100/ton	$ 165/ton
Alfalfa meal	$ 36/ton	$ 64/ton
Wheat bran	$ 35/ton	$ 60/ton
Distiller's dried solubles	$ 80/ton	$ 84/ton
Dried whey	$ 92/ton	$ 150/ton
Dried skim milk	$ 316/ton	$ 464/ton
Dicalcium phosphate	$ 88/ton	$ 88/ton
Steamed bone meal	$ 75/ton	$ 130/ton
Defluorinated rock phosphate	$ 67/ton	$ 71/ton
Ground limestone	$ 8/ton	$ 8/ton

Table 7

Breakeven yield of high-lysine corn needed as a percent
of regular yellow corn yield related to high-protein sources
(Mann and Scott, 1973)

Feed ingredient and price sets	Variety No. 1 opaque-2 corn	Variety No. 2 opaque-2 corn
Corn with all protein sources		
Low price set (Table 6)	91.9	95.3
High price set (Table 6)	92.0	95.4
Corn with soybean meal only as the high-protein source		
Low price set (Table 6)	90.2	94.2
High price set (Table 6)	90.6	94.5

Table 7 shows the breakeven points in yield above which it
would be profitable for a corn grower to produce that variety of
high lysine corn. No differences in per acre production costs were
assumed for the high lysine varieties. It should be noted that the
better quality high-lysine variety No. 1 has yield reduction breakeven points that are in the range of the yielding capabilities of
many opaque-2 varieties. A 10% yield reduction compared to normal
corn would be almost at the calculated breakeven point. Due to
the poorer quality of high lysine variety No. 2, less of a yield
reduction could be profitably tolerated.

It seems unlikely that many commercial opaque-2 varieties
would yield well enough to be profitable at this time. In a survey
of commercially grown opaque-2 corn grown in 1972, 1973, and 1974
in several locations, Kornegay (Kornegay et al., 1975) found protein and lysine values to be more like variety No. 2 than variety
No. 1. Nutritional values less than variety No. 2 were common. It
can be concluded that the 10% yield reduction of opaque-2 varieties
is still too great to allow profitable production under the
assumptions used in Mann's study.

Table 8

Breakeven yields of high-lysine corn as a percent of regular corn at selected higher prices of soybean meal
(Mann and Scott, 1973)

soybean meal	Variety No. 1 percent	Variety No. 2 percent
$120 per ton	88	93
$150 per ton	84	90
$175 per ton	80	88

The value of the protein source in normal corn rations for
swine has a bearing on the substitution values of high lysine
varieties in the diet. Table 8 considers the change in yield
reduction breakeven points when the cost of soybean meal rises.
Only under conditions of a high soybean meal cost to corn cost
ratio does it become realistically profitable for the swine feeder
to grow high lysine maize varieties (Mann and Scott, 1973).

Price premiums for high lysine corn in the market place are
really not relevant to current discussions of the profitability of
raising such maize. The massive problems of administering such
a premium will likely preclude such a program for quite some time.
The testing and identification of high lysine corn lots and their
subsequent separate handling and storage does not profitably lend
itself to current U.S. corn marketing procedures. Even if yields
of opaque-2 varieties were consistently equivalent to normal maize
varieties, only the swine feeder is likely to find growing high
lysine maize a profitable management practice.

The acceptance of opaque-2 varieties in the developing countries has also been very limited. It would seem that countries
with such a well-demonstrated protein-calorie malnutrition problem
would turn to those types of maize that offer the greatest possibility for improving the quality of the traditional diets. Such
has not been the case on a widespread scale. Yield reduction, insect and disease susceptibility, and the floury kernel phenotype
have all contributed to the reluctant use of opaque-2 maize. Sub-
sistence farmers are not easily convinced that nutritionally superior corn is worth a yield trade-off. Only in certain regions of
the Andean highlands is maize with a chalky endosperm phenotype
commonly used, so the unacceptability of the floury endosperm tex-

ture limits the acceptance of opaque-2 maize in areas traditionally accustomed to normal vitreous kernels. The researchers at CIMMYT believe that there will be no widespread acceptance of opaque-2 varieties or other nutritionally superior maize varieties until their agronomic characteristics and yielding capabilities are equivalent to maize varieties already being grown. The improved protein quality would be a bonus (CIMMYT, 1976).

In summary, several general comments can be made about the current status of breeding maize with improved nutritional quality. Maize breeders have shown the ability to dramatically alter the nutritional characteristics of maize. The opaque-2 gene has been the principle vehicle of this improvement but modifier complexes of the opaque-2 gene as well as other endosperm mutants are utilized to improve the agronomic characteristics of traditional opaque-2 varieties. Selection for improved protein quality in normal corn populations as well as new methods in the field of cell and tissue culture techniques may allow plant breeders to intensify the search for plants with nutritionally improved grain.

The negative association between yield and nutritional quality must be broken by plant breeders if improved maize varieties are to be widely accepted. Recent work has shown that this association may be very difficult to break and that additional inputs may be necessary to achieve high yielding, nutritionally superior maize varieties. Additional insight into the protein-calorie trade-off problem is provided by Hornstein and Leng of AID (Hornstein and Leng, 1976). They report that AID's Task Force on Corn, Sorghum and Millet recommended that breeders place primary emphasis on improving yields (Dudley, Alexander, and Lambert, 1975).

The need for nutritionally superior varieties of maize exists in much of the maize-eating areas of the developing world. Cut off from what we consider normal marketing and distribution patterns by poverty and ignorance, these people could benefit significantly by a nutritional improvement in the diet to which they are accustomed. They must decide for themselves what yield trade-offs will be acceptable for improved nutrition.

REFERENCES

Bhatia, C.R. and Rabson, R. (1976). Bioenergetic considerations in cereal breeding for protein improvement. Sci., 194, 1418-21.

Brock, R.D., Friederich, E.A. and Langridge, J. (1973). The modification of amino acid composition of higher plants by mutation and selection. In, 'Nuclear Techniques for Seed Protein Improvement', International Atomic Energy Agency, Vienna.

Brown, William L. (1975). Worldwide seed industry experience with opaque-2 maize. In, 'High-Quality Protein Maize', Dowden, Hutchinson and Ross, Inc., Stroudsburg, Pennsylvania.

Centro Internacional de Mejoramiento de Maize y Trigo (CIMMYT). (1976). CIMMYT Review 1976. El Batan, Mexico.

Dudley, J.W. (1973). Seventy generations of selection for oil and protein content in the corn kernel. Proceedings of the 28th Annual Corn and Sorghum Res. Conf., American Seed Trade Assoc., Washington, D.C.

Dudley, J.W., Alexander, D.E., and Lambert, R.J. (1975). Genetic improvement of modified protein maize. In, 'High-Quality Protein Maize', Dowden, Hutchinson and Ross, Inc., Stroudburg, Pennsylvania.

Dudley, J.W., Lambert, R.J. and de la Roche, I.A. (1976). Genetic analysis of crosses among corn strains divergently selected for percent oil and protein. Crop Sci., 17, 111-117.

Eggum, B.O. (1977). The nutritive quality of cereals. Cereal Res. Comm. 5, 153-157.

Frey, K.J. (1973). Improvement of quantity and quality of cereal grain protein. In, 'Alternative Sources of Protein for Animal Production', National Academy of Sciences, Washington, D.C.

Glover, D.V. (1976). Improvement of protein quality in maize. In, 'Improving the Nutrient Quality of Cereals. II. Report of Second Workshop on Breeding and Fortification', Agency for International Development, Washington, D.C.

Green, C.E. (1974). Application of tissue and cell culture techniques to corn breeding. Proceedings of the 29th Annual Corn and Sorghum Res. Conf., American Seed Trade Assoc., Washington, D. C.

Hanson, H. (1974). The role of maize in world food needs to 1980. In, 'Symposium Proceedings. Worldwide Maize Improvement in the 70's and the Role for CIMMYT', Centro Internacional de Mejoramiento de Maiz y Trigo. El Batan, Mexico.

Hornstein, I. and Leng, E. (1976). Opening remarks. In, 'Improving the Nutrient Quality of Cereals. II. Repeat of Second Workshop on Breeding and Fortification', Agency for International Development, Washington, D.C.

Kornegay, E.T., Hedges, J.D., Webb, K.E., Jr., Thomas, H.R., Baker, D.H., Carlisle, G.R., Harmon, B.G. and Jenson, A.H. (1975). Protein and amino acid evaluation of commercially grown opaque-2 corn. J. of Anim. Sci., 41, 1546-1554.

Mann, T.L. and Scott, J.T., Jr. (1973). An estimate of the aggregate demand for high-lysine corn by swine. University of Illinois Agricultural Experiment Station.

Mertz, E.T. (1976). Interactions between yield, protein and lysine in cereals. In, 'Improving the Nutrient Quality of Cereals. II.Report of Second Workshop on Breeding and Fortification', Agency for International Development, Washington, D.C.

Mertz, E.T., Bates, L.S., and Nelson, O.E. (1974). Mutant gene
    that changes protein composition and increases lysine content
    of maize endosperm. Sci., 145, 279-280.
Nelson, O.E. (1975). Breeding for protein quality in maize:
    current issues and problems. In, High-Quality Protein Maize',
    Dowden, Hutchinson and Ross, Inc., Stroudburg, Pennsylvania.
Singh, J. and Asnani, V.L. (1975). Present status and future
    prospects of breeding for better quality in maize through
    opaque-2. In, 'High-Quality Protein Maize', Dowden,
    Hutchinson and Ross, Inc., Stroudsburg, Pennsylvania.
United Nations, Protein Advisory Group. (1973). The protein
    problem. PAG Statement No. 20, March 1, 1973.
Vasal, S.K. (1974). Nutritional quality in maize. In,'Symposium
    Proceedings. Worldwide Maize Improvment in the 70's and the
    Role for CIMMYT', Centro Internacional de Mejoramiento de
    Maiz y Trigo. El Batan, Mexico.
Zuber, M.S. (1976). Breeding maize for protein quantity and
    quality. In, 'Improving the Nutrient Quality of Cereals.
    II. Report of Second Workshop on Breeding and Fortification',
    Agency for International Development, Washington, D.C.
Zuber, M.S. (1975). Protein quality improvement in maize. Proceed-
    ings of the 30th Annual Corn and Sorghum Res. Conf., American
    Seed Trade Assoc., Washington, D.C.
Zuber, M.S. and Helm, J.L. (1975). Approaches to improving protein
    quality in maize without the use of specific mutants. In,
    'High-Quality Protein Maize', Dowden, Hutchinson and Ross, Inc.,
    Stroudsburg, Pennsylvania.

16

IMPROVEMENT OF WHEAT PROTEIN QUALITY AND QUANTITY BY BREEDING

V. A. Johnson and P. J. Mattern

USDA, ARS, North Central Region and Agronomy Department

University of Nebraska, Lincoln, Nebraska 68583

ABSTRACT

Substantial genetic variability for grain protein content in wheat has been identified. In appropriate combinations known genes can increase protein content of wheat grain by 5 percentage points. Productive high protein experimental lines with good agronomic traits and satisfactory processing attributes have been identified. A high protein hard red winter variety developed in Nebraska was released for commercial production in 1975 under the name "Lancota". The high protein of Lancota resides entirely in the starchy endosperm portion of the kernel and is fully transmissible to white milled flour. The high protein of Lancota results from elevated NO_3 reductase activity, increased N-absorption by the roots, and more complete translocation of N to the grain. Despite strong environmental influence on wheat protein level, genes for high protein have been demonstrated to effectively increase protein content in many different production environments. Lysine % of protein decreases but lysine % of grain increases as protein is increased. Genetic variability for lysine of sufficient magnitude to overcome the normal depression of lysine % of protein as protein is increased has been uncovered. Experimental lines have been developed in the ARS-Nebraska program in which genes for high protein and high lysine were combined. The lines have been widely distributed for use in other breeding programs.

INTRODUCTION

Cereal grains comprise the most important source of calories and protein for mankind. Five cereal species, wheat, rice, corn, sorghum and millet, are especially important. Wheat and rice, according to estimates, together constitute dietary mainstays for nearly two-thirds of the world's four billion people.

Wheat protein has an imbalance of essential amino acids for its full utilization when wheat is the sole source of protein in human diets. Lysine is in shortest supply. Gliadin and glutenin which comprise most of wheat protein, are notably poorer in lysine than the albumins and globulins which constitute the remaining 10-15% of the wheat protein. The proportions of these 4 solubility fractions largely account for differences in the amino acid composition of the cereal grains (Neurath and Bailey, 1954).

Genes that affect the amount of protein and/or its amino acid composition have been identified in all the major cereal food species. Associated significant enhancement of nutritional quality has been demonstrated for these genetic changes in quantity and composition of the protein in most cases. Progress in improving the quantity and quality of protein in the grain of wheat at the University of Nebraska since the authors last reported to the American Chemical Society in 1971 at its symposium on seed proteins, will be reviewed (Johnson et al., 1972).

GENETIC VARIABILITY FOR PROTEIN AND LYSINE

The World Wheat Collection maintained by the U. S. Department of Agriculture contains more than 20,000 entries. Common and durum wheats (<u>Triticum</u> <u>aestivum</u> L. and <u>Triticum</u> <u>durum</u>), the cultivated economically important species, comprise most of the collection. The University of Nebraska Wheat Quality Laboratory has systematically analyzed all wheats in the Collection, except the most recent accessions, for protein and lysine. The genetic component of total variation for protein was determined to be 5 percentage points (Vogel et al., 1975). In contrast to the substantial amount of protein variation, genetic variation for lysine per unit protein was only 0.5 percentage point, approximately 1/3 of the 1.5 percentage points increase needed to bring lysine into reasonable balance with other essential amino acids in wheat protein.

Genes with major effect on lysine have been identified in maize, barley, and sorghum, all of which are diploid species. Our failure to uncover similar genes in hexaploid common wheats suggested possible genomic masking of such genes. We have now

largely ruled out this possibility based on our analyses of wheats
in the T. durum and T. monococcum collections. The range of variation for lysine in these tetraploid and diploid groups was similar to that demonstrated for the hexaploid common wheats.

RELATIONSHIP OF PROTEIN AND LYSINE

The amount of lysine in wheat protein is influenced by the
level of protein (Vogel et al., 1973). The relationship is negative and non-linear. The protein content of wheat commonly varies
from 8% to as much as 20%. Lysine per unit protein ranges from
2.5% to 3.5%. Increases in protein content from 8% to 15% are
associated with pronounced depression of lysine per unit protein
(Figure 1). Further increases of protein above 15% produce little,
if any, further depression of lysine. We have determined that 52%
of the variation in lysine per unit protein among the common wheats
in the World Collection can be attributed to variation in protein
content. Clearly then, unadjusted lysine comparisons among wheats
that differ significantly in protein content (in the 8-15% range)
would be invalid for detection of genes controlling lysine level.

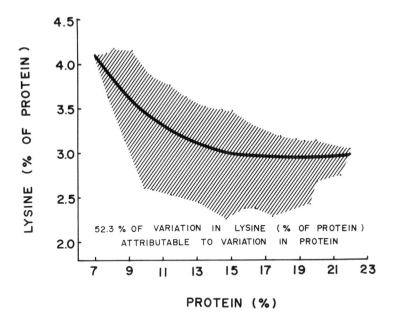

Figure 1. Curvilinear regression of lysine per unit protein
on protein and the range of dispersion of lysine values about the
regression line computed from the analyses of 12,613 common wheats
in the USDA World Collection.

In contrast to the depression of lysine per unit protein associated with increased protein content, lysine expressed as % of
grain weight increases with increased protein level (Figure 2).
This suggests that the depression of lysine per unit protein associated with higher protein content is not proportionate to the
lysine increase in wheat grain directly attributable to increased
protein content. On the basis of the relationship shown in figure
2 it is readily apparent that the lysine content of wheat grain
can be effectively increased by increasing its protein content.

Valid comparisons of lysine among wheats that differ in protein content require the removal of the effect of protein level on
lysine per unit protein. We now routinely utilize the curvilinear
negative regression of lysine per unit protein on protein shown in
figure 1 to adjust the lysine values to a common protein level.
The procedure largely removes the direct effect of level of protein on lysine per unit protein. It has permitted us to effectively select for elevated lysine among hybrid progenies differing significantly in protein content.

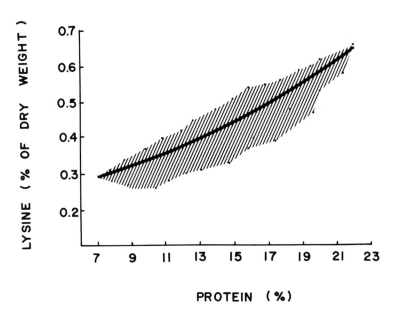

Figure 2. Curvilinear regression of lysine per unit grain
weight on protein and the range of dispersion of lysine values
about the regression line computed from the analyses of 12,613
common wheats in the USDA World Collection.

Changes in the protein content of wheat grain result in shifts in the 4 protein solubility fractions that comprise the protein. The proportion of water- and salt-soluble albumins and globulins is highest in low protein wheats. Higher protein content results in larger proportions of the glutenin and gliadin fractions. The albumin and globulin fractions contain significantly higher lysine than do the latter fractions. We believe this to largely account for observed depression of lysine per unit total protein with increased protein content.

Known genetic variation for lysine in wheat, although limited, is of sufficient magnitude to fully compensate for the lysine depression normally associated with increases in protein content. We have successfully developed experimental high protein wheats in which the lysine per unit protein is equal to that of low protein varieties by utilizing known genetic sources of elevated lysine in our hybridization program (Table 1). Note that there is no depression of actual lysine in 3 lines that are 1.8-4.6 percentage points higher in protein than the check variety 'Centurk'.

GENETIC SOURCES OF HIGH PROTEIN AND HIGH LYSINE

Genetic potential for elevated protein has been identified in numerous wheats. They include:

TABLE 1

Experimental lines with combined high protein and normal lysine grown at Lincoln, Nebraska in 1975.

Variety or line	Plot no.	Plot yield g	Seed rating	Protein content %	Lysine per unit protein %
Centurk	9081	309	Good	14.5	2.9
CI13447//Lcr/At 66/Cmn	9075	258	Good	17.3	3.0
At 66/Cmn//CI13449	9147	309	Good	16.3	3.0
Nap Hal/Atlas 66	9167	200	Medium	19.1	3.0

<u>Growth habit</u>

Atlas 50 (CI12534)   intermediate
) same genes
Atlas 66 (CI12561)   intermediate
Male Fertility Restorer (NB542437)   winter
Nb/4/Agrus/7*Thatcher/3/2*Hume (SD69106)   "
Hybrid English (CI6225)   "
Nap Hal (PI176217)   spring
Cirpiz (PI166859)   winter
Velvet (PI283864)   "
Favorit (Romania)   "

Only a few wheats with proven potential for elevated lysine
have been identified. Those most prominently used in the ARS-
Nebraska program are:

    Nap Hal (PI176217)   spring
    Norin 10/Brevor//50-3 (CI13449)   winter
    Norin 10/Brevor//25-15//Rex/Rio (CI13447)   "

Nap Hal is of particular interest for its combined elevated protein and lysine.

BREEDING PROGRESS FOR HIGH PROTEIN

We have successfully transferred genes for high protein from
Atlas 66 to productive, agronomically acceptable high quality hard
red winter wheat varieties. One such variety 'Lancota' was released to growers in 4 states in 1975. In Nebraska performance
trials in 1973 and 1974 'Lancota' was equal in yield to the popular 'Centurk' and 'Scout 66' varieties and it produced grain with
1.5 percentage points higher protein content than Centurk and
Scout 66 (Table 2).

Lancota has the genetic potential to produce grain with 2
percentage points higher protein than most other varieties grown
in the hard winter wheat region. Lancota and Centurk were evaluated in 16 paired test plots at Lincoln, Nebraska in 1975. Lancota was consistently somewhat higher in yield than Centurk and
produced grain with 2 percentage points higher protein content
than Centurk (Table 3). Because Lancota carries no genes for
elevated lysine its higher protein content results in an average
lysine depression of 0.2 percentage point -- the approximate depression that would be predicted from the regression of lysine on
protein shown in Figure 1.

Nap Hal also has been used extensively in crosses at Nebraska
as a genetic source for high grain protein. The cross of Nap Hal/

TABLE 2

Performance of Lancota in Nebraska
statewide trials in 1973 and 1974.

Variety	C.I. No.	Grain yield (q/ha)			Protein content (%)[1]		
		1973	1974	2-yr. $\bar{x}$	1973	1974	2-yr. $\bar{x}$
Lancota	17389	28.6	32.6	30.6	15.5	15.0	15.3
Centurk	15075	29.3	32.6	31.0	13.9	13.7	13.8
Scout 66	13996	29.3	31.3	30.3	13.9	13.8	13.9

[1]Dry weight basis

Atlas 66 produced progeny rows significantly higher in protein
content than either parent variety and much higher in protein than
ordinary varieties (Table 4). This suggests different genes for
high protein in Atlas 66 and Nap Hal which function additively
(Johnson et al., 1973). Note that progeny rows were recovered
that approach the Atlas 66 parent in yield and are 3 to 4 percentage points higher in protein content than either Atlas 66 or Nap
Hal. They range from 4 to 7 percentage points higher in protein
than the Centurk variety but are less productive than Centurk.
In each of the progeny rows the elevated lysine of the Nap Hal
parent was recovered in combination with very high protein.

Other hybrid combinations also have provided evidence of the
existence of many different genes for high protein in wheat. One
of these, Favorit/5/Cirpiz//Jang Kwang/4/Atlas 66/Comanche/3/Velvet
produced highly promising progeny rows shown in Table 5. The
progeny rows exceeded Centurk and Lancota in yield. They produced
grain that averaged 19% protein compared with only 15.6% for Centurk and 17.5% for Lancota. Additionally, they were substantially
shorter in height than the check varieties and produced excellent
seed with good dough-mixing properties. The same lines grown under irrigation at Yuma, Arizona in 1976 again were comparable in
yield, were higher in protein content and produced larger seed
than Centurk, Lancota and CI13449 (Table 6). Lysine content of
the lines was 3.0% or higher.

Early protein research at Nebraska implicated the internal
nitrogen transport system of the wheat plant in the high grain

TABLE 3

Grain yield and protein content of Centurk and
Lancota winter wheat varieties in paired
plot comparisons at Lincoln, Nebraska, 1975.

	Centurk				Lancota		
Protein	Lysine		Yield	Protein	Lysine		Yield
	Adj.	Unadj.			Adj.	Unadj.	
%	%	%	q/ha	%	%	%	q/ha
15.3	3.3	3.1	40.7	16.6	3.0	2.8	45.7
15.6	3.1	2.9	36.2	17.6	2.9	2.7	40.8
16.1	3.1	2.9	37.0	17.8	2.9	2.6	37.7
16.1	3.1	2.9	33.8	17.1	2.9	2.7	38.0
16.1	3.0	2.9	34.1	17.9	2.9	2.7	33.5
15.3	3.2	3.0	36.6	17.9	2.9	2.7	39.2
15.9	2.9	2.7	33.2	17.4	2.9	2.7	38.2
15.4	3.2	3.0	35.2	17.1	2.9	2.7	35.2
16.0	2.8	2.6	35.3	17.7	3.0	2.8	34.9
15.8	3.2	3.0	32.4	17.7	2.9	2.7	28.9
15.3	3.3	3.1	38.3	16.7	3.0	2.8	43.0
15.6	3.2	3.0	35.6	17.7	2.9	2.6	37.3
15.0	3.1	3.0	37.9	17.3	2.8	2.5	40.0
15.6	3.2	3.0	38.8	17.6	2.9	2.7	36.5
14.9	3.0	2.9	37.6	17.8	2.9	2.7	38.7
15.2	3.2	3.1	42.9	17.7	2.8	2.6	39.9
16.2	3.1	2.9	34.7	17.6	2.7	2.5	37.3
15.6	3.2	3.0	25.2	17.5	2.9	2.7	29.9
$\bar{x}$=15.6	3.1	2.9	35.9	17.5	2.9	2.7	37.5

protein phenomenon. Our data indicated that high protein lines
from Atlas 66 crosses translocated foliage nitrogen to the grain
more efficiently and more completely than ordinary varieties
(Johnson et al., 1969). We postulated that, if elevated grain
protein content results from more efficient and complete nitrogen
translocation, phenotypic expression of high protein genes could
be expected on low fertility as well as high fertility soils. We
have been able to substantiate this in subsequent Nebraska and international experimentation (Table 7) (Johnson et al., 1973). In
trials on low fertility soils of central and western Nebraska conducted over a 3-year period, high protein CI14016 (derived from
an Atlas 66 cross) was equal to in yield and maintained a 2 percentage points protein advantage over the 'Lancer' variety in a
wide array of soil fertility levels.

TABLE 4

Grain yield, protein, and lysine content of
selected varieties and F_7 lines from Nap Hal/Atlas 66
grown at Yuma, Arizona in 1975.

Population	No.	Protein (%)	Adj. lysine (% of protein)	Grain yield (q/ha)
Nap Hal/Atlas 66	13	16.8 (16.7-19.7)	3.3 (3.2-3.4)	38 (27-60)
Nap Hal	3	13.0 (12.7-13.4)	3.3 (3.2-3.4)	29 (17-35)
Atlas 66	3	14.4 (14.0-14.7)	3.1 (3.0-3.1)	63 (53-72)
Centurk	3	10.5 (10.0-10.8)	2.9 (2.7-3.0)	58 (40-68)
Lancota	3	13.9 (12.9-15.3)	3.0 (3.0-3.1)	78 (44-96)

Both Atlas 66 and Nap Hal exhibit elevated foliage nitrate reductase activity compared to varieties with ordinary grain protein
content. The reduction of NO_3 is believed to be a rate-limiting
step in plant nitrogen metabolism. If so, high protein wheat varieties also must exhibit high capability for NO_3 reduction. We
have recently determined that the high protein Lancota variety derived from Atlas 66 combines elevated NO_3 reductase activity with
higher soil nitrogen absorption and the capability to translocate
a higher percentage of the absorbed nitrogen to its grain than the
Lancer variety with which it was compared.

BREEDING PROGRESS FOR ELEVATED LYSINE

The ARS-Nebraska breeding program has mainly utilized Nap Hal
and CI13449 as genetic sources of elevated lysine. Each variety
consistently produces lysine levels that average from 0.3 to 0.5
percentage point or 10 to 15% higher than that of ordinary varieties.
The elevated lysine of CI13449 resides mainly in the starchy endosperm of the grain whereas that of Nap Hal is in the aleurone layer
(Table 8) (Johnson, 1976).

TABLE 5

Promising high protein experimental winter wheats grown
in unreplicated plots at Lincoln, Nebraska in 1975.

Pedigree or name	Plot no.	Plant height (cm)	Seed rating[1]	Grain yield (q/ha)	Grain protein content (%)	Mixing Time (min)	Mixing Tolerance
Centurk (check)	x̄ of 18 plots	102	G	35.9	15.6	3-2/3	4
Lancota (check)	"	97	VG	37.5	17.5	3-1/3	3
Favorit/5/Cirpiz// Jang Kwang/4/At 66/ Cmn/3/Velvet	11345	86	VG	39.6	19.1	3-2/3	4
"	12288	84	VG	41.4	18.9	3	4
"	12291	81	G-VG	41.0	19.8	3-2/3	4
"	12293	84	VG	41.1	19.3	3-2/3	4
"	12297	81	VG	42.0	19.1	3	3+
"	12312	81	VG	39.0	19.1	4	4
"	12327	86	VG	41.0	18.7	4	4
"	12332	84	VG	41.6	18.9	4	4-
"	12335	86	Exc.	41.9	18.5	4	4-

[1]G, VG, and Exc. = good, very good, and excellent, respectively.

TABLE 6

Performance of promising new high protein lines
evaluated in duplicate nursery plots at Yuma, Arizona in 1976.

Variety or Pedigree	Plot number	Yield	100-kernel weight	Protein	Lysine (% of protein)	
					Unadj.	Adj.
		q/ha.	g	%	%	%
Centurk	x̄ of 14 plots	54	3.6	11.6	3.3	3.2
Lancota	"	45	3.7	12.9	3.2	3.2
CI13449	"	50	3.1	12.1	3.3	3.4
Favorit/Cirpiz/ Jang Kwang/At 66/ Comanche/Velvet	343	51	4.5	14.3	3.2	3.3
"	436	48	4.5	14.3	3.2	3.3
"	437	48	4.5	14.6	3.1	3.2
"	439	49	4.6	14.2	3.2	3.3
"	444	51	4.6	14.1	3.2	3.4
"	457	50	4.3	14.3	3.1	3.2
"	459	49	4.6	14.6	3.0	3.2
"	460	54	4.5	14.2	3.0	3.1
LSD .05		12.3	--	--	--	--

TABLE 7

Mean yield and protein responses of CI14016 and
Lancer wheats to nitrogen fertilizer at
selected low fertility test sites in Nebraska
in 1969 and 1970.

Nitrogen applied	Grain yield		Protein content	
	Lancer	CI14016	Lancer	CI14016
kg/ha	q/ha	q/ha	%	%
0	25.9	25.8	10.8	12.5
22.5	29.9	27.4	11.2	13.3
45.0	31.4	29.5	11.8	14.0
67.5	31.1	30.6	12.6	14.9
90	31.1	30.3	13.2	15.4
112.5	30.7	30.5	13.6	15.8
135	30.2	31.1	14.0	16.3
LSD$_{.05}$	1.1	1.1	0.3	0.3

We have identified selections from the cross Nap Hal x
CI13449 higher in lysine than either parent variety (Table 9).
In several lines the elevated lysine was combined with the Nap
Hal grain protein level and with high grain yield.

The Nap Hal x CI13449 lines were evaluated internationally
in 1975 and 1976 as entries in a High Protein-High Lysine International Observation Nursery. Seed from harvested rows was analyzed for protein and lysine in the Nebraska laboratory. If
sites were used as replications, highly significant varietal differences both in protein and lysine were demonstrable (Table 10)
(Johnson et al., 1977). The Nap Hal/CI13449 lines also were the
highest in lysine and the most productive lines in a replicated
nursery at Yuma, Arizona.

TABLE 8

Protein and lysine contents of whole grain, endosperm, and non-endosperm fractions of 4 wheat varieties grown at Yuma, Arizona in 1973.

Variety	Protein content[1](%)			Lysine content (% protein)		
	Whole grain	Endosperm fraction	Non-endosperm fraction	Whole grain	Endosperm fraction	Non-endosperm fraction
Nap Hal	19.6	18.9	24.5	3.1	2.5	4.6
Atlas 66	19.4	19.3	19.8	2.8	2.5	4.4
CI13449	15.5	14.5	19.6	3.1	2.8	4.4
Centurk	15.4	15.0	19.6	3.0	2.5	4.5
LSD.05	1.0	0.9	1.0	NS	NS	NS

[1]Dry weight basis

TABLE 9

Grain yield, protein, and lysine content of
selected varieties and F$_6$ lines from Nap Hal/
CI13449 grown at Yuma, Arizona in 1975.

Population	No.	Protein (%)	Adj. lysine (% of protein)	Grain yield (q/ha)
Nap Hal/CI13449	18	12.7 (12.0-14.8)	3.5 (3.4-3.6)	58 (25-84)
Nap Hal	4	13.0 (12.7-13.6)	3.3 (3.2-3.4)	25 (16-32)
CI13449	4	10.5 (10.2-11.3)	3.2 (3.1-3.3)	62 (51-79)
Centurk	4	10.1 (9.8-10.4)	2.9 (2.8-3.1)	46 (33-55)
Lancota	5	13.1 (12.7-14.2)	3.1 (2.9-3.3)	84 (81-90)

TABLE 10

Average protein and lysine content of selected
high protein-high lysine experimental lines
grown at 11 test sites in 10 countries in 1975.

Variety or Pedigree	Plot no.	Protein %	Lysine % of protein
Centurk	$\bar{x}$ of 2 plots	14.3	3.0
Nap Hal/At 66	219	17.5	3.0
"	180	17.5	3.0
"	220	16.9	3.0
Nap Hal/CI13449	171	16.8	3.2
"	194	16.4	3.2
"	173	16.2	3.2
"	207	16.0	3.2
LSD$_{.05}$		1.2	0.11

OUTLOOK

The bio-energy implications of changing cereal grain protein concentration by plant breeding recently has been examined by researchers at the IAEA in Vienna, Austria (Bhatia and Rabson, 1976). They have shown that increased imputs of carbon assimilates and nitrogen are necessary to increase protein concentration in cereal grains while maintaining high yields. Presumably, such imputs would be increasingly difficult to achieve in the new high yielding varieties when the environment for full expression of their high yield potential is provided. However, most of the world's wheat production is from rain-fed areas where environmental constraints cause yields to be relatively low and the genetic yield potential of the varieties grown is seldom fully expressed. We believe that in these sub-optimal environments, increased bio-energy requirements of higher grain protein would not constitute a breeding barrier.

Insurmountable genetic linkages of high protein genes in wheat with undesirable agronomic and quality traits have not been uncovered in our research. Within the yield ranges normally encountered in the bread wheat area of the U. S. A. higher grain protein content has not proven to be incompatible with high yield. Lancota is an example. Neither have we found incompatibility of the protein genes from Atlas 66 with acceptable milling and bread-making characteristics. Again the Lancota variety serves as an example. Commercial millers and bakers have rated the processing qualities of Lancota as entirely acceptable to excellent in all respects. It has been suggested that short stature in wheat may be incompatible with high protein (McNeal et al., 1971). We have been unable to demonstrate this within the plant height range of our experimental materials. Note in Table 5 that the very high protein selections from Favorit//Cirpiz/Yang Kwang/Atlas 66/Cmn/ Velvet all have shorter straw than Lancota and Centurk.

The utility of genes for high protein with which we are working in Nebraska appears to be high. Baked products and pasta, the forms in which most wheat is consumed in the U. S., are prepared from white milled flour which carries the starchy endosperm fraction of the wheat kernel. We find that the effect of the protein genes from Atlas 66 resides entirely in the starchy endosperm and, therefore, is transmitted in its entirety to white milled flour (Table 8). In the case of Nap Hal the effect is found both in the starchy endosperm and non-endosperm (bran) milling fractions. Since endosperm constitutes more than 80% of the wheat kernel, it is unlikely that high protein from any source, as measured by whole kernel analysis, would be confined to the bran milling fraction.

REFERENCES

Bhatia, C. R. and Rabson, R. (1976). Bio-energetic considerations
    in cereal breeding for protein improvement. Science, 194, 1418.

Johnson, V. A. (in press) Wheat protein. Proc. Int. Symposium
    on Genetic Control of Diversity in Plants, Lahore, Pakistan,
    1976.

Johnson, V. A., Dreier, A. F., and Grabouski, P. H. (1973). Yield
    and protein responses to nitrogen fertilizer of two winter
    wheat varieties differing in inherent protein content of their
    grain. Agron. J. 65:259-263.

Johnson, V. A., Mattern, P. J., and Schmidt, J. W. (1972). Genetic
    studies of wheat protein. Chapter 9. In 'Symposium: Seed
    Proteins', G. E. Inglett (Editor). Avi Publishing Company,
    Inc.

Johnson, V. A., Mattern, P. J., Schmidt, J. W., and Stroike, J. E.
    (1973). Genetic advances in wheat protein quantity and com-
    position. Proc. 4th Int. Wheat Genetics Symposium. Missouri
    Agr. Exp. Sta., Columbia, MO. 547-556.

Johnson, V. A., Mattern, P. J., Whited, D. A., and Schmidt, J. W.
    (1969). Breeding for high protein content and quality in
    wheat. Proc. IAEA/FAO Panel on New Approaches to Breeding
    for Plant Protein Improvement, Rostanga, Sweden. 29-40.

Johnson, V. A., Mattern, P. J., Wilhelmi, K. D., and Kuhr, S. L.
    (in press). Seed protein improvement in common wheat (Triti-
    cum aestivum L.): opportunities and constraints. Proc. 4th
    Res. Coordination Meeting, FAO/IAEA/GSF Seed Protein Improve-
    ment Program, Baden, Austria, 1977.

McNeal, F. H., Berg, M. A., Brown, P. L., and McGuire, C. F. (1971).
    Productivity and quality response of five spring wheat geno-
    types, Triticum aestivum L. to nitrogen fertilizer. Agron.
    J. 63:908-910.

Neurath, H., and Bailey, K. (1954). Proteins. 1st edition.

Vogel, K. P., Johnson, V. A., and Mattern, P. J. (1973). Results
    of systematic analyses for protein and lysine composition of
    common wheats (Triticum aestivum L.) in the USDA World Col-
    lection. Nebr. Res. Bul. 258. 27 pages.

Vogel, K. P., Johnson, V. A., and Mattern, P. J. (1975). Re-
    evaluation of common wheats from the USDA World Wheat Col-
    lection for protein and lysine content. Nebr. Res. Bul. 272.
    36 pages.

17

PROTEIN QUALITY OF INDUCED HIGH LYSINE MUTANTS IN BARLEY

Bjørn O. Eggum

National Institute of Animal Science

Rolighedsvej 25, DK-1958, Copenhagen, Denmark

ABSTRACT

Evidence of high-lysine gene sources in barley derived from spontaneous and induced mutations has been presented. In addition barley sources considered to be "normal" also differ in lysine content. Changes in lysine concentrations invariable results in changes in other amino acids in barley protein. Protein fractions are altered in several mutant barleys and differ also in so called "normal barleys". The fractions in the normal barleys are probably more dependent upon environmental conditions than in mutant barleys.

It is clearly demonstrated with chemical analyses and biological experiments with rats, poultry and pigs that high-lysine cultivars are superior in nutritive quality than their low-lysine isotypes. However, it appears that most of the lysine genotypes possess reduced grain weight and lower grain yield. This is of course unfortunate as an adequate supply of food appears to be the number one nutritional priority in the world today. This does not mean, however, that protein improvement would be of no practical value under conditions of marginal energy deprivation. The literature reviewed suggests that protein improvement would likely be of value under these conditions.

INTRODUCTION

Concerted efforts on the genetic upgrading of the nutritional quality of cereal protein were initiated only during the last decade following the discoveries of Opaque-2 (Mertz et al. 1964) and Floury-2 genes (Nelson et al. 1965) in maize. The lead given by the

Purdue group was soon followed by an exclusive search for nutritionally superior genotypes in the world cereal germ plasm collections.
This resulted in the identifications of Opaque-7 (McWhirter, 1971)
and brittle genes (Misra et al. 1972) in maize, Hily and Hiproly
genes conferring higher lysine or/and higher protein barley (Munck
et al. 1970) and high lysine genes in two Ethiopian sorghum lines
possessing higher protein (Singh and Axtell, 1973).

Studies with different varieties of barley (Eggum, 1970; Munck
et al. 1971; Thomke, 1970; Toft Viuf, 1972) have shown that there
is a negative correlation between the amount of protein in the seed
and the lysine content of the protein. If the lysine content is expressed on a dry matter or grain basis the amounts of protein and
lysine are positively correlated. Items of this major group are
conveniently termed normal lysine barleys. A high lysine barley is
defined as one deviating positively from this general relationship
between protein and lysine contents, or stated in another way, one
having a higher lysine content than ordinary varieties with the
same protein content. This definition implies that the recognition
of the high lysine property requires knowledge of both the lysine
and protein content. Also, it follows that certain high lysine types with a high protein content may actually have less lysine in
their protein than a normal lysine type with a low protein content.

Since lysine is the first limiting amino acid in cereal grain
proteins, an improvement in the level of lysine consequently results
in improved nutritional quality. However, high protein and/or high
lysine strains and mutants have been found to be associated with
reduced grain weight resulting in lower yields. Lysine, in addition
to being usually the most limiting amino acid for monogastric animals, is also found to be the least available amino acid from cereal grains when determined by the faecal analysis method (Eggum,
1973a; Olsen et al. 1968; Poppe and Meier, 1971; Sauer et al. 1974).
Several workers suggest the relatively high concentration of lysine in aleurone protein to be responsible for its low availability from cereal grains (Eggum, 1973a; Munck, 1964; Sauer et al.
1974; Thomke and Widstrømer, 1975). Protein in aleurone cells (albumin and globulin) may be of limited digestibility since the thick
cellulosic cell wall of these cells is thought to interfere with
digestion of the protein that is contained in these cells (Eggum,
1977). A certain amount of this protein may also be tightly bound
to the cellulosic matrix of the aleurone cells (Saunders and Kohler, 1972). Postel (1957) suggested that since barley has a multi-
cellular aleurone layer, it should be higher in aleurone protein
as a percentage of total protein than e.g. wheat, which has a single aleurone layer.

This paper, however, will review research efforts in chemical and biological evaluation of some of the high-lysine barley
cultivars.

TABLE 1

Nutritional studies of a high-lysine barley (Hiproly)
compared with a low-lysine reference barley with a
comparable amount of nitrogen in seed
(Munck et al. 1970)

	Lysine (g/16gN)	14 days male CBA x Swiss mice growth test		9 days male rat nitrogen-balance test			
		Gain (g)	PER	TD (%)	BV (%)	NPU (%)	TD of lysine (%)
Hiproly	4.08	8.9	1.72	85.2	76.0	64.8	78.7
Reference	3.13	7.8	1.54	82.0	71.1	59.2	69.5

HIPROLY

Hiproly barley was found in the world barley collection by
Hagberg and Karlson (1969) and Munck et al. (1971). Lysine, threonine, valine, methionine, isoleucine, alanine, glycine and aspartic acid were higher in Hiproly barley, whereas cystine, glutamic
acid, proline and NH_3 (after hydrolysis) were lower than other varieties having comparable protein contents (16-18% of dry matter)
(Munck et al. 1971). The question arose as to what extent the changed amino acid composition of Hiproly could be used to produce high-
yielding barley varieties.

Feeding trials were made with Hiproly grown in Sweden (Munck
et al. 1970) and a reference mixture of four naked six-row lines
(see Table 1). The N% in Hiproly was 2.69 and in the reference mixture 2.76%. Mice were fed individually ad libitum (Munck, 1964)
and rats were fed individually but restricted (Eggum, 1973a). In
the mice experiments were determined gain and protein efficiency
ratio (PER) while in the experiments with rats were measured true
protein digestibility (TD), biological value (BV), net protein utilization (NPU) and true lysine digestibility.

In mice PER was increased with the Hiproly diet, and in rats
TD, BV and NPU were likewise improved. True digestibility for lysine in rats, as measured with the faecal analysis method (Kuiken
and Lyman, 1948) was significantly increased on the Hiproly diet.
These values are in agreement with work on pigs carried out by

Thomke and Widstrømer (1975). It is interesting to note that some
of the limiting amino acids in the protein and lysine rich varieties were digested better than those from the Ingrid barley variety. In contrast to the higher digestibility of crude protein, lower digestibility values were found for organic matter, nitrogen
free extracts and crude carbohydrates.

In another work of Munck (1972) was compared the nutritional
quality of high-lysine morphological deviates showing no starch-
protein adherence with those of normal high-lysine barley controls.
A related normal-lysine barley control also was included (Table 2).

NPU was increased to about 70% in the high-lysine lines, compared with 60% in the normal control. The starch-protein adherence
trait of the high-lysine lines did not appear to affect TD, BV or
NPU. Consequently the morphological character associated with the
high lys gene in barley seems to have no effect on protein quality.
Elwinger (1973) in work with broilers also observed the superiority
of Hiproly barley when compared with normal barley.

TABLE 2

Nutritional quality in feeding tests with rats,
displaying different lys lines of barley
(Munck, 1972)

Sample	N in seed (%)	Lysine (g/16gN)	TD (%)	BV (%)	NPU (%)
Normal (control)	2.02	3.25	84.0	71.2	59.8
High-lysine starch-protein adherent	2.06	4.05	85.9	79.2	69.0
High-lysine starch-protein nonadherent	2.00	4.07	85.8	78.9	67.7

RISØ MUTANTS

Hiproly and high-amylose Glacier were exciting discoveries in the research for improved nutritive quality in barley. However, these cultivars were overshadowed by the discovery of the Bomi mutant, Bomi/Risø 1508 (Ingversen et al. 1973). The mutant 1508 was found in 1970 in the Danish two-rowed spring variety Bomi treated with ethyleneimine. The lysine content of the protein varied from 5.18 to 5.42% in four replications of 1508 compared with 3.64 to 3.82% in Bomi. A 36% increase in threonine was also found along with a considerable increase in histidine, arginine, aspartic acid, glycine and alanine. Glutamic acid and proline and to a lesser extent cystine and phenylalanine were decreased. Albumins/globulins increased from 27% in Bomi to 46% in 1508 while prolamines decreased from 29 to 9%, respectively. Glutelin was not altered. The lysine content of the prolamines and of the glutelins, respectively, were 192 and 36% above the respective value for the parent while the amino acid composition of the mutant albumin/globulin fraction was similar to that of Bomi. The mutant is further characterized by a 10% reduction in seed size and a reduction in yield per unit area of 28% (Doll and Køie, 1973).

In addition to Bomi/Risø 1508 twelve mutants have been discovered from mutagenically treated material (Doll, 1973). These have 10 to 40% more lysine in the seed protein than the parent varieties. The productivity and seed composition of mutant 1508 and the parent variety Bomi are shown in Table 3.

TABLE 3

Productivity and seed composition of mutant 1508
and the parent variety Bomi
(Doll and Køie, 1973)

	Bomi	Mutant 1508	Relative value of mutant
Lysine content, g/16 g N	3.75	5.20	139
Lysine yield, g/plot	10.4	13.7	132
Protein content, 6.25 x N%	9.7	11.0	113
Protein yield, g/plot	278	263	95
Seed size, mg	40.8	37.5	92
Number of seeds/plot x 10^{-3}	70.7	63.4	90
Grain yield, kg/plot	2.88	2.38	83

TABLE 4

Grain yield and composition of the series I and II mutants,
the parent varieties and established high lysine barleys
(Doll et al. 1974)

Variety or line	Grain yield g/plot	Seed size mg	Protein content of grain (%)	g lysine per 16 g N
Carlsberg II	438	42	9.5	3.90
Mutant 29	320	30	11.6	4.09
Line 29[+]	412	37	10.9	4.19
Mutant 86	251	26	12.9	3.98
Line 86[+]	345	35	11.6	4.19
Mutant 56	232	30	12.4	4.39
Bomi	492	45	10.4	3.73
Mutant 440	316	30	12.8	4.32
Mutant 527	369	39	11.5	4.18
Mutant 1508	434	41	11.1	5.30
Hily 71/669	292	35	12.3	4.31
Hily 82/3	439	39	11.5	4.32
Standard error	19	1	0.3	0.05

Selected mutants from the work of Doll et al. (1974) were tested in field micro plots together with their parents and established high lysine lines.

The high lysine property of the mutants and the Hily lines is reflected in their higher lysine content in the protein as compared with the two normal varieties. In the evaluation of the lysine property it should be noted, as discussed above, that the lysine content of the protein is generally negatively correlated with the protein content. Since the protein content of the mutants and Hily lines is 1-3% higher than that of the normal varieties, the increase in lysine of the mutants and lines would be somewhat higher if they were compared with normal barleys having the same protein content as the high lysine barleys.

All the six mutants have a lower grain yield than their parent variety (Table 4). However, there is no clear relation between the decrease in yield and the increase in lysine content, since the mutant with the highest lysine content, No. 1508, is also the one having the highest grain yield. The lower grain yield of the mutants is mainly caused by a reduced seed size (Table 3). Mutant 1508 is also exceptional with respect to the yield of lysine, which is more than 30% higher than that of the parent variety, Bomi. Also, the two lines 29 and Hily 82/3 have a higher lysine yield, i.e. about 15%, than their respective normal lysine parents. Only line 29 is superior to its parent, Carlsberg II, with respect to protein yield. However, Hily 82/3 is nearly equal to Bomi in protein production and mutant 1508 is less than 10% inferior to Bomi in this respect.

The nutritional value of the seed protein of some of the mutants and varieties was tested on rats. The results appear in Table 5.

TABLE 5

Nutritional value of high lysine mutants and lines,
and the parent varieties
(Doll et al. 1974)

Variety or line	True digestibility (%)	Biological value (%)	Net protein utilization (%)
Carlsberg II	78	78	61
Mutant 29	77	87	66
Line 29[+]	75	88	66
Mutant 56	82	79	64
Bomi	83	76	63
Mutant 1508	78	90	70
Hily 71/669	85	83	71
Hily 82/3	84	82	69

The very high lysine content of the mutant 1508 protein leads to a nearly 20% increase in BV compared with Bomi. However, due to a reduced TD, the NPU in mutant 1508 is only improved about 10%. Mutant 29 has about the same improvement in NPU as mutant 1508, but the BV and TD are less changed in No. 29 than in No. 1508. The similarity of line 29 and mutant 29 shows that the backcross to Carlsberg II had no effect on protein quality.

Mutant 56 seems to have a better TD than the parent variety, Carlsberg II. It is puzzling that the substantially increased lysine content of mutant 56 apparently has no effect on BV of the protein. The lines Hily 71/669 and 82/3 have about the same increase in NPU as the mutants 29 and 1508. There is no indication of a reduced digestibility in the Hily lines, which is in accordance with results of feeding tests with Hiproly (Munck et al. 1970).

Bomi and mutant 1508 were grown at different N-fertilizer levels (Andersen and Køie, 1975).

The BV values of the seed samples from the pot experiment with the most extreme protein contents are shown in Table 6, together with the nitrogen, lysine and methionine + cystine concentrations.

TABLE 6

Concentrations of lysine and methionine + cystine
and biological value of seed samples
grown at different N-fertilizer levels
(Køie et al. 1976)

Cultivar	Fertilizer (gN/pot)	N in seed (%)	BV (%)	de-crease (%)	Lysine (g/16gN)	de-crease (%)	Meth.+cyst. (g/16gN)	de-crease (%)
Bomi	2	1.5	78		4.0		2.8	
	6	2.5	69	12	3.4	15	2.5	11
M 1508	2	1.7	93		5.4		2.8	
	6	2.6	83	11	5.2	4	2.4	14

A significant negative correlation between percentage N in the seed and levels of lysine, methionine + cystine and BV was found for both Bomi and mutant 1508. All other essential amino acids decreased less than these three when more N-fertilizer was used. It should be noted that the decrease in lysine is more pronounced for Bomi than for M 1508.

The results of the studies of the Risø mutants in Denmark agree very well with the work of Newman and Eslick (1976) in America. All the Risø mutants showed a significant increase (12-56%) in percentage lysine over the parent Bomi and Carlsberg II with the exception of Bomi Risø 9.

It was further shown by Newman and Eslick (1976) that a rise in percentage lysine was accompanied by a decrease in the percentage of glutamic acid and proline in the proteins. Arginine, threonine and the two nonessential amino acids, alanine and aspartic acid appeared to be increased in the mutant barley proteins. The Bomi/Risø 1508 mutant evidenced the greatest percentage increase (55.6%) of lysine over the parent followed by the Bomi Risø 8 (32.5%) and Bomi Risø 13 (30.5%) mutants.

Newman and Eslick (1976) further showed that fractionation of the protein from Bomi/Risø 1508 indicated variance due to location. The results of their work are shown in Table 7.

TABLE 7

Correlation of animal performance with lysine and protein fraction of Bomi and Bomi/Risø 1508
(Newman & Eslick, 1976)

Location	Cultivar	PER	BV (%)	Lys (%)	Al/Glo (%)	Glu (%)	Hord (%)	Res (%)
Huntley	Bomi	1.82	65.0	3.62	36	32	20	11
	Bomi/Risø 1508	2.19	78.8	4.41	45	25	15	16
Bozeman 1	Bomi	1.95	70.7	3.53	39	28	21	13
	Bomi/Risø 1508	2.15	72.8	4.45	49	19	15	18
Bozeman 2	Bomi	2.13	75.1	3.61	37	24	25	13
	Bomi/Risø 1508	2.48	91.7	5.60	55	24	5	15

The percentage of hordeins in two samples of Bomi/Risø 1508 were idential (15%). The levels of the salt soluble albumin/globulin fractions were nearly similar (45 and 49%). The third sample of Bomi/Risø 1508 had only 5% hordein and showed a large increase in the albumin/globulin fraction (55%). The Bomi cultivars did not vary in this respect but contained considerable more hordein and less of the albumin/globulin fraction than the Bomi/Risø 1508 mutants. Animal performance appeared to be influenced to a greater extent by the total percentage of lysine in the seed protein than by content of the separate Osborne fractions. However, there was a negative correlation(P<0.05) between the percentage of hordein and the percentage of lysine in the seed protein (r = -0.79).

NOTCH-1 AND NOTCH-2 MUTANTS

Two barley mutants, named Notch-1 and Notch-2, possessing higher protein and lysine were identified at the Indian Agricultural Research Institute by the Dye Binding Capacity (DBC) method from ethyl, methanesulphonate (EMS) treated populations of the variety NP-113 (Bansal, 1970). The kernels of these mutants carried a dorsal depression and hence the name Notch. Preliminary analysis showed that these mutants possessed increased protein and lysine contents of about 40% and 20%, respectively, over the parent (Bansal, 1970, 1972).

Balaravi et al. (1976) reported the chemical characterisation and protein quality of the Notch mutants along with their parent NP-113. Alterations in the Osborne solubility fractions of the seed protein and in the amino acid profiles of whole seed meal from the mutants and the parent were studied to understand the basic mechanism of induced change. Investigations into the composition of carbohydrates were made to determine the influence of increased protein content on carbohydrate accumulation. The biological superiority of the mutants was evaluated with rat feeding experiments.

Grain samples of Notch-1, Notch-2 and their parent variety NP-113 and Hiproly (CJ 3947) came from the spring harvest of 1974. Hiproly was used as the reference high protein and high lysine genotype.

Whole seed chemical composition of Notch mutants, NP 113 and Hiproly is given in Table 8. The mutants Notch-1 and Notch-2 had 34 and 25% more seed protein, respectively, than their parent variety NP-113. Hiproly which was used to compare the nutritional standard of the mutants contained only about 7% more protein than Notch-1. Protein content per grain was also increased over the parent by 12.6% in the Notch-1 and only slightly in Notch-2. It may be noted that while a maximum decrease of 18.5% in 100 seed weight occurred in Notch-2, the reduction in seed weight in Notch-1 was 16%. Hiproly had 43% more protein than in NP-113.

TABLE 8

Chemical composition of whole grain samples or parent variety
NP-113, Notch-1 and Notch-2 mutants and Hiproly
(Balaravi et al. 1976)

	NP-113	Notch-1	Notch-2	Hiproly
Protein (% of sample)	11.69	15.69	14.62	16.81
(mg/seed)	4.43	4.99	4.52	5.80
Lysine (g/16 g N)	3.38	4.00	3.96	4.08
(% of sample)	0.395	0.587	0.579	0.686
(mg/seed)	0.15	0.20	0.18	0.24
100 seed weight (g)	3.79	3.18	3.09	3.45
Percentage of germ	3.12	5.20	4.64	3.77
100 germ weight (mg)	120	150	130	130
Reducing sugars (%)	0.22	0.36	0.43	0.14
Non-reducing sugars (%)	0.86	2.10	3.10	0.70
Starch (%)	66.2	39.6	41.4	64.8
Crude fibre (%)	7.0	10.4	12.8	5.0
Total carbohydrates[a] (%)	74.3	52.5	57.7	70.6
Free amino acids (mg/g grain weight)	1.3	2.1	2.3	2.3

a Excluding water-soluble polysaccharides which were not estimated.

Lysine content expressed as g per 16 g N showed very little
difference between Notch mutants and Hiproly. However, in comparison to NP-113, the Notch mutants had nearly 18% more lysine. Lysine per seed was about 30 and 60% higher in Notch mutants and Hiproly, respectively, than in NP-113. The increased lysine per unit
weight of flour in the mutants was about 50% more than in NP-113.

The proportion of embryo and endosperm in cereal grains is another parameter determining the protein content and quality. Our
study on this relationship in the four genotypes revealed that the
mutants possessed an increased embryo/endosperm ratio (Table 8).
Increase in the weight of 100 embryos over NP-113 was 25% in the
Notch-1 but much lower in Notch-2 and Hiproly. Estimation of total

TABLE 9

Amino acid composition of whole seed protein of NP-113 (parent),
Notch-mutants and Hiproly
(Balaravi et al. 1976)

	NP-113		Notch-1		Notch-2		Hiproly[a]	
	g/16gN	g/100g flour	g/16gN	g/100g flour	g/16gN	g/100g flour	g/16gN	g/100g flour
Asp.	5.95	0.64	6.51	0.89	6.63	0.90	6.2	1.06
Tre.	3.15	0.34	3.06	0.42	3.09	0.42	3.5	0.60
Ser.	3.55	0.38	3.32	0.46	3.42	0.46	4.6	0.79
Glu.	22.95	2.45	21.03	2.39	20.47	2.79	24.0	4.13
Pro.	10.11	1.08	9.04	1.24	8.45	1.16	12.0	2.06
Gly.	3.88	0.41	4.13	0.57	4.02	0.55	3.7	0.64
Ala.	3.79	0.40	4.38	0.60	4.69	0.64	4.2	0.72
Val.	4.69	0.50	5.12	0.70	5.06	0.69	5.3	0.91
Ileu.	3.39	0.36	3.57	0.49	3.46	0.47	3.9	0.67
Leu.	6.49	0.69	6.54	0.90	6.36	0.87	7.0	1.20
Tyr.	3.12	0.33	3.37	0.46	3.26	0.44	2.9	0.50
Phe.	4.63	0.49	4.87	0.67	4.50	0.61	6.0	1.03
Lys.	3.38	0.36	4.00	0.55	3.95	0.54	4.0	0.69
His.	2.23	0.24	2.15	0.29	2.32	0.31	2.1	0.36
NH_3	2.64	0.28	2.30	0.32	2.18	0.30	3.3	0.57
Arg.	5.30	0.57	5.41	0.74	5.29	0.72	4.4	0.76
Met.	2.01	0.21	1.56	0.21	1.66	0.23	2.0	0.34
Cys.	3.33	0.35	1.89	0.26	2.13	0.29	1.7	0.29
Trp.	1.14	0.12	1.07	0.15	1.08	0.15	1.2	0.21
N%	1.71		2.20		2.18		2.75	

a Munck et al. 1970.

free amino acids as mg equivalent of leucine in the sample meal
showed that both the mutants and the Hiproly contained about 75%
more free amino acids than that in NP-113.

The mutants showed major differences from NP-113 and Hiproly in seed carbohydrate composition. The two mutants contained almost double the amount of reducing sugars (RS) present in NP-113. A similar trend was also observed in the case of non-reducing sugars (NRS). Starch which is the major chemical constituent of seed underwent a drastic decrease in the Notch mutants. This reduction in relation to the percentage of starch present in NP-113, was about 42% in Notch-1 and 37% in Notch-2. No reduction in starch content was, however, apparent in Hiproly. The percentage of crude fibre in the sample meal was highest in the mutants, a little over twice that present in Hiproly.

Amino acid analyses of whole grain meal of NP-113, mutants and Hiproly presented in Table 9 revealed differences in the amino acid composition between NP-113 and Notch mutants, and Notch mutants and Hiproly. Compared with NP-113, the mutants had an increased amount of essential amino acids (EAAs) such as lysine, isoleucine, tyrosine and valine. Only Notch-1 showed an increase in the level of leucine and phenylalanine. The decrease in the amount of threonine in the mutants was only marginally different from that of NP-113. Of the two mutants, Notch-2 had the higher level of sulphur-containing amino acids, 40% less than that in NP-113. Aspartic acid, glycine and alanine are the only non-essential amino acids (NEAAs) which were found to have increased in the mutants. A notable reduction in the level of NEAAs in the Notch mutants was that of 10-16% in proline. This is of importance due to their reduced prolamin fraction.

All amino acids except cystine showed higher levels in the mutants in comparison to NP-113 when expressed as percentage of sample. This increase was highest in Hiproly. For lysine content in the sample, Notch mutants and Hiproly were superior to NP-113 by about 40 and 65%, respectively. These larger differences arose not only because of a *per se* increase in the percentage of some amino acids in the protein but also because of an increase in the percentages of sample protein in the mutants and Hiproly.

The proportions of total essential to non-essential amino acids (E/N "ratio") in the Notch mutants were higher than those of NP-113 and Hiproly. This improvement in the amino acid profile of the mutants was due to a reduction in the amount of total non-essential amino acids per gram nitrogen. The increased levels of essential amino acids in the Hiproly, on the other hand, could not influence its E/N ratio owing to a compensatory increase in the amount of non-essential amino acids. In spite of the improvement in the amount of lysine, threonine, isoleucine and leucine in the Notch mutants and Hiproly, these essential amino acids continue to be still limiting in them (Table 10). The milligram amounts of these limiting amino acids per gram N in NP-113, Notch-1, Notch-2 and Hiproly were 1025.6, 1073.0, 1054.3 and 1149,9, respectively. How-

TABLE 10

Chemical score with reference to FAO (1973) pattern
(Balaravi et al. 1976)

Amino acid	NP-113	Notch-1	Notch-2	Hiproly
Lysine	63.3	75.6	75.9	70.7
Threonine	80.4	78.5	80.5	84.0
Isoleucine	86.5	91.8	90.3	93.8
Leucine	94.0	95.5	94.0	95.5

ever, the Notch mutants were superior to both NP-113 and Hiproly
with regard to the chemical score for lysine. These changes, coupled with enhanced protein content in the mutants, assures an increased availability of these limiting amino acids per unit weight of
flour and thus improved biological utilization of their protein.

Seed protein was fractionated as salt-soluble (albumin-globulin), aqueous-ethanol-soluble prolamin, dilute acetic acid soluble,
glutelin I and dilute alkali soluble glutelin II (Table 11). About
20% of seed protein was extracted as albumin-globulin in NP-113. A
significant increase in their proportion was observed in the Notch
mutants and Hiproly. In the three high-lysine genotypes the prolamin content was significantly reduced. While Notch-1 was comparable
to Hiproly, Notch-2 fell between Hiproly and NP-113 on the basis of
prolamin content.

Glutelin I formed the smallest fraction in which no recogni-
sable differences between the low and high protein genotypes were
observed. Maximum seed protein was extracted as Glutelin II. A reduction in the amount of this protein fraction was observed in
Notch-2

The data in Table 12 show that both mutants Notch-1 and Notch-2
have a much higher protein quality than the parent variety NP-113.
This is especially the case with the high lysine content of Notch-2.
The biological value (BV) is 11.8 units higher than in NP-113. This
brings the net protein utilization above 70 - even higher than for
Hiproly. Notch-1 has a rather low true protein digestibility which
leads to a significantly lower NPU value compared with Notch-2.

TABLE 11

Protein solubility fractionation profile of NP-113, Notch mutants
and Hiproly (percentage of total seed protein)
(Balaravi et al. 1976)

Genotype	Salt-soluble (albumin-globulin)	Alcohol-soluble (Prolamin)	Acid-soluble (Glutelin I)	Alkali-soluble (Glutelin II)	Total seed protein extracted (%)
NP-113	20	29	9	36	94
Notch-1	29	22	11	38	99
Notch-2	28	25	10	31	94
Hiproly	25	22	8	37	92

Two Notch mutants evaluated broaden the scope for improving
the protein content and quality in barley. Unlike Hiproly these
mutants are six-rowed, hulled types and give a higher yield which,
however, is 30% lower than their parent variety. In addition to
their superiority over Hiproly in certain nutritional aspects discussed here, these mutants by virtue of their better yield give
rise to hopes of transferring their quality traits to the cultivars.

TABLE 12

Protein quality of the parent variety NP-113,
Notch-1 and Notch-2 mutants as determined in
N-balance experiments with rats
(Balaravi et al. 1976)

	TD (%)	BV (%)	NPU (%)
NP-113	86.6±0.7	75.8±1.8	65.5±1.8
Notch-1	78.9±1.4	86.4±1.7	68.2±1.8
Notch-2	83.6±0.6	87.6±1.5	73.3±1.3

$$B_1$$

In other Indian work (Bansal et al. 1977) the biological superiority of a high protein strain B_1 possessing bold and plump grains with high 1000 grain weight (46g) was studied and compared with the high lysine mutant Notch-2, its parent NP-113 and a standard variety Jyoti.

Protein quantity and quality and yield characteristics of B_1, Notch-2, NP-113 and the cultivar Jyoti are presented in Table 13. Crude protein content on percentage basis was respectively 24 and 19% higher in Notch-2 than its parent NP-113 and Jyoti. Protein content in B_1 was higher by about 8, 28 and 34%, respectively, compared to Notch-2, Jyoti and NP-113. On per grain basis also B_1 had 39-55% higher protein over other strains. Protein content per grain did not show many differences among the three strains, Notch-2, NP-113 and Jyoti.

TABLE 13

Protein, lysine, DBC values and yield characteristics
of barley strains
(Bansal et al. 1977)

	B_1	Notch-2	NP-113	Jyoti
Macro-Kjeldahl protein				
(% of sample)	16.75	15.50	12.50	13.06
(mg/grain)	7.72	5.13	4.97	5.56
Lysine				
(g/16 g N)	3.56	3.96	3.38	2.93
(mg/grain)	0.27	0.20	0.17	0.16
(% of sample)	0.596	0.614	0.422	0.383
Chemical score[a]	64.7	72.0	61.5	53.3
DBC value (absorbance units)	0.235	0.281	0.219	0.196
1000 grain weight (g)	46.1	33.1	39.8	42.6
Grain yield/m^2 (g)	282.0	265.5	270.7	267.7

a Based on lysine as the first limiting amino acid and 5.5 g
lysine/16 g N in the FAO 1973 reference amino acid pattern.

Lysine (g/16gN) content was 11-35% higher in Notch-2 as compared to the other three genotypes (Table 13). The amount of lysine per grain in Notch-2 was higher (17%) than in NP-113 while it was lower (35%) than in B_1. The level of lysine per unit weight of flour in B_1 was slightly lower than that of Notch-2, whereas both these genotypes contained 40-60% more lysine than NP-113 and Jyoti on flour basis. DBC value which has a good correlation with protein and lysine content was the highest for Notch-2 followed by B_1, NP-113 and Jyoti.

Though there were significant differences among the four genotypes in respect of 1000 grain weight, the grain yield per square metre did not show significant differences (Table 13). B_1 possessed the highest while Notch-2 had the lowest grain weight.

Protein fractionation data presented in Table 14 show that the proportion of albumin in Notch-2 was higher by about 20-25% in comparison to B_1, NP-113 and Jyoti. Prolamin content was higher (16-20%) in NP-113 than the other three genotypes which did not differ much among themselves. Globulin was similar in Notch-2, NP-113 and Jyoti whereas it was higher in B_1. Glutelin was found to be the major fraction and constituted 41-48% of the total grain protein. Although the percentage of glutelin was almost similar in NP-113, Jyoti and Notch-2, B_1 had substantially higher glutelin proportion. Because of the higher amount of protein/grain, the proportions of all the fractions in B_1 on per grain basis were higher than in the other genotypes.

TABLE 14

Grain protein fractions (%) in four genotypes of barley[a]
(Bansal et al. 1977)

Genotype	Albumin	Globulin	Prolamin	Glutelin	Residue
B_1	21.5	12.9	12.6	48.3	8.3
	(1.66)	(0.99)	(0.97)	(3.73)	(0.64)
Notch-2	26.0	11.0	13.1	43.5	9.2
	(1.33)	(0.56)	(0.67)	(2.23)	(0.47)
NP-113	20.8	11.2	15.2	42.1	11.0
	(1.03)	(0.56)	(0.75)	(2.09)	(0.55)
Jyoti	20.5	10.1	13.6	41.1	16.2
	(1.14)	(0.56)	(0.76)	(2.28)	(0.90)

a Numbers in parentheses () = mg/grain

TABLE 15

Nutritional quality of four barley strains
(Bansal et al. 1977)

	B_1		Notch-2		NP-113		Jyoti	
	(%)	s	(%)	s	(%)	s	(%)	s
True digestibility (TD)	91.5	0.7	82.3	0.4	86.6	1.8	87.0	0.5
Biological value (BV)	82.3	2.7	85.3	1.8	75.8	1.8	67.5	1.0
Net protein utilization (NPU)	75.0	2.4	70.1	1.8	65.6	1.0	58.7	0.9
Utilizable protein (UP)	13.2	0.4	10.9	0.3	7.7	0.1	7.7	0.1
Protein in dry matter (%)	17.50		15.50		11.69		13.06	
Digestible energy (%)	81.2	0.4	71.9	1.8	–	–	77.1	0.6

In order to test the nutritive values of the four strains, rat feeding experiments were conducted and the results of nitrogen balance and digestible energy studies are given in Table 15. TD of B_1 was the highest (91%) whereas it was the lowest (82%) for Notch-2, NP-113 and Jyoti had intermediate TD values. BV of Notch-2 mutant and B_1 were much higher than the BV for NP-113 and Jyoti. NPU which indicates the actual nitrogen retention by body was the highest for B_1 followed by Notch-2. NPU for NP-113 and Jyoti were considerably lower. The utilizable protein (UP) which combines both quantity and quality of protein in the samples was also the highest for B_1 indicating that B_1 is superior to the other three strains as protein source. Notch-2 also had a considerably higher UP compared to Jyoti and NP-113. The digestible energy values reveal that the percentage digestible energy was the highest (81%) for B_1 and the lowest (72%) for Notch-2.

Barley strain B_1 has higher protein content without any reduction in the grain weight unlike Hiproly (Cl 3947) from which it was selected. The higher protein content in bold and plump grains with higher 1000 grain weight indicates that B_1 possesses inherent higher protein synthesizing capacity without affecting starch synthesis.

Though protein percentage in Notch-2 was substantially higher than that in NP-113 and Jyoti, protein content on per grain basis was more or less the same. Therefore, the increased protein percentage is a direct result of reduced grain weight. Studies on grains of Notch-2 during development show that there is a premature cessation of starch accumulation (unpublished) and desiccation of grains during later stages results in the formation of a uniform depression on the dorsal side of the grain. Hence for breeding purposes protein content per kernel and protein yield per unit area should be taken into consideration rather than protein as per cent sample.

Higher NPU values for Notch-2 compared to its parent NP-113, indicate a change in the type of protein in the former. The increase in protein quantity together with the high quality of B_1 cause the highest UP values (Table 15) of this genotype.

The lower BV of B_1 compared to Notch-2 was mainly due to the lower lysine content but the higher digestibility as well as higher protein content ultimately resulted in the higher UP value of B_1. It was found that the poor digestible energy content of Notch-2 was not due to presence of higher proportion of husk. This may be due to some other factors.

Protein quality of Notch-2 was improved due to the increased level of lysine as a result of a higher proportion of albumin and reduced amount of prolamin (Table 14).

Based on chemical as well as biological tests it can be concluded that B_1 is a high protein quantity and better quality genotype while Notch-2 is a better protein quality genotype compared to NP-113 and Jyoti.

CI 7115

Toft Viuf (1972) used the negative relationship of crude protein and the amide content of barley protein to locate a high-lysine cultivar, CI 7115. This barley displayed an increased lysine content of 15% compared to normal barleys. Lysine (g/16gN) is rather constant in CI 7115 at various levels of nitrogen fertilizer (Toft Viuf, 1972) and resembles Hiproly in this respect. Ingversen and Køie (1973) have studied the composition of the salt-soluble proteins of this cultivar while Eggum (1973b) carried out the amino acid analyses and a N-balance experiment with rats. The results appear in Table 16.

It is to be seen that CI 7115 has a very high N-content, almost twice that of Bomi. In spite of this the lysine content (g/16gN) is very much the same as in Bomi. The negative relation-

TABLE 16

Protein quality of CI 7115 and Bomi expressed as amino acid
composition and TD, BV, NPU and UN determined in experiments
on rats
(Eggum, 1973b)

	CI 7115 (g/16gN)	Bomi (g/16gN)
Lysine	3.61	3.63
Methionine	1.77	1.60
Cystine	2.06	2.02
Aspartic acid	5.78	5.74
Threonine	3.47	3.10
Serine	4.38	4.26
Glutamic acid	25.37	25.11
Proline	11.23	10.89
Glycine	4.04	3.71
Alanine	3.89	4.01
Valine	4.80	5.02
Isoleucine	3.41	3.44
Leucine	7.10	7.16
Tyrosine	2.49	1.52
Phenylalanine	5.31	5.05
Histidine	2.28	2.18
Arginine	4.88	4.11
N in dry matter (%)	2.75	1.98
TD (%)	86.1	83.0
BV (%)	71.8	76.0
NPU (%)	61.8	63.1
UN	1.70	1.25

ship discussed earlier between N-content and protein quality does not seem to hold for CI 7115. This has thus caused the BV of CI 7115 at approximately the same level as for normal barley. Furthermore, TD in this variety is high (86.1). This together with the high BV and the high N-content has caused a very high UN-value, 1.70 compared to 1.25 for a normal Bomi variety.

Madsen and Mortensen (1974) showed that the relatively high content of protein, lysine and threonine in CI 7115 was equivalent to approximately 5% soybean meal in the diet to bacon pigs. On a CI-7115-diet without soybean meal the pigs were able to grow quite well but produced carcasses of poor quality. Lysine supplementation improved results considerably.

COMMENTS

Obtaining an adequate supply of food would appear to be the number one nutritional priority in the world today. This does not mean, however, that protein improvement would be of no practical value under conditions of marginal energy deprivation. The literature reviewed suggests that protein improvement would likely be of value under these conditions (Jansen and Verburg, 1977). Several other considerations lend additional support to these suggestions. One is that under conditions of protein and energy deprivation, energy needs can be reduced by level of bodily activity whereas this is not likely to be the case for protein. Jansen and Verburg (1977) also wonder if it is possible that voluntary energy intake for young children fed poor quality cereal diets might be increased marginally by improving the dietary protein supply as occurs in rats, possibly via an effect of the plasma amino acid pattern on the food intake regulatory mechanism in the brain (Harper et al. 1970).

Results of Jansen and Monte (1977) confirm that addition of lysine or lysine and threonine to bread fed to rats during pregnancy and lactation significantly increases growth and brain development of the offspring at the time of weaning. It is of interest that dams fed unfortified white bread at 70% of ad libitum intake were not able to deliver and raise viable youngs, in contrast to the results with lysine fortified bread at only a slightly higher level of food intake.

Results of Jansen and Monte (1977) demonstrate clearly that amino acid fortification of bread improved growth and brain development in the offspring of dams fed diets through pregnancy and lactation in which the bread was sole protein source, even when total protein and energy intake were 13% to 15% less than the amounts consumed by dams fed unfortified bread. These results are consistent with results obtained with postweaning rats in which growth and nitrogen utilization were significantly improved by amino acid fortification of bread fed substantially below the energy need (Jansen and Chase, 1976). These improvements, which have been demonstrated to occur both during pregnancy and lactation, and in the postweaning period suggest that protein quality improvement of cereals is of definite value even if food intake is marginally deficient (Jansen and Verburg, 1977). This conlcusion would appear to have relevance for quality improvement through plant breeding programs and possibly other improvement programs as well as for quality through amino acid fortification.

In interpreting rat growth experiments in terms of their implications in human nutrition, a major factor to consider is that the human infant grows at a slower rate than does the weanling rat. In comparing early development in the human with that in the rat, it is important to consider that rat growth occurs more in the postnatal period than is the case for the human (Chase, 1973). However, Dobbing and Sands (1973) have presumed that cellular development in the human brain continues well into the second year and that the rat may resemble the human infant more closely in postnatal brain development than was initially recognized.

As discussed by Jansen and Monte (1977), two important issues have to be resolved concerning the practical value of protein quality improvement of cereals: namely the extent to which the beneficial effects of protein quality improvement are maintained under conditions of marginal inadequacy in the supply of dietary energy. The results of Jansen and Monte (1977) demonstrate the value, for the rat, of protein quality improvement under these conditions. It seems likely that such improvement would also be of value for the slower growing infant even if dietary energy was not completely adequate, but Jansen and Monte (1977) conclude that this point has to be demonstrated yet. The fact that energy need can be reduced by decreasing the level of bodily activity whereas the protein requirement cannot, would lend support to their suggestion.

REFERENCES

Andersen, A.J. and Køie, B. (1975). N fertilization and yield response of high lysine and normal barley. Agronomy J. 67, 695–698.

Balaravi, S.P., Bansal, H.C., Eggum, B.O. and Bhaskaran, S. (1976). Characterisation of induced high protein and high lysine mutants in barley. J. Sci. Fd. Agric. 27, 545–552.

Bansal, H.C. (1970). A new mutant induced in barley. Curr. Sci. 39, 494.

Bansal, H.S. (1972). Stability for high protein content in barley mutants. ESNA Newsletter 2, 10–11.

Bansal, H.C., Srivastava, K.N., Eggum, B.O. and Mehta, S.L. (1977).
    Nutritional evaluation of high protein genotypes of barley.
    J. Sci. Fd. Agric. 28, 157-160.
Chase, H.P. (1973). The effects of intrauterine and postnatal un-
    dernutrition on normal brain development. Ann. N.Y. Acad. Sci.
    205, 231-244.
Dobbing, J. and Sands, J. (1973). Quantitative growth and develop-
    ment of human brain. Arch. Dis. Child. 48, 757-767.
Doll, H. (1973). Inheritance of the high-lysine character of a
    barley mutant. Hereditas 74, 293-294.
Doll, H. and Køie, B. (1973). Evaluation of high lysine barley mu-
    tants. In "Breeding for Seed Protein Improvement using Nuclear
    Techniques". IAEA, Vienna. p. 55-59.
Doll, H., Køie, B. and Eggum, B.O. (1974). Induced high lysine mu-
    tants in barley. Radiation Botany 14, 73-80.
Eggum, B.O. (1970). Über die Abhängigkeit der Proteinqualität vom
    Stickstoffgehalt der Gerste. Zt. Tierphysiol., Tierernähr.
    Futtermittelk. 26, 65-71.
Eggum, B.O. (1973a). A study of certain factors influencing pro-
    tein utilization in rats and pigs. Beretn. 406. Institute of
    Animal Science. Copenhagen, Denmark.
Eggum, B.O. (1973b). Kornarternes værdi som proteinkilde. Tolv-
    mandsbladet 45, 2-8.
Eggum, B.O. (1977). The nutritive quality of cereals. Cereal Res.
    Communications 5, 153-157.
Elwinger, K. (1973). Rapport om forsök med korn av Hiproly-typ till
    broiler. I. 1-10. Lantbrukshögskolan, Uppsala, Sweden.
Hagberg, A. and Karlsson, E. (1969). Breeding for high protein con-
    tent and quality in barley. In "New Approaches to Breeding for
    Improved Plant Protein". IAEA, Vienna. p. 17-21.
Harper, A.E., Benevenga, N.J. and Wohlhueter, R.M. (1970). Effects
    of ingestion of disproportionate amounts of amino acids.
    Physiol. Rev. 50, 428-558.
Ingversen, J., Køie, B. and Doll, H. (1973). Induced seed protein
    mutant of barley. Experientia 29, 1151-1152.
Jansen, G.R. and Chase, H.P. (1976). Effect of feeding lysine and
    threonine fortified bread during gestation and lactation on
    growth of the offspring in rats. J. Nutr. 106, 33-40.
Jansen, G.R. and Monte, W.C. (1977). Amino acid fortification of
    bread fed at varying levels during gestation and lactation in
    rats. J. Nutr. 107, 33-309.
Jansen, G.R. and Verburg, D.T. (1977). Amino acid fortification of
    wheat at varying levels of energy intake to rats. J. Nutr. 107,
    289-299.
Kuiken, K.A. and Lyman, C.M. (1948). Availability of amino acids
    in some foods. J. Nutr. 36, 359-368.
Køie, B., Ingversen, J., Andersen, A.J., Doll, H. and Eggum, B.O.
    (1976). Composition and nutritional quality of barley protein.
    In "Evaluation of Seed Protein Alterations by Mutation Breed-
    ing". IAEA, Vienna. p. 55-61.

Madsen, A. and Mortensen, H.P. (1974). Feeding pigs with varieties
    of barley possessing differing protein levels. In "Cereal Sup-
    ply and Utilisation". U.S.Feed Grains Council, London, p.39-65.
McWhirter, K.S. (1971). A floury endosperm, high lysine locus on
    chromosome 10. Maize Genetics Newsletter 45, 184.
Mertz, E.T., Bates, L.S. and Nelson, O.E. (1964). Mutant gene that
    changes protein composition and increases lysine content in
    maize endosperm. Science 45, 279-280.
Misra, P.S., Jambunathan, R., Mertz, E.T., Glover, D.V., Barbosa,
    H.M. and McWhirter, K.S. (1972). Endosperm protein synthesis
    in maize mutants with increased lysine content. Science 176,
    1425-1427.
Munck, L. (1964). The variation of nutritional value in barley. I.
    Variety and nitrogen fertilizer effects on chemical composi-
    tion and laboratory feeding experiments. Hereditas 52, 1-35.
Munck, L. (1972). High-lysine barley; a summary of the present re-
    search development in Sweden. Barley Genetics Newsletter 2,
    54-59.
Munck, L., Karlsson, K.E., Hagberg, A. and Eggum, B.O. (1970).
    Gene for improved nutritional value in barley seed protein.
    Science 168, 985-987.
Munck, L., Karlsson, K.E. and Hagberg, A. (1971). Selection and
    characterization of a high-protein, high-lysine barley variety
    from the world barley collection. In "Barley Genetics II"
    (R.A. Nilan ed.). Pullman, Washington. p. 544-558.
Nelson, O.E., Mertz, E.T. and Bates, L.S. (1965). Second mutant
    gene affecting the amino acid pattern of maize endosperm pro-
    teins. Science 150, 1469-1470.
Newman, C.W. and Eslick, R.F. (1976). Gene sources for high-lysine
    barley breeding. In "Improving the Nutrient Quality of Cereals
    II". Agency for International Development, Washington D.C.
    p. 154-182.
Olsen, E.M., Summers, J.D. and Slinger, S.J. (1968). Evaluation of
    protein quality in wheat by-products: Digestibility of protein
    and absorption of amino acids by the rat. Can. J. Animal Sci.
    48, 215-220.
Poppe, S. and Meyer, H. (1971). Vergleichende Betrachtungen der
    Aminosäurenresorption bei verschiedenen Tierarten. Arch. Tier-
    ernähr. 21, 531-542.
Postel, W. (1957). Studien über exogene Aminosäuren in differen
    tierten Zonen von Gerstencaryopsen, ökologischer verschiedener
    Standorte. Zt. Pflanzenz. 37, 113-126.
Sauer, W.C., Giovannetti, P.M. and Stothers, S.C. (1974). Avail-
    ability of amino acids from barley, wheat, triticale and soy-
    bean meal for growing pigs. Can. J. Animal Sci. 54, 97-105.
Saunders, R.M. and Kohler, G.O. (1972). In vitro determination of
    protein digestibility in wheat millfeeds for monogastric ani-
    mals. Cereal Chem. 49, 98-103.

Singh, R. and Axtell, J.D. (1973). High lysine mutant gene (hl) that improves protein quality and biological value of grain sorghum. Crop. Sci. 13, 535-539.

Thomke, S. (1970). Über die Veränderung des Aminosäuregehaltes der Gerste mit steigendem Stickstoffgehalt. Zt. Tierphysiol., Tierernähr. Futtermittelk. 27, 23-31.

Thomke, S. and Widstrømer, B. (1975). Nutritional evaluation of high lysine barley fed to pigs. In "Protein Nutritional Quality of Foods and Feeds". (Mendel Friedman, ed.). Marcel Dekker - New York. p. 79-100.

Toft Viuf, B. (1972). Varietal differences in nitrogen content and protein quality in barley. Royal Vet. & Agric. University, Copenhagen, Denmark. Yearbook. 1972. p. 37-61.

18

POTENTIAL FOR IMPROVING COTTONSEED QUALITY BY GENETIC AND

AGRONOMIC PRACTICES

John P. Cherry and Joseph G. Simmons

Southern Regional Research Center[1]
P. O. Box 19687
New Orleans, La. 70179

and

Russell J. Kohel

Agronomy Field Laboratory[1]
College Station, Texas 77843

ABSTRACT

Potential utilization of cottonseeds as edible food sources accentuated the need for research on their composition. Studies included evaluation of cottonseed composition; e.g., seed grade, protein, amino acids, free fatty acids, oil, fatty acids, cyclopropenoid fatty acids, total gossypol, differential settling as an indicator of potential performance of cottonseed in the liquid cyclone process, and extractability of nonstorage and storage proteins and their gel electrophoretic properties. These extended studies were used to develop a data base on composition of various cottonseed cultivars grown in different locations of Texas that resemble environmentally most of the regions of the United States cotton belt. Tests showed that most constituents of cottonseed vary; statistically significant variables include cultivar, location, and their interaction term, cultivar x location. These

[1] Facilities of Science and Education Administration,
    U.S. Department of Agriculture.

data suggest that breeding and agronomic practices could be used to alter cottonseed composition. Although protein quantity of cotton- seed from various cultivars differ and can be influenced by agro- nomic practices, this variability is not reflected in quality of cottonseed protein as detected by gel electrophoretic techniques. Analyses showed that both genetic and agronomic factors influenced formation of edible flour with high protein and low free gossypol content.

INTRODUCTION

Economic factors and research on cotton have been controlled by fiber yield and quality; however, the economic value of cotton- seed oil and protein products has increased to a point where these commodities are a source of income to the grower. In addition, research goals have been broadened due to the development of gland- less cotton cultivars and to the liquid cyclone process that lowers gossypol levels in cottonseed and flour, yielding food grade pro- ducts (Hess, 1976; Gardner et al., 1976). Advancing technology for the development of food-grade cottonseed products has provided a major incentive to improve cottonseed composition while maintaining optimum cotton fiber properties.

Through the cooperative efforts of chemists, engineers, geneticists, and agronomists, there is potential for improving cottonseed composition that will meet world nutritional and functional demands for food and feed. Percentages of protein, oil, and gossypol in cottonseed are extremely important in the processing and consumption of seeds as food or feed (Rathbone, 1977). For example, an increase of just 2% of oil content of cottonseed, while improving its unsaturated fatty acid profile, would yield approximately 40 pounds more oil per ton of seed, depending on cultivar and growing location (oil content of cotton- seed averages between 17% and 22%). A 0.5% increase in protein content of cottonseed would improve the yield of 41% protein meal by over 10 pounds per ton of processed seed. Reducing total gos- sypol in cottonseed would correspondingly benefit the production of both cottonseed oil and protein.

Earlier studies have shown that genetic and environmental factors affect oil, nitrogen, and gossypol content in cottonseed (Pope, 1945; Stansbury et al., 1953a,b, 1954, 1956). Cultivars no longer in production in commercial acreage were included in these reports. Recent investigations, undertaken to assess current seed quality, suggest that these sources exhibit the same type of response as those of the older cultivars (Cherry et al., 1977; Lawhon, et al., 1977; Turner et al., 1976a,b). Research on com- positional differences among seed can help to determine the extent of genetic variability in cultivated varieties. Additionally, genetic, environmental, and agronomic factors that affect seed composition should be assessed for their effect on processing

techniques and on functional properties used as criteria for making food ingredients. For example, peanuts grown under different
agronomic conditions differed widely in roasted flavor characteristics (Cobb and Swaisgood, 1971), and exhibited varying protein
extractability properties during moist heat processing (Cherry and
McWatters, 1975). The research discussed in this paragraph can
assist in finding reserve germ plasm needed to solve many of the
new agricultural problems brought on by pollution, dwindling water
supplies, and biological control of insects and plant pathogens
(Cherry, 1977).

This chapter presents the initial results of a study to update
understanding of cottonseed composition as it relates to genetic,
environmental, and agronomic factors. A number of characteristics
of cottonseed quality are evaluated more extensively than in past
studies. Quality factors include seed grade, protein (N x 6.25),
amino acids, oil, free fatty acids, fatty acids, cyclopropenoid fatty acids, total gossypol, nonstorage and storage protein extractability, gel electrophoretic properties of protein fractions, and protein
and free gossypol in flour prepared by the differential settling
method that simulates the liquid cyclone processed product. Four
National Standard cotton cultivars were included in this research:
Acala 1517-70, Coker 310, Deltapine 16, and Lockett 4789. Eight
growing locations in Texas were selected to represent, environmentally, most of the United States cotton belt. These locations were
College Station (Central Texas—Brazos Valley); Chillicothe, Lubbock,
and Lamesa (North—High Plains and Rolling Plains); Pecos and El Paso
(West—dry); and Weslaco and Corpus Christi (South—Subtropical and
Coastal Bend). The cultivars and their locations are shown in
Figure 1.

QUALITY CHARACTERISTICS OF COTTONSEED

Analysis of variance for quality. Analysis of variance shows
that the cultivar and location effects for seed grade, protein,
oil, free fatty acids, total gossypol, and cyclopropenoid fatty
acids of cottonseeds were highly significant (Table 1). These
quality factors all had highly significant interaction effects,
suggesting that the response to the genetic characteristics of
cotton are not the same for each growing location, or vice versa.
The protein and free gossypol percentages in the overflow fraction
from differential settling tests (Vix et al., 1949) of cottonseed
meals were highly significant for the cultivar, location, and
interaction effects; only the F test for the cultivar effect on
protein content in the overflow fraction was nonsignificant. The
ability to separate nonstorage and storage proteins from cottonseed
kernels with water and 0.01N NaOH, respectively, was only affected
significantly by location.

Seed grade. Standards (National Cottonseed Products Association, 1977-78) specify that all offers and acceptances of cottonseed

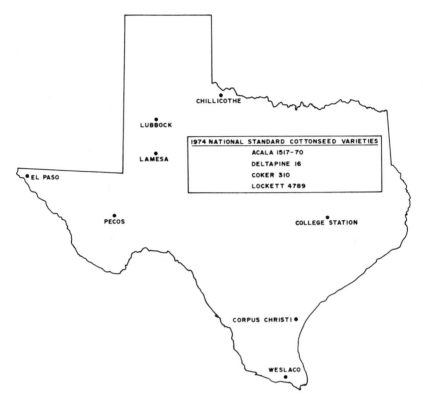

Figure 1. 1974 National Standard cottonseed varieties and growing locations.

shall be based on their classification as prime, below prime, off quality, and below grade quality. This is accomplished through a series of mathematical numbering systems that results in a basis grade of cottonseed set at 100; high and low grades, respectively, are set above and below this value. The basis formula for the seed grade of cottonseed includes two factors: (1) quantity index, which involves percentage oil and ammonia; and (2) quality index, which involves percentage of foreign matter, moisture and free fatty acids. Seed grade is equal to quantity index x quality index, divided by 100.

Seed grade did not significantly differ among cultivars at most locations, ranging between 80% and 110% (Figure 2). Exceptionally high seed grades (120% to 130%) were noted for all cultivars harvested at Corpus Christi. Off quality grades, ranging between 30% and 60%, were observed for cottonseed from College Station. At this latter location, Acala 1517 was significantly higher than the other varieties in the test, which did not vary statistically from each other. These low grade values were

Table 1. F test for each percentage quality factor of cottonseed.

Quality Factor	Cultivars(C)	Locations(L)	C x L
	Source of Variation[1]		
Seed grade	12.69**	294.75**	2.67**
Protein	15.98**	6.76**	3.32**
Oil	14.81**	23.38**	4.03**
Free fatty acids	24.08**	585.59**	9.38**
Total gossypol	29.10**	15.86**	11.13**
Cyclopropenoid fatty acids	2.78**	26.14**	7.22**
Differential settling overflow:			
Protein	1.9	7.3**	2.2*
Free gossypol	35.7**	40.7**	9.3**
Protein extractability:			
Non-storage proteins	1.6	0.5	0.9
Storage proteins	0.2	2.5*	1.3

[1]Cultivar, location, interaction and error had degrees of freedom of 3,7,21, and 32, respectively, for seed grade, protein, oil, and free fatty acids, and total gossypol, and 3,6,18, and 28 for cyclopropenoid fatty acids, differential settling overflow and protein extractability. The Pecos location was not included in the latter tests because of insufficient samples.

*Significant at the 0.05 level of probability; **significant at the 0.01 level of probability.

due mainly to high free fatty acid content (11.0%-18.5%) of the cottonseed (Figure 3). The excessively high free fatty acid values were the result of two factors that combined to reduce seed quality in the field. They were (a) a prolonged period of rainfall delayed harvesting the cotton; and (b) unusually warm temperatures that prevailed during this period of high moisture that caused germination in the bolls and seed deterioration. Variables included in seed grade determinations of all cultivars ranged as follows: Moisture--5.4% to 10.1%; foreign matter--0% to 12.5%; fatty acids, 0.4-18.5% (Figure 3); oil, 21.4%-26.8% (Figure 4); and protein, 23.5-29.5% (Figure 5).

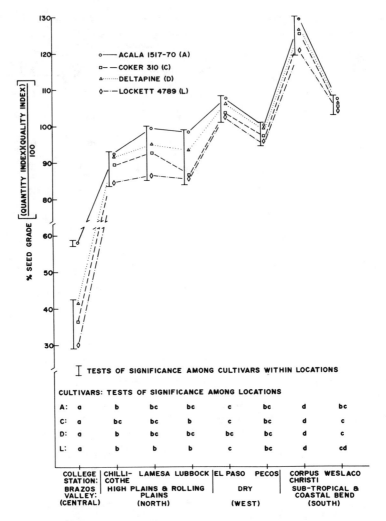

Figure 2. Mean values of cottonseed grade. Tests of significance in Figures 2-7, 8-9, and 12-13 are at the 0.05 level of
probability, according to the Newman-Keuls multiple range test.

Free fatty acids. Except for the high values noted for
College Station cottonseed, free fatty acids for all cultivars
grown at the other Texas locations ranged between 0.4% and 4.0%
(Figure 3). Significant differences among cultivars were not
noted for cottonseed from the Subtropical and Coastal Bend (South)
region of Texas. Variability in fatty acid content was observed
in cottonseed among cultivars within the other locations. In the
High Plains and Rolling Plains (North) area, Acala 1517-70 and

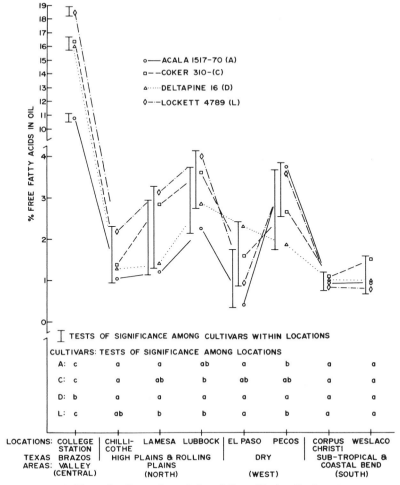

Figure 3. Mean values of free fatty acids in oil of cotton-seed. Methods of analysis for free fatty acids and for oil, protein and total and free gossypol were officially published by the American Oil Chemists' Society (1976).

Figure 3. Mean values of free fatty acids in oil of cotton-seed. Methods of analysis for free fatty acids and for oil, protein and total and free gossypol were officially published by the American Oil Chemists' Society (1976).

Deltapine 16 had relatively low percentages compared to the other two cultivars. Cottonseeds from the Dry (West) area were variable, containing free fatty acid amounts ranging from 0.4% to 3.8%. The high free fatty acid content of cottonseed from College Station was discussed in the previous section on seed grade.

Oil. In general, Acala 1517-70 maintained the highest percentage of oil among cultivars in most locations; Lockett 4789

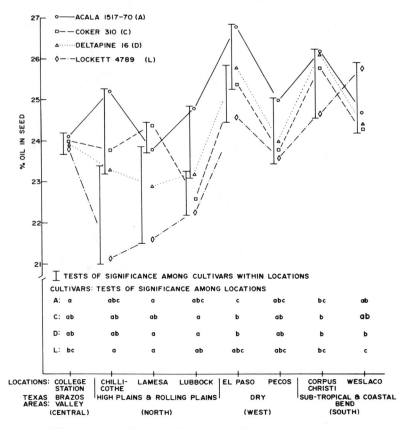

Figure 4. **Mean values of oil in cottonseed.**

generally had the lowest values, and the other two cultivars varied between these two extremes (Figure 4). Percentage oil values
among cultivars were highest at the Dry (West) and Subtropical and
Coastal Bend (South) locations. Cottonseed of all cultivars grown
at College Station contained similar amounts (23.7% to 24.2%) of
oil. Significant variability in percentages were noted for cottonseed from Chillicothe, Lamesa, Lubbock, and El Paso (21% to
26.8%).

Proteins. Protein remained between 24% and 29% (Figure 5).
Deltapine 16 showed the greatest amount of differences among locations, while Lockett 4789 displayed the least detectable
variability.

Total gossypol. Lockett 4789 cottonseed from the High Plains
and Rolling Plains (North) and Dry (West) regions maintained the
lowest total gossypol percentages (0.8% to 0.9%) among cultivars
grown in Texas (Figure 6). Within each location of these two

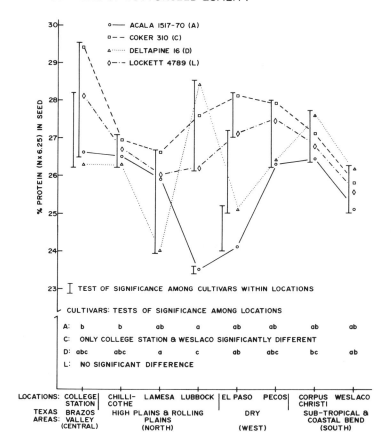

Figure 5. Mean values of protein (macroKjeldahl nitrogen x 6.25) in cottonseed.

regions, the gossypol values of the other cultivars did not vary significantly from each other, but did differ between growing areas ranging from 0.88% to 1.1%. At College Station, the cultivars could be separated into high and low gossypol-containing groups of 1.1% (Deltapine 16, Coker 310) and 0.8% to 0.9% (Acala 1517-70, Lockett 4789), respectively. Similar variations were noted for cottons grown in the Subtropical and Coastal Bend region; gossypol ranged from a low of 0.8% (Acala 1517-70, Deltapine 16) to highs between 1.0% and 1.04% (Deltapine 16, Coker 310, Lockett 4789).

Cyclopropenoid fatty acids. The cyclopropenoid fatty acids in cottonseed oil varied widely among cultivars and between locations (Figure 7). Values ranged from a low of 0.71% for Lockett 4789 (El Paso) to a high of 1.38% for Coker 310 (Lubbock). Nonsignificant differences among cultivars were noted at Chillicothe, El Paso and Corpus Christi. Cyclopropenoid fatty

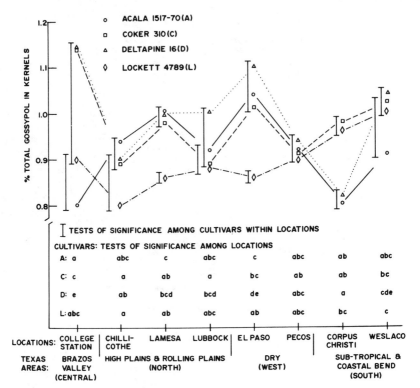

Figure 6. Mean values of total gossypol in cottonseed.

acid content of cottonseed oil from Lockett 4789 and Coker 310 varied significantly at the High Plains and Rolling Plains growing location; values ranged between 1.0% and 1.38%. The values for these cultivars were as low as 0.71% (Lockett 4789 at El Paso) and 0.78% (Coker 310 at Weslaco). At College Station, Deltapine 16 was significantly lower (0.77%) than the other three cultivars (1.1% to 1.21%), which did not differ from one another.

Amino acid profile. All amino acids except alanine, proline, and phenylalanine had significant F tests for at least one or more of the variables of cultivar, location, and their interaction effect, cultivar x location (Table 2). Glycine, serine, and the total amino acid composition were significantly affected by the cultivar factor. Glutamic acid and arginine were affected only by the location effect. Both cultivar and location effects were significant for leucine, threonine, aspartic acid, tyrosine, and lysine. Valine, isoleucine, methionine, histidine, and half-cystine had significant interaction terms.

The Newman-Keuls multiple range test showed differences for only leucine, threonine, serine, and half-cystine content among

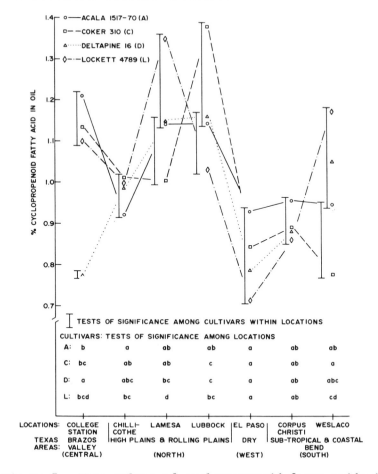

Figure 7. Mean values of cyclopropenoid fatty acids in cottonseed. Method of analysis was that of Brown (1969).

cottonseeds of cultivars. Examining the ranges of low and high values for amino acids showed that among cultivars, Deltapine 16 had the greatest number (10) of amino acids of low content, and Coker 310 had the greatest number (8) of high content; among locations, cottonseed grown at Lamesa contained the greatest number (5) of amino acids of low content, and that grown at Corpus Christi, the greatest number (8) of high content. Many of the high quantities of amino acids in cottonseed were noted for Coker 310 grown at Chillicothe.

Fatty acid profile. Except for the cultivar x location interaction effect for stearic acid, all fatty acid levels of oil varied significantly for cultivar, location, and their interaction effects (Table 3). In most cases, Lockett 4789A of Corpus Christi had the highest value for each fatty acid; the percentage 0.82% for

Table 2. Amino acid composition[1] of cultivars averaged across locations.[2]

Amino Acid	Mean Amino Acid Content[3] (g/100g flour) of Cultivars from all Locations				Range of Amino Acids		F Test[4] for Percentage Amino Acids		
	Acala 1517-70	Coker 310	Deltapine 16	Lockett 4789	Low	High	Cultivars(C)	Locations (L)	C x L
Alanine	2.12	2.13	2.08	2.17	2.00 C-W[5]	2.26L-EP	2.31	0.43	1.14
Valine[6]	2.25	2.25	2.12	2.20	1.66 D-CS	2.61 A-CC	2.69	4.14*	3.01**
Glycine	2.18	2.24	2.16	2.25	2.08A-Lu	2.35L-EP	3.11*	1.61	0.97
Isoleucine[6]	1.61	1.63	1.51	1.60	1.20D-CS	1.86A-C	2.23	2.91*	2.40*
Leucine[6]	3.09a	3.27b	3.00a	3.13ab	2.88D-La	3.84C-W	3.42*	3.50*	1.97
Proline	1.97	2.02	1.93	1.93	1.83L-Lu	2.13A-CC	1.46	1.48	0.61
Threonine[6]	1.66a	1.79b	1.71ab	1.79b	1.42A-W	1.98C-C	6.41**	2.64*	1.80
Serine	2.31a	2.48b	2.36ab	2.44ab	2.14D-La	2.59D-C	3.97*	2.14	1.2
Methionine[6]	0.68	0.78	0.77	0.72	0.59A-W	0.96C-W	3.20*	1.39	2.2*
Phenylalanine[6]	2.82	2.88	2.76	2.84	2.62C-W	3.02L-Lu	2.00	0.72	0.99
Aspartic acid	4.86	5.03	4.82	5.01	4.5ED-EP	5.25L-La	3.15*	3.77**	0.81
Glutamic acid	10.47	10.76	10.31	10.58	9.46D-CC	11.15C-CC	2.01	2.95*	1.13
Tyrosine	1.49	1.58	1.48	1.50	1.29D-La	1.68C-CC	4.04*	4.13**	1.75
Lysine[6]	2.45	2.47	2.42	2.52	2.28D-EP	2.63L-EP	3.83*	6.59**	1.79
Histidine[6]	1.42	1.44	1.39	1.40	1.12L-CS	1.62D-Lu	0.63	2.47*	4.99*
Arginine	5.65	5.49	5.20	5.38	4.39D-La	6.42C-CC	2.10	5.38**	0.90
Half Cystine	0.86ab	0.92b	0.92b	0.82a	0.70L-EP	1.08C-CC	8.04**	7.75**	2.13*
Total	47.91	49.03	46.86	48.30	44.34D-La	50.82C-CC	3.12*	2.38	1.11

1　Method of Kaiser et al. (1974).
2　College Station, Chillicothe, Lamesa, Lubbock, El Paso, Pecos, Corpus Christi, Weslaco.
3　Amino acids having same superscript are not significantly different according to the Newman-Keuls multiple range test; values
　　without superscripts are not different.
4　*Significant at the 0.05 level of probability; **significant at the 0.01 level of probability.
5　Cultivar-location: Acala 1517-70, A; Coker 310, C; Deltapine 16, D; Lockett 4789, L;College Station, CS;
　　El Paso, EP; Weslaco, W; Lamesa, La; Chillicothe, C; Lubbock, Lu; Corpus Christi, CC.
6　Essential amino acids.

Table 3. Fatty acid composition[1] of cultivars averaged across locations[2].

	Mean Fatty Acid Content (% of oil) of Cultivars of all Locations				Range of Fatty Acids		F Test for Percentage Fatty Acids		
Fatty Acid	Acala 1517-70	Coker 310	Deltapine 16	Lockett 4789	Low	High	Cultivars(C)	Locations(L)	C x L
Myristic (C14:0)	0.85^{b3}	0.73^a	0.81^b	0.91^c	0.68C-Lu	1.16L-CC	102.71**[3]	81.94**	4.81**
Palmitic (C16:0)	23.65^a	23.30^a	23.76^a	23.99^a	21.63A-Lu	26.18L-CC	8.71**	96.80**	2.73**
Palmitoleic (C16:1)	0.70^b	0.61^a	0.62^a	0.67^{ab}	0.56D-CS	0.82A-CC	29.79**	21.53**	2.33**
Stearic (C18:0)	2.50^a	2.59^a	2.64^a	2.45^a	2.27L-C	2.88C-W	3.54*	12.30**	1.62
Oleic (C18:1)	18.62^b	16.29^a	16.36^a	18.35^b	15.17D-CS	19.94L-CC	356.91**	79.99**	6.89**
Linoleic (C18:2)	53.31^a	56.20^b	55.35^b	53.32^a	49.07A-CC	57.64C-Lu	238.39**	229.04**	10.08**

1 Method of Amer. Oil Chem. Soc. (1976).
2 See Table 2 for list of locations.
3 See Table 2 for explanation of postscripts.

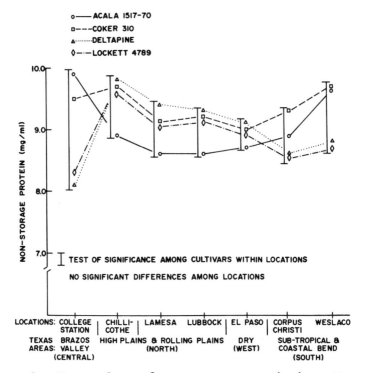

Figure 8.   Mean values of nonstorage protein in cottonseed.

palmitoleic acid in oil of Acala 1517-70 from Corpus Christi was
only 0.06% higher than that of Lockett 4789 grown in the same location.   Low percentages were scattered among all cultivars and most
locations.   The greatest amount of unsaturated fatty acids were
noted among oils of cottonseed grown in the High Plains and Rolling
Plains region.

Newman-Keuls multiple range analysis among cultivars showed
the following: (a) no significant differences for palmitic and
stearic acids, (b) Acala 1517-70 and Lockett 4789 were not different in oleic acid composition but were significantly higher than
Coker 310 and Deltapine 16 (the latter two were not different),
(c) Coker 310 and Deltapine 16 were higher in linoleic acid than
Acala 1517-70 and Lockett 4789, and (d) myristic acid had much more
significant variability among cultivars than the other fatty acids.

Extraction of nonstorage and storage proteins.   Berardi et al.
(1969) showed that nonstorage and storage proteins could be
extracted separately from cottonseed products with water and
0.015N NaOH.   These methods were used to test cottonseed from the

various cultivars grown at different locations. Quantities of
nonstorage proteins, determined by the method of Lowry et al.
(1951), ranged between 8.5 and 9.8 mg/ml for all cultivars grown
in every location except College Station (Figure 8); no statistically significant differences were noted among cultivars. Although
these values were not significantly different, quantities of
extractable nonstorage protein in Acala 1517-70 cottonseed was
lower than those of Deltapine 16, Coker 310 and Lockett 4789 in the
North and West regions. At the Central and South areas, Acala
1517-70 cottonseed had high quantities of extractable nonstorage
protein. Experimental variability was high in these analyses and
probably masked any potentially significant differences among cultivars. The Neuman-Keuls analysis showed no differences for cultivars compared among growing locations.

Differences in extractability of storage protein from seed of
cultivars grown in College Station, Chillicothe, and Lamesa were

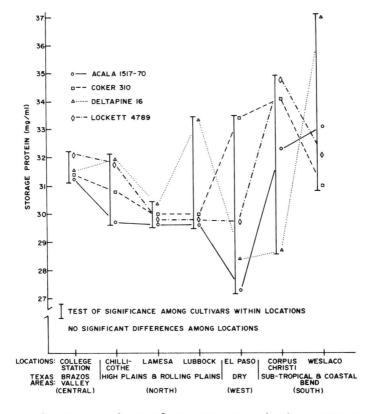

Figure 9. Mean values of storage protein in cottonseed.

small (Figure 9). On the other hand, much variation was noted for data accumulated from Lubbock, El Paso, Corpus Christi, and Weslaco. Due to variability in the extraction of these proteins, the Newman-Keuls multiple range test showed that no statistically significant differences existed among cultivars and locations, and no consistent pattern (high or low values) was observed for any cultivar; the F test indicated that the location effect was marginally significant at the 0.05 level of probability (Table 1).

Gel electrophoretic patterns of proteins. Although there was significant variability in total quantity of protein in cottonseed among cultivars grown in various Texas locations, gel electrophoretic patterns of their nonstorage and storage proteins lacked variability (Figure 10). Thus, quantity of protein of cottonseed from various cultivars differs and can be influenced by environment and agronomic practices. This variability, however, is not reflected in the individual components of seed protein.

Protein and free gossypol in cottonseed flour prepared by the differential settling method. A fractionation process described as differential settling was developed to separate oil, pigment glands, and hull fragments from cottonseed flour (Vix et al., 1949). The method uses the principle of mixed solvent (hexane) flotation to

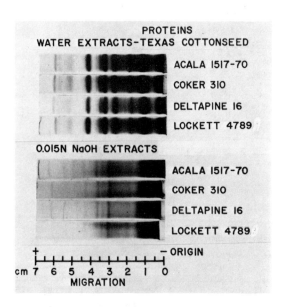

Figure 10. Typical polyacrylamide disc-gel electrophoretic patterns of cottonseed proteins. Method of gel electrophoresis was that of Cherry (1977).

separate a low weight, high protein fraction from oil, gossypol glands, and other coarse material. The product is edible grade cottonseed flour with free gossypol levels of less than 0.045% (Food and Drug Administration approval, Federal Register, 1973, 1974). The method has been engineered to pilot plant scale as the liquid cyclone process (Gardner et al., 1976). A flow diagram is presented in Figure 11. The underflow fraction noted in this figure contains most of the gossypol, some protein, and hull materials. Differential settling is now used to determine how efficiently gossypol can be removed from a cottonseed meal to form a high protein food-grade flour.

The protein levels in flour made by the differential settling method from cottonseed of different cultivars varied both within and between locations (Figure 12). Differentially fractionated flour with 67% to 70% protein was obtained from cottonseed of most

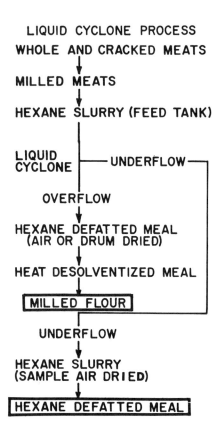

Figure 11. Steps in the liquid cyclone process for making edible flour from glanded cottonseed.

cultivars grown in College Station, Chillicothe, Lubbock, and
Corpus Christi; Coker 310 and Acala 1517-70 from El Paso and
Weslaco, respectively, were also in this percentage range. Flours
with significantly low protein content were mainly obtained from
cottonseed harvested in Lamesa, El Paso, and Weslaco. Overall,
cottonseed from Acala 1517-70 and Coker 310 had greatest potential
for producing high protein flour among the cultivars examined in
this study; Deltapine 16 cottonseed from Lubbock also formed an
excellent protein product.

Except for cottonseed of Acala 1517-70 and Coker 310 from
College Station, processed flour from cottonseed of all cultivars
collected at the different locations had free gossypol levels ranging between 0.010% and 0.045% (<u>Figure 13</u>); cottonseed of the former

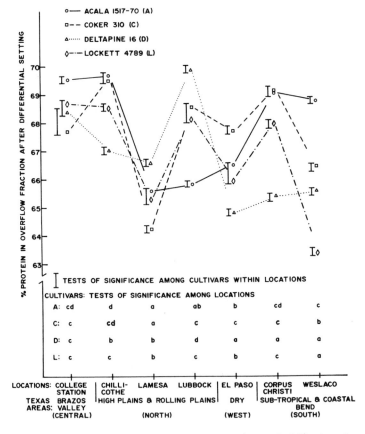

Figure 12. Mean values of protein (N x 6.25) in the edible
flour formed by differential settling of cottonseed meal.

two cultivars produced flours with 0.08% to 0.09% free gossypol.
Tests made to determine statistical significance among locations
showed little variation, except for the high percentages noted at
College Station for Acala 1517-70 and Coker 310, and the low value
of Lockett 4789 from Corpus Christi. The high values of cultivars
from College Station are probably related to the poor quality cottonseed obtained from this location, as indicated by high free
fatty acid and poor seed grade percentages. Interestingly, none of
the other quality factors of the cottonseed from cultivars grown at
College Station were affected by the adverse location effects discussed earlier in the section on seed grade. On the average, free
gossypol was highest in flour of Coker 310 and was lowest for that
of Lockett 4789. Cottonseed of the other two cultivars produced
flours ranging somewhere between the extremes of these two

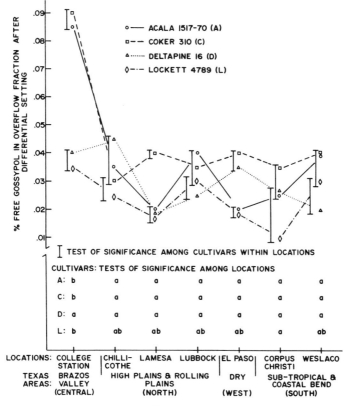

Figure 13. Mean values of free gossypol in the edible flour
formed by differential settling of cottonseed meal.

DISCUSSION

Ideally, cottonseed for food use should have high percentages of seed grade, oil, and protein, and low quantities of free fatty acids, gossypol, and cyclopropenoid fatty acids. Free fatty acids should be kept at a minimum by harvesting mature cottonseeds and maintaining optimum storage and handling conditions to minimize seed deterioration during preprocessing periods. Low levels of gossypol in cottonseed would make techniques such as the liquid cyclone process more readily applicable than is possible under present conditions. Consistency in the extractability of nonstorage and storage proteins from cottonseed would improve yields of isolate and enhance their use as food ingredients. Cyclopropenoid fatty acids have been suggested to cause physiological disturbance in animals, thus, it would be advantageous to maintain low limits of these substances in cottonseed products. In addition, cottonseed should have a high percentage of essential amino acids, especially lysine and methionine, to improve quality of nonstorage and storage protein isolates, and unsaturated fatty acids should be low enough to minimize rancidity during storage. These constituents, however, should be in high enough quantities to maintain liquidity of the oil.

In 1945, Pope examined eight replicates of cottonseed from 10 cultivars grown at a number of locations throughout the cotton belt for protein, oil, and linters. He noted large differences in these constituents within each year. Values remained consistent among cultivars, but, location variation was significant, suggesting that weather conditions influenced cottonseed composition. The data suggested further that oil, protein, and linters were dependent on genetic constitution of the cultivar and that a consideration of these variables in breeding programs should result in the isolation of superior lines in any one or all of these characteristics. In addition, protein and oil were substantially independent relative to genetic constitution, but negatively associated when the environmental effects were considered. These observations were substantiated further in studies by Stansbury and coworkers (1953a, b, 1954, 1956) and by Bailey et al. (1966), who included phytin, gossypol, fatty acid, and cyclopropenoid fatty acid analyses in their studies. More recently, Turner and coworkers (1976a,b), Lawhon, et al. (1977), and Pandey and Thejappa (1975) showed that cottonseed from present-day gossypol glanded and glandless commercial cultivars also varied in composition due to genetic and agronomic factors.

Both the earlier and present studies showed negative correlation coefficients for protein, oil, and gossypol content in cottonseed, suggesting that the potential existed for specifically improving percentages of each constituent. Moreover, research has shown that application of fertilizers containing nitrogen will increase protein and decrease oil content of cottonseed (Sood et al., 1976).

The data presented in this paper support many of the conclusions of past researchers; i.e., cultivar, location, and the cultivar times location effects on cottonseed are statistically significant. Preliminary evaluation of the correlation coefficients for oil and protein, cyclopropenoid fatty acids and protein, and free gossypol and protein in the flour from differential settling tests were negative and statistically significant at the 10% level of probability. The correlation coefficient of total gossypol and protein was nonsignificant, but showed a negative relationship; oil related to either total gossypol or cyclopropenoid fatty acids had positive correlations but were nonsignificant. No doubt the genetic and agronomic variability exists for all these factors, and what remains is selection of the most ideal conditions to improve cottonseed quality.

REFERENCES

American Oil Chemists' Society (1976). Official and tentative methods (third edition-additions and revisions). Aa-4-38, Aa-5-38, Aa-6-38, Ba-7-58, Ba-8-55, Ce 1-62. The Society: Chicago, Ill.

Bailey, A. V., Harris, J. A., and Skau, E. L. (1966). Cyclopropenoid fatty acid content and fatty acid composition of crude oils from twenty five varieties of cottonseed. J. Amer. Oil Chem. Soc. 43, 107-110.

Berardi, L. C., Martinez, W. H. and Fernandez, C. J. (1969). Cottonseed protein isolates: two step extraction procedure. Food Technol. 23, 75-82.

Brown, L. E. 1969. Methods for the determination of cyclopropenoid fatty acids: VII. The HBr titration method applied to small samples. J. Amer. Oil Chem. Soc. 46, 654-656.

Cherry, J. P. (1977). Potential sources of peanut seed proteins and oil in the genus Arachis. J. Agric. Fd. Chem. 25, 186-193.

Cherry, J. P., Simmons, J. G. and Tallant, J. D. (1977). Cottonseed protein composition and quality of Gossypium species and cultivars. Proc. Beltwide Cotton Conf. 31, 46-49.

Cherry, J. P. and McWatters, K. H. (1975). Solubility properties of proteins relative to environmental effects and moist heat treatment of full-fat peanuts. J. Food Sci. 40, 1257-1259.

Cobb, W. Y. and Swaisgood, H. E. (1971). Roasted peanut flavor and its relation to growth environment. J. Food Sci. 36, 538-539.

Federal Register. (1973). Title 21, Part 2. Food Additives 39 (159): 22241.

Federal Register. (1974). Title 21, Part 2, Food Additives 39 (177): 32725.

Gardner, H. K., Hron, R. J. and Vix, H. L. E. (1976). Removal of pigment glands (gossypol) from cottonseed. Cereal Chem. 53, 549-560.

Hess, D. C. (1976). Prospects for glandless cottonseed. Oil Mill
    Gaz. 81, 20–26.
Kaiser, F. E., Gehrke, C. W., Zumwalt, R. W. and Kuo, K. C. (1974).
    Amino acid analysis. Hydrolysis ion–exchange cleanup,
    derivatization, and quantitation by gas–liquid chromatography.
    J. Chromatog. 94, 113–133.
Lawhon, J. T., Cater, C. M. and Mattil, K. F. (1977). Evaluation
    of the food use potential of sixteen varieties of cottonseed.
    J. Am. Oil Chem. Soc. 54, 75–80.
Lowry, O. H., Rosebrough, N., Farr, A. L. and Randall, R. J.
    (1951). Protein measurement with the Folin phenol reagent.
    J. Biol. Chem. 193, 265–275.
National Cottonseed Products Association. (1977–78). Rules of the
    National Cottonseed Products Association. Ann. Session of the
    Assoc. 81, 57–61.
Pandey, S. N. and Thejappa, N. (1975). Study on relationship
    between oil, protein, and gossypol in cottonseed kernels.
    J. Am. Oil Chem. Soc. 52, 312–315.
Pope, O. A. (1945). Effect of variety, location, and season on
    oil, protein, and fuzz of cottonseed and on fiber properties
    of lint. Tech. Bull. 903, U. S. Dept. Agric. pp. 1–41.
Rathbone, C. R. (1977). Development of cottonseed products.
    Proc. Beltwide Cotton Prod.–Mech. Conf. 36, 32–33.
Sood, D. R., Kumar, V. and Dhindsa, K. S. (1976). Composition
    of cottonseed as affected by N, P and K application.
    Agrochimica 20, 77–81.
Stansbury, M. F., Pons, W. A. and Hoffpauir, C. L. (1953a).
    Influence of variety of cottonseed and environment. Phospho-
    rus compounds in cottonseed kernels. J. Agric. Fd. Chem. 1,
    75–78.
Stansbury, M. F., Hoffpauir, C. L. and Hopper, T. H. (1953b).
    Influence of variety and environment on the iodine value of
    cottonseed oil. J. Am. Oil Chem. Soc. 30, 120–123.
Stansbury, M. F., Cucullu, A. F. and Den Hartog, G. T. (1954).
    Influence of variety and environment on oil content of cotton-
    seed kernels. J. Agric. Fd. Chem. 2, 692–696.
Stansbury, M. F., Pons, W. A. and Den Hartog, G. T. (1956).
    Relations between oil, nitrogen, and gossypol in cottonseed
    kernels. J. Am. Oil Chem. Soc. 33, 282–286.
Turner, J. H., Ramey, H. H. and Worley, S. (1976a). Influence of
    environment on seed quality of four cotton cultivars. Crop
    Sci. 16, 407–409.
Turner, J. H., Ramey, H. H. and Worley, S. (1976b). Relationship
    of yield, seed quality, and fiber properties in Upland
    cotton. Crop Sci. 16, 578–580.
Vix, H. L. E., Spadaro, J. J., Murphey, C. H., Persell, R. M.,
    Pollard, E. F. and Gastrock, E. A. (1949). Pilot–plant
    fractionation of cottonseed. II. Differential settling.
    J. Am. Oil Chem. Soc. 26, 526–530.

19

THE NUTRITIVE VALUE OF MIXED PROTEINS

Anthony A. Woodham

From The Rowett Research Institute

Bucksburn, Aberdeen AB2 9SB

ABSTRACT

Mixtures of protein foods given to chickens or rats frequently result in better growth than would be expected from the performance obtained with each component of the mixture given on its own. Mixing often results in the provision of a better amino acid balance in the diet and the improved growth can be attributed to the minimising of deficiencies of particular essential amino acids in the diet. This explanation is not always possible however. Some mixtures which give better growth have lower levels of some important amino acids than the better component of the mixture, and in such cases it is suggested that the improvements are due to the achievement of better overall amino acid balance. In particular it seems clear that amino acid excesses may have a deleterious effect, and diet balancing should be designed not merely to minimise deficiencies of essential amino acids, but also to cut down excesses.

INTRODUCTION

More than a century ago at Rothamsted, England, Lawes and Gilbert carried out a feeding experiment with pigs which was of crucial significance in indicating that proteins differed in their nutritional value (Lawes and Gilbert, 1866). A pig fed lentils excreted twice as much urea nitrogen as one fed barley, clearly indicating that very different proportions of the nitrogenous material of these two foods were being converted into body protein. Fifty years were to elapse before the work was carried further and in the first two decades of the 20th Century the chemical differences between the proteins of various feeds were noted and studied, and the concepts of the "essential" amino acid and the "limiting" amino acid were developed.   Some maintained even then that the most economical use of food protein was achieved when it was similar in composition to the body protein of the animal fed (Abderhalden, 1912).   The general principle of balancing the protein constituents of the diet in order to achieve improved protein utilisation dates from this same period.   The inadequecy of zein as a source of food nitrogen for example was recognised, and its improvement by combining with gliadin was proposed and experimentally achieved by Osborne and Mendel in 1914.   McCollum and various of his collaborators extended this work, feeding many combinations of legumes and cereals to rats and deducing from the results that certain amino acids were limiting in the diets.   Mixtures of wheat, maize or oats with gelatin, wheat gluten or zein were given to experimental animals and it was noted that while zein and gelatin were good supplements for oats neither enhanced the value of maize.   Wheat was improved by the addition of gelatin but not by zein.   It was concluded from the results that neither lysine nor tryptophan was limiting in oats but that lysine was probably the limiting amino acid in wheat, and these conclusions were based upon the supposition that the improvements in oat growth observed with some mixtures was due to an increase in the quantities of particular amino acids known to be well provided by the particular supplement used (McCollum, Simmonds and Pitz, 1916).   Similar experiments demonstrated the high quality of combinations of cereals with legumes, while mixtures of legumes alone or of cereals alone were little, if at all, better than the individual components (McCollum, Simmonds and Parsons, 1921).   Anomalies were however evident.   Neither flax-seed nor millet were significantly improved by combination with cereals, peas or soyabean, and the authors concluded that it was not possible from their experiments to conclude which amino acids were limiting (McCollum, Simmonds and Parsons, 1919).

AMINO ACID COMPOSITION AND THE QUALITY OF PROTEIN MIXTURES

Analytical procedures for estimating the contents of amino acids in proteins were of course subject to considerable errors in these early days, and the knowledge of the amino acid requirements of the different animal species was very limited. Nevertheless the results achieved corresponded at least approximately to the information that was available and there seemed no reason to doubt that given accurate analytical data the formulation of ideal diets by combining protein foods appropriately was a logical development.   Block and Mitchell

(1946) tabulated the excesses and deficiencies in amino acid
composition for a number of foods including milk, wheat flour,
beef muscle, maize, oats and cottonseed meal.   Whole egg protein
was taken as the standard protein against which the others were
compared.   They then showed that the calculated benefits to be
obtained by mixing, for example, beef and cereals were indeed
borne out in biological tests with rats.   Conversely they were
able to show that no benefit was obtained on mixing cottonseed
and maize and this was attributed to the fact that both were
limited by deficiencies of the same amino acid, lysine.   An
arginine deficiency in a lactalbumin-cereal diet was corrected by
the calculated addition of meat scraps (Ott and Boucher, 1944) and
it was also reported that a mixture of 7 parts of sesame and 13
parts of soyabean meal, as well as being theoretically optimal
from the point of view of contributing the maximum possible
amounts of lysine and methionine, did in fact give better weight
gains in chicks than did mixtures of the two protein foods in
other proportions (Grau and Almquist, 1944).   For mixtures of
sesame with groundnut it has been similarly shown that while the
protein efficiency ratio of each is respectively 1.7 and 1.6,
a 50:50 mixture has a PER of 2.0 (Tasker, Joseph, Narayana Rao,
Rajagopalan, Sankaran and Swaminathan, 1960).   These appear to
be good examples of the successful use of supplementation to
achieve the best possible combination of given pairs of protein
concentrates when added to a cereal-based diet for poultry.
More recently mixtures of cow pea with maize were found to give
higher protein efficiency ratios (PER) than diets containing
either component alone (Bressani and Scrimshaw, 1961).   Equal
parts of both gave a value of 1.84, one part maize to three parts
of cow pea gave a value of 1.82, and maize and cow pea by themselves gave respectively PERs of 1.22 and 1.41.   Bressani and
Elias (1968) reviewed the position and from an examination of all
of the published work concluded that when two or more protein
sources are mixed the results follow one of four patterns.   The
nutritional value of a mixture of two materials of differing
nutritive value may lie between the two and be predictable by
calculation from the relative proportions of each component in
the mixture.   A second pattern, which is really a special case of
this one, concerns the combination of two materials having the
same nutritional value to give a mixture which is equivalent to
each of the components.   The remaining two patterns are of much
greater nutritional and economic significance.   Substantial
amounts of a relatively poor quality protein source may be
combined with a superior one and the mixtures may be equal in
nutritive value to that of the better component alone.   In such
a case the sparing action of the poorer material could be
explained by the hypothesis that the better component is itself
providing a luxus diet and dilution is still allowing optimum
performance to be achieved.   The final pattern is not always so

easy to explain.   Here, combination of a poor and a good protein
source may actually yield mixtures which are superior to the
better component, and the maize-cow pea system mentioned above is
an example of such fruitful complementation.

     Bressani and Elias pointed out that though it was usually
assumed that the observed results depend upon the absolute and
relative amounts of the available essential amino acids,
particularly lysine and methionine, insufficient studies had been
made at that time, and they further suggested that other possible
factors could include the ratios of essential to non-essential
amino acids in the protein components of the mixtures, and their
digestibilities.   Further complications could arise if the
mixing of a relatively good and relatively poor quality protein
source led to the establishment of amino acid antagonism by
producing for example an undesirable ratio of lysine to arginine.
This possibility cannot be disregarded in circumstances where
combinations are designed to increase dietary lysine content
without taking due note of the effect upon other amino acid levels.
Similarly one can envisage the achieving of growth depressing
levels of methionine, particularly small excesses of which are
known to be deleterious (Russell, Taylor and Hogan, 1952).

     Block and Mitchell (1946) proposed that protein foods might
be ranked in order of nutritive value on the basis of the
essential amino acid which was in greatest deficit when compared
with a reference protein such as whole egg.   Some, including
ourselves have used as a reference protein a hypothetical mixture
of amino acids thought to meet the optimum requirements of the
animal concerned.   The value obtained by dividing the percentage
of the most deficient amino acid - the limiting amino acid - by
the percentage of the same amino acid in the chosen reference
protein, is called the Chemical Score.   In the majority of cases
the limiting amino acid will be either lysine or methionine +
cystine and when consideration is deliberately restricted to these
amino acids the expression has been termed the Simplified Chemical
Score.

     Although it has been suggested that account should be taken
of all of the essential amino acids and not merely of that one
which is first limiting (Oser, 1951; UN Protein Advisory Group,
1974) many still argue that the extent to which a protein may be
utilised is solely dependent upon the limiting amino acid
(e.g. Bender, 1973).   While parameters such as the Essential
Amino Acid Index - EAAI (Oser, 1951) may assume importance under
conditions where protein sources are being evaluated at the low
levels of overall protein demanded by standard tests such as
Protein Efficiency Ratio (PER) and Net Protein Utilisation (NPU),
under practical and near-practical conditions such as those used

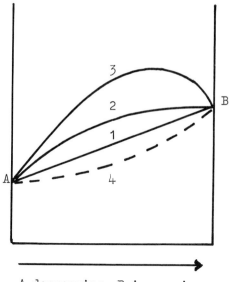

A decreasing, B increasing

Figure 1.   Possible curves representing the nutritional value of
mixtures of a relatively poor protein concentrate A with a
superior one B.

in the Total Protein Efficiency (TPE) method in which the protein
source is combined with a basal cereal, it is very likely that the
majority of essential amino acids will be in adequate supply or
even in excess of requirement.   Indeed in many cases the only amino
acid in deficit will be the limiting one, usually lysine or
cystine + methionine, and then the appropriate measure is clearly
the Chemical Score.   Even when other essential amino acids fall
below requirement level, the deficits are usually small so that the
effect of allowing for them adds little to the measure provided by
the limiting amino acid alone.   In fact the application of the
EAAI calculation to such practical or near-practical diets
provides a range of values all of which approach 100 and are
insufficiently separated to provide a useful discriminatory
measure (Woodham and Deans, 1977).

     Examination of a wide variety of protein pairs has shown that
all provide patterns corresponding to a straight line (1) or convex
curves (2 or 3) in Fig. 1.   From this it follows that all mixtures
are as good as, or better than, the value which would be predicted
from a knowledge of the nutritive value of each component.   It
could well be asked why there are no instances where a mixture is
poorer than the predicted value.   Why no concave curves such as 4
(Fig. 1)?

If we agree that convex curves such as 2 and 3 are evidence of complementation between the amino acid patterns of the two protein-containing constituents then the better of the two will be contributing quantities of those amino acids which are inadequately provided by the poorer material, and as we have seen, these will frequently be lysine and cystine + methionine.   One must assume that the effect of raising the levels of these important amino acids outweighs other effects concomitant upon these combinations.

There is a greater tendency nowadays to appreciate that overall amino balance is important in determining protein quality and that ideally foods should not merely contain adequate quantities of each of the amino acids, but also that excesses should be avoided whenever possible.   When chickens are provided with quantities of amino acids which, though excessive, are not such as to cause overt toxic symptoms, feed intake and growth are impaired, especially if the environmental conditions impose a stress (Waldroup, Mitchell, Payne and Hazen, 1976; Miller, 1976). Using purified diets and a dual feeding technique, Robel concluded in 1973 that excessive levels of the essential amino acids were a distinct disadvantage in the efficient utilisation of protein by the chick.   It is perhaps fortunate that those amino acids which produce deleterious effects in relatively small excess are indeed those which are least likely to be found in excess under practical conditions.   A total dietary methionine level of 0.7% was reported to produce growth retardation in rats (Russell, Taylor and Hogan, 1952) and a level of 1.05% of dietary lysine was found to be detrimental to rat growth (Fau, 1975).   Excesses of other amino acids appear to be less harmful and this could explain the failure to detect the depressed concave curve in mixtures of protein pairs.

EVALUATION OF PROTEIN PAIRS BY CHICK AND RAT TESTS

We have carried out a considerable number of studies into the effects of mixing pairs of protein foods in diets for growing rats and chickens.   A typical series of results for chick feeding trials of the total protein efficiency (TPE) type (Woodham and Deans, 1968) are presented in Table 1.   Five protein concentrates - fish, meat, soyabean, groundnut and sunflower seed meals - were combined in all of the 10 possible pairs, and the proportions of protein contributed by the components of each pair were varied from 100% of one and none of the second, to none of the first and 100% of the second.   All diets provided the same total amount of protein and energy and all contained 6% of cereal protein in addition to 12% from the protein concentrates being examined.   Full experimental results have been published elsewhere (Woodham and Deans, 1977).

TABLE 1

Total protein efficiency (TPE) of diets consisting of cereal

mixed with pairs of protein concentrates combined

in various proportions

Components of mixture	Relative amounts of components						
	120 0	100 20	80 40	60 60	40 80	20 100	0 120
Fishmeal– Soyabean meal	3.10	3.14	3.14	3.16	3.08	2.98	2.69
Fishmeal– Meat meal	3.01	2.95	2.75	2.68	2.54	2.34	2.08
Fishmeal– Sunflower seed meal	2.92	2.98	2.95	2.94	2.80	2.59	2.27
Fishmeal– Groundnut meal	2.88	3.02	3.03	2.93	2.71	2.49	2.09
Soyabean– Sunflower seed meal	2.56	2.70	2.74	2.67	2.67	2.51	2.33
Soyabean– Meat meal	2.74	2.84	2.81	2.69	2.57	2.38	2.22
Soyabean– Groundnut meal	2.69	2.63	2.55	2.54	2.44	2.32	2.12
Sunflower– Meat meal	2.42	2.49	2.45	2.39	2.39	2.29	2.15
Sunflower– Groundnut meal	1.94	2.21	2.29	2.24	2.21	2.15	2.13
Groundnut– Meat meal	2.15	2.25	2.33	2.33	2.31	2.18	2.09

The TPE curves for each of the 10 pairs are presented in
Fig. 2 and it will be seen that in every case a convex curve is
produced. In nine cases the nutritive value of the best mixture
is greater than that of the better component, and in the

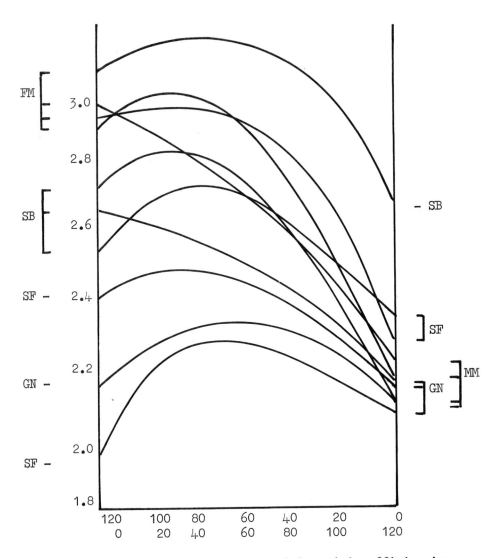

Figure 2.   Curves representing the total protein efficiencies
(TPE) for mixtures in varying proportions, of all possible pairs
from the series of 5 protein concentrates including fishmeal (FM),
soyabean (SB), sunflower seed (SF), groundnut (GN) and meat meal
(MM).

remaining case - the mixtures of soyabean with groundnut meal -
all of the mixtures give values which lie above the straight line
joining the TPE of the two components.   In other words all of the
mixtures examined exhibit beneficial synergistic effects.

Comparison of the growth curves for one of the pairs – fishmeal and sunflower seed meal – with the amino acid compositions of the various mixtures of the two components indicates that all of the essential amino acids are provided in adequate amounts in all of the mixtures with the single exception of lysine. Mixtures in which sunflower seed predominates are lysine-deficient and the chick's requirements are not met until the proportions of fishmeal and sunflower seed are equal (Fig. 3). However the fact that mixtures containing higher proportions of fishmeal give somewhat better growth than that given by the 50:50 mixture or by the fishmeal-cereal diet alone is not explicable on the basis of the diet's Chemical Score.

It must be concluded that Chemical Score, which is a measure of the adequacy of the most limiting amino acid in the diet, cannot predict differences in nutritive value between diets found under the near-practical conditions of the TPE trial. Overall amino acid balance is important, and it has been pointed out that the TPE test is capable of distinguishing between chick diets all of which have Chemical Scores around 100 (Woodham, 1976). This indicates that growth depression must be attributable to the provision of certain amino acids in excess of requirement, and not merely to a deficiency of one or more essential amino acids.

While these chick tests are near-practical in that total dietary protein levels are only slightly less than those used in commercial practice, the standard rat tests mentioned earlier employ decidedly sub-optimal levels of protein and amino acids. With these tests the synergistic effects are much less marked and the only striking deviations from a straight line relationship were exhibited by three of the sunflower seed mixtures (sunflower-soyabean, sunflower-fishmeal and sunflower-meat meal) (Woodham and Clarke, 1977). It seems that when the amino acid provision falls well below requirement, as in the case of standard tests such as the estimation of net protein utilisation (NPU) or protein efficiency ratio (PER), the amino acid level is critical and has a major influence upon the results of the growth test. When however the provision of essential amino acids is adequate or nearly so as in the case of the chick total protein efficiency (TPE) test, the precise level of individual amino acids is no longer the over-riding factor, and other influences including overall amino acid balance, growth inhibitors and amino acid excesses could combine to determine the growth response.

So far it has not proved possible to formulate an expression which would predict nutritional value from total amino acid composition. Decreasing levels of lysine and sulphur-containing amino acids in the diet are frequently accompanied by increases in arginine and glycine in particular. In the series referred to

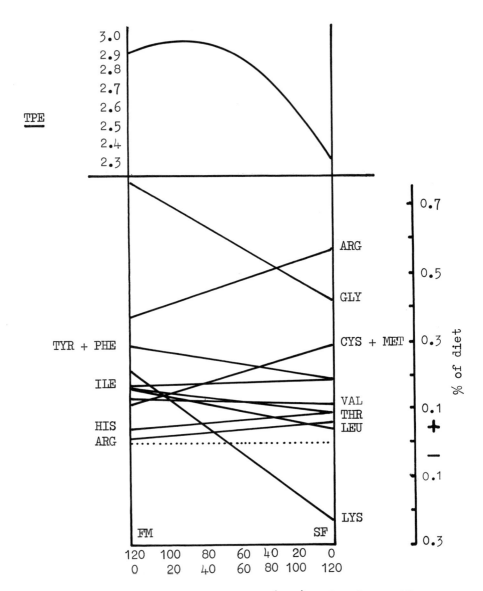

Figure 3.   Total protein efficiency (TPE) and amino acid
composition expressed in relation to the chicks' requirements, for
5 mixtures containing varying proportions of fishmeal (FM) and
sunflower seed (SF).   The dotted line indicates the amino acid
requirements for the chicken.

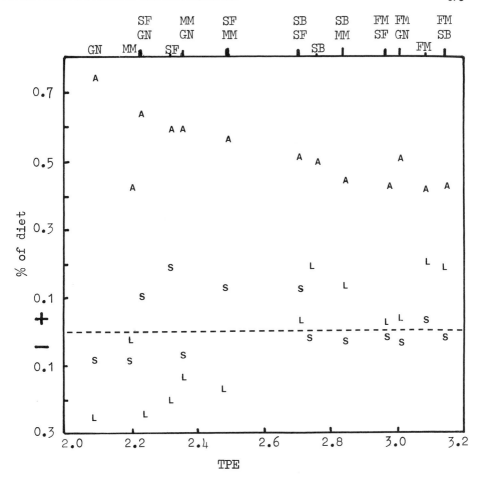

Figure 4.   Provision of arginine (A), lysine (L) and methionine +
cystine (S) by groundnut (GN), meat meal (MM), sunflower seed (SF),
soyabean (SB) and fishmeal (FM) and optimum pairs, in 18% crude
protein chick diets containing a constant amount of cereal protein,
expressed as surplus or deficit in relation to the chickens'
requirements and plotted against the total protein efficiency (TPE)
of the diets.

above, TPE values for the individual single protein concentrates
and those of the optimum mixtures correlate fairly well with
dietary lysine content.   If the 12% meat meal protein diet is
excluded the negative correlation between TPE and arginine content
is almost as good (Fig. 4) and the correlation with the dietary
lysine-arginine ratio is slightly better than both.   It is
conceivable that the poor result for the meat meal diet could be

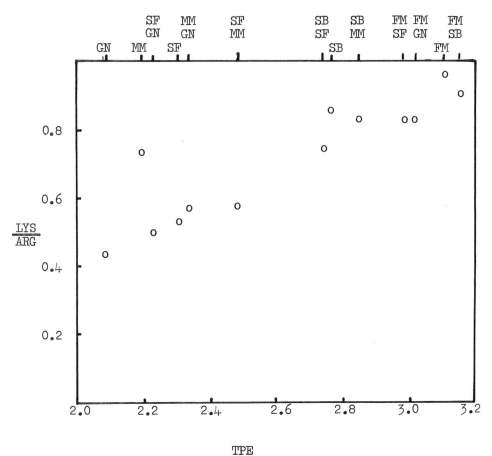

Figure 5.   The ratio of the total amounts of lysine and arginine
in 18% crude protein chick diets containing the same protein
concentrates as in Fig. 4, plotted against the total protein
efficiency (TPE) of the diets.

attributable to its exceptionally high glycine content but
whether this imbalance is indeed the reason requires further
experimental testing.   The relative growth depressant effects
of excesses of different amino acids are not understood and it
appears likely that these effects are not additive.   Whether
there is any relationship between the growth-depressant effects
of relatively small excesses of amino acids and their toxicities
at higher levels of inclusion remains to be shown.

REFERENCES

Abderhalden, E. (1912). Synthese der Zellbausteine in Pflanze
    und Tier. Berlin p. 85.

Bender, A. E. (1975). Chemical Scores and availability of amino
    acids. In 'Proteins in Human Nutrition'. J. W. G. Porter
    and B. A. Rolls (Editors). Academic Press: London.

Block, R. J. and Mitchell, H. H. (1946). The correlation of the
    amino acid composition of proteins with their nutritive value.
    Nutr. Abst. Rev., 16, 249-278.

Bressani, R. and Elias, L. G. (1968). Processed vegetable protein
    mixtures for human consumption in developing countries.
    Adv. Fd Res. 16, 1-103.

Bressani, R. and Scrimshaw, N. S. (1961). Pubs. Natn. Res. Counc.
    Wash. No. 843 p. 35.

Fau, D. (1975). Déséquilibre par exces de lysine et correction
    par un supplement de thréonine en fonction des modalités
    alimentaires. Ann. Nutr. Aliment. 29, 321-335.

Grau, C. R. and Almquist, H. J. (1944). Sesame protein in chick
    diets. Proc. Soc. Exp. Biol. Med. 57, 187-9.

Lawes, J. B. and Gilbert, J. H. (1866). Food in its relations to
    various exigencies of the animal body. Phil. Mag. 32, 55-64.

McCollum, E. V., Simmonds, N. and Parsons, H. T. (1919).
    Supplementary relationships between the proteins of certain
    seeds. J. Biol. Chem. 37, 155-177.

McCollum, E. V., Simmonds, N. and Parsons, H. T. (1921).
    Supplementary protein values in foods. 4. The supplementary
    relations of cereal grain with cereal grain; legume seed
    with legume seed; and cereal grain with legume seed with
    respect to improvement in the quality of their proteins.
    J. Biol. Chem. 47, 207-234.

McCollum, E. V., Simmonds, N. and Pitz, W. (1916). Is lysine the
    limiting amino acid in the proteins of wheat, maize or oats?
    J. Biol. Chem. 28, 483-6.

Miller, R. F. (1976). The effect of excess amino acids on feed
    intake and performance of chickens. Proc. 36th ann.
    meeting, AFMA Nutrition Council, Memphis. pp 24-6.

Osborne, T. B. and Mendel, L. B. (1914). Amino acids in nutrition and growth. J. Biol. Chem. 17, 325-349.

Oser, B. L. (1951). A method for integrating essential amino acid content in the nutritional evaluation of protein. J. Amer. Dietet. Ass. 27, 396-402.

Ott, W. H. and Boucher, R. V. (1944). Lactalbumin as a protein supplement for growing chickens. Poult. Sci. 23, 497-506.

Robel, E. J. (1973). Amino acid intake of chickens: effects of feeding excess amino acids. Poult. Sci. 52, 1981.

Russell, W. C., Taylor, M. W. and Hogan, J. H. (1952). Effect of excess essential amino acids on growth of the white rat. Arch. Biochem. 39, 249-253.

Tasker, P. K., Joseph, K., Narayana Rao, M., Rajagopalan, R., Sankaran, A. N. and Swaminathan, M. (1960). Supplementary value of the proteins of sunflower (Helianthus annus) and sesame seeds to groundnut and Bengal gram (Cicer arietinum) proteins. Ann. Biochem. exp. Med. (India) 20, 37-40.

U.N. Protein Advisory Group (1974). P.A.G. guideline (No. 6) for preclinical testing of novel sources of protein. P.A.G. Bulletin No. 4, 17-31.

Waldroup, P. W., Mitchell, R. J., Payne, J. R. and Hazen, K. R. (1976). Performance of chicks fed diets formulated to minimize excess levels of essential amino acids. Poult. Sci. 55, 243-253.

Woodham, A. A. (1968). A chick growth test for the evaluation of protein quality in cereal-based diets. 1. Development of the method. Brit. Poult. Sci. 9, 53-63.

Woodham, A. A. (1976). The relationship between amino acid composition and nutritive value for plant and animal protein concentrates. Qual. Plant. 25, 311-316.

Woodham, A. A. and Clarke, E. M. W. (1977). Nutritive value of mixed proteins. 2. As determined by net protein utilization and protein efficiency ratio tests. Br. J. Nutr. 37, 309-319.

Woodham, A. A. and Deans, P. S. (1977). Nutritive value of mixed proteins. 1. In cereal-based diets for poultry. Br. J. Nutr. 37, 289-308.

20

SOME THOUGHTS ON AMINO ACID SUPPLEMENTATION OF PROTEINS IN

RELATION TO IMPROVEMENT OF PROTEIN NUTRITURE

N. J. Benevenga and D. G. Cieslak

Departments of Nutritional Science and Meat and

Animal Science, University of Wisconsin, Madison 53706

ABSTRACT

Supplementation of diets with free amino acids has not routinely been beneficial and poses a potential risk. Thus, mixing proteins to increase the quality of the dietary protein is attractive. The slope-ratio technique for evaluation of protein quality has serious drawbacks, because the growth response is not linear and animals appear to adapt to the diet and thus make more efficient use of diets low in protein or low in protein quality. Apparently, the relative value of proteins is not constant, but varies with the amino acid spectrum as well as intake. Thus, evaluation of proteins or protein mixtures should be determined under the conditions (e.g. maintenance or maximum gain) of their potential use. This approach could lead to the development of a protein replacement equivalents system similar to the starch equivalents system in the evaluation of the net energy of animal feeds.

INTRODUCTION

Fortification of diets with amino acids or proteins so that the requirement for amino acids can be met within levels of consumption which are physiologically reasonable or do not lead to excessive intakes of energy, is obviously possible given the availability of single amino acids or proteins of widely differing amino acid composition. The problem of fortification of human diets with amino acids or mixtures of proteins is complex, especially when it is considered from the point of view of the family food supply. Supplementation of the infant diet within the framework of the contemporary American family is somewhat

simplified, because the infant is not dependent upon the general
family menu. The complexity of amino acid supplementation within
the age and sex spectrum of the "typical" 4-6 member family is
seen when it is realized that the requirement for protein falls
from 2.2 g/kg to 1.5 g/kg over the first six months of life and
declines further to 1.0 g/kg at 1 year of age. The decline in
protein requirement falls further to about 0.7 g/kg at the age
of 10 (Williams et al., 1974). The decline in the requirement
of the individual amino acids is greater than that of protein,
so that the fraction of the total amino acids classified as
indispensable falls from 48% of the total for 4-6 months old
children to 30% of the total for children at the age of 10 and
to 17% of the total for the adult (Williams et al., 1974).

One of the problems encountered in the determination of the
level of supplementation of amino acids or protein required to
obtain an "ideal" or acceptable amino acid pattern of a diet, is
simply the determination of the amino acid spectrum of the diet.
Two of the amino acids that are often thought to be limiting in
diets (methionine and tryptophan) are among the most difficult to
determine accurately. The magnitude of this problem with respect
to the sulfur amino acids at least, is seen in a report by
Jamalian and Pellett (1968). They showed that the estimation of
the cystine content of proteins was increased by an average of
32% when the sample was oxidized with performic acid, but that of
methionine was more variable and was only 88% of that of samples
not treated. The problem of estimation of the tryptophan content
of the protein of foods is no less challenging since it is destroyed during typical acid hydrolysis procedure and hence requires alkaline hydrolysis along with considerable care in order
to obtain satisfactory estimates (Hugli and Moore, 1972). Additional problems encountered in evaluating the nutritional value
of proteins with known amino acid compositions relates to the
bioavailability of the amino acids in the diet. The terms availability or bioavailability conceptually have been used to convey
the idea that amino acids may not be released and absorbed during
the digestion process. De Muelenaere and associates (1967, 1967a)
showed that the estimation of the availability of amino acids was
dependent not only on the level of the amino acid of interest,
but the level of energy (fat), type of carbohydrate, level of
protein and amino acid balance. These general relationships were
further amplified in a recent report from Baker's laboratory at
the University of Illinois (Teeter, Baker and Becker, 1977).
They used the young growing chick assay to test the availability
of lysine in soybean meal. The availability of lysine in soybean meal when compared to a crystalline amino acid standard
growth curve was 80%, however, when compared to a standard curve
developed with an amino acid diet simulating soy protein, the
bioavailability approached 100%. Hence, it is again quite clear

that the amino acid pattern of the diet affects the estimation
of the availability of lysine and that in this case, the bioavailability of lysine in soybean meal approached 100%.

It must be obvious from the preceeding discussion that considerable judgment must come in to play when supplementation of
dietary protein is considered. The majority of the rest of this
presentation will emphasize the child (20 kg) rather than the
infant or adult, because it appears to the authors, that the
greatest likelihood of a nutritional deficiency rests with the
rapidly growing child. Comparison of the best estimate of an
amino acid pattern that will meet the need of the child with
three cereals used as a source of dietary energy, is seen in
table 1. It is evident from this table that the amino acid concentrations of the proteins in some of the cereals are lower than
the reference pattern for the infant in relation to lysine,
tryptophan, isoleucine and threonine. Similar analysis of the
protein supplements of plant origin would reveal that soybean
and black bean proteins are low in the sulfur amino acids. Obviously, addition of crystalline amino acids to the diet would
improve the amino acid pattern and, theoretically, the quality
of the "protein". However, when this has been tried, it has not,
in general, lead to a readily detectable improvement (Harper and
Hegsted, 1974). One risk seldomly pointed out when considering
supplementation of low protein diets with amino acids, is the
real possibility of depressed growth due to the addition of relatively high level of the sulphur amino acids or tryptophan. The

TABLE 1

Comparison of cereal amino acid patterns

	Infant Reference Pattern[1]	Maize[2]	Wheat Flour (60/70)[2]	Rice[2]
		mg/g Nitrogen		
Ile	262	230	217	262
Leu	438	783	400	514
Lys	319	167	113	226
TSA	163	217	229	229
TAAA	456	544	423	503
Thr	219	225	153	207
Trp	69	44	58	84
Val	300	303	240	361

1 From Williams et al., 1974, pg. 56.
2 From amino acid content of foods and biological data on proteins
   F.A.O., Pub. #24, 1970.

relationship between the amino acid requirement for the rat and
the level of individual amino acids which result in a discernable
depression in performance is presented in table 2. It is important to note that the difference between the level required and
that which causes adverse effects, is rather narrow for methionine, which is one of the amino acids often supplemented. Although there is a slight depression in growth of rats consuming a
diet containing 75% casein (Anderson, Benevenga and Harper, 1968),
the level of the individual amino acids consumed when the diet
contains 70% casein, is in excess of that causing adverse effects
when added to a low protein diet alone. While it is clear that
glycine and serine specifically alleviate the toxicity of excess
levels of methionine (Benevenga and Harper, 1967), it is not clear
that it is the concentration of these two amino acids in a diet
containing 70% casein that results in no marked depression in
growth.

    Although the authors could find no evidence in the litera-
ture, it would be expected that free amino acids added to a diet
containing intact protein, may be used less efficiently for
protein synthesis than if the amino acids were absorbed along
with the bulk of the amino acids from the protein. The magnitude
of the difference in the absorption of methionine (^{35}S or ^{75}Se)
when it was in dried egg white, versus that when it was in free
form (^{75}Se or ^{35}S) is seen in table 3. Early in the experiment
(15-60 minutes), from 25-40% more of the free than the protein-
bound methionine was absorbed. This again points to the potential problems that can be anticipated when diets are supplemented
with free amino acids.

    Because of the basic question of the beneficial affects of
supplementation of the diet with free amino acids and the potential risks in the addition of the free amino acids to mixed diets
the remainder of this presentation, will emphasize the potential

TABLE 3

Percent of dietary methionine apparently absorbed[1]

Time After Feeding Min.	Protein Bound Met	Free Met	Free Bound
15	29.1	36.5	1.25
30	33.2	43.6	1.39
60	40.9	54.0	1.32
120	62.2	77.3	1.24
240	95.7	96.1	1.00

1 Adapted from Canolty and Nasset (1975).

TABLE 2

Level at which individual amino acids result in adverse effects in rats fed a low protein diet in relation to the requirement of the amino acid and its content in a high protein diet[1]

Amino Acid	Requirement % of the Diet	Dietary Level Which Results in Depressed Growth %	Multiple Requirement Which Results In Adverse Effects	Amounts in a 70% Casein Diet %
Methionine	.5	1.5	3.0	2.3
Cystine	-	3.0	-	0.3
Tryptophan	.12	2.0	16.6	1.1
Threonine	.5	5.0	10.0	3.2
Leucine	.7	2.5	3.6	7.0
Isoleucine	.55	5.0	9.0	4.7
Valine	.55	5.0	9.0	5.2
Phenylalanine	.9	4.0	4.4	4.1
Tyrosine	-	3.0	-	4.5
Lysine	.9	5.0	5.5	5.8
Histidine	.26	2.0	7.7	2.1

1 Modified from Harper, A. E.; 1974, Effects of disproportionate amounts of amino acids, o. 156-7 in National Research Council Committee on Amino Acids. Improvement of Protein Nutriture.

benefits of mixing natural ingredients.   In approaching this
question, the potential for the use of maize, wheat flour or rice
in concert with soybean, pork or chicken as sources of the indispensable amino acids and nitrogen, was investigated.   The amino
acid pattern for the infant fed at a level of 0.75 g CP/kg body
weight (Williams et al., 1974) was selected as a basis for estab-
lishing the amounts of the cereals alone or supplemented with
soybean, pork or chicken required to meet the amino acid and
nitrogen requirement of a 20 kg child.   The amount of maize protein or maize protein supplemented with various combinations of
soybean and pork or soybean and chicken required to meet the amino
acid and nitrogen requirement of the child is shown in table 4.
The theoretical dry matter consumption of a 20 kg child (360 gm)
was estimated by assuming that an average diet contains 5 Kcal
M.E./gm and that the M.E. requirement of a 20 kg child is 1,800
Kcal (Nat. Acad. Sci., 1974).   Substitution of 10% of the maize
protein with soybean protein reduces the amount of protein required to meet the need for indispensable amino acids and nitrogen by 12%.   Use of pork instead of soybean resulted in a reduction of 20% in the amount of crude protein needed to meet the
child's requirement.   The most important point to note is that
even with maize protein alone, the "protein" requirement can be
met with only 78% of the theoretical dry matter consumption.
However, this level of consumption provides only 58% of the
energy needed.   The deficiency in energy can be overcome by a
high energy foodstuff (e.g. fat).   When similar calculations were
made for wheat flour (table 5), it became clear that wheat flour
alone could not meet the amino acid and nitrogen requirement of
of the child within normal levels of dry matter consumption.
While replacement of 10% of the wheat protein with soybean, pork
or chicken protein does depress the amount of the mixture required to meet the amino acid needs, the energy requirement
cannot be met.   Replacement of 20% of the wheat flour protein
with soybean, pork or chicken protein gives rise to a dietary
combination that meets both the protein and energy requirements.
Calculations made using rice (table 6) revealed again that the
protein requirement of the child could be met with rice alone
when the dry matter consumption was 88% of the theoretical maximum.   At this level of intake only 65% of the energy requirement was met.   Replacement of 10% of the rice protein with soybean
protein approximated and replacement with 10% of pork or chicken
protein allowed the protein and energy requirement to be met
within the theoretical dry matter consumption limits.   The protein and energy requirement could be more easily met if the dry
matter consumption limitation was based on a dietary energy value
of 4 Kcal/g rather than 5 Kcal/g used here.   The "bulk" limit
would be raised to 450 g (1,800 Kcal ÷ 4 Kcal/gm = 450 gm).
Should this be the case, then only 10% of the wheat flour protein
would have to be replaced and rice could theoretically meet both

TABLE 4

Theoretical calculation of the amount of maize protein alone or supplemented with soybean, pork or chicken required to meet the amino acid & nitrogen requirement of the child

Diet[1]				gm C.P./kg[2]	% Theoretical D.M. Consumption[3]	Intake Kcal/kg	% Energy Requirement[4]
Maize	Soy	Pork	Chicken				
100	-	-	-	1.37	78	52	58
90	10	-	-	1.21	64	42	47
90	-	10	-	1.09	61	40	44
90	-	-	10	1.13	62	40	44
80	20	-	-	1.09	53	35	39
80	-	20	-	0.87	48	30	34
80	-	-	20	0.96	49	31	35
80	10	10	-	0.99	52	33	37
80	10	-	10	1.02	51	33	37
75	25	-	-	1.03	46	30	34
75	15	10	-	0.94	47	30	34
75	15	-	10	0.97	47	30	33
75	-	25	-	0.83	45	28	32
75	-	-	25	0.89	44	28	31

1 Amino acid data from Amino Acid Content of Foods and Biological Data on Proteins. F.A.O. No. 24, 1970 and Orr and Watt. Amino Acid Content of Foods, Home Econ. Res. Report #3. 1966.

2 Based on Ile 42, Leu 70, Lys 51, TSA 26, TAAA 73, Thr 35, Trp 11, Val 48, mg/gm protein and 0.75 g of this protein per kg body weight. Taken from Nat. Acad. Sci. Comm. on Amino Acids, 1975, pg. 52 and 56 Improvement of Protein Nutriture.

3 Based on energy requirement of 1800 Kcal for a 20 kg child. Taken from N.R.C. recommended dietary allowances. 8th Edition, 1974, and assuming an average of 5 Kcal (ME)/gm diet at 90% D.M.

4 Based on an energy requirement of 1800 Kcal for a 20 kg child.

TABLE 5

Theoretical calculation of the amount of wheat flour[1] protein alone or supplementation with soybean, pork or chicken required to meet the amino acid & nitrogen requirement of the child

Diet[2]							
Wheat	Soy	Pork	Chicken	gm C.P./kg[3]	% Theoretical D.M. Consumption[4]	Intake Kcal/kg	% Energy Requirement[5]
100	-	-	-	2.13	129	86	95
90	10	-	-	1.69	94	62	69
90	-	10	-	1.46	86	56	62
90	-	-	10	1.53	88	57	63
80	20	-	-	1.41	72	47	53
80	-	20	-	1.11	64	41	45
80	-	-	20	1.20	64	41	46
80	10	10	-	1.24	67	44	48
80	10	-	10	1.29	67	44	49
75	25	-	-	1.30	63	42	46
75	15	10	-	1.16	61	39	43
75	15	-	10	1.20	61	39	43
75	-	25	-	0.99	57	36	39
75	-	-	25	1.08	57	35	39

1 60-70% extraction.

2 Amino acid data from Amino Acid Content of Foods and Biological Data on Proteins. F.A.O. No. 24, 1970 and Orr and Watt. Amino Acid Content of Foods, Home Econ. Res. Report #3, 1966.

3 Based on Ile 42, Leu 70, Lys 51, TSA 26, TAAA 73, Thr 35, Trp 11, Val 48, mg/gm protein and 0.75 g of this protein per kg body weight. Taken from Nat. Acad. Sci. Comm. on Amino Acids, 1975, pg. 52 and 56 Improvement of Protein Nutriture.

4 Based on energy requirement of 1800 Kcal for a 20 kg child. Taken from N.R.C. recommended dietary allowances. 8th Edition, 1974, and assuming an average of 5 Kcal (ME)/gm diet at 90% D.M.

5 Based on an energy requirement of 1800 Kcal for a 20 kg child.

TABLE 6

Theoretical calculation of the amount of rice proteins alone or supplemented with soybean, pork or chicken required to meet the amino acid & nitrogen requirement of the child

| Diet[1] | | | | gm C.P./kg[2] | % Theoretical D.M. Consumption[3] | Intake Kcal/kg | % Energy Requirement[4] |
Wheat	Soy	Pork	Chicken				
100	–	–	–	1.06	88	58	65
90	10	–	–	0.99	76	50	55
90	–	10	–	0.90	72	47	52
90	–	–	10	0.93	72	47	52
80	20	–	–	0.92	64	42	47
80	–	20	–	0.78	59	38	42
80	–	–	20	0.82	59	38	42
80	10	10	–	0.85	61	40	44
80	10	–	10	0.87	61	40	44
75	25	–	–	0.89	59	39	43
75	15	10	–	0.82	57	37	41
75	15	–	10	0.84	56	37	41
75	–	25	–	0.74	54	35	39
75	–	–	25	0.78	54	34	38

1 Amino acid data from Amino Acid Content of Foods and Biological Data on Proteins. F.A.O. No. 24, 1970 and Orr and Watt. Amino Acid Content of Foods, Home Econ. Res. Report #3, 1966.

2 Based on Ile 42, Leu 70, Lys 51, TSA 26, TAAA 73, Thr 35, Trp 11, Val 48, mg/gm protein and 0.75 g of this protein per kd body weight. Taken from Nat. Acad. Sci. Comm. on Amino Acids, 1975, Pg. 52 and 56 Improvement of Protein Nutriture.

3 Based on energy requirement of 1800 Kcal for a 20 kg child. Taken from N.R.C. recommended dietary allowances. 8th Edition, 1974, and assuming an average of 5 Kcal (ME)/gm diet at 90% D.M.

4 Based on energy requirement of 1800 Kcal for a 20 kg child.

the energy and protein requirements. These examples demonstrate
rather clearly the point that the protein gap is really one of
total food intake (Harper, Payne and Waterlow, 1973; McLaren,
1974; Whitehead, 1974).

   The concept of mixing proteins of differing amino acid composition so that the mixture meets the requirement at a lower total
crude protein intake, is not new. The difference between protein
complimentation and protein supplementation has been recently
reviewed (Bressani, 1974). In cases where the total protein
content of the diet is derived from two sources so that the
ratios of the two proteins may vary, i.e. 100:0; 90:10 ...;
10:90; 0:100, one would expect a measure of protein quality such
as PER or NPU to change as follows. In cases where one protein
has a surplus of an indispensable amino acid, it can be diluted
by a protein which is limited in that amino acid. The amount of
a protein mixture needed to meet the requirement would be diminished relative to that of the deficient protein, but would not be
expected to be lower than that of the protein with the surplus of
the indispensable amino acid. This would be an example of a
protein supplementation. Protein complimentation on the other
hand, would be a condition where the proteins are mutually supplementary so that addition of protein A to protein B enhances
performance relative to B and likewise addition of B to A performance relative to A. Obviously, the majority of protein interactions will be supplementary in nature. This was clearly
demonstrated in a recent paper of Woodham and Deans (1977). In
their work with chickens, they used a basal diet made up of
cereal, so that the crude protein content derived from cereals
was 6%. To this basal diet they added alone, or in specific
combinations, two different protein concentrates (soybean meal,
sunflower-seed meal, groundnut meal, meat meal, and fish meal)
so that the total crude protein of the diet was 18%. As a measure of protein quality, they calculated the total protein
efficiency (TPE) which is defined as the grams of weight gain/g
protein consumed. The results of two series of experiments are
shown in figure 1. The difference in series 1 and 2 may be due
to the different strains of chickens used. Note that in general,
the trends obtained within both experiments are nearly identical.
As suspected, there is no evidence of protein complimentation.
Although some may suggest that this is so for the sunflower-
seed-groundnut meal results from the series 2 experiments, this
notion can easily be dispelled, because all of the other values
for sunflower-seed meal varied from 2.2 - 2.5 at the 120 level.
It is clear from this figure, that fish meal supplements groundnut meal, sunflower-seed meal, soybean meal and meat meal. A
similar association is seen between soybean meal and meat meal
and groundnut meal. The total protein content of the fish meal
combinations can probably be decreased, because a TPE of 3 was
maintained over a number of mixtures, suggesting that the growth
rate of the chicken limited the response. This illustrates one

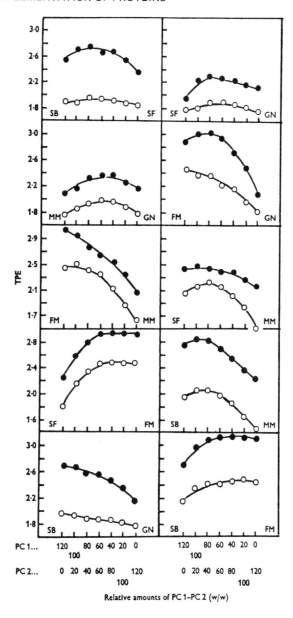

Figure 1. Total protein efficiency (g weight gain/g protein consumed; TPE) of diet with 180 g crude protein (nitrogen x 6.25)/kg, containing cereals (60 g protein/kg) in addition to pairs of protein concentrates (PC_1, PC_2) mixed in varying proportions contribute 120 g protein/kg; (0), series 1; (●) series 2. SB, soya-bean meal; SF, sunflower-seed meal; GN, groundnut meal; MM, meat meal; FM, fish meal. Taken from Woodham and Deans (1977).

of the problems in evaluating protein quality within a dietary
framework with a fixed protein level.

The obvious alternative approach would be to test the minimum level of a variety of protein combinations that would result
in nitrogen balance or maximum growth. This approach is much
more demanding and tedious than those previously reviewed, but
does allow for more accurate evaluation of protein mixtures since
they can be evaluated for the function intended, e.g. maintenance
or growth. The most extensive series of experiments in which
numerous combinations of proteins have been tested in order to
minimize the amount required for nitrogen balance, have come from
Kofrányi's Laboratory (Kofrányi, 1972, 1973; Kofrányi, Jekat and
Müller-Wecker, 1970). This work has been carried out with adult
human males. At the beginning of all tests and between each
treatment, a "normal" mixed diet was used which resulted in a
nitrogen balance of + 1.0-1.5 g/day. With this approach, the
"labile protein pool" was considered replenished and the subject
then received the test diet. The nitrogen balance over the first
10-12 days was generally strongly negative, therefore, adjust-
ments were made both in the energy and nitrogen level of the diet
until slightly negative nitrogen balances were achieved. Only
when the minimum value had been maintained for 10 or so days, was
the information used to calculate the minimum nitrogen required
to maintain balance.

Because the amount of nitrogen required for nitrogen balance
for each subject varied, each was given whole egg protein and
the minimum nitrogen required for balance determined. The amount
of egg nitrogen/kg required for a balance averaged about 0.5 g/
kg, but varied from 0.37-0.62 g over the 27 subjects tested. This
value was somewhat greater than the 0.38 g/kg which can be calculated from the information presented by Young (1972). The
values for each of Kofrányi's subjects were adjusted to a common
0.5 g/kg average. A composite of the results of a number of the
protein-protein combinations is shown in figure 2. Note that
with the exception of the beef-potato combination, the minimum
amount of nitrogen required for maintenance is less than that
required for either of the single food stuffs alone. These
responses should be considered as examples of complimentation
rather than supplementation. Probably the most interesting observation is that with one exception, the minimum nitrogen required to maintain nitrogen balance with all of the other protein
combinations is lower than that for whole egg protein alone. That
the amino acid pattern itself was responsible for the low nitrogen
requirement for achieving N-balance was revealed in another experiment in which an amino acid mixture patterned after the egg-
potato proteins replaced the protein combination.

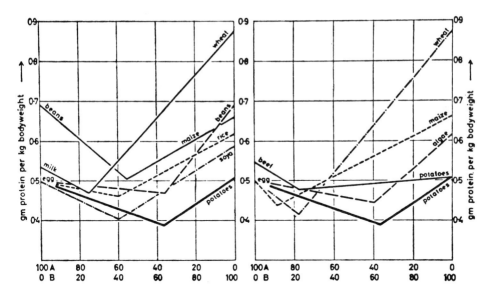

Figure 2.   The standardized diagrams for the minimum requirement of protein mixtures.   The abscissae show in percentages the
proportions of the mixtures of two proteins; the ordinates show
the daily minimum amounts of protein per kg body weight needed
to maintain the balance.   All ten mixtures have been normed to
egg = 0.50 g protein/kg body weight.   (A) protein from milk, egg
or beef.   (B) protein from potatoes, soya, beans, rice, wheat,
maize or algae.   Taken from Kofrányi (1972).

As pointed out earlier, the amount of energy and protein
were varied in order to determine the minimum amount of nitrogen
required to achieve balance.   The only information that the
authors found (Kofrányi, 1970), indicated that the range of energy
values used varied from 37.9-41.1 or 36.1-47.6 Kcal/kg/body
weight.   While these values would be expected to influence the
amount of nitrogen required to achieve balance, the alteration
in energy levels throughout any single evaluation did not follow
a pattern such that the highest energy intake coincided with the
minimum nitrogen requirement.   The role of energy intake in the
attainment of nitrogen balance with the FAO/WHO safe level of egg
protein intake has recently been discussed (Garza, Schrimshaw and
Young, 1976, 1977, 1977a).   In their studies, nitrogen balance
could be obtained with energy intakes that were increased 10%
(e.g. to 47-50 Kcal/kg).   These values are considerably higher
than those reported by Kofrányi (1970).   Differences of this magnitude are probably not explainable by the differences in assumptions or tabular energy values used.   Some of the apparent

inconsistencies may be explained by the adaptation of an amino
acid conserving mechanisms or the depression in protein synthesis
described by Waterlow (1968, 1975) in animals fed diets low in
protein.

A question arises as to the validity of applying results of
zero nitrogen balance studies to the needs of rapidly growing
animals. One wonders whether or not the amino acid spectrum which
would be ideal for maintenance is in fact ideal for growth. Although the authors are not aware that such a comparison has been
made, it is implied from published requirements that there may
indeed be differences (Williams et al., 1974). It has also been
suggested that there may be differences in the ability to conserve protein at very low intakes of specific amino acids (Said
and Hegsted, 1970; Said, Hegsted and Hayes, 1974). Therefore,
although protein quality may be accurately ascertained for animals
in a maintenance state from nitrogen equilibrium studies, it is
not clear that this is equally sufficient for young growing
animals receiving substantially larger amounts of protein. The
slope ratio assay has been suggested as one of the more effective
means whereby proteins can be evaluated in this context (Hegsted,
1974).

In assays of this type the response of the organism to graded
levels of an essential nutrient has long been known to be a
saturation phenomena. This is the theory behind the so-called
"break point" analysis of nutrient requirements. In a broader
perspective, this suggests that the efficiency of utilization is
a function of the level of nutrient intake. Previous efforts to
evaluate protein quality by dose response assays, have largely
ignored the changing efficiency of utilization by rigidly ad-
hering to predetermined nutrient levels. The evaluations are
made under an assumed linear response. However, for a given
protein or protein mixture which has not been previously evaluated, it may be difficult to determine which level of intake
will fall into a linear range. For example, decreases in efficiency of utilization of high quality proteins may be observed
with dietary levels as low as 12-15% protein (Hegsted and Chang,
1965). Substantially greater amounts of poor quality proteins
would be required to maximize growth. A method of evaluation of
protein quality which depends upon a growth response that is
proportional to the amount of nitrogen consumed, has been proposed
by Hegsted (Hegsted and Chang, 1965; Hegsted, Neff and Worcester,
1968; Hegsted and Neff, 1970; Hegsted and Juliano, 1974). In
his initial work, (Hegsted and Chang, 1965) it was evident that
the response was not linear with nitrogen intake and in some
cases, the response could be described by a sigmoidal curve. The
sigmoidal response was dealt with by comparing values with different proteins only over the linear proteins of the dose response

curve (Hegsted, Neff and Worcester, 1968; Hegsted and Juliano, 1974). A more versatile approach (Morgan, Mercer and Flodin, 1975; Mercer et al., 1977; Flodin, Mercer and Morgan, 1977; Flodin, Morgan and Mercer, 1977) which is based on a mathematical model capable of describing the entire dose response curve, appears to be more promising. The development of the entire curve allows almost limitless comparisons of two or more protein mixtures.

We were interested in using this model to evaluate the effect of corn and corn-whey protein mixtures. One hundred twenty male Holtzman rats (70 g) were equally divided among 4 protein treatments. Within each treatment, five rats were assigned to each of the six (2, 5, 10, 15, 18, or 22-27%) crude protein levels. The reason for the range in the highest levels was due to variation in the protein sources so that the range represent the maximum amount of crude protein that could be incorporated into a given treatment. The proteins used consisted of 100% "corn protein" made up from a mixture of corn processing by-products (table 7); 90% corn protein and 10% sweet cheddar cheese whey protein (table 7); 75% corn protein and 25% whey protein; 40% corn protein and 60% whey protein. Diets were offered ad libitum for three weeks and animal weights and food intake were determined on all alternate days. An attempt to fit response curves to the data used a procedure similar to that of Mercer et al., 1977, except that it has been adapted to use a non-linear regression fitting program available through MADISON ACADEMIC COMPUTING CENTER for their UNIVAC 1110 computer. Unfortunately, curves could not always be generated. Even when levels of crude protein of the diet exceeded 25%, this level of protein was insufficient to generate the expected maximum gain of the rat (approximately 7 g/day. Since a maximal response is one of the essential components of the saturation equation, an adequate regression could not be generated. The response curve for one of the diets (40/60) in which a maximum gain could be obtained is shown in figure 3. If the response is assumed to be a linear function of the protein consumption, as for example in the slope ratio approach taken by Hegsted, the least squares estimate of the ordinate intercept would be very close to zero ($Y = -0.9 + 17.2$ x; $r = 0.93$). This would suggest that maintenance of body weight could be achieved with a protein free diet, which is an obvious overestimation. If the same approach was taken with the gains over the last two weeks of the experiment, the intercept ($Y = 9.2 + 12.5$ x; $r = 0.90$) was actually positive. Even though maximum gains could be obtained, it appears that evaluation of protein over the linear portion of the response curve, can be very misleading. When the data from the three week experiment was summarized over the first and second week or the second and third week, it became clear that the animals underwent some type of adaptation. For example, the performance of animals fed the maximum level of protein increased

TABLE 7

Composition of corn-whey protein diets

Ingredient	% of Diet
Protein Source[1]	Variable
Corn Starch	to 100
Vitamin Mix[2]	0.5
Salt Mix[2]	5.0
Choline Cl	0.2
Corn Oil	10.0

1 The corn "protein" mixture was made up of the following materials, corn flour 36.25; corn fermentive extractives 37.47; corn gluten 15.56; corn germ 10.72 and contained 26% crude protein. These were a gift from Dave Schroeder, Corn Products Co., Argo, Illinois. The Cheddar cheese whey protein concentrate contained 39% crude protein and was a gift from Mr. Frank Thomas, Thomas Technical Service, Greenwood, Wisconsin.

2 See Rogers, Q. R. and A. E. Harper, 1965, Amino acid diets and maximal growth in the rat. J. Nutr. 87: 273-287.

some 50-100% from the first to the second and third weeks. Because there was no clear cut maximum obtained, a curve was hand-drawn so that a maximum (130 g) and minimum (-10 g) response was obtained over the two-week experiment. With these limits artificially imposed, the program could be used on the raw data. Results of the treatment of the data in this fashion are seen in figure 4. It is important to note that the response of animals fed the higher quality proteins (40/60 and 75/25) is sigmoidal and that those of animals consuming the poorer quality proteins are linear. While it would surely be premature to suggest that this difference in response would be the case in general, each treatment does involve a total of 30 rats and hence, this information should be given some weight. The different response of the rats fed the high and low quality proteins, should it hold up under further testing, will have relatively serious consequences. The amount of nitrogen required to obtain 0, 45, 60 and 90% of the theoretical Rmax are shown in table 8. Note that the relative efficiency of the poorer quality proteins becomes similar to that of the higher quality proteins as either zero or the Rmax is approached. This was unexpected as it was assumed by us and certainly by others (Flodin, Mercer and Morgan, 1977), that the shape of the response curve (gain versus N-consumed) is similar over widely varying protein qualities and that a constant relationship would be expected between the nitrogen required for gain at 1/2 Rmax and requirement to obtain the maximum gain. Additionally, one would expect that the "lag" in growth seen in

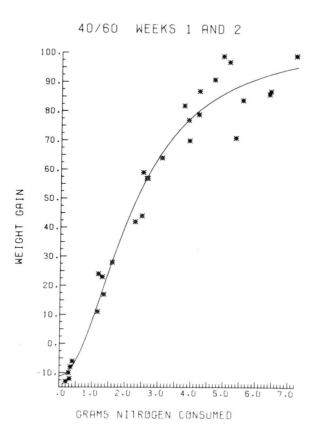

Figure 3. Growth response of rats fed the 40/60 diet over the first two weeks of the experiment. Each point represents a single rat. The curve was fit by a procedure similar to that described by Mercer et al. (1977).

the sigmoidal growth response curves, also would be related to the quality of dietary protein so that it would be proportionately longer when lower quality proteins were fed. Hence, the relative value of proteins determined at a low protein level may seriously overestimate the value of high quality proteins used to attain maximum gains or alternatively their requirement for maintenance. An alternative approach would be to develop a protein replacement equivalents system. The results from Kofrányi

TABLE 8

Relative efficiency of high quality and low quality proteins at different rates of growth

Diet[1]	0% of R max[2]		45% of R max		60% of R max		90% of R max	
	N req.	Rel. eff.	N req.	Rel. eff.	N req.	Rel. eff.	N req.	Rel. eff.
100/0	1.1	64	6.5	49	8.7	53	12.2[3]	78
90/10	1.0	70	6.1	52	8.0	58	11.3[3]	84
75/25	0.8	88	3.9	82	5.7	81	10.1	94
40/60	0.7	100	3.2	100	4.6	100	9.5	100

1 Relative percentage of corn "protein" and whey "protein" in the diet.

2 R_{max} assumed to be 130 g gain over 2 weeks.

3 Extrapolated values the maximum N intake of these groups was approximately 9 gm.

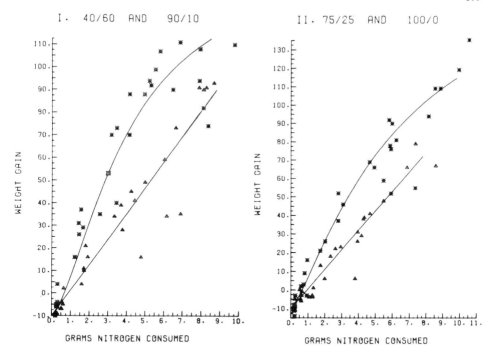

Figure 4.   Growth response over the last two weeks of the three week experiment of rats fed the 40/60 (*) or 90/10 (Δ) panel I or 75/25 (*) or 100/0 (Δ) panel II diets.   Each point represents the food intake and growth response of a single rat over the last two weeks of the three week experiment.   Curves were drawn as in figure 3 after an artificial minimum (-10 g) and maximum (130 g) values were assigned so that the program could generate this figure.

experiments on the minimum amount of a variety of protein mixtures necessary for maintenance of nitrogen balance in man, is in
essence available for use in the development of a protein replacement equivalents system.   Similar replacement equivalents should
be developed for young growing animals.   From our results (figure
4), it is clear that at a maximum rate of gain, the mixture of
25% whey protein and 75% corn protein is equivalent to the mixture of 60% whey protein and 40% corn protein.   The concept of
protein replacement equivalents deserves more consideration.
For example, a gain of 90 g over the last two weeks of the experiment (i.e. after the animals adapted) required a consumption of
5.5 g of N from the 40/60 mixture, 6.5 g from the 75/25 mixture,
8.8 g from the 90/10 mixture and 9.5 g (estimated) for the corn
"protein" alone.

REFERENCES

Anderson, H. L., Benevenga, N. J. and Harper, A. E. (1968). Associations among food and protein intake, serine, dehydratase and plasma amino acids. Am. J. Physiol. 214, 1008-1013.

Benevenga, N. J. and Harper, A. E. (1967). Alleviation of methionine and homocystine toxicity in the rat. J. Nutr. 93, 44-52.

Bressani, R. (1974). Complimentary amino acid patterns. 149-166. in Nutritients in processed foods - proteins. Ed. P. L. White and D. C. Fletcher. Publishing Sciences Group Inc. Action, Massachusetts.

Canolty, N. L. and Nasset, E. S. (1975). Intestinal absorption of free and protein-bound dietary methionine in the rat. J. Nutr. 105, 867-877.

De Muelenaere, H. J. H., Chen, M-L. and Harper, A. E. (1967). Assessment of factors influencing estimation of lysine availability in cereal products. Ag. & Food Chem. 15, 310-316.

De Muelenaere, H. J. H., Chen, M-L. and Harper, A. E. (1967a). Assessment of factors influencing estimation of availability of threonine, isoleucine, and valine in cereal products. Ag. & Food Chem., 15, 318-323.

Flodin, N. W., Mercer, L. P. and Morgan, P. H. (1977). Protein quality assay by rat growth, based on a saturation kinetics model. Nutr. Rep. Int., 16, 1-9.

Flodin, N. W., Mercer, L. P. and Morgan, P. H. (1977). The problem of human protein requirements: some kinetic and metabolic considerations. Med. Hypoth., 3, 94-110.

Garza, C., Scrimshaw, N. S. and Young, V. R. (1976). Human protein requirements: the effect of variations in energy intake within the maintenance range. Am. J. Clin. Nutr., 29, 280-287.

Garza, C., Scrimshaw, N. S. and Young, V. R. (1977). Human protein requirements: a long-term metabolic nitrogen balance study in young men to evaluate the 1973 FAO/WHO safe level of egg protein intake. J. Nutr., 107, 335-352.

Garza, C., Scrimshaw, N. S. and Young, V. R. (1977a). Human protein requirements: evaluation of the 1973 FAO/WHO safe level of protein intake for young men at high energy intakes. Br. J. Nutr., 37, 403-419.

Harper, A. E., Payne, P. R. and Waterlow, J. C. (1973). Assessment of human protein needs. Am. J. Clin. Nutr., 26, 1168-1169.

Harper, A. E. and Hegsted, D. M. (1974). Improvement of protein nutriture. p. 184-200. National Research Council Committee on Amino Acids. Improvement of protein nutriture.

Hegsted, D. M. and Chang, Y-O. (1965). Protein utilization in growing rats. I. Relative growth index as a bioassay procedure. J. Nutr., 85, 159-168.

Hegsted, D. M., Neff, R. and Worcester, J. (1968). Determination of the relative nutritive value of proteins factors affecting precision and validity. J. Agr. Food Chem., 16, 190-195.

Hegsted, D. M. and Neff, R. (1970). Efficiency of protein utilization in young rats at various levels of intake. J. Nutr., 100, 1173-1180.

Hegsted, D. M. and Juliano, B. O. (1974). Difficulties in assessing the nutritional quality of rice protein. J. Nutr., 104, 772-781.

Hegsted, D. M. (1974). Assessment of protein quality. 64-88. National Research Council - Committee on Amino Acids. Improvement of protein nutriture.

Hugli, T. E. and Moore, S. (1972). Determination of the tryptophan content of proteins by ion exchange chromatography of alkaline hydrolysates. J. Biol. Chem. 247, 2828-2834.

Jamalian, J. and Pellett, P. L. (1968). Nutritional value of Middle Eastern food stuffs. IV. - Amino acid composition. J. Sci. Fd. Agric. 19, 378-382.

Kofrányi, E., Jekat, F. and Müller-Wecker, H. (1970). The determination of the biological value of dietary proteins, XVI. The minimum protein requirement of humans, tested with mixtures of whole egg plus potato and maize plus beans. H-S. Z. Physiol. Chem., 351, 1485-1493.

Kofrányi, E. (1972). Protein and amino acid requirements. A. Nitrogen balance in adults. In International Encyclopedia of Food and Nutrition, Vol. II. Protein and amino acid functions, Ed. E. J. Bigwood. Pergamon Press-Oxford.

Kofrányi, E. (1973). Evaluation of traditional hypotheses on the biological value of protein. Nutr. Rev. Int. 7, 45-50.

McLaren, D. S. (1974). The great protein fiasco. The Lancet, July 13, 93-96.

Mercer, L. P., Farnell, K. E., Morgan, P. H., Longenecker, H. E., Jr. and Lewis, J. R. (1977). Mathematical analysis of nutrient-response data. Nutr. Rep. Int., 15, 1-7.

Morgan, P. H., Mercer, L. P. and Flodin, N. W. (1975). General model for nutritional responses of higher organisms. Proc. Nat. Acad. Sci., USA, 72, 4327-4331.

National Research Council. Food and Nutrition Board. Recommended dietary allowances. 8th Edition, 1974.

Said, A. K. and Hegsted, D. M. (1970). Response of adult rats to low dietary levels of essential amino acids. J. Nutr., 100, 1363-1376.

Said, A. K., Hegsted, D. M. and Hayes, K. C. (1974). Response of adults rats to deficiencies of different essential amino acids. Br. J. Nutr., 31, 47-57.

Teeter, R. G., Baker, D. H. and Becker, D. E. (1977). Amino Acid Bioavailability: Methodology as Applied to Lysine. Fed. Proc. 36, 1098.

Waterlow, J. C. (1968). Observation on the mechanism of adaptation to low protein intakes. The Lancet, Nov. 23, 1091-1097.

Waterlow, J. C. (1975). Adaptation to low-protein intakes. 23-35, In protein-calorie malnutrition, Ed. by R. E. Olson, Academic Press, New York.

Whitehead, R. G. (1974). Protein requirement. The Lancet, Aug. 3, 280.

Williams, H. H., A. E. Harper, D. M. Hegsted, G. Arroyave, and L. E. Holt, Jr. (1974). Nitrogen and amino acid requirements in National Research Council - Committee on Amino Acids. Improvement of protein nutriture, 23-63.

Woodham, A. A. and Deans, P. S. (1977). Nutritive value of mixed proteins. 1. In cereal-based diets for poultry. Br. J. Nutr. 37, 289-308.

Young, V. R. (1975). Recent advances in evaluation of protein quality in adult humans. Proc. 9th Int. Congr. Nutr., 3, 348-362.

21

NUTRITIONAL EVALUATION OF DRY-ROASTED NAVY BEAN FLOUR AND MIXTURES

WITH CEREAL PROTEINS

N. R. Yadav and Irvin E. Liener

Department of Biochemistry, College of Biological

Sciences, University of Minnesota, St. Paul, MN 55108

ABSTRACT

A navy bean flour prepared by dry roasting in a salt bed as a medium of heat exchange was found to have a higher PER than beans which had been autoclaved in the conventional manner. This difference was attributed to a small but significant improvement in the digestibility of the protein. The PER of the roasted beans was higher than the autoclaved beans even in the presence of supplemental methionine. When various proportions of roasted beans and corn were fed at a level of 8.3% protein in the diet, a mixture in which 40% to 60% of the protein was provided by either beans or corn had a PER essentially the same as casein. Diets containing roasted beans and various cereal grains (oats, barley, buckwheat, wheat germ, and rice) were formulated in proportions calculated to give the highest chemical scores. In most cases the PER's were not significantly different from that of casein, and, in the case of rice, the PER was higher than that of casein. Supplementation of such diets with their first limiting amino acid failed to produce a further enhancement of the PER.

INTRODUCTION

Legumes constitute an important potential source of dietary protein which has yet to be fully exploited (Milner, 1972). Although their protein content is high (18-32%) and they already have a high level of consumer acceptance in many parts of the world, their use is restricted by the fact they contain a number of antinutritional factors and are deficient in the S-containing amino acids. By properly soaking and cooking beans, however, one can produce a very palatable dish which, when eaten in combination with cereal grains, is also highly nutritious. Nevertheless, the use of beans would be considerably expanded if there were available a product of greater stability and uniformity and in such a form that it could be incorporated directly into other food dishes without the tedious time-consuming steps of presoaking and cooking. For example, pre-cooked dehydrated whole beans or bean flour would extend the util-ity of beans by permitting their incorporation into mixed blends with cereal proteins for use as a weanling food, in the formulation of baked goods, pancake flour, pizza, tortilla, and as a meat ex-tender. Bean flours have been usually prepared in the past by soaking the beans in water, cooking for an appropriate period of time, and finally dehydrating by drum or roller drying (Elias et al., 1973; Bakker et al., 1973). To introduce water only to remove it again is obviously a wasteful and expensive process. Another disadvantage of such a cooking process is the fact that free amino acids, which constitute as much as 10% of the weight of the bean (Bell et al., 1977), may be leached out into the cooking water and lost unless the latter is recovered. The alternative of dry roasting beans in the absence of moisture has been generally regarded as an ineffective means of improving the nutritive value of beans (Klose et al., 1948; DeMuelenaere, 1964), although more recent studies have shown that the dry roasting of soybeans (Harper and Lorenz, 1974; Olsen et al., 1975) and navy beans (Carvalho et al., 1977) can effectively enhance the nutritional value of the protein.

This paper will deal with the nutritional evaluation of a navy bean flour which has been prepared by dry roasting in a bed of granular salt as a medium of heat exchange. Data are also presented which indicate that the nutritive value of such a product may be significantly enhanced by complementation with a wide variety of cereal proteins.

DRY-ROASTING PROCESS

A schematic drawing of the equipment used for the dry-roasting process is shown in Figure 1. This process is based on the use of a heated bed of granular salt as a medium of heat exchange. The design of the equipment is similar to that originally described by Benson (1966) and later used by Harper and Lorenz (1974). In this process whole navy beans (Sanilac or Seafarer variety, Phaseolus vulgaris), which have been rejected for use as canned beans because they are split or otherwise damaged, are introduced into a hopper and become mixed with granular salt being introduced into an in-clined, rotating drum ("contactor") via a screw conveyor. Gas burners are used to apply heat to the outside of the contactor, and the mixture of beans and salt are conveyed forward by the action of helical flights within the contactor. The speed of the rotation of the contactor is such that the beans are in contact with the heated

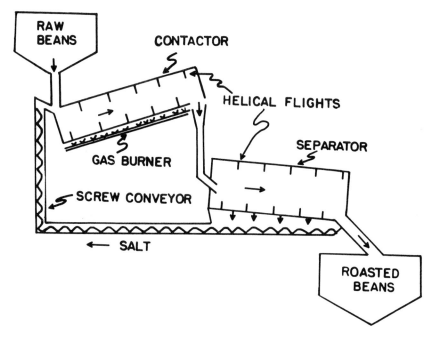

Figure 1. Schematic drawing of equipment used for the dry-roasting of navy beans.

salt for 20 to 25 sec at a temperature of 196 to 204°. From the contactor the mixture of beans and salt flows into a rotating screen drum ("separator") which allows the salt to fall onto a screw conveyor which serves to recycle the salt. The whole roasted beans are eventually collected in a suitable receptacle and finally ground into a flour with a hammer mill. As a result of the roasting process the moisture content of the bean is re-duced from 8-10% to 3-4%. This equipment is capable of processing approximately 2 tons of beans per h.

NUTRITIONAL STUDIES

Comparison of Dry-Roasted Beans with Autoclaved Beans

In all of the studies to be described, protein quality was assessed by the standard AOAC (1975) assay for protein efficiency ratio (PER). The basal diet contained 6% corn oil, 4% salt mixture (Hubbell et al., 1937), 1% vitamin mix (Kakade et al., 1970), 1% cellulose, and corn starch to 100%. The various sources of protein were incorporated into the basal diet at the expense of corn starch so as to provide a final level of 8% to 9% protein (N x 6.25). Casein was used as the reference protein, and all PER values were adjusted to a value of 2.5 for casein. Male weanling rats (Holtzman) were randomly divided into groups of 6 animals, and individually housed in wire cages with free access to food and water. The experimental period ranged from 21 to 28 days. Apparent protein digestibility was calculated from data on the quantity and N-content of food intake and feces collected during the course of the PER experiment, using the equation:

$$\text{(N intake-N in feces/N intake)} \times 100$$

Of immediate interest was a comparison of the nutritive value of the protein of the roasted navy bean flour with that obtained by the more conventional technique of autoclaving. In order to insure that a maximum response was obtained by autoclaving, raw navy bean flour which had been autoclaved (pressure, 1.03 kg/cm^2; temperature, 121°) for various periods of time was compared with the roasted navy bean product. As shown in Table 1 the highest PER that could be obtained by autoclaving was 1.69, the value achieved after 15 min. This value, however, was significantly

Table 1

Comparison of PER's and Digestibilities of Autoclaved (121°C) and Dry Roasted Navy Beans

Diet	PER[1]	Digestibility[1]
Autoclaved navy beans		%
0 min	-0.87^a	44.3^a
3 min	1.11^b	56.2^b
5 min	1.30^c	54.6^b
8 min	1.51^d	56.2^b
15 min	1.69^e	66.0^c
30 min	1.46^d	66.4^c
60 min	1.15^{bc}	62.8^d
Dry roasted navy beans	1.92^f	69.2^e
Casein	2.50^g	92.0^f

[1]Mean values for 6 rats per group. Those values not sharing a common superscript were significantly different at P < 0.05.

lower than the PER value of 1.92 which was obtained with the
roasted bean flour.

Autoclaving also increased the apparent digestibility of the
bean protein presumably due to the destruction of the trypsin inhibitor and perhaps because of the greater digestibility of the
heat-denatured protein (Kakade et al., 1973). Maximum digestibility was obtained under the same conditions that resulted in the
highest PER by autoclaving; however, the value so obtained (66%)
was slightly, but significantly, less than that obtained with the
roasted beans (69%). This difference in digestibility between the
autoclaved and roasted beans cannot be attributed to any difference
in trypsin inhibitor activity since, as shown in Table 2, the
roasted beans actually had a somewhat higher level of the trypsin
inhibitor than beans which had been autoclaved for 15 min. The
destruction of the phytohemagglutinins, which are also known to be
a factor contributing to the poor nutritive value of raw legumes
(Liener, 1974), was virtually complete in both the autoclaved and
roasted means. Amino acid analysis, shown in Table 3, likewise
revealed no essential difference in the amino acid composition of
the autoclaved and roasted bean powders. It is of particular interest to note that the lysine content of the protein had not been
affected either by autoclaving for 15 min or by roasting. Thus
the only explanation for the nutritional superiority of the roasted
bean product, as measured by PER, must reside in the somewhat

Table 2

Trypsin Inhibitor and Hemagglutinating Activities of
Autoclaved and Roasted Navy Beans

Treatment	Trypsin Inhibitor[1] units/g x 10^{-3}	Hemagglutination[2] units/g x 10^{-3}
Autoclaved		
0 min	16.5	35.5
3 min	11.1	0.3
5 min	7.4	0.3
8 min	3.8	0.2
15 min	2.5	0.2
30 min	0	0
60 min	0	0
Roasted	4.1	0.2

[1]Assayed according to Kakade et al. (1969).

[2]Assayed according to Liener (1955).

Table 3

Essential Amino Acid Composition of Autoclaved and Dry
Roasted Navy Beans (Expressed as g/16g N)

Amino Acid	Raw	Autoclaved[1]	Roasted
Threonine	3.7	4.0	4.1
Valine	4.6	5.0	4.9
Methionine	1.0	1.0	1.0
Cystine	0.7	0.8	0.9
Methionine + Cystine	1.7	1.8	1.9
Isoleucine	4.1	4.4	4.2
Leucine	7.5	7.9	7.8
Tyrosine	3.0	3.0	3.1
Phenylalanine	4.9	5.2	5.2
Histidine	2.3	2.4	2.4
Lysine	5.9	6.1	5.9
Tryptophan	0.9	1.1	1.2

[1]Autoclaved at 121° for 15 min.

better digestibility of the protein from the roasted beans. The
reason for this small but significant difference in digestibility,
however, remains obscure at the present time.

Because of the well-known deficiency of beans in the S-containing amino acids, an experiment was carried out to determine the
effect of supplementary methionine (0.6% of diet) on both the autoclaved and roasted bean powders. As shown in Figure 2, methionine
supplementation markedly enhanced the protein value of both products. Also confirmed in this experiment was the nutritional
superiority of the roasted bean, both in the presence and absence
of supplemental methionine. Thus, the availability of methionine
itself does not appear to be a cause for the differences in PER
observed here. The fact that the roasted navy bean was more digestible than the autoclaved beans either in the presence or absence
of supplemental methionine would suggest that there was a greater
availability of other amino acids in the roasted product. This
would serve to enhance the effectiveness of supplemental methionine
to a greater extent in the roasted beans compared to the autoclaved
beans.

Complementation of Roasted Navy Beans with Corn

It is well known that the nutritive value of legume proteins
can be significantly enhanced by complementation with cereal grains

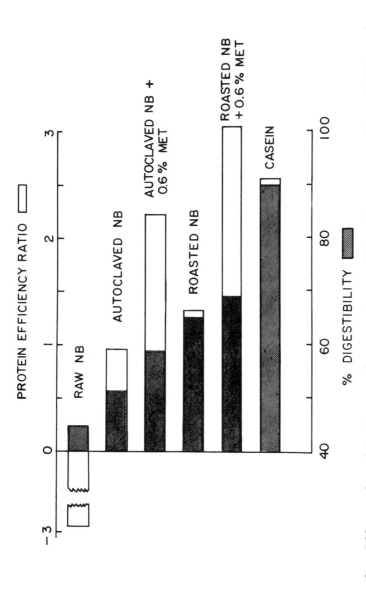

Figure 2. Effect of methionine supplementation on PER and apparent digestibility of autoclaved (121° for 15 min) and dry-roasted navy beans.

due to the mutual supplementary effect of the S-containing amino
acids and the lysine provided by these two protein sources
(Bressani and Valienti, 1962; Bressani et al., 1962; DeSouza et al.,
1972; Oke, 1975; Kardjati, 1976). Experiments were therefore conducted to ascertain the effect of complementing the roasted bean
product with lime-treated corn ("masa harina"). Diets were formulated to provide various proportions of the protein from beans and
corn at a fixed level of 8.3% protein. The results of this experiment are shown in Figure 3. The combinations producing the highest
PER's were those which provided 40-60% of the protein from either
the roasted beans or the corn. The maximum PER's obtained with
these combinations were not significantly different from casein.
Although other workers (Bressani et al., 1962; Sirinit et al.,
1965; Oke, 1975) have reported that the protein value of beans is con-

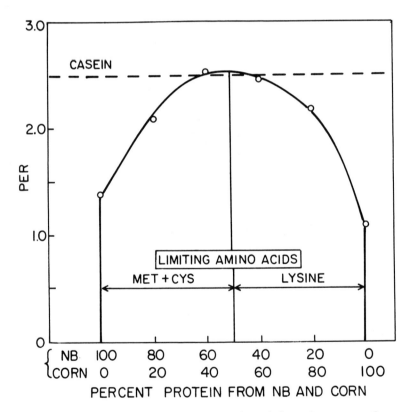

Figure 3. Complementary effect produced by mixtures of roasted
navy beans and corn. Protein level, 8.3%.

siderably enhanced by complementation with corn protein, the increases so obtained generally fell short of casein.

Calculation of the chemical scores of the various combinations of beans and corn based on the 1973 FAO pattern revealed, as might have been anticipated, that those combinations in which navy beans contribute over one-half of the protein are limiting with respect to the S-containing amino acids, whereas, lysine becomes limiting when over one-half of the protein is derived from corn. As shown in Figure 4 there was in fact a high degree of correlation ($r = +0.95$; $P < 0.01$) between the PER's recorded in Figure 4 and their chemical scores. These results confirm the conclusion reached by Kaba and Pellett (1975) that the 1973 FAO pattern, which is based on the needs of preschool age children, affords an accurate means for predicting the true limiting amino acid for test diets in which the first limiting amino acid is either lysine or methionine.

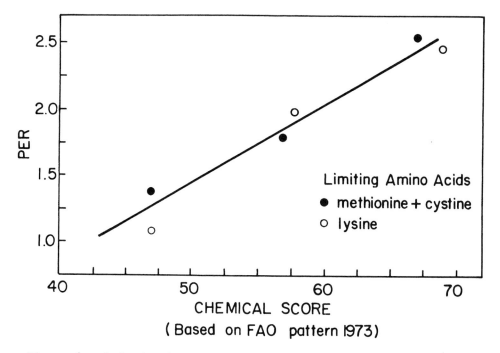

Figure 4. Relationship between PER of various combinations of roasted navy beans and corn and their chemical score based on the 1973 FAO reference pattern.

Complementation of Roasted Navy Beans with Other Cereal Proteins

Based on the foregoing considerations, complementation studies
of the navy bean protein were extended to several other cereal
grains including oats, rice, barley, buckwheat, and wheat germ.
Combinations with beans were formulated so that the mixture of the
two proteins would give the highest possible chemical score based
on the amino acid composition and the 1973 FAO reference pattern.
The results of this study are summarized in Figure 5. These data
show that, when navy beans are combined with various cereal proteins

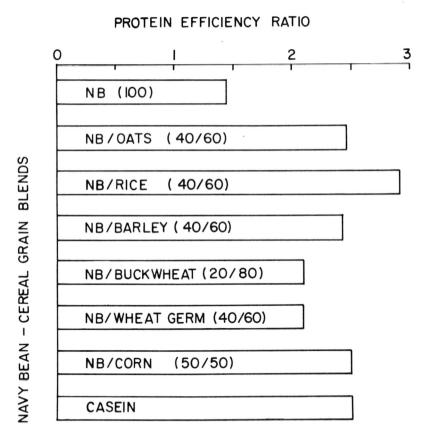

Figure 5. Complementation of roasted navy beans with various cereal grains. Ratios in parentheses denote the percent of total
protein in the diet (8.3%) which is derived from roasted navy
beans (NB) to that which is derived from the cereal indicated.

in the proportion designed to give the highest chemical score, the PER's so obtained were in general not significantly different from casein. A statistical comparison of the various blends, however, revealed that a combination of beans and rice was nutritionally superior to the combination of beans with all of the other sources of cereal protein. Kardjati (1976) has similarly reported that the PER of a rice-green gram diet was higher than that of casein, and DeSouza et al. (1973) found that a mixture of rice and beans produced higher nitrogen retention in preschool children than a mixture of beans and corn.

An attempt was made to improve further the nutritional value of the navy bean/corn and navy bean/rice mixtures by supplementation with lysine or methionine plus lysine, the amino acids which would be predicted from their chemical score to be first limiting. From the data shown in Table 4 it is evident that supplementation with lysine alone or in combination with methionine failed to increase the PER to any significant extent. Thus, it would appear that growth under these conditions must still be limited by the unavailability or deficiency of other essential amino acids. No attempt was made, however, to identify these other amino acids.

CONCLUSION

The results presented here indicate that it is possible to produce a dry navy bean powder which, when combined with various

Table 4

The Effect of Amino Acid Supplementation on the Nutritive Value of Mixtures of Roasted Navy Beans with Corn and Rice.

Protein source	Limiting Amino Acids	Chemical Score	Supple- ment	PER
Navy beans/corn (50:50)	Lys + Met + Cys	67	None	2.31
			0.35% Lys	2.39
			0.35% Lys + 0.40% Met	2.42
Navy beans/rice (40:60)	Met + Cys	72	None	2.75
			0.35% Lys	2.85
			0.35% Lys + 0.40% Met	2.87
Casein				2.50

cereal proteins, particularly with rice, has a PER value which is
at least equivalent to that of casein. The availability of such
a nutritious protein in a dry, stable form offers much opportunity
and flexibility for the formulation of blends with cereal proteins
which could be used in a wide variety of food products. The principle advantage of such mixtures would be that conventional sources
of cereal proteins could be used to improve local diets without
necessitating drastic changes in food habits.

ACKNOWLEDGMENTS

The authors wish to thank Mr. Charles Brown of Protein Products, Inc., Olivia, Minn., for providing us with the dry roasted
navy bean flour used in these studies. This work was supported by
Grant No. AM 18324 awarded by the National Institutes of Health,
DHEW.

REFERENCES

A.O.A.C. (1975). Biological Evaluation of Protein Quality. Asso-
    ciation of Official Agricultural Chemists, Washington, D. C.,
    857-860.
Bakker, F. W., Patterson, R. J. and Bedford, C. L. (1973). Pro-
    duction of instant bean powders. In, 'Nutritional Aspects of
    Common Beans and Other Legume Seeds as Animal and Human Foods',
    W. G. Jaffé (Editor). Arch. Latinoamer. Nutr., Caracas,
    Venezuela.
Bell, E. A., Quereshi, M. Y., Charlwood, B. V., Pilbeam, D. J. and
    Evans, C. S. (1978). The variability of free amino acids and
    related compounds in legume seeds. Phytochemistry, in press.
Benson, J. D. (1966). Puffing food products. U.S. Patent No.
    3,253,533.
Bressani, R. and Valienti, T. (1962). All-vegetable protein mix-
    tures for human feeding. VII. Protein complementation between
    polished rice and cooked black beans. J. Food Sci., 27, 401-
    412.
Bressani, R., Valienti, A., and Tejada, C. E. (1962). All-vegetable
    protein mixtures for human feeding. VI. The value of combina-
    tions of lime-treated corn and cooked black beans. J. Food
    Sci., 27, 394-400.
Carvalho, C.C.C., Jansen, G. R., and Harper, J. M. (1977). Protein
    quality evaluation of an instant bean powder produced by dry
    heat processing. J. Food Sci., 42, 553-554.
DeMuelenaere, H.J.H. (1964). Effect of heat treatment on the
    hemagglutinating activity of legumes. Nature, 201, 1029-1030.
DeSouza, N., Santo, J. E., and Dutra de Oliviera, J. E. (1973).
    Clinical and experimental studies on common beans. In, 'Nutri-
    tional Aspects of Common Beans and Other Legume Seeds for Animal

and Human Foods', W. G. Jaffé (Editor). Arch. Latinoamer. Nutr., Caracas, Venezuela, 241–248.

Elias, L. G., Bressani, R. and Flores, M. (1973). Problems and potentials in storage and processing of food legumes in Latin America. In, 'Potentials of Field Beans and Other Food Legumes in Latin America'. Centro Internacional de Agricultura Tropical, Cali, Columbia, 52–87.

FAO/WHO Technical Report Series No. 522 (1973). Energy and Protein Requirements. World Health Organization, Geneva, Switzerland.

Harper, J. M. and Lorenz, K. (1974). Production and evaluation of salt-bed roasted full-fat soy flour. Lebensmitt.-Wiss. U.-Technol., 7, 268–272.

Hubbell, R. B., Mendel, L. B., and Wakeman, H. J. (1937). A new salt mixture for use in experimental diets. J. Nutr., 14, 273–277.

Kaba, H. and Pellett, P. L. (1975). Prediction of true limiting amino acids using available protein scoring systems. Ecol. Food Nutr., 4, 109–116.

Kakade, M. L., Simons, N., and Liener, I. E. (1969). An evaluation of natural versus synthetic substrates for measuring the antitryptic activity of soybean meals. Cereal Chem., 46, 518–526.

Kakade, M. L., Simons, N., and Liener, I. E. (1970). Nutritional effects induced in rats by feeding natural and synthetic inhibitors. J. Nutr., 100, 1003–1008.

Kardjati, M. S. (1976). Protein quality of rice-soya bean and rice-green gram mixtures. Nutr. Rep. Int., 13, 463–470.

Klose, A. A., Hill, B., and Fevold, H. L. (1948). Food value of soybeans as related to processing. Food Technol., 2, 201–206.

Liener, I. E. (1955). The photometric determination of the hemagglutinating activity of soyin and crude soybean extracts. Arch. Biochem. Biophys., 54, 223–231.

Liener, I. E. (1974). Phytohemagglutinins: their nutritional significance. J. Ag. Food Chem., 22, 17–22.

Milner, M. (1972). Nutritional Improvement of Food Legumes by Breeding. Food and Agricultural Organization, Rome, Italy.

Oke, O. L. (1975). A method for assessing optimum supplementation of a cereal-based diet with grain legumes. Nutr. Rep. Int., 11, 313–321.

Olsen, E. M., Young, L. G., Ashton, G. C., and Smith, G. C. (1975). Effects of roasting and particle size on the utilization of soybeans by pig and rats. Can. J. Animal Sci., 55, 431–440.

Sirinit, K., Soliman, A.-G.M., van Loo, A. J., and King, K. W. (1965). Nutritional value of Haitian cereal-legume seeds. J. Nutr., 86, 415–423.

22

NUTRITIONAL EVALUATION OF OILSEEDS AND LEGUMES AS PROTEIN SUPPLEMENTS TO CEREALS

G. Sarwar[1], F.W. Sosulski and J.M. Bell,
College of Agriculture, University of
Saskatchewan, Saskatoon, Saskatchewan
and
J.P. Bowland, Faculty of Agriculture and Forestry,
University of Alberta, Edmonton, Alberta

ABSTRACT

Several oilseed and legume protein products were fed to rats as the sole source of dietary protein, and in blends with cereals for the determination of protein efficiency ratio (PER) and biological availability of amino acids. In addition oilseed protein isolates were fed to mice for the determination of PER. Results of the mouse study revealed that the adjusted PER (casein=100) for Target rapeseed isolate (108) was higher than those of sunflower (74), safflower (77), soybean (86) or flax (92) isolates.

Results of the rat trials revealed that the adjusted PER for Tower rapeseed meal (88) was higher than those of fababean (21), field pea (59) and soybean meal (72). Supplementation with methionine (0.2%) resulted in improved PER for fababean (84), field pea (101) and soybean meal (97). Mustard flour and rapeseed flour gave PER of 109 and 106, respectively, while the value of sunflower flour was low (56). Protein isolates of Tower rapeseed and soybean gave PER of 92 and 80, respectively. Blending of legumes and oilseeds with wheat flour (PER=28) gave high PER

[1]Present address (G.S.): Bureau of Nutritional Sciences, Health Protection Branch, National Health and Welfare, Ottawa, Ontario, K1A 0L2.

values (60-85), as also occurred in rice blends (71-88).
Supplementation of wheat-legume blends with lysine
(0.4%), methionine (0.2%) and threonine (0.1%) brought
all PER values above 100. It appeared that differences
in PER of the diets paralleled the levels of the first
limiting amino acid for rat growth. Results of balance
trials indicated that the availability of the limiting
amino acid(s) was lower than other essential amino
acids for each protein source.

INTRODUCTION

The world-wide shortage of plant and animal protein
for human nutrition has been given high priority in
development programs sponsored by the WHO, FAO and other
agencies of the United Nations. In the heavily popu-
lated regions of the world, the protein problems arise
from an excessive dependence on cereal grains and root
crops for most of the dietary calories. Oilseeds and
grain legumes are higher in protein content than
cereals, and contain moderate to high levels of lysine
to balance deficiencies of cereal-based diets. Although
their protein contents are high, most oilseed meals are
fed to livestock because of dark colours, unpalatability
and higher crude fibre levels. However, dehulling prior
to solvent extraction of oilseeds results in protein
flours (ca. 50% protein) which in turn can be used to
obtain protein concentrates (ca. 70% protein) and
isolates (ca. 90% protein). In the United States, the
processing technology for soybean has been developed
for the production of food grade protein flours,
concentrates and isolates and their textured products,
and more recently cottonseed, peanut and sunflower
have received substantial attention. There is on-going
research in Canada to develop food grade protein
products from rapeseed, mustard, field pea, fababean,
and many other Canadian crops. The establishment of
the POS Pilot Plant Corporation in Saskatoon, Saskatchewan, to provide physical facilities for technology
development in processing various crops to the level of
food and feed grade products, is generating considerable
interest and impetus to the establishment of a plant
protein industry in Canada.

Extensive research has been done on the functional
and nutritional properties of soybean flour, concentrate
and isolate. Similar studies on the protein products
from other oilseeds and legumes are of current interest
in many research centres. The objectives of this

presentation were to evaluate nutritive value of oilseeds (rapeseed, mustard, sunflower, safflower, flax)
and legumes (field pea, field bean, lentil, broad bean,
fababean) as protein supplements to cereals (wheat and
rice).

MATERIALS AND METHODS

The ANRC casein; polished rice; white wheat flour,
straight grade, 72% extraction rate; milling wheat,
Neepawa; utility wheat, Glenlea; and seeds of Tower
(low glucosinolate-low erucic acid) rapeseed (Brassica
napus), Target (high glucosinolate) rapeseed (B. napus),
yellow mustard (B. hirta), Altona soybean (Glycine max),
Commander sunflower (Helianthus annuus), Gila safflower
(Carthamus tinctorius) and Redwing flax (Linum usita-
tissimum) were purchased from commercial sources.

The seeds were ground and the oil extracted with
n-hexane and a Soxhlet apparatus. The meals were
desolventised in a vacuum oven at 45C for 24 hours.
Isolated proteins were extracted from the oilseed meals
with 0.2% sodium hydroxide and precipitated by adjusting
the pH to the isoelectric point of proteins (Sosulski
and Bakal, 1969). The pH of a minimum solubility for
the extracted proteins was 4.5 for soybean, 4.7 for the
rapeseed species, 4.4 for flax, 4.4 for sunflower and
4.4 for safflower. The protein isolates were washed
and freeze dried before conducting amino acid analyses,
and feeding trials.

Sunflower flour was prepared by dehulling and
defatting of the seed, while the Tower rapeseed and
yellow mustard flours were prepared by dehulling, wet-
heat treating to inactivate myrosinase, washing in
water, drying, and finally extracting the Brassica
meats with hexane (Tape et al., 1970).

Seed samples of Century field pea (Pisum sativum
arvense), Limelight field bean (Phaseolus vulgaris),
lentil (Lens culinaris), Windsor broad bean (Vicia
faba major) and Schledemer fababean (Vicia faba minor)
were obtained from experimental plots. Antinutritive
factors in the grain legumes were destroyed by dipping
the seed in boiling water for 2 minutes, soaking in hot
water for 1 hour and, after drainage, autoclaving at
103K Pa (120C) for 10 minutes. The wheat flour, rice,
soybean meal (SBM) and soybean isolate were also autoclaved at 103K Pa (120C) for 15 minutes before feeding.

Proximate analyses (Table 1) were determined by the A.O.A.C. (1970) procedures using the nitrogen-to-protein factor of 6.25. The amino acid analyses (Table 2) were conducted on a Beckman Model 120C Analyzer with separate hydrolyses for the sulphur-containing amino acids and tryptophan determinations (Sosulski and Sarwar, 1973). The method of Youngs and Wetter (1967) was used in determining the oxazolidinethione and isothiocyanate contents of the rapeseed products. The p-hydroxy-benzyl isothiocyanate contents of the mustard products were determined by an unpublished method of Wetter (L.R. Wetter, NRC-PRL, 110 Gymnasium Road, University Campus, Saskatoon, Saskatchewan).

Experiment 1 (Nutritional evaluation of oilseed isolates by mice)

The protein isolates were fed at a 10% protein (Nx6.25) level in all diets including the casein control (Table 3). The protein sources were incorporated into the diets at the expense of a protein-free basal mixture containing 33% corn starch, 38% cerelose, 9% sucrose, 10% corn oil and 10% cellulose. Each diet contained the 5% vitamin premix and 5% mineral premix. (Sarwar et al., 1973). The experimental design for the feeding trial was a randomized complete block with eight replications of one mouse each. The diets were fed to individually caged mice originating from the Carworth Farms No.1 strain. The weanling male mice at initial weights of 10-12 g were fed the experimental diets and water ad libitum for 14 days. Weights of mice and their feed intakes were recorded weekly.

Experiments 2 (Nutritional evaluation of wheat flour, oilseed products and wheat-oilseed blends by rats), 3 (Effects of amino acid supplementation on the nutritive value of legumes and wheat-legume blends), and 4

(Nutritional evaluation of cereal-legume blends).

The experimental diets in these three rat growth studies (Tables 4, 5 and 6) were formulated to be isocaloric, and to contain 10% protein, 10% fat, 5% crude fibre, 4% minerals and 1% vitamins (AOAC, 1970). In the case of cereal-oilseed or legume blends, each source supplied 50% of the total dietary protein. In the case of amino acid supplementation, ℓ-lysine, ℓ-methionine and ℓ-threonine were added at 0.4, 0.2 and

Table 1. Proximate composition of casein, cereals, oilseeds and legumes (% dry basis).

Protein source	Crude protein	Fat	Crude fibre	Ash
Casein (control)	96.0	0.2	0.2	1.3
Cereal				
Rice	9.1	0.4	0.3	0.5
Wheat flour	15.0	1.2	0.2	0.5
Oilseed				
Soybean meal	52.3	2.3	2.7	6.8
Mustard meal	45.5	2.1	8.3	5.9
Rapeseed meal	42.5	3.2	11.8	7.4
Mustard flour	70.6	2.0	5.0	7.2
Rapeseed flour	61.3	1.0	5.3	9.7
Sunflower flour	58.3	3.3	3.6	8.2
Soybean isolate	94.7	0.2	0.2	3.7
Rapeseed isolate	86.9	0.5	0.5	2.8
Sunflower isolate	95.7	1.6	0.4	1.3
Safflower isolate	93.7	1.0	0.3	1.4
Flax isolate	84.9	0.7	0.4	2.1
Legume				
Field pea	21.1	1.1	6.2	3.1
Field bean	24.5	1.4	4.8	5.2
Lentil	21.3	0.9	4.9	3.5
Broad bean	26.9	1.1	6.5	3.7
Fababean	27.8	1.2	8.0	3.3

Table 2. Essential amino acid distribution in casein, cereals, oilseeds and legumes.

(g amino acid/16 g nitrogen)

Essential amino acids	Arg	His	Ile	Leu	Lys	Met	Met+cys	Phe	Thr	Try	Val
Protein source											
Casein (control)	3.4	2.6	4.9	8.7	7.8	2.7	3.2	5.0	3.8	2.9	6.2
Cereal											
Rice	9.1	2.4	4.5	8.9	3.9	2.8	4.8	5.5	3.8	0.9	6.4
Wheat flour	3.5	2.1	3.3	6.2	2.0	2.5	4.9	4.8	2.4	1.5	3.6
Oilseed											
Soybean meal	7.3	2.5	4.4	7.6	6.4	1.5	2.6	5.2	3.8	1.8	4.9
Mustard meal	5.5	2.6	3.8	6.7	5.2	1.7	3.0	4.2	4.1	1.3	4.9
Rapeseed meal	5.8	2.4	4.1	6.9	5.6	2.0	3.6	4.1	4.1	1.5	4.9
Mustard flour	6.2	2.9	4.0	7.5	6.1	2.0	4.0	3.9	4.2	1.4	5.0
Rapeseed flour	6.5	2.5	4.0	7.3	5.6	2.1	3.8	3.5	4.2	1.5	5.6
Sunflower flour	8.2	2.2	3.9	6.0	3.1	2.1	3.6	4.3	3.2	1.3	4.8
Soybean isolate	8.6	2.3	4.6	7.9	6.0	1.4	3.1	5.3	3.5	1.5	6.7
Rapeseed isolate	7.7	2.6	4.1	7.6	5.4	2.2	4.0	3.8	4.4	1.6	5.2
Sunflower isolate	9.6	2.2	3.9	6.0	3.1	2.1	3.6	4.3	3.2	1.3	4.8
Safflower isolate	10.6	2.1	4.2	6.9	2.4	1.7	3.3	4.9	3.1	1.2	5.3
Flax isolate	10.2	1.9	4.3	8.4	3.1	2.0	4.0	4.7	3.4	1.4	5.5
Legume											
Field pea	8.8	2.5	4.4	7.4	7.7	1.3	2.4	4.9	3.8	1.3	4.9
Field bean	5.8	2.7	4.9	8.7	7.0	1.5	2.2	6.1	4.4	1.0	5.7
Lentil	7.1	2.5	4.5	7.4	8.1	1.3	2.1	5.0	3.8	0.8	5.0
Broad bean	8.7	2.4	4.0	7.0	6.3	1.3	2.0	4.0	3.4	0.7	4.6
Fababean	8.4	2.3	3.9	6.9	6.1	1.0	2.0	4.0	3.3	1.0	4.3

Table 3. Effects of protein isolates on weight gain, food consumption and protein utilization by mice (two weeks study).

Protein isolate	Gain g	Food g	PER	PER (casein=100)
Casein (control)	10.4	55	1.89	100
Soybean[1]	8.9	55	1.62	86
Rapeseed[2]	12.1	59	2.05	108
Flax	9.3	53	1.75	92
Sunflower	7.7	55	1.40	74
Safflower	8.4	58	1.45	77
LSR minimum (P=0.05)	1.2	5	0.16	
maximum	1.4	6	0.19	

[1]Autoclaved

[2]Target

Table 4. Effects of oilseed proteins and blends with wheat flour on weight gain, food consumption and protein utilization by rats (two weeks study).

Protein sources	Lys	Met⁺cys	Thr	Try	gain	Food	PER	Modified PER	PER	Modified PER
	% of rat requirements				g	g			(casein=100)	(casein=100)
Casein (control)	78	48[1]	68	170	45	113	3.98	5.01	100	100
Wheat flour	20	73	43	88	5	73	0.68	2.15	28	43
Oilseed proteins										
Rapeseed meal	56	54	73	88	41	117	3.50	4.72	38	94
Mustard flour	61	60	75	82	56	131	4.27	5.46	108	109
Rapeseed flour	56	57	75	88	54	132	4.09	5.31	104	106
Sunflower flour	31	53	57	76	27	121	2.23	3.43	56	68
Soybean isolate	60	46	62	88	43	135	3.18	4.26	80	85
Rapeseed isolate	54	60	78	94	45	121	3.72	4.91	92	98
Wheat flour + protein supplements										
Casein	49	60	55	129	55	138	3.98	5.11	100	102
Rapeseed meal	38	63	58	88	21	96	2.19	3.35	55	67
Mustard flour	40	61	59	85	39	130	3.00	4.00	75	80
Rapeseed flour	38	65	59	88	31	116	2.67	3.86	67	77
Sunflower flour	25	63	50	82	23	117	1.96	2.99	49	60
Soybean isolate	40	59	52	83	32	126	2.54	3.69	63	74
Rapeseed isolate	37	66	60	91	25	103	2.43	3.64	61	73
LSR minimum					6	12	0.34	0.80		
maximum					7	15	0.41	0.96		

[1]First limiting amino acid(s) is underlined.

Table 5. Effects of protein sources and amino acid supplementation on food consumption, weight gain and protein utilization by rats (four weeks study).

Protein sources	Ile	Lys	Met+cys	Thr	Try	Gain g	Food g	PER	Modified PER	PER	Modified PER
	% of rat requirement[1]					g	g			(casein=100)	(casein=100)
Protein supplement											
Casein (control)	80	78	48	68	170	119	344	3.44	4.10	100	100
Soybean meal	72	64	39	68	82	68	274	2.49	3.28	72	80
Field pea	72	77	36	68	76	36	181	2.02	3.04	59	74
Fababean	64	61	30	59	59	10	140	0.72	1.50	21	36
Protein supplement+met											
Casein	80	78	78	63	170	153	357	4.26	4.98	124	121
Soybean meal	72	64	69	68	82	127	378	3.35	3.97	97	97
Field pea	72	77	66	68	76	142	407	3.48	4.08	101	99
Fababean	64	61	60	59	59	100	343	2.90	3.50	84	85
Wheat-protein supplement blend											
Casein	67	49	60	55	129	141	405	3.49	3.95	98	96
Soybean meal	64	42	56	55	85	74	291	2.55	3.06	72	75
Field pea	64	48	54	55	79	84	303	2.78	3.29	79	80
Fababean	59	40	51	51	70	80	323	2.47	3.05	72	74
Wheat-protein supplement blend+lys, met and thr											
Casein	67	89	90	75	129	168	388	4.33	5.02	126	122
Soybean meal	64	82	86	73	85	150	392	3.82	4.46	111	109
Field pea	64	88	84	73	79	145	365	3.96	4.44	115	108
Fababean	59	80	81	69	70	136	372	3.66	4.30	106	105
LSR minimum (P=0.05)						20	42	0.08	0.16		
maximum						24	50	0.10	0.18		

[1]First limiting amino acid(s) is underlined.

Table 6. Effects of cereal-legume blends on weight gain, food consumption and protein utilization by rats (four weeks study).

Protein sources	Lys	Met+cys	Thr	Try	Gain g	Food g	PER	BV %	PER	BV
	% of rat requirement								(cereal-casein blend = 100)	
Wheat-legume blend										
Casein (control)	49[1]	60	55	129	134	410	3.45	60	100	100
Soybean meal	42	56	55	97	83	338	2.81	46	81	77
Field pea	48	54	55	82	85	318	2.94	52	85	87
Field bean	45	53	61	73	96	360	2.70	51	78	85
Lentil	50	52	55	68	75	298	2.60	57	75	95
Broad bean	41	51	52	65	68	294	2.51	49	73	82
Fababean	40	51	51	72	63	293	2.37	44	69	73
Rice-legume blend										
Casein	58	60	68	111	152	420	3.61	63	100	100
Soybean meal	51	55	68	79	137	424	3.16	63	87	100
Field pea	58	54	68	64	120	376	3.19	61	88	97
Field bean	54	52	73	56	88	321	2.74	58	76	92
Lentil	60	51	68	50	94	351	2.68	54	74	86
Broad bean	51	51	63	47	92	340	2.71	55	75	87
Fababean	50	51	63	56	90	350	2.57	56	71	89
LSR minimum (P=0.05)					10	33	0.15	4		
maximum					11	37	0.18	5		

[1]First limiting amino acid is underlined.

0.1%, respectively. The diets were fed ad libitum to
individually caged weanling (40-50g) male Wistar rats.
Weekly records of food consumption and body weight were
kept during the two weeks (experiment 2) and the four
weeks (experiment 3, Sarwar et al., 1975a; and
experiment 4, Sarwar et al., 1975b) feeding trials.
Protein efficiency ratio (PER) and modified PER
(McLaughlan and Keith, 1975) values were calculated.

In experiments 3 and 4, the collected feces were
pooled and analysed for chromic oxide and protein
contents to calculate protein digestibility coefficients
(Sarwar et al., 1975a; 1975b). In experiment 4 true
biological value (BV) was calculated by a modified
Thomas-Mitchell equation in which the retained nitrogen
was estimated directly by carcass analyses (Sarwar et
al., 1975b).

Experiments 5 and 6 (Amino acid availability determinations)

Availability of amino acid in wheat (Sarwar and
Bowland 1975; 1976); rapeseed proteins (Sarwar et al.,
1975); legumes and wheat-legume blends (Sarwar et al.,
1977), as determined by the balance trial was calculated
using the following equation:

$$\text{Availability \%} = \frac{AAI - (FAA - MFAA)}{AAI} \times 100$$

where, AAI = Total intake of amino acid, FAA =
fecal excretion of amino acid, MFAA = Metabolic
fecal amino acid.

Estimates of metabolic fecal nitrogen and metabolic
amino acids were made by analyzing the feces of rats fed
the nitrogen-free diet.

Statistical analyses

The data for weight gain, food consumed, PER,
Modified PER, protein digestibility, BV, availability
of nitrogen and amino acids were subjected to analysis
of variance and Duncan's multiple range test (Duncan,
1955). The least significant range (LSR) test was
utilized to demonstrate the significant differences
between means. When the means were ranked in increasing
order, the minimum LSR is used to test the differences

between adjacent means while the maximum LSR is
applied to differences between the extreme values.

Results and Discussion

Chemical composition

Rice was much lower in protein concentration than
wheat flour, while SBM contained twice as much protein
as the non-oilseed legumes (Table 1). The legumes,
including SBM, contained 1-2, 3-7 and 3-6% fat, ash and
fibre, respectively, except for fababean which
contained 8% fibre.

Tower rapeseed meal (RSM) and mustard meal were
lower in protein and higher in crude fibre than SBM
(Table 1). Rapeseed and sunflower flours contained
about 60% protein, while mustard flour contained about
70% protein, but the differences among the flours in
fat, crude fibre and ash levels were relatively small.

The protein isolates were washed only once before
freeze drying and a wide range in protein contents
(84.9-95.7%) were obtained due to varying compositions
of non-protein constituents (Table 1). The isolates
were almost free of crude fibre, and their ash contents
were substantially lower than the levels in the flours
or meals.

In the present investigation the yield of the
rapeseed isolate was much lower than those of soybean,
sunflower or safflower. But recently procedures have
been developed where as much as 94% of the RSM nitrogen
was extracted (El Nockrashy et al., 1977). A two step
precipitation, first at pH 6.0 and then at pH 3.6,
washing and drying resulted in two highly purified
rapeseed isolates containing well above 90% protein.

Two species of rapeseed are commonly grown in
Canada, B. Campestris or turnip rape (Polish type) and
B. napus or Argentine rape. Rapeseed, in common with
other members of Brassica, contains glucosinolates
which may be hydrolysed by the enzyme myrosinase to
yield oxazolidinethione and isothiocyanate. Oxazolidinethione has long been recognized as a goitrogenic
substance but isothiocyanates also affect thyroxine
synthesis and possibly liver enzyme functions
(Bowland et al., 1965; Appelqvist and Ohlson, 1972).
The commercial practice in Canadian processing plants

is to inactivate the myrosinase in the rapeseed by heating the crushed seed to 80-90C as rapidly as possible before moisture is added during cooking (Bowland et al., 1965). However, this process does not remove or destroy the glucosinolates, consequently metabolic problems may still arise.

RSM is used extensively in feed manufacturing in Canada, but under more restrictive conditions than apply to SBM because of the potential problem associated with the glucosinolates. Feeding guidelines have been carefully developed for all major classes of farm animals (Bowland et al., 1965) and if these are followed, normal performance usually will be obtained. The introduction of low glucosinolate varieties such as Tower (B. napus), which contains only 1/10th the level of glucosinolates present in established varieties of rapeseed, should largely eliminate this quality problem in RSM.

Although not commercially feasible, the preparation of rapeseed flour by dehulling, enzyme inactivation, water washing, drying and solvent extraction, results in a high quality, low glucosinolate product (Bell et al., 1976; Loew et al., 1976; Tape et al., 1970).

Mustard meal resembles RSM in most respects (McKenzie, 1973) but it does not contain glucosinolates that yield oxazolidinethione. However, it contains relatively high levels of isothiocyanates which differ in structure, depending upon the species of mustard involved. The isothiocyanates are responsible for the bitter taste and characteristic pungent odour, hence both palatability and potential toxicity may become of concern in feeding mustard meal. Several patented processes are available for removal or destruction of glucosinolates in mustard.

Glucosinolate analyses of the Brassica products used in the present investigation (Table 1) revealed that Tower RSM contained 0.9 and 0.5 mg/g of oxazolidinethione and isothiocyanates, respectively, but the values for Tower flour were very low (0.02 and 0.01 mg/g of oxazolidinethione and isothiocyanates, respectively). Isolation of protein from Tower RSM resulted in complete removal of the glucosinolates. Yellow mustard meal contained a high level (33.5 mg/g) of p-hydroxybenzyl isothiocyanate, but the value was less than 1 mg/g in the case of the mustard flour.

Amino acid composition

    The cereals were good sources of methionine +
cystine, but were deficient in lysine (Table 2). The
deficiency in lysine was more marked in wheat flour.
Legumes in general were rich sources of lysine and
contained fair amounts of threonine, but were
deficient in methionine + cystine and tryptophan
(Table 2). SBM and field pea contained higher amounts
of the deficient amino acids while broad beans and
fababeans tended to be lower in essential amino acids
(EAA) than other legumes. Although lentil and field
bean exhibited high levels of lysine and threonine,
respectively, lentil was seriously deficient in
tryptophan.

    Sunflower, safflower and flax isolates were
substantially higher in arginine than the other oilseed proteins (Table 2). On the other hand these
three isolates contained about one half the level of
lysine found in soybean, rapeseed and mustard products.
Mustard and rapeseed products were also excellent
sources of sulphur amino acids. In general, it appeared
that the Brassica products contained the better balance
of EAA, while sunflower, safflower and flax products
were definitely inferior to the other oilseed products.

Experiment 1 (Nutritional evaluation of oilseed isolates
by mice)

    Diets containing the plant protein isolates were
consumed at about the same level as the casein control
(Table 3). In the case of soybean isolate the gain and
PER data from about the same level of intake were
significantly lower than the data for rapeseed isolate
and casein. Only sunflower isolate gave lower gain
than soybean isolate, but PER values for both sunflower
and safflower isolates were lower. Although the
safflower, sunflower and flax isolate were quite low
in lysine (Table 2), their PER values were 74-92% of
the control (Table 3). This observation may suggest
that lysine requirement of the growing mouse may be
lower than that specified by NAS (Bell, 1972). Similar
observations have been made more recently by John and
Bell (1976), who obtained maximum growth and protein
utilization responses when the dietary dry matter
contained around 0.4% lysine.

Experiment 2 (Nutritional evaluation cf wheat flour, oilseed products and wheat-oilseed blends by rats)

The diet containing 10% protein from wheat flour was a good source of methionine + cystine, but was seriously deficient in lysine for rat growth, therefore, food intake, gain and PER data on this diet were very low (Table 4).

The diet containing 10% protein from soybean isolate supplied a fair amount of lysine, but was mainly deficient in methionine + cystine (Table 4). On the other hand, the sunflower flour diet was a good source of S-amino acids, but was deficient in lysine. However, the diets containing mustard or rapeseed products supplied moderate levels of both lysine and S-amino acids, and their chemical scores were equivalent to, or higher than, the score for casein control.

Mustard and rapseed flours supported higher weight gains and food intakes, and showed higher PER values than the other oilseed proteins and casein in most cases (Table 4). The sunflower flour diet was significantly lower in weight gains, consumption and PER data than the other protein sources. Nutritional values for Tower RSM and isolate were similar to the casein control but soybean isolate showed a lower PER than casein.

When wheat flour provided one-half of the protein in blends with the oilseed products, its nutritive value was substantially improved (Table 4). In most cases except with sunflower flour, the chemical score of wheat flour protein was doubled, with lysine being the first limiting amino acid in each blend. Rat gains data for the blends were intermediate between the data for wheat flour and oilseed proteins but food intake data approached that of oilseed proteins and casein. Therefore, PER values for the wheat-oilseed blends varied between 2.0-3.0 with mustard flour being the best supplement for wheat proteins and sunflower flour the poorest. As supplements to a cereal flour such as wheat, the PER values ranked the supplements in the order of casein > mustard flour > rapeseed flour = soybean isolate = rapeseed isolate = RSM = sunflower flour.

PER versus modified PER

     PER is a simple, convenient, widely used measure
of protein quality, and is the official method in
Canada and the United States. The most serious drawback of the PER method is that it makes no allowance
for maintenance requirements. A protein may be adequate
for maintenance, but its PER could be close to zero.
Such a protein would supply the amino acid requirements
for adults and might have a marked supplementary effect
on the utilization of other proteins in the diet.   In
order to have a measure of protein used for both growth
and maintenance, the modified PER (McLaughlan and Keith,
1975) was determined also by the equation:

$$\text{Modified PER} = \frac{\text{Wt. gain of test group} + 0.1\ (\text{initial} + \text{final wt. of test group})}{\text{Protein consumed}}$$

The factor 0.1 (initial + final weight) is considered
similar in magnitude to the weight loss of nonprotein
group in the net protein ratio (NPR) method of Bender
and Doell (1957), however, unlike NPR, modified PER
does not overestimate the protein quality of lysine
deficient proteins (McLaughlan and Keith, 1975).

     Although both the PER methods ranked the protein
sources in the same order, the modified method proved
more beneficial for the poor quality proteins (Table
4).   The modified PER for the diet containing 10%
protein from wheat flour was three times higher than
its PER.   Sunflower flour was more benefited (54%),
by the use of modified PER method, than the other oilseed proteins (about 35%).   Among the blends, the
modified method proved more beneficial for RSM and
sunflower flour (52%) than for mustard flour (33%),
while rapeseed flour, soybean isolate and rapeseed
isolate occupied an intermediate position.   When the
two PER values were expressed as a % of casein control,
the modified values for the lysine deficient diets were
10-15 percentage units higher than the conventional
ones, and this improvement appeared to be proportional
to the degree of lysine deficiency.

Experiment 3 (Effects or amino acid supplementation on the nucritive value of legumes and wheat-legume blends)

Relative to rat requirements, the diets containing 10% protein from legumes or casein were deficient in the S-amino acids (methionine + cystine), and the SBM, field pea and fababean diets were progressively lower than casein in this first limiting amino acid (Table 5).

Differences in food intake and weight gains of rats paralleled the levels of S-amino acids in the diets and ranked the protein sources in the order of casein> SBM> field pea> fababean (Table 5). The protein digestibility of fababean (80%) was also significantly lower than those of SBM (87%) and field pea (85%) which were, in turn, much lower than the 99% recorded for casein. The PER values for the fababean diet were, therefore, very low while the field pea diet was significantly lower in protein utilization than SBM.

Methionine supplementation of the diets increased the chemical scores by 35-100% (Table 5). In these supplemented diets, the first limiting amino acids were threonine in casein, lysine in SBM, methionine + cystine in field pea, and four essential amino acids in fababean diet. Food intake of all legume diets were equal or better than the casein control, but their weight gain data were significantly lower. The weight gain on the fababean diet was also significantly lower than the other legume diets, which may reflect the influence of a low protein digestibility. The PER values were relatively high in all methionine-supplemented diets and only the values for fababean were not equal to the values for the unsupplemented casein control.

The diets containing equal proportions of protein from wheat and legumes or casein were more deficient in lysine than sulphur amino acids (Table 5). The chemical scores of field pea and fababean blends were sub-stantially. improved over those of the legumes alone and this was reflected in the rat growth and protein utilization data. There were no significant differences among the three wheat-legume blends in food intake or weight gain data, but the wheat-field pea diet was superior to the other two in PER rating. It appeared that the improved protein digestibility of the blends of wheat with SBM (92%), field pea (94%) and fababean (90%) was due to the high digestibility of the wheat protein.

Supplementation of the wheat-legume blends with
three essential amino acids provided over 80% of the
rat requirements for lysine and sulphur amino acids
(Table 5). The chemical scores averaged only 63
because isoleucine became the first limiting amino acid
in each diet. The feeding results were very high for
each supplemented wheat-legume blend. Most of the amino
acid deficiencies in fababean appear to have been overcome in this treatment, and its PER values exceeded
those of the unsupplemented casein.

PER vs. modified PER

Consistent with the results of previous experiment
(Table 4), both the PER methods ranked the diets in the
same order (Table 5). The modified PER values for most
of the diets were about 20% higher than their PER values,
but this improvement was much higher in the case of the
diets containing 10% protein from fababean (200%), field
pea (50%) and SBM (30%). It was evident that PER
method had penalised the diets deficient in S-amino acids,
and the extent of penalty was proportional to the degree
of the deficiency in methionine + cystine.

Experiment 4 (Nutritional evaluation of cereal-legume
blends).

Wheat-legume blends

Lysine was the first limiting amino acid in all the
wheat-containing blends (Table 6). The blends of wheat
with SBM, broad bean and fababean were lower in lysine
than those with lentil, casein and field pea. Most of
the wheat blends also supplied only 50-60% of the rat
requirements for methionine + cystine and threonine,
but tryptophan levels were quite high. Despite the
similarity in EAA composition, wheat-casein diet gave
much higher results, for food intake, gain, and PER,
than any wheat-legume blend. Protein digestibility of
the wheat-casein diet (96%) was also higher than the
values for blends of wheat with lentil (84%), fababean
(87%), field bean (88%), broad bean (90%), SBM (92%)
and field pea (94%). Among the wheat-legume blends,
field pea and SBM were superior to lentil, broad bean
and fababean diets in rat growth, protein digestibility
and PER. Differences in food intake were not large
but wheat-field bean diet was more acceptable than the
other blends, and showed a higher gain despite an
intermediate protein digestibility and PER.

Rice-legume blends

Rice protein contained more lysine and threonine, but less tryptophan, than wheat protein (Table 6). The net effect was a more uniform balance of EAA in relation to rat requirements. Therefore, two or more amino acids were near the first limiting amino acid level in most rice based diets. While lysine or S-amino acids appeared to be the most deficient amino acids in other diets, tryptophan was apparently first limiting in the rice-broad bean blend.

Food intake of the rice-legume diet averaged about 40 g higher than the wheat-legume blends, and only rice-field bean showed a significant reduction in the rate of consumption (Table 6). The weight gains ranked the rice blends in the same order as food intake with casein > SBM > field pea > other legumes. While significantly lower than casein, SBM and field pea were significantly higher than the other rice-legume diets in PER. Protein digestibility of the SBM (91%) and the field pea (92%) blend were also higher than the values for the other blends (81-88%). As in the wheat based diets, rice-broad bean diet was intermediate in protein digestibility (88%), while rice-lentil blend was particularly low (81%). While significantly higher than the wheat-legume blends in most cases, the PER values of the rice blends were ranked in the same general order of casein> SBM = field pea> field bean = lentil = broad bean> fababean.

In blends with wheat, casein was substantially superior in BV to all the legumes except lentil (Table 6). SBM and fababean were particularly low in BV when combined with wheat flour. All the legumes except lentil were significantly improved in BV by blending with rice. The blends of rice with SBM or field pea were equal to rice-casein diet in BV, although the other rice-legume blends were still significantly lower than the control. These BV results in general confirm the PER data but, more specifically, reflect the chemical scores that predicted a low nutritive value for wheat-SBM blend and a high value for wheat-lentil diet.

Correlation coefficients

For the combined data from the three rat growth trials (Tables 4, 5 and 6), the correlation coefficients were highly significant in most cases (Table 7).

Table 7. Correlation coefficients among protein nutritive
          indices obtained in rat growth trials in Tables
          4, 5 and 6 (n = 45).

Parameter[1]	Chemical score	Food intake	Weight gain
Food intake	0.58**		
Weight gain	0.78**	0.91**	
PER	0.85**	0.31*	0.60**

*Significant at P = 0.05

**Significant at P = 0.01

Chemical score gave reasonably good prediction of food
intake, weight gain and PER. The correlation between
chemical score and PER was especially high. The
correlations show that the levels of the most limiting
amino acid(s) were the principal factors controlling
protein utilization by rats for these particular diets.

Experiment 5 (Availability of amino acids in wheat and
oilseed proteins).

     The availability values of nitrogen and amino acids
in the two types (milling, Neepawa; utility, Glenlea)
of wheats were similar (Table 8). Although the availability values for lysine (83-85%) were low, the values
for nitrogen (93-95%) and other amino acids (91-96%)
were high.

     The nitrogen and lysine in SBM were about 88%
available and availability of other amino acids varied
between 84-95% (Table 8). Isolation of proteins from
SBM decreased the loss of nitrogen and most amino acids
in the feces. The nitrogen, lysine and methionine
availability values of soybean isolate were 5-7
percentage units higher than those of SBM.

Table 8. Nitrogen and essential amino acid availability values[1] (%) of wheat and rapeseed proteins as determined by balance trials with rats.

Protein source	Nitrogen	Arg	His	Ile	Leu	Lys	Met	Phe	Thr	Try	Val
Wheat											
Neepawa	93	94	92	93	94	83	94	95	91	96	94
Glenlea	95	95	93	93	94	85	94	95	92	96	95
Soybean											
Meal	87	94	95	85	87	88	84	90	85	94	86
Isolate	94	98	95	98	96	93	90	95	92	96	89
Rapeseed[2]											
RSM	85	90	88	85	88	83	91	85	84	90	83
ARSM, 2h	83	89	83	83	86	74	86	84	83	90	69
ARSM, 4h	70	73	74	68	68	45	67	66	65	72	49
RSM, DE	85	89	90	86	89	83	92	86	86	89	85
RSI	93	97	96	99	97	93	97	96	96	91	93

[1] The LRS minimum and maximum for the availability values were 2 and 3, respectively.

[2] RSM = rapeseed meal; ARSM = autoclaved rapeseed meal; DE = diffusion extracted; RSI = rapeseed isolate.

Table 9. Effects of amino acid supplementation on the availability[1] (%) of nitrogen and amino acids in legumes and wheat-legume blends.

Protein source	Nitrogen	Arg	His	Ile	Leu	Lys	Met	Phe	Thr	Val	Cys
Legume											
Soybean meal	87	94	95	85	88	88	84	90	85	86	85
Field pea	85	95	96	82	86	91	75	89	80	84	76
Fababean	80	90	90	78	82	85	70	82	78	80	70
Legume+methionine											
Soybean meal	90	98	97	89	91	92	98(94)[2]	93	85	89	88
Field pea	88	99	96	86	89	94	96(90)	91	82	86	80
Fababean	83	98	92	80	85	87	96(89)	86	80	80	75
Wheat-legume blend											
Soybean meal	92	94	93	88	90	84	90	93	86	90	90
Field pea	94	94	94	87	90	86	85	91	85	88	86
Fababean	90	94	91	85	88	82	81	90	84	86	84
Wheat-legume blend+lys, met and thr											
Soybean meal	92	96	94	93	95	98(92)	97(95)	98	95(89)	92	96
Field pea	91	96	94	93	94	97(94)	95(93)	96	92(89)	91	92
Fababean	91	95	95	90	94	93(91)	93(91)	97	92(90)	90	93

[1] The LSR minimum and maximum for the availability values were 3 and 4, respectively.

[2] Expected availability values denoted by brackets were calculated by assuming 100% availability of the supplemental met, lys or thr.

The amino acids in Span RSM were 83-90% available
with lysine and threonine being particularly low
(Table 8). Autoclaving the RSM for two hours had little
or no effect on the availability of nitrogen and amino
acids except lysine and valine. The value for lysine was
lowered from 83 to 74%. Autoclaving the RSM for four
hours reduced the availability of nitrogen and most
amino acids by about 20%, but caused a reduction of
over 40% in lysine and valine availability. Diffusion
extraction with 0.01N NaOH designed to remove glucosinolate had little or no effect on the nitrogen and
amino acid availability values of the RSM but isolation
of protein generally improved the values by about 10%.

Experiment 6 (Availability of amino acids in legumes and
wheat-legume blends).

Fababean was inferior to SBM and field pea in
availability of nitrogen and all amino acids (Table 9).
Lysine in the field pea was more available than in SBM,
however, SBM was superior to field pea in terms of the
availability values for isoleucine, mehtionine, threonine
and cystine.

When the legumes were fed as sole source of dietary
protein, methionine and cystine were low in availability,
especially in fababean, while high values were obtained
for arginine and histidine (Table 9). The low
availability of S-amino acids may seriously limit
the nutritional value of legume protein because methionine
was the first limiting amino acid in legume proteins
(Table 5). In addition, the average availability values
of the S-amino acids were 85, 75, and 70% respectively,
in SBM, field pea and fababean (Table 9), and the
level of sulphur amino acid contents ranked SBM>
field pea> fababean (Table 5). Apparently the availability was positively correlated with level of these
amino acids, which may explain why the PER of fababean
was only 0.5 as compared to 1.5 and 1.8 for field pea
and SBM, respectively (Tables 5 and 9).

Methionine supplementation of the legume diets
improved availability of most amino acids uniformly by
3-4 percentage units (Table 9). Methionine availability
values were particularly high. Most of the improvement
would be due to complete availability of supplemental
crystalline methionine. However, after correcting for
100% utilization of l-methionine, there was still an
increase of 4-7 percentage units in the utilization of
methionine in the legumes. This observation is in

accordance with reports that the rate of absorption of
amino acids is accelerated by the feeding of a balanced
diet instead of a deficient one (Squibb, 1968; Tao et
al., 1971).

Blending of the legumes with wheat flour protein
caused increases in amino acid availability but the
average effects were greater in the fababean than in
the SBM (Table 9). In addition, the availability values
of methionine and cystine were improved markedly
especially in fababean, but that of lysine decreased
significantly. The availability of lysine in wheat
proteins was lower than other amino acids including
S-amino acids (Table 8). Apparently the differences
in availability between legume and wheat-legume blends
were due, in part, to protein species differences in
availability, but complementary effects in the blends were
also evident (Tables 8 and 9); it appeared that there
may be interactive effects between the legume and the
cereal proteins within the digestive tract.

Lysine, methionine and threonine were low in
availability in the wheat-legume blends, and these amino
acids were added as supplements to these diets (Table 9).
As with methionine supplementation of the legume diets,
the availability values of most amino acids were
increased by 4-5 percentage units. After correcting for
100% utilization of crystalline lysine, methionine and
threonine, it was observed that the supplementation
improved the availability of lysine by 3-7, methionine
by 2 and threonine by 2-7 percentage units in the wheat-
legume blends.

The low availability values for S-amino
acids (first limiting amino acid) in the legumes and
for lysine (first limiting amino acid) in the wheat and
wheat-legume blends, obtained in the present investigation, and the substantial improvement noted in the
availability of the deficient amino acids by supplementation with the crystalline amino acids would indicate that
the first limiting amino acid is inferior to other
essential amino acids with regards to availability
(Tables 8 and 9). Similar observations about low
availability of methionine in SBM and of lysine in
cereals have previously been made (Eggum, 1968). Slump
and Beek (1975) also reported that those amino acids
which have a low true protein digestibility coefficient
usually occur in relative low levels in the dietary
protein.

ACKNOWLEDGMENTS

The authors are grateful for the assistance provided by H.W. Braitenbach, M.J. Farmer, P.H.L. Larsen, A. John and V. Kneisly. Financial assistance was provided by the National Research Council of Canada, the Department of Industry, Trade and Commerce under the Rapeseed Utilization Assistance Program of the Rapeseed Association of Canada, and the Hantelman Agricultural Research Fund.

REFERENCES

A.O.A.C. official methods of analysis. 1970. 9th ed. Association of Official Agricultural Chemists, Washington, D.C.

Appelqvist, L.A. and Ohlsón, R. 1972. Rapeseed cultivation, composition, processing and utilization. Elsevier Publ. Co., Amsterdam.

Bell, J.M. 1972. Nutrient requirements of the laboratory mouse. In Nutrient Requirements of Laboratory Animals. 2nd ed. National Academy of Sciences, Washington, D.C.

Bell, J.M., Giovannetti, P., Sharby, T.F., and Jones, J.D. 1976. Digestibility and protein quality evaluation of rapeseed flour. Can. J. Anim. Sci. 56:763-768.

Bender, A.E., and Doell, B.H. 1957. Biological evaluation of proteins; a new aspect. Br. J. Nutr. 11:140-148.

Bowland, J.P., Clandinin, D.R., and Wetter, L.R. 1965. Rapeseed meal for livestock and poultry - a review. Can. Dept. Agric. Publ. 1257.

Duncan, B.D. 1955. Multiple range and multiple F tests. Biometrics 11:1-42.

Eggum, B.O. 1968. Nutritional evaluation of proteins by laboratory animals. In Bender, A.E., Kihlberg, R., Lofquist, B., and Munck, L. (Ed.) Evaluation of Novel Protein Products. Proc. of International Biological Programme (IBP) and Wenner-Gren Centre Symposium, Stockholm, Sweden. Pergamon Press, New York.

El Nockrashy, A.S., Mukherjee, K.D., and Mangold, H.K. 1977. Rapeseed protein isolates by countercurrent extraction and isoelectric precipitation. J. Agr. Food Chem. 25:193-197.

John, A., and Bell, J.M. 1976. Amino acid requirements of the growing mouse. J. Nutr. 106:1361-1367.

Loew, F.M., Doige, C.E., Manns, J.G., Searcy, G.P., Bell, J.M., and Jones, J.D. 1976. Evaluation of dietary rapeseed protein concentrate flour in rats and dogs. Toxicol. Appl. Pharmacol. 35: 257-267.

McKenzie, S.L. 1973. Cultivar differences in proteins of oriental mustard (Brassica juncea L. Cross). J. Am. Oil Chem. Soc. 50:411-414.

McLaughlan, J.M., and Keith, M.O. 1975. Bioassays for protein quality. In Friedman, M. (Ed.) Protein Nutritional Quality of Foods and Feeds. Part 1. Assay Methods - Biological, Biochemical and Chemical. Marcel Dekker, Inc. New York.

Sarwar, G., and Bowland, J.P. 1975. Availability of amino acids in wheat cultivars used in diets for weanling rats. Can. J. Anim. Sci. 55:579-586.

Sarwar, G., and Bowland, J.P. 1976. Availability of tryptophan in wheat and oilseed proteins for weanling rats. Can. J. Anim. Sci. 56:433-437.

Sarwar, G., Shannon, D.W.F., and Bowland, J.P. 1975. Effects of processing conditions on the availability of amino acids in soybean and rapeseed proteins when fed to rats. Can. Inst. Food Sci. Technol. J. 8:137-141.

Sarwar, G., Sosulski, F.W., and Bell, J.M. 1973. Nutritional evaluation of oilseed meals and protein isolates. Can. Inst. Food Sci. Technol. J. 6:17-21.

Sarwar, G., Sosulski, F.W. and Bell, J.M. 1975a. Nutritive value of field pea and fababean proteins in rat diets. Can. Inst. Food Sci. Technol. J. 8:109-112.

Sarwar, G., Sosulski, F.W., and Bell, J.M. 1977.
Availability of amino acids in legumes and legume-
wheat blends. Can. Inst. Food Sci. Technol. J.
10:31-35.

Sarwar, G., Sosulski, F.W., and Holt, N.W. 1975b.
Protein nutritive value of legume-cereal blends.
Can. Inst. Food Sci. Technol. J. 8:170-174.

Slump, P., and Beek, V. 1975. Amino acids in feces
related to digestibility of food proteins. In
Friedman, M. (Ed.) Protein nutritional quality
of foods and feeds. Part 1. Assay Methods –
Biological, Biochemical and Chemical. Marcel Dekker,
Inc. New York.

Sosulski, F.W., and Bakal, A. 1969. Isolated
proteins from rapeseed, flax and sunflower
meals. Can. Inst. Food Technol. J. 2:28-32.

Sosulski, F.W., and Sarwar, G. 1973. Amino acid
composition of oilseed meals and protein isolates.
Can. Inst. Food Sci. Technol. J. 6:1-5.

Squibb, R.L. 1968. Effect of a dietary imbalance
of lysine on protein metabolism in the chick.
Poult. Sci. 47:199-204.

Tao, R., Belzile, R.J., and Brisson, G.J. 1971.
Amino acid digestibility of rapeseed meal fed
to chickens. Effects of fat and lysine
supplementation. Can. J. Anim. Sci. 51:705-709.

Tape, N.W., Sabry, Z.I., and Eapen, K.E. 1970.
Production of rapeseed flour for human consumption.
Can. Inst. Food Technol. J. 3:78-81.

Youngs, C.G., and Wetter, L.R. 1967. Microdetermination of major indiviual isothiocyanates
and oxazolidinethiones in rapeseed. J. Am. Oil
Chem. Soc. 44:551-554.

23

AMINO ACID SUPPLEMENTATION OF ISOLATED SOYBEAN PROTEIN IN MILK REPLACERS FOR PRERUMINANT LAMBS

Rodrigo Pelaez, David D. Phillips and Donald M. Walker

Department of Animal Husbandry, University of Sydney

Sydney, N.S.W. 2006, Australia

ABSTRACT

The growth of preruminant calves and lambs fed on milk replacers containing vegetable proteins is generally inferior to that of preruminants given cows' milk. The inferior performance has variously been attributed to an amino acid imbalance, to heat damage in preparation, and to the presence of growth-retarding substances. Soybean products that have been treated to remove, or destroy, growth-retarding substances are now available commercially.

An experimental design is described that has been used to determine the order of limiting amino acids in soy protein isolates, and which may also be used to estimate requirements for individual amino acids. The design allows an economy in time and in experimental animals, and gives results that are not significantly different from those determined in classical balance experiments.

INTRODUCTION

The proteins of cows' milk form the basis of the majority of milk replacers now used commercially to rear calves and lambs. The use of vegetable proteins in diets for pigs and poultry is widely accepted as a means of sparing animal protein, but it is only in recent times that they have been used in milk replacers to spare cows' milk proteins. However, the substitution of milk protein by vegetable protein in the diets of preruminants has not been very successful until quite recently, when commercial methods of preparation have been adopted that remove or destroy many of

the growth-retarding substances present in vegetable oil seeds.
Soybean products have been most widely used in milk replacers,
since the soybean is a readily available source of vegetable
protein with a relatively well-balanced amino acid composition.
However, the amino acid imbalance which exists in soy proteins
is a relatively minor problem, when compared with those problems
associated with the removal or destruction of the many substances
in the soybean which may have growth-retarding effects. It has
been noted with milk replacers containing soy products that, in
general, the cruder the product, the worse the performance of the
calves or lambs, though a number of protein isolates have also
given poor results.

PREPARATION OF SOY PRODUCTS

The raw soybean has the following average composition: crude
protein, 41%; fat, 22%; carbohydrates, 27%; crude fibre, 5%;
ash, 5%. After selection of clean, whole seeds, processing starts
by removing the hulls and extracting the fat. The soybean meal or
flour from the dehulled, defatted soybeans contains about 56%
protein, about 15% water soluble carbohydrates (mainly sucrose,
raffinose and stachyose; Yoshida et al, 1969) and 15% insoluble
carbohydrates (mainly neutral arabinogalactans, acidic polysaccharides and arabinan). The preruminant is unable to utilize carbohydrates other than glucose, galactose and lactose (Huber, 1969;
Walker, 1959), whilst moderate intakes of sugar, which would be
well tolerated by most monogastric animals, will lead to diarrhoea
(Blaxter and Wood, 1953; Walker and Faichney, 1964). Thus, a
milk replacer in which soyflour provides all the protein may also
contain excess soluble carbohydrates. In preparing a protein
concentrate the soyflour is extracted with a hot ethanol, water
mixture, not only to remove the soluble carbohydrates, but also to
remove or destroy certain unidentified substances, which have been
shown to lead to gastrointestinal allergic reactions, and to the
production of antibodies against soy protein in the blood of calves
fed on milk replacers containing soy products (van Adrichem and
Frens, 1965; van Leeuwen et al, 1969; Smith and Sissons, 1975).
The soy concentrate that remains after removal of the soluble
carbohydrates contains between 70 and 72% protein in the dry
matter. This protein may contain up to ten different antitrypsins.
Although these antitrypsins have not been shown experimentally
with preruminants to have a growth-retarding effect, they have
been shown to decrease pancreatic protease activity (Gorrill and
Nicholson, 1971). They are destroyed by careful heating of the
soy concentrate, without reducing the nutritive value of the main
proteins. The insoluble carbohydrates which remain in the soy
concentrate are indigestible in the small intestine of the pre-

ruminant, and seem to be resistant to breakdown by microbial enzymes in the large intestine. However, they may have a beneficial effect by absorbing water and reducing the incidence of diarrhoea.

A common procedure for preparing isolated soy proteins is to extract the defatted, dehulled soybeans with water at an alkaline pH, followed by acidification with hydrochloric acid to precipitate the globulin fraction. The curd is then washed with water, dispersed at neutral pH with alkali, and spray dried. The product contains from 90 - 96% protein and has a low carbohydrate and lipid content, but may still contain phytic acid, which could reduce the availability of various ions such as calcium, phosphorus, magnesium, iron and zinc. The isolate may also contain antitrypsins, together with those substances, mentioned above, which are responsible for the production of antibodies to soy protein in the blood of calves. There is considerable variability between different isolates in their physical and functional properties (Mattil, 1974); many of these differences are intentional and provide diversity required in the food industry.

FEEDING TRIALS WITH SOY PRODUCTS

The results of feeding trials with soy products in milk replacers for preruminants have been variable. In the past this was not surprising, since the *in vitro* tests to determine the presence of growth-retarding substances, or the availability of certain essential amino acids, were inadequate, so that the feeding trials with preruminants were, in themselves, biological assays. It was not possible to rely on tests with small laboratory animals, since there is evidence that different species react differently to the antitrypsins in soy products and probably to other growth-retarding substances. For example, Gorrill and Nicholson (1971) observed a decrease in protease activity in calves fed on whole milk with added soybean trypsin inhibitor, whereas in chickens and rats there is pancreatic hypertrophy and hypersecretion of enzymes (Mickelsen and Yang, 1966; Gertler et al, 1967). Nevertheless, in the experiments of Gorrill and Nicholson (1971) no evidence was given to show that the protease activity, although decreased, led to a reduction in the apparent digestibility of the dietary protein. The experiments of Nitsan et al (1971) with calves are also inconclusive, in determining whether the reduction in nitrogen digestibility of unheated soy protein concentrate (71% protein) is attributable to the antitrypsins, or to other inhibitors which are also destroyed by heating. Until recently, very few experiments had been carried out with preruminants in which soy products provided the sole source of protein in the milk replacer.

EVALUATION OF PROTEIN QUALITY

The value of a protein in the diet of a growing animal is determined by its ability to promote nitrogen retention. The classical methods of estimating nitrogen retention, namely, by balance and comparative slaughter methods, are time consuming and expensive in terms of labour and experimental animals. Thus, in recent years, many attempts have been made to develop indirect methods for assessing protein quality. These methods are based on the changes in composition that occur in blood and urine when the quality of the dietary protein is changed. For example, Eggum (1970) has demonstrated a close relationship between protein quality and plasma urea nitrogen concentration (PUN). However, as Kirk and Walker (1976b) have stated "a simple acceptance of the general relationship between PUN and nitrogen balance" (as a measure of protein quality)....." can be misleading, and ...... individual values for PUN, taken without reference to the source and amount of dietary protein given, cannot be used to predict nitrogen balance with any precision". The same comments would apply to the measurement, and use in prediction, of any other single component of the blood or urine. Furthermore, Kirk and Walker (1976b) concluded "that no further increase in the precision of predicting protein quality from PUN (or urinary nitrogen constituents) was possible, unless an experimental design was used in which the values for individual lambs were compared before and after a change in dietary treatment".

Soybean protein is known to be deficient in sulphur-containing amino acids when compared with milk protein (Orr and Watt, 1968) and, although soybean flours and isolates have been used in milk replacers for calves and lambs (Benevenga and Ronning, 1963; Gorrill and Nicholson, 1969, 1972; Nitsan et al, 1972; Porter 1969), there have been few attempts to assess, with preruminants, the requirements for supplementary amino acids, or to determine the order of limiting amino acids in vegetable proteins.

EXPERIMENTAL DESIGN

Kirk and Walker (1976a) demonstrated with lambs that when the dietary protein concentration of a milk replacer was changed from low (0.10 of total energy as protein) to medium (0.25), and back to low, the PUN concentration, estimated on successive days, reflected the change in the protein content of the diet within 3 - 4 days. This observation is in accord with the findings of Das and Waterlow (1974) with rats, that the response to a change in dietary protein concentration is complete in 30 hours, as measured by the change in urinary nitrogen excretion, or of Brown and Cline (1974), who showed with growing pigs that the response to a change in lysine intake is complete in 2 - 3 days, as measured by the urinary urea excretion. Thus, in the growing animal, much shorter dietary periods than are usually acceptable in classical balance experiments may be suitable for comparative studies of protein quality. However, some carry-over effect may be present if the diets to be compared differ considerably in amino acid composition. A change-over design has been adopted in our recent experiments to reduce the carry-over effect. In this design an even number of lambs (six, eight or ten), equal in number to the dietary treatments, are each given all diets in a particular order so that each diet is preceded once by all other diets (Figure 1). Four-day periods were adopted. The statistical analysis of the balanced change-over design was according to Patterson and Lucas (1962). Nitrogen balance was determined by one day, or two day, collections of urine and faeces on the third and fourth days of each period. The purpose of these experiments was to determine the limiting amino acids in two samples of isolated soy protein (ISP), but the change-over design has also been used to estimate the requirements of preruminants for individual amino acids. The commercial samples (ISP (A) and ISP (B)) were similar in chemical composition and apparently, also, in their methods of preparation. However, sample A was poorly accepted by the lambs when included in the diet as the sole source of protein, to supply 10% of the total energy as protein. Energy intake was controlled in all experiments at about twice the amount required to maintain energy balance in the lambs but, with sample A, it was not possible to persuade the lambs to consume greater amounts. On the other hand, sample B was readily accepted in a milk replacer of similar chemical composition, and there was no difficulty in persuading the lambs to consume additional milk, so that the energy intake was more than three times the maintenance requirement.

		Lamb no.					
		1	2	3	4	5	6
Period	1	C	D	E	B	A	F
	2	A	B	C	F	E	D
	3	B	C	D	A	F	E
	4	E	F	A	D	C	B
	5	D	E	F	C	B	A
	6	F	A	B	E	D	C

Figure 1. A 6 x 6 change-over design chosen to reduce carry over effects. Dietary treatments A - F.

TABLE 1

Experimental treatments

Treatment	Experiment 1	Experiment 2
1	ISP* + met (SM)	ISP + met, lys, isol, thr, val, try (SAA)
2	SM + lys	SAA - lys
3	SM + isol	SAA - isol
4	SM + thr	SAA - thr
5	SM + val	SAA - val
6	SM + try	SAA - try

*ISP = isolated soy protein, sample A or B .

All diets were supplemented with DL-methionine (met). Other amino acids were added in amounts sufficient to raise their concentrations in the diet to those in whole egg proteins (g amino acid per 16g nitrogen; Walker, 1975). The possible second-limiting amino acids (after methionine) were lysine (lys), isoleucine (isol), threonine (thr), valine (val) and tryptophane (try). Thus, there were six dietary treatments. The supplementary amino acids, L-forms, were added singly in experiment 1, or as a mixture in experiment 2, with one amino acid omitted in each of the other five diets (see Table 1). Glycine was added to make all diets isonitrogenous, and the ratio of essential : dispensible amino acid nitrogen was maintained at approximately 1:1, similar to that in cows' milk.

Nitrogen balance was measured on the last two days of each period. A summary of the results is given in Table 2 with nitrogen balances in treatments 2 - 5 expressed relative to the balance (expressed as 100) in treatment 1.

The results in experiment 1 show that the addition of single amino acids, in addition to methionine, did not lead to a significant improvement in nitrogen balance. In experiment 2, the performances of the lambs given diets 2 and 4 (minus lysine or threonine) were significantly inferior to those given diet 1. It was concluded that the amino acids lysine and threonine were equally second-limiting. Previous experiments had shown that the addition of

TABLE 2

Nitrogen balances of the lambs expressed
relative to treatment 1 (=100).

Treatment	Experiment 1		Experiment 2	
	ISP (A)*	ISP (B)	ISP (A)	ISP (B)
1	100	100	100^a	100^a
2 (+ lys)	93	107	76^b	77^b
3 (+ isol)	90	97	97^a	97^a
4 (+ thr)	92	93	83^b	85^b
5 (+ val)	93	93	93^a	97^a
6 (+ try)	-	93	100^a	100^a

*Walker and Kirk (1975b);   [ab]Values in the same column
with different superscripts differ significantly (P = 0.05).

methionine to ISP led to a significant increase in liveweight gain
and nitrogen balance (Walker and Kirk, 1975a) and, since the sulphur-
containing amino acids in ISP are most deficient, relative to their
content in whole egg proteins, methionine was regarded as the
first-limiting amino acid in soybean protein, as it is in other
monogastric animals (Berry et al, 1962; Snetsinger and Scott, 1958).

The experimental change-over design gave a reliable estimate
of the second-limiting amino acids in ISP with only six lambs, in
a period of 24 days (or 18 days if sub-periods were 3 days each).
Thus, 144 lamb-days (or a minimum of 108) were required. With the
classical nitrogen balance method the same result would have
required 432 lamb-days (6 lambs x 6 treatments x 12 days). These
results do not, however, illustrate clearly the superiority of ISP
(B) over ISP (A). Although the apparent digestibilities of
nitrogen in the two samples were similar, we have observed considerable variation in digestibility between batches of the same product,
particularly with ISP (A). In this product the digestibilities of
nitrogen may vary from 75 - 90%, and utilization of the apparently
digested nitrogen from <40 to >55%, in milk replacers providing
10% of the total energy as protein (Walker and Kirk, 1975a,b).
These values for nitrogen digestibility are not changed markedly

by amino acid supplementation, and the main effect of supplementation is on improved utilization.

Comparing milk protein and soy protein diets and using re-
entrant ileal cannulae, we have observed considerable differences
between diets in the amounts of nitrogen reaching the terminal
ileum. With a milk protein diet, 90% of the nitrogen ingested
was absorbed anterior to the terminal ileum, compared with 82%
with a soy protein diet. A proportion of this undigested nitrogen
was further degraded in the large intestine and did not appear in
the faeces. It was shown that the concentration of ammonia nitrogen
in the large intestine contents was significantly higher in lambs
given the soy protein diet.

Recent experiments with soy flours and isolates suggest that
the products now available commercially, for use in milk replacers,
have a much higher nutritive value than the soy isolate (sample A)
used in our earlier experiments, though it should be noted that
ISP - sample A was not intended by the manufacturers as a protein
to be used in milk replacers, but was produced as a functional
protein, with gelling properties, for use as a food additive.
Nevertheless, this isolate has proved invaluable in our experiments,
to demonstrate the importance of defining more clearly those methods
of processing which are important in improving the nutritive value
of vegetable proteins, and the need for rapid indirect methods of
assessing protein quality and detecting the presence of growth-
retarding substances.

REFERENCES

Benevenga, N.J. and Ronning, M. (1963). Response of calves to
     high fat milk replacer diets. J. Anim. Sci., 22, 832.
Berry, T.H., Becker, D.E., Rasmussen, O.G., Jensen, A.H. and
     Norton, H.W. (1962). The limiting amino acids in soybean
     protein. J. Anim. Sci., 21, 558-561.
Blaxter, K.L. and Wood, W.A. (1953). Some observations on the
     biochemical and physiological events associated with
     diarrhoea in calves. Vet. Rec., 65, 889-892.
Brown, J.A. and Cline, T.R. (1974). Urea excretion in the pig:
     an indicator of protein quality and amino acid requirements.
     J. Nutr., 104, 542-545.
Das, T.K. and Waterlow, J.C. (1974). The rate of adaptation of
     urea cycle enzymes, aminotransferases and glutamic dehydrogenase
     to changes in dietary protein intake. Br. J. Nutr., 32, 353-
     373.
Eggum, B.O. (1970). Blood urea measurement as a technique for
     assessing protein quality. Br. J. Nutr., 24, 983-988.

Gertler, A., Birk, Y. and Bondi, A. (1967). A comparative study of the nutritional and physiological significance of pure soybean trypsin inhibitors and of ethanol-extracted soybean meals in chicks and rats. J. Nutr., 91, 358-370.

Gorrill, A.D.L. and Nicholson, J.W.G. (1969). Growth, digestibility and nitrogen retention by calves fed milk replacers containing milk and soybean proteins, supplemented with methionine. Canad. J. Anim. Sci., 49, 315-321.

Gorrill, A.D.L. and Nicholson, J.W.G. (1971). Effect of soybean trypsin inhibitor, diarrhoea and diet on flow rate, pH, proteolytic enzymes, and nitrogen fractions in calf intestinal digesta. Canad. J. Anim. Sci., 51, 377-388.

Gorrill, A.D.L. and Nicholson, J.W.G. (1972). Alkali treatment of soybean protein concentrate in milk replacers : its effects on digestion, nitrogen retention, and growth of lambs. Canad. J. Anim. Sci., 52, 665-670.

Huber, J.T. (1969). Development of the digestive and metabolic apparatus of the calf. J. Dairy Sci., 52, 1303-1315.

Kirk, R.D. and Walker, D.M. (1976a). Plasma urea nitrogen as an indicator of protein quality. I. Factors affecting the concentration of urea in the blood of the preruminant lamb. Aust. J. Agric. Res., 27, 109-116.

Kirk, R.D. and Walker, D.M. (1976b). Plasma urea nitrogen as an indicator of protein quality. II. Relationships between plasma urea nitrogen, various urinary nitrogen constituents, and protein quality. Aust. J. Agric. Res., 27, 117-127.

Mattil, K.F. (1974). Composition, nutritional, and functional properties, and quality criteria of soy protein concentrates and soy protein isolates. J. Am. Oil Chemists Soc., 51, 81A-84A.

Mickelsen, O. and Yang, M.G. (1966). Naturally occurring toxicants in foods. Fed. Proc., 25, 104-123.

Nitsan, Z., Volcani, R., Gordin, S. and Hasdai, A. (1971). Growth and nutrient utilization by calves fed milk replacers containing milk or soybean protein-concentrate heated to various degrees. J. Dairy Sci., 54, 1294-1299.

Nitsan, Z., Volcani, R., Hasdai, A. and Gordin, S. (1972). Soybean protein substitute for milk protein in milk replacers for suckling calves. J. Dairy Sci., 55, 811-821.

Orr, M.L. and Watt, B.K. (1968). Amino acid content of foods. U.S. Dep. Agric. Home Econ. Res. Rep. No. 4. U.S. Govt. Printing Office, Washington.

Patterson, H.D. and Lucas, H.L. (1962). Change-over Designs. Tech. Bull. no. 147. North Carolina Agric. Expt. Sta.

Porter, J.W.G. (1969). Digestion in the preruminant animal. Proc. Nutr. Soc., 28, 115-121.

Smith, R.H. and Sissons, J.W. (1975). The effect of different feeds, including those containing soya-bean products, on the passage of digesta from the abomasum of the preruminant calf. Br. J. Nutr., 33, 329-349.

Snetsinger, D.C. and Scott, H.M. (1958). The adequacy of soybean oil meal as a sole source of protein for chick growth. Poultry Sci., 37, 1400-1403.

van Adrichem, P.W.M. and Frens, A.M. (1965). Soya protein as a feed antigen for fattening calves. Tijdschr. Diergeneesk., 90, 525-530.

van Leeuwen, J.M. Weide, H.J. and Braas, C.C. (1969). Feeding value of soyabean oilmeal compared with dried skimmed milk. Versl. landbouwk. Onderz. Ned., no. 732.

Walker, D.M. (1959). The development of the digestive system of the young animal. III. Carbohydrase enzyme development in the young lamb. J. Agric. Sci., 53, 374-386.

Walker, D.M. (1975). Utilization of whole egg and its components in milk replacers for preruminant lambs. Aust. J. Agric. Res., 26, 599-614.

Walker, D.M. and Faichney, G.J. (1964). Nutritional diarrhoea in the milk-fed lamb and its relation to the intake of sugar. Br. J. Nutr., 18, 209-215.

Walker, D.M. and Kirk, R.D. (1975a). The utilization by preruminant lambs of milk replacers containing isolated soya bean protein. Aust. J. Agric. Res., 26, 1025-1035.

Walker, D.M. and Kirk, R.D. (1975b). The utilization by preruminant lambs of isolated soya bean protein in low protein milk replacers. Aust. J. Agric. Res., 26, 1037-1052.

Yoshida. A., Umai, A., Kurata, Y. and Kawamura, S. (1969). Utilization of soybean oligosaccharides by the intact rat. J. Jap. Soc. Fd. Nutr., 22, 262-265. (quoted in Nutr. Abstr. Rev., 1970, 40, Abstr. 676).

24

THE NUTRITIVE VALUE OF FABA BEANS AND LOW GLUCOSINOLATE RAPESEED MEAL FOR SWINE

F.X. Aherne and A.J. Lewis

Department of Animal Science, University of Alberta

Edmonton, Alberta, Canada   T6G 2E3

ABSTRACT

Faba beans may be effectively used as a partial replacement for other protein supplements in swine diets. Breeding swine appear to be particularly sensitive to the level of faba beans in their diets. The lack of a response to autoclaving faba beans suggests that the trypsin inhibitor level and condensed tannin content of faba beans do not significantly influence the performance of growing-finishing swine. Supplementation of diets containing faba beans with lysine and/or methionine has not improved pig performance.

The scientific selection and commercial production of low glucosinolate varieties of rape constitutes a major advance for swine nutrition. All swine experiments that have compared low glucosinolate rapeseed meal with regular rapeseed meal have demonstrated the superiority of the low glucosinolate material as a protein source. Substantially larger proportions of the low glucosinolate material may be fed to all classes of swine without any significant depression in performance.

INTRODUCTION

The demand for protein for human and animal nutrition is increasing and is likely to continue to do so due to an ever increasing world population and an increase in the economic development of both the developed and less industrialized countries. This increased demand for protein is likely to lead to increased protein

453

scarcity and cost, particularly in animal and poultry production.
It is desirable, if not essential that we fully explore the potential of any or all protein feeds that can be grown in Canada. In
recent years faba beans (Vicia faba L.) and rapeseed (Brassica
napus and Brassica campestris) have shown considerable potential
as alternatives to soybeans as protein sources in poultry and
animal feeds (Blair, 1977). The objective of this paper is to
review the literature related to the evaluation of the nutritive
value of faba beans and rapeseed meal in the diets of. pigs.

Composition

     A comparison of the composition of faba beans, rapeseed meal
and soybean meal is shown in Tables 1 and 2. These tables have
been compiled from data presented by Clarke (1969), Hansen and
Clausen (1969), Allen (1976), Bowland (1976), NRC (1973) and from
analyses conducted at the University of Alberta. The most striking
difference in composition between faba beans and soybean meal is
the protein and amino acid composition. Faba beans contain approximately 26% protein and are considerably lower in the sulphur
amino acids than is soybean meal. The lysine level of faba beans
compares well with that of soybean meal, being approximately 6.7%
of the protein in both cases. The mineral composition of both
compare reasonably well but faba beans are lower in most vitamins
than soybean meal.

     Rapeseed meal contains approximately 38% protein. Relative
to soybean meal it is a rich source of methionine, but contains
less lysine. Rapeseed meal is quite high in mineral content. The
substantial contents of phosphorus and selenium may be of practical
significance in swine ration formulation.

FABA BEANS

     The multiplicity of names used for Vicia faba and its sub-
species has tended to confuse any evaluation of its nutritive
value. In this review only Vicia faba L. var minor will be discussed. Some of the vernacular names used to describe Vicia faba
L. var minor are: horse bean, tick bean, field bean, faba bean,
feverole, ackerbohnen and hestebonner. For the purpose of this
report the name faba bean will be used. This appellation is in
accordance with the genuine botanical name and represents an attractive and simple designation for Vicia faba L. var minor
(Presber, 1972).

TABLE 1

Proximate and amino acid composition of
faba beans, rapeseed meal and soybean meal.

Ingredients	Faba beans	Rapeseed meal	Soybean meal
International feed number	5-09-262	5-08-135	5-04-604
Dry matter (%)	89	91	89
Digest. energy (kcal/kg)	3263	2900	3130
Metab. energy (kcal/kg)	3083	2700	2825
Protein (%)	25.7	38.0	44.0
Ether extract (%)	1.4	2.0	0.8
Crude fiber (%)	8.2	10.9	7.3
Ash (%)	6.0	7.2	6.0
Arginine (%)	2.5	2.3	3.3
Cystine (%)	0.2	0.4	0.7
Histidine (%)	0.2	1.0	1.2
Isoleucine (%)	1.1	1.4	2.4
Leucine (%)	1.9	2.6	3.5
Lysine (%)	1.72	2.11	2.93
Methionine (%)	0.2	0.7	0.7
Phenylalanine (%)	1.2	1.4	2.3
Tyrosine (%)	0.7	0.9	1.3
Threonine (%)	0.96	1.75	1.81
Tryptophan (%)	0.24	0.39	0.62
Valine (%)	1.2	1.8	2.3

Nutritive Value for Growing-Finishing Pigs

One of the first reported studies of the use of faba beans in pig diets was that of Aherne and McAleese (1964). They included 10, 20 or 30% faba beans in the diets of growing-finishing pigs. There was no significant difference in average daily gain or feed conversion efficiency of pigs fed the control diet or diets containing 10 or 20% faba beans. However, average daily gain and feed conversion efficiency were significantly (P<0.05) better for pigs fed the control diet than for pigs fed the 30% faba bean diet.

These results were confirmed by Hansen and Clausen (1969) in a series of 42 experiments involving 736 pigs. They observed no significant differences in average daily gain or feed conversion efficiency of pigs fed a soybean-meat meal supplemented diet or diets containing 5, 10 or 15% faba beans. When faba beans constituted the only protein supplement in the pigs diet, average daily

TABLE 2

Mineral and vitamin composition of faba beans,
rapeseed meal and soybean meal.

Ingredient	Faba beans	Rapeseed meal	Soybean meal
Calcium (%)	0.14	0.60	0.29
Chlorine (%)	-	-	0.05
Copper (mg/kg)	4.1	5.5	36.3
Iron (mg/kg)	70	155	120
Magnesium (%)	0.13	0.52	0.27
Manganese (mg/kg)	8.4	47.5	29.3
Phosphorus (%)	0.54	1.05	0.65
Potassium (%)	1.20	1.09	2.00
Selenium (mg/kg)	-	0.98	0.10
Sodium (%)	0.80	-	0.34
Sulfur (%)	-	-	0.43
Zinc (mg/kg)	42	60	27
Biotin (mg/kg)	0.09	-	0.32
Choline (mg/kg)	1670	6700	2794
Folacin (mg/kg)	-	-	0.5
Niacin (mg/kg)	22	188	60
Pantothenic acid (mg/kg)	3.0	12.5	13.3
Pyridoxine (mg/kg)	-	-	8.0
Riboflavin (mg/kg)	1.6	3.1	2.9
Thiamin (mg/kg)	5.5	1.8	1.7
Vitamin E (mg/kg)	1	-	2.1

gain and feed conversion efficiency were significantly reduced.
Up to 30% faba beans in the pigs' diet did not significantly influence carcass quality or taste of the meat. In a review article,
Clarke (1969) cites the results of some experiments by Luscombe
(1969) in which partial or complete replacement of soybean meal by
faba beans in pig diets produced no significant reduction in average
daily gain or feed conversion efficiency. Methionine supplementation of the diets gave no improvement in pig performance compared
with control diets. From Germany, Feist, Hofmann, Kirchgessner and
Schwarz (1974) reported that replacement of some or all of the
fish meal in the diets of pigs from 25 to 97 kg liveweight by 15
or 30% faba beans did not significantly affect average daily gain,
feed conversion efficiency or carcass quality of pigs. Cole,
Blades, Taylor and Luscombe (1971) compared the performance of
pigs fed a soybean-fish meal control diet with that of pigs fed
diets containing 10 or 20% faba beans during the growing period

and 20 or 30% faba beans in the finishing period. There were no significant differences between treatments in growth rate, feed conversion efficiency or carcass quality. Castell (1976) reported no significant reduction in growth rate or feed to gain ratio when pigs were fed 18% protein diets ad libitum, which contained 0, 7.5, 15 and 30% faba beans, over the growth period from 25 to 90 kg liveweight. However, the linear component of the treatment effect was significant (P<0.05) indicating that an increase in the faba bean content of the diet produced a linear reduction in growth rate and feed conversion efficiency. Fowler and Livingstone (1972) reported that when faba beans were used as the only protein supplement, they fell well below their theoretical exchange ratio of 3.75% beans to 1% fish meal based on their crude protein or lysine.

In recent years several experiments involving faba beans have been conducted in Canada. Two of these experiments conducted at The University of Alberta (Bowland, Aherne and Egbuiwe, 1975) were designed to evaluate faba beans and rapeseed meal from a low erucic acid-low glucosinolate rapeseed (B. napus cv 1788) as protein supplements alone or in combination with soybean meal or meat meal in the diets of growing-finishing pigs. With pigs from 7 kg to market weight, there were no significant (P>0.05) differences in daily feed intake, daily gain, efficiency of feed conversion or carcass measurements when isonitrogenous diets containing soybean, rapeseed meal, faba beans or various combinations of these protein supplements were fed. In the second experiment there were no significant differences in daily feed intake, daily gain or carcass measurements of pigs fed isonitrogenous diets containing 9.0% soybean meal, 21.0% faba beans, 15% faba beans+2.5% soybean meal, 15.0% faba beans+3.5% rapeseed meal, 15% faba beans+2% meat meal or 10% faba beans+7.5% rapeseed meal during the period 44 kg to slaughter at 85 kg liveweight. However feed efficiency was significantly lower for pigs fed 15% faba beans+3.5% rapeseed meal than for those fed faba beans alone or 10% faba beans+7.5% rapeseed meal. The results indicate that replacement of soybean meal by ground unprocessed faba beans or by rapeseed meal (from low glucosinolate, low erucic acid rapeseed meal) or 50/50 combinations of these supplements will not depress growth rate or feed efficiency of growing-finishing pigs.

Though there is some disagreement as to the maximum level of faba beans that may be included in pig diets without reducing the growth and feed efficiency of growing-finishing pigs the majority of the reports suggest that no significant reduction in pig performance might be expected, when faba beans are included in the diets of growing pigs at levels of up to 20% of the diet, while total replacement of other protein supplements by faba beans in the finishing period is unlikely to reduce growth rate, feed conversion efficiency or carcass quality.

Heat Treatment of Faba Beans

The effects of autoclaving faba beans on energy and nitrogen digestibility of diets containing faba beans has been reported by Aherne, Lewis and Hardin (1977). The rations fed to pigs included a control diet (no faba beans added) and five diets containing 25% faba beans that had been autoclaved for either 0, 15, 30, 45 or 60 min at 121°C. There were no significant differences in digestible nitrogen or digestible energy between the control diet or the diets containing 25% unheated or autoclaved faba beans. However both digestible energy and digestible nitrogen were lower in the faba bean diets than the control diet and digestible energy tended to decrease progressively as the autoclaving time increased. In a second experiment by Aherne, Lewis and Hardin (1977) pigs with an average initial weight of 10.0 kg were allotted to diets containing 0, 10, 15, 20 or 25% unheated faba beans or 25% faba beans that had been autoclaved for 30 min at 121°C. The results of this experiment are shown in Table 3. For the starter, grower and finisher phases and for the whole study, there was a slight but definite reduction in average daily feed intake and average daily gain as the level of faba beans in the diet was increased above 15%. Feed conversion efficiency was not consistently influenced by either the level of faba beans in the diet or by autoclaving the beans. Autoclaving the beans encouraged a slightly higher feed intake but did not improve growth rate or feed conversion efficiency. Using re-entrant cannulas in the terminal ileum of 35 kg pigs, Ivan and Bowland (1976) reported that autoclaving faba beans for 30 or 60 min had no significant effect on digestibility of dry matter, gross energy, nitrogen and individual amino acids, except arginine, which was significantly increased.

Faba Beans for Breeding Swine

The effects of including faba beans in the diets of pregnant and lactating sows has received little attention. Nielsen and Kruse (1974) reported a significant reduction in milk yield and litter size at birth and weaning when faba beans were included in the diets of gestating and lactating sows. In a recent experiment, Etienne (1977) observed no significant effects on conception rate, ovulation rate, weight gain or total embryonic mortality of sows fed 15 or 20% faba beans in their diets throughout gestation compared to sows fed a soybean meal control diet. However, sows fed the diets containing faba beans had lighter foetuses and lighter placentas. The factors in the faba beans responsible for the reduction in the weight of foetuses was not determined.

TABLE 3

Performance of pigs fed diets containing four levels of faba beans.

	Control	10	15	20	25	25A+	SEx̄
				Faba bean levels (%)			
Number of pigs	12	12	12	12	12	12	
Starter (10-25 kg)							
Daily feed (kg)§	1.27	1.24^a	1.20^a	1.11^b	1.17^{ab}	1.21^{ab}	0.05
Daily gain (kg)	0.55^a	0.54^a	0.54^a	0.48^b	0.51^{ab}	0.52^{ab}	0.02
Feed/gain	2.31	2.31	2.22	2.31	2.30	2.34	0.08
Grower (25-43 kg)							
Daily feed (kg)	2.02	2.00	1.97	1.82	1.86	1.94	0.07
Daily gain (kg)	0.69	0.66	0.65	0.63	0.64	0.66	0.02
Feed/gain	2.91	3.01	3.03	2.87	2.90	2.96	0.06
Finisher (43-89 kg)							
Daily feed (kg)§	3.09^{ab}	3.21^a	2.88^{bc}	2.80^c	2.75^c	2.87^{bc}	0.08
Daily gain (kg)	0.80	0.78	0.76	0.72	0.75	0.73	0.02
Feed/gain	3.89	4.12	3.82	3.89	3.70	3.97	0.11
Whole experiment							
Daily feed (kg)§	2.38^{ab}	2.44^a	2.26^{bc}	2.19^c	2.17^c	2.27^{bc}	0.05
Daily gain (kg)§	0.71^a	0.70^{ab}	0.68^{abc}	0.65^c	0.67^{abc}	0.66^{bc}	0.01
Feed/gain	3.35	3.50	3.34	3.37	3.26	3.43	0.07

+Faba beans were autoclaved for 30 min at 121°C.

§Means within rows followed by different letters were significantly different (P<0.05). Comparisons (using Duncan's, 1955 multiple range test) were made only when the treatment F value was significant (P<0.05).

Digestibility Studies

Livingstone, Fowler and Woodham (1970) reported the apparent digestibility coefficient for the nitrogen of faba beans to be 83 to 87% for spring and winter varieties, respectively. Liveweight gain was reduced as the level of beans in the diet increased. They suggested that the dietary substitution ratio (% beans:% fishmeal) is clearly higher than the theoretical rate of 2.4 to 1 calculated using the total lysine of the diets as the criterion of equivalence. Nitrogen digestibility (77.7%) and nitrogen retention (25.8 g N/100 g N intake) was reported by Whittemore and Taylor (1973) to be significantly lower for diets containing 25% faba beans than for a control soybean meal supplemented diet, even though the amino acid content of the diets were very similar. They suggested that the role of trypsin inhibitor activity in faba beans may warrent further investigation. Aherne and McAleese (1964) obtained digestibility coefficients for faba bean nitrogen of 81% in diets containing 10, 20 and 30% faba beans. Using semi-purified diets, Pastuszewska, Duee, Henry, Burdon and Jung (1974) reported that the digestibility coefficient of the protein of faba beans (78.80%) was significantly lower than that of soybean meal (88.49%). The digestible energy coefficient of the faba beans was also significantly lower than that of soybean meal, but the differences were not as great as observed for protein (89.79 vs 84./9%). Shelling the faba beans improved the digestibility for both nitrogen and energy. Whether this improvement in digestibility is a reflection of a reduction in the fiber level or growth inhibitor level of the diet is not clear. They obtained apparent digestibility coefficients for cystine, methionine, lysine and threonine that were 10 to 15% lower for faba beans than for soybean meal. Their value of 77.93% for lysine digestibility is very similar to the 78% digestibility figure obtained with purified diets containing 20% faba beans by Sarwar and Bowland (1974). Walz (1974) fed diets containing 30% raw or toasted (3 hr, 80°C) faba bean meal as the sole source of protein for pigs of 20 to 23 kg liveweight. He reported that the biological value of the protein of the normal and toasted faba bean meal to be 54.5% and 57%, respectively. The higher biological value of the toasted meal was attributed to a 9% higher nitrogen digestibility.

Amino Acid Supplementation

Aherne and McAleese (1964) calculated that diets supplemented with 10, 20 or 30% faba beans contained 0.52, 0.41 and 0.33% methionine plus cystine. Thus all three diets were lower than the level of 0.6% recommended by the National Research Council at that time (1959). In spite of the apparent sulphur amino acid deficiency in these diets there was no significant improvement in pig performance when dietary methionine was raised to a level of 0.6% with supplemental methionine. Hansen and Clausen (1969) also reported no

significant response in pig growth or feed efficiency when diets
containing 5, 10 or 15% faba beans were supplemented with methionine. Cole, Blades, Taylor and Luscombe (1971) added methionine
to diets containing 20% faba beans during the growing period or 30%
faba beans in the finishing period and observed no improvement in
growth rate, feed utilization or carcass quality whether the methionine was included during the finishing period or throughout the
whole experiment. Fowler and Livingstone (1972) also reported
that the addition of methionine to faba bean supplemented diets did
not improve the nutritive value of such diets. However, the response to methionine was much greater in diets in which faba beans
were used in combination with fish meal. Balboa, Zurita and Guedas
(1966) and Feist, Schwarz, Hofmann and Kirchgessner (1974) reported
a significant increase in growth rate of pigs when faba bean diets
containing 0.43% or 0.45% sulphur amino acids were supplemented
with methionine.

Poppe, Schlage, Scheider and Weisemuller (1975) reported the
results of three experiments conducted in Germany in which faba
beans were used to replace some or all of the soybean meal, fish
meal or meat meal in the diets of pigs from 35 to 115 kg liveweight.
Levels of 10 to 30% faba beans in the diets, with or without lysine
supplementation, did not significantly affect the average daily
gain, feed conversion efficiency or carcass quality of the pigs.
Onaghise and Bowland (1977) observed that when pigs of 5.9 kg
were fed diets in which soybean meal was replaced by up to 21%
faba beans there was no significant reduction in average daily feed
intake, growth rate or efficiency of feed conversion. Total replacement of soybean meal by faba beans, even when supplemented with
lysine and methionine produced a significantly (P<0.01) lower feed
intake, average daily gain and feed conversion efficiency.

In spite of the apparent deficiency of sulphur amino acids in
diets containing 20 to 30% faba beans and the reported low digestibility of these amino acids in faba beans (Pastuszewska, Duee,
Henry, Burdon and Jung, 1974) there has been a general lack of
response from supplementing such diets with methionine. These data
support the suggestion that the sulphur amino acid requirements
established by the National Research Council (1973) may be too high
(Allee and Trotter, 1974; Brown, Harmon and Jensen, 1974) or that
some other factor in the faba bean diets is limiting the response
to methionine supplementation. Why methionine supplementation of
diets containing faba beans has shown an improvement in pig performance under certain circumstances is not clear.

Growth Depressing Factors in Faba Beans

The poor utilization of faba beans relative to soybean meal
observed in several studies when faba beans were fed at levels of

greater than 20% of the diet of growing pigs could be attributed
to the presence of certain growth depressing factors in the faba
beans. Kadirvel and Clandinin (1974) reported that the tannin
content of four varieties of faba beans was 0.34 to 0.50%. The
testa contained a greater proportion of the total tannins (phen-
lics) than the embryo. However, they suggested that the level of
tannins in diets containing up to 35% faba beans would not likely
be detrimental to growth of chicks or turkey poults. Support for
this contention is provided by Wilson and McNab (1972) who obtained no improvement in the growth of chicks fed diets containing
faba beans from which the tannins had been removed by extraction
with 75% ethanol. However, Marquardt, Campbell and Ward (1976) and
Marquardt, Ward, Campbell and Cansfield (1976) reported that the
principal chick-growth depressing factor in faba beans is located
primarily in the hull (testa) portion of the bean and is a thermo-
labile condensed tannin. They suggested that its mode of action is
to reduce appetite and reduce nutrient retention. These results
could explain the demonstrated improvement in rate of growth and
efficiency of feed utilization in chicks fed diets containing
autoclaved faba beans compared with raw faba beans (Wilson and
McNab, 1972; Marquardt and Campbell, 1973; Marquardt and Campbell,
1974; Marquardt, Campbell, Stothers and McKirdy, 1974). Subsequent
experiments by the Manitoba researchers (Olaboro, Campbell and
Marquardt, 1977) have shown that egg production equivalent to
controls was evident among hens receiving high (25-30% of the diet)
levels of ground faba beans, although a consistent depression in
egg weight was apparent. Heat treatment (autoclaving) of the
faba beans did not aleviate the egg weight depression. They suggested that the factor(s) causing the egg weight depression was
associated with the protein portion of the cotyledon of the faba
bean and not with the condensed tannin content of the hull. These
results with laying hens are more consistent with the lack of response to autoclaving faba beans observed in the experiments with
swine (Aherne, Lewis and Hardin, 1977). In many of the experiments
in which faba beans were fed to swine feed intake was not reported.
However, Hansen and Clausen (1969) reported that feed intake was
reduced when faba beans constituted the only protein supplement in
swine diets. They suggested that the reduction in feed intake may
have resulted from the high tannic acid content of the faba beans.
Aherne, Lewis and Hardin (1977) observed a slight but definite
reduction in average daily feed intake as the level of faba beans
in the diet was increased above 15%. Autoclaving the beans encouraged a slightly higher feed intake but did not improve growth
or feed conversion efficiency.

Kadirvel and Clandinin (1974) recorded trypsin inhibitor
activity of crude raw, extract of faba beans as being 4% of the
inhibitor activity of raw soybean. Wilson, McNab and Bentley (1972
a, b) using a different method of analysis reported one fifth as much

inhibitor activity in raw faba beans as in raw soybean. Kadirvel and Clandinin (1974) suggest that the reason for the lack of agreement in the two studies on trypsin inhibitor activity may be related to the differences in the methods of measurement used. In a recent study Marquardt, Campbell and Ward (1976) reported a level of 1.8 mg/g of trypsin inhibitor in faba beans, while the hemaglutinin activity was 2700 units. Autoclaving reduced the trypsin inhibitor level to 0.2 mg/g and the hemaglutinin activity to 40 units.

Autoclaving or infrared radiation of faba beans may improve their metabolizable energy values (Edwards and Duthie, 1973 and McNab and Wilson, 1974) though Marquardt, Campbell and Ward (1976a) suggest that the influence of heat treatment on the nutritional quality of faba beans is confined primarily to the protein component as compared to the starch component of the faba beans.

From the above review of the literature it can be seen that there are some limitations to the use of faba beans in swine diets. It may be concluded that when each 5% faba beans added to the diet replaces 2.8% grain and 2.2% soybean, a reduction in gain of approximately 0.01-0.02 kg/day might be expected. Average daily feed intake may be reduced slightly but feed conversion efficiency and carcass quality is unlikely to be affected by inclusion of faba beans in swine diets at levels of 10 to 25%. No advantage in digestibility or pig performance is to be gained by heat treatment of the beans, or by supplementing diets containing faba beans with methionine and/or lysine.

LOW GLUCOSINOLATE RAPESEED MEAL

The use of rapeseed meal in rations for swine has been restricted by its content of glucosinolates, substances which when hydrolyzed by enzymes that occur naturally in rapeseed give rise to products that may reduce the performance of growing pigs and adult swine. Canadian guidelines (Bowland and Bell, 1972) recommend that the amount of rapeseed meal in rations should not exceed 5% for young pigs and 3% for gestating and lactating females. The basis for these recommendations was reviewed by Bowland (1976).

The limitations imposed by glucosinolates have provided a major incentive for plant breeders to develop varieties of rape with reduced amounts of these compounds. Remarkable progress has been made, and a variety, Tower, containing low levels of glucosinolates, is now commercially available in Canada. Most of the data discussed in this review are derived from experiments to evaluate the use of low glucosinolate rapeseed meal in rations for swine.

Low Glucosinolate vs Regular Rapeseed Meal for Growing Pigs

Glucosinolates and related compounds occur in many different types of plants, but among the agriculturally important species they are found particularly in the Cruciferae. It is the products of glucosinolates that are responsible for the well-known goiter problems associated with this family of plants. Characteristic symptoms of ingestion of substantial amounts of glucosinolates are reduced performance, enlarged thyroid glands, and reduced levels of circulating thyroid hormones.

Traditionally, rapeseed meal has contained from 5 to 10 mg/g total glucosinolates, depending largely on what variety it was derived from. In 1967, however, plant breeders in Canada and Sweden, working independently, found a particular rape vareity, Bronowski, that has a glucosinolate content which is much lower than average. Since 1974, most published material relating to the nutritive value of rapeseed meal for swine has dealt with either Bronowski (0.3-0.7 mg/g total glucosinolates) or varieties derived from it, particularly Tower (0.9-1.5 mg/g total glucosinolates).

All swine experiments that have compared low glucosinolate rapeseed meal with regular rapeseed meal have demonstrated the superiority of the low glucosinolate material as a protein source for pigs (Bowland, 1974; Bell, 1975; Bowland, 1975; McCuiag and Bell, 1976; McKinnon and Bowland, 1976; Moody, Slinger and Summers, 1976; Castell, 1977a). This work has established unequivocally the progress that has been made in improving nutritional quality by selecting for low glucosinolate content.

Most of the experiments referred to above, and also those of Omole and Bowland, 1974; Grandhi, Slinger, Brown and Hacker, 1976; Grandhi, Bowman and Slinger 1977; Pearson and Bowland, 1977 and Lewis and Aherne, 1977 have shown that at least half of the supplemental protein in starting and growing pig rations (up to about 10% of the total diet) can be provided by low glucosinolate rapeseed meal without significantly reducing performance. For finishing pigs (55-90 kg), most of the studies have demonstrated that low glucosinolate rapeseed meal can be used to provide all of the supplemental protein without any significant reduction in performance relative to pigs fed soybean meal. The only experiment showing a contrary result seems to be that of Castell (1977b). In this experiment pigs fed 7.5% Tower rapeseed meal during the starting phase, and 12.5% Tower rapeseed meal during the growing and finishing phase grew more slowly (P<0.05 and P<0.01, respectively) than pigs fed the same amount of soybean meal.

Thus work published during the last three years has established that substantially larger amounts of rapeseed meal than formerly recommended can be included in rations for growing pigs provided the meal is of the low glucosinolate type. Despite this welcome situation, most experiments with very young pigs (initial weight less than 25 kg) have indicated that when low glucosinolate rapeseed meal provides the sole source of supplemental protein the performance of this class of pig will be reduced relative to animals fed an equivalent amount of soybean meal. Much of the current rapeseed research, both plant breeding and nutritional evaluation, is directed towards this situation.

The new types of rapeseed meal still contain measurable amounts of glucosinolates (Tower contains 0.9-1.5 mg/g), and there is evidence that at least part of the depressed performance in young pigs may still be due to goitrogenic activity. Thus Bowland (1974) reported that serum thyroxine and protein-bound iodine concentrations were lower in young pigs fed Tower rapeseed meal than in control pigs fed a diet based on soybean meal. Slinger (1977) found that the relative thyroid weight (mg thyroid/kg body weight) of pigs fed Tower rapeseed meal was greater than that of control pigs fed a soybean meal diet, but the increase (46%) was much less than that found in pigs fed the high glucosinolate rapeseed meal, Target, (251%).

Several authors have suggested that there may be a sex (barrows vs gilts) difference in the way that growing pigs respond to dietary inclusion of rapeseed meal. Bowland (1971) found that including whole ground rapeseed (high glucosinolate) in the ration reduced weight gain in gilts more than in barrows. The same effect was observed in a later experiment (Bowland, 1974), that included low glucosinolate rapeseed meal (Bronowski). This same trend has also been noticed in our recent experiments at Alberta (Lewis and Aherne, 1977; Pearson and Bowland, 1977). In contrast, the opposite effect was recorded by Castell (1977b), who found that the growth rate of barrows, but not gilts was depressed when Tower rapeseed meal was included in the ration. The reason for this discrepancy is not apparent and it is not known whether there is some factor other than glucosinolates present in rapeseed meal that may affect the sexes differently. Various rapeseed meal x sex interactions on swine carcasses (McCuaig and Bell, 1976) and on metabolic parameters in rats (Loew, Doige, Manns, Searcy, Bell and Jones, 1976) have also been observed.

The suitability of the amino acid pattern of rapeseed meal for swine has been examined; particularly by the addition of synthetic amino acids. Bell (1975) added 0 or 0.1% methionine hydroxy analog and 0, 0.05 or 0.1% lysine in a factorial arrangement to diets containing Bronowski rapeseed meal for growing pigs. He found a 15% improvement in growth rate due to supplemental methionine, but essentially no response to lysine. This was a somewhat surprising result as, relative to an isonitrogenous amount of soybean meal, rapeseed meal is a little low in lysine, but rich in sulfur amino acids (see Table 1). Furthermore, there is evidence that the lysine of rapeseed meal may be less available than that of soybean meal (Cho and Bayley, 1972). Moody, Slinger and Summers (1976) added 0, 0.125 or 0.250% lysine to diets based on Tower rapeseed for young pigs, and found a tendency for performance to improve with the addition of 0.125% lysine, but this was not statistically significant.

As gilts seem to be more susceptible to a lysine deficiency than barrows (Meade, Hanke and Rust, 1974) we (Lewis and Aherne, unpublished) recently examined the effect of lysine addition to Tower rapeseed meal in the diets of young growing (20-60 kg) gilts. Seventy two gilts were allotted to one of three treatments (1) a soybean meal control diet (2) a Tower rapeseed meal diet isonitrogenous with diet 1 (3) a diet similar to diet 2 but with added lysine to provide an available lysine level equal to that of diet 1. Performance of gilts fed the Tower rapeseed meal diets was lower than that of those fed soybean meal (confirming our earlier results, Lewis and Aherne, 1977), but there was no response to the added lysine.

It is difficult, therefore, to draw conclusions regarding which amino acid is potentially first limiting in diets for swine based on rapeseed meal. On the basis of chemical analyses this seems most likely to be lysine, but the experimental data to this time show that a response is more likely to be obtained from supplementing methionine than lysine. Of course, the nature of the rest of the diet (i.e. corn or wheat/barley based) may affect this conclusion.

Rapeseed meal contains a substantially higher crude fiber level than soybean meal (see Table 1), and this may contribute to the lower performance observed when rapeseed meal contributes all of the supplemental protein for starting pigs. As a consequence, Canada's plant breeders are attempting to select varieties with lower fiber content. It has been shown (Stringam, McGregor and Pawlowski, 1974) that reduced fiber content is associated with yellow seedcoat. A reduction of about 4% in fiber is potentially possible through the introduction of yellow seeded cultivars. Tests at the University of Alberta (Aherne and Lewis, unpublished) with one such cultivar, variety 1821, have not proved encouraging. In an experiment with growing (20-60 kg) barrows and gilts, animals fed diets containing variety 1821 did not outperform those fed Tower, and both of these groups grew more slowly than those fed soybean meal. We have also observed a similar result in young rats.

Breeding Animals

In the past, considerable caution has been necessary when feeding rapeseed meal to gestating and lactating sows and gilts. Experiments with rapeseed meals derived from the older rape varieties demonstrated reduced conception rates and smaller litter size if rapeseed meal was included in the diet at levels of 6-8% or greater. Consequently, Canadian guidelines (Bowland and Bell, 1972) recommend an upper limit of 3% rapeseed meal in the total diet for gestating and lactating females. The advent of low glucosinolate rapeseed meal should allow considerable relaxation of this restriction. Data, as yet unpublished, from three research centers (Lennoxville, Quebec; MacDonald College, Quebec; and The University of Alberta) indicate that it should be possible to include at least 10% and possibly supply all of the supplemental protein from rapeseed meal, in gestation and lactation rations, provided a low glucosinolate type is used.

General Recommendations

Based on the extensive work on low glucosinolate rapeseed meal during the last three years, it is evident that this is a satisfactory source of protein for swine. For young pigs during the starting and growing periods up to 10% of the rations may be composed of low glucosinolate rapeseed meal. For finishing pigs it can be used as the sole protein supplement. Preliminary data with gilts and sows during gestation and lactation indicate no reduction in reproductive performance from using low glucosinolate rapeseed meal as the sole protein supplement.

REFERENCES

Aherne, F.X. and McAleese, D.M. (1964). Evaluation of tick beans (Vicia faba L.) as a protein supplement in pig feeding. Proc. R. Dubl. Soc. B., 1, 113-121.

Aherne, F.X., Lewis, A.J. and Hardin, R.T. (1977). An evaluation of faba beans (Vicia faba) as a protein supplement for swine. Can. J. Anim. Sci., 57, 321-328.

Allee, G.L. and Trotter, R.M. (1974). Sulfur amino acid requirement of the finishing pig. J. Anim. Sci. 36, 974 (Abstr).

Allen, R.D. (1976). Feedstuffs ingredient analysis table. Feedstuffs Yearbook Issue, 47, No. 38, 33-38.

Balboa, J., Zorita, E. and Rodriquez Guedas, J. (1966). Beanmeal (Vicia faba L.) as a protein supplement for growing pigs. Rev. Nutricion Animal, Madrid, 4, 41-46.

Bell, J.M. (1975). Nutritional value of low glucosinolate rape-
    seed meal for swine. Can. J. Anim. Sci., 55, 61-70.
Blair, R.B. (1977). Faba beans: An improved crop for animal
    feeding. Feedstuffs, July 18, Vol. 49, No. 29, p. 15.
Bowland, J.P. (1971) Rapeseed as an energy and protein source in
    diets for growing pigs. Can. J. Anim. Sci., 51, 503-510.
Bowland, J.P. (1974). Comparison of low glucosinolate rapeseed
    meal, commercial rapeseed meal and soybean meal as protein
    supplements for growing pigs. Can. J. Anim. Sci., 54, 679-685.
Bowland, J.P. (1975). Evaluation of low glucosinolate-low erucic
    acid rapeseed meals as protein supplements for young growing
    pigs, including effects on blood serum constituents. Can.
    J. Anim. Sci., 55, 409-419.
Bowland, J.P. (1976). The use of rapeseed meal in pig and poultry
    rations. In, 'Feed Energy Sources for Livestock'. H. Swan
    and D. Lewis (Editors). Butterworths, London.
Bowland, J.P., Aherne, F.X. and Egbuiwe, A.M. (1975). Faba beans
    and low glucosinolate rapeseed meal as supplemental protein
    sources for growing-finishing pigs. The 54th Annual Feeders'
    Day Report, Univ. Alberta, Edmonton, Alta. p. 9-12.
Bowland, J.P. and Bell, J.M. (1972). Rapeseed meal for pigs. In,
    'Canadian Rapeseed Meal in Poultry and Animal Feeding'.
    Rapeseed Association of Canada, Winnipeg, Manitoba.
Brown, H.W., Harmon, B.G. and Jensen, A.H. (1974). Total sulfur-
    containing amino acids, isoleucine and tryptophan requirements
    of the finishing pig for maximum nitrogen retention. J. Anim.
    Sci., 38, 59-63.
Castell, A.G. (1976). Comparison of faba beans (Vicia faba) with
    soybean meal or field peas (Pisum sativum) as protein supple-
    ments in barley diets for growing-finishing pigs. Can. J.
    Anim. Sci., 56, 425-432.
Castell, A.G. (1977a). Effects of cultivar on the utilization of
    ground rapeseed in diets for growing-finishing pigs. Can. J.
    Anim. Sci., 57, 111-120.
Castell, A.G. (1977b). Effects of virginiamycin on the performance
    of pigs fed barley diets supplemented with soybean meal or
    low-glucosinolate rapeseed meal. Can. J. Anim. Sci., 57,
    313-320.
Cho, C.Y. and Bayley, H.S. (1972). Amino acid composition of
    digesta taken from swine receiving diets containing soybean
    or rapeseed meals as sole source of protein. Can. J. Physiol.
    Pharmacol., 50, 513-522.
Clarke, H.E. (1969). The evaluation of the field bean (Vicia faba
    L.) in animal nutrition. Nutr. Soc. Proc., 28, 64-73.
Cole, D.J.A., Blades, R.J., Taylor, R. and Luscombe, J.R. (1971).
    Field beans (Vicia faba L.) in the diets of bacon pigs.
    Exp. Husb., 20, 6-11.
Edwards, D.G. and Duthie, I.R. (1973). Processing to improve the
    nutritive value of field beans. J. Sci. Food Agric., 24,
    496-498.

Etienne, M. (1977). Possibilities d'introduction de la feverole dans le regime des truies en gestation. Journees Rech. Porcine en France, 199-203, In Ra-ITP Ed., Paris.

Feist, E. von., Hofmann, P., Kirchgessner, M. and Schwarz, F.J. (1974). Ackerbohnen als Fischmehlersatz in Schweinemastfutter. Zuechtungskunde, 46, 50-54.

Feist, E. von., Schwarz, F.J., Hofmann, P. and Kirchgessner, M. (1974). DL-Methionin-zulagen zu einen Ackerbohnen. Getreideration in der Schweinemast. Das Wirtschaftseigene Futter. p. 229-235.

Fowler, V.R. and Livingstone, R.M. (1972). Evaluation of field beans (Vicia faba) in pig diets by slope-ratio assay. Proc. Br. Soc. Anim. Prod. (Abstr). p. 138.

Grandhi, R., Slinger, S.J., Brown, R.G. and Hacker, R.R. (1976). Thyroid hormone synthesis in rapeseed meal fed pigs. J. Anim. Sci., 43, 252 (Abstr).

Grandhi, R., Bowman, G.H. and Slinger, S.J. (1977). Effect of feeding Tower rapeseed meal on carcass quality of heavy weight hogs. In, Proceedings of the Nutrition Conference for Feed Manufacturers. University of Guelph, Guelph, Ontario.

Hansen, V. and Clausen, H. (1969). Hestebønner (Vicia faba) som foder til slagterisvin. 374. beretning fra forsøgslaboratoriet Udgivet af Statens Husdyrbrugsudvalg, Kobenhavn.

Ivan, M. and Bowland, J.P. (1976). Digestion of nutrients in the small intestine of pigs fed diets containing raw and autoclaved faba beans. Can. J. Anim. Sci., 56, 451-456.

Kadirvel, R. and Clandinin, D.R. (1974). The effect of faba beans (Vicia faba L.) on the performance of turkey poults and broiler chicks from 0-4 weeks of age. Poultry Science, 53, 1810-1816.

Lewis, A.J. and Aherne, F.X. (1977). Performance of growing gilts fed Tower rapeseed meal. The 56th Annual Feeders' Day Report, Univ. Alberta, Edmonton, Alta. p. 10-11.

Livingstone, R.M., Fowler, V.R. and Woodham, A.A. (1970). The nutritive value of field beans (Vicia faba) for pigs. Proc. Nutr. Soc., 29, 46A-47A.

Loew, F.M., Doige, C.E., Manns, J.G., Searcy, G.P., Bell, J.M. and Jones, J.D. (1976). Evaluation of dietary rapeseed protein concentrate flours in rats and dogs. Toxicol. Appl. Pharmacol., 35, 257-267.

Marquardt, R.R. and Campbell, L.D. (1973). Raw and autoclaved faba beans in chick diets. Can. J. Anim. Sci., 53, 741-746.

Marquardt, R.R. and Campbell, L.D. (1974). Deficiency of methionine in raw and autoclaved faba beans in chick diets. Can. J. Anim. Sci., 54, 437-442.

Marquardt, R.R., Campbell, L.D., Stothers, S.C. and McKirdy, J.A. (1974). Growth responses of chicks and rats fed diets containing four cultivars of raw or autoclaved faba beans. Can. J. Anim. Sci., 54, 177-182.

Marquardt, R.R., Campbell, L.D. and Ward, T. (1976). Studies with chicks on the growth depressing factor(s) in faba beans (Vicia faba L. var. minor). J. Nutr., 106, 275-284.

Marquardt, R.R., Ward, T., Campbell, L.D. and Cansfield, P. (1976). Purification of the growth inhibitor in faba beans (Vicia faba). Proc. West. Sec. Amer. Soc. Anim. Sci., 27, 138-141.

McCuaig, L.W. and Bell, J.M. (1976). Rapeseed meal x sex interaction on swine carcasses. Proc. West. Sec. Amer. Soc. Anim. Sci., 27, 112-114.

McKinnon, P.J. and Bowland, J.P. (1976). Evaluation of Tower rapeseed meal for young pigs. The 55th Annual Feeders' Day Report, Univ. Alberta, Edmonton, Alta. p. 21-73.

McNab, J.M. and Wilson, B.J. (1974). Effects of micronising on the utilization of field beans (Vicia faba L.) by the young chick. J. Sci. Food Agric., 25, 395-400.

Meade, R.J., Hanke, N.E. and Rust, J.W. (1974). Protein levels and supplemental lysine for finishing swine. I. Feedlot performance. J. Anim. Sci., 39, 979 (Abstr).

Moody, D.L., Slinger, S.J. and Summers, J.D. (1976). Value of Tower rapeseed products for pigs and turkeys. Nutr. Conf. for Feed Manufacturers, Univ. Guelph, Guelph, Ontario.

National Academy of Sciences - National Research Council (1959). Nutrient requirements of domestic animals. No. 2, Nutrient requirements of swine, (4th Rev. Ed.), Washington, D.C.

National Academy of Sciences - National Research Council (1973). Nutrient requirements of domestic animals. No. 2, Nutrient requirements of swine, (7th Rev. Ed.), Washington, D.C.

Nielsen, H.E. and Kruse, P.E. (1974). Effect of dietary horse beans (Vicia faba) on colostrum and milk composition and milk yield in sows. Livest. Prod. Sci., 1, 179-185.

Olaboro, G., Campbell, L.D. and Marquardt, R.R. (1977). The nutritive value of faba beans for laying hens. Proc. Can. Soc. Anim. Sci., 27th Annual Conf., Aug. 14-18, p. 59.

Omole, T.A. and Bowland, J.P. (1974). Copper, iron and manganese supplementation of pig diets containing either soybean meal or low glucosinolate rapeseed meal. Can. J. Anim. Sci., 54, 481-493.

Onaghise, G.T.U. and Bowland, J.P. (1977). Influence of dietary faba beans and cassava on performance, energy and nitrogen digestibility and thyroid activity of growing pigs. Can. J. Anim. Sci., 57, 159-167.

Pastuszewska, B., Duee, P.H., Henry, Y., Bourdon, D. et Jung, J. (1974). Utilisation de la feverole entiere et decortiquee par le porc en croissance: Digestibilite et disponibilite des acides amines. Ann. Zootech., 23, 537-554.

Pearson, G. and Bowland, J.P. (1977). Comparative nutritive values of Tower rapeseed meal, meat meal, and soybean meal for growing pigs. The 56th Annual Feeders' Day Report, Univ. Alberta, Edmonton, Alta. p. 12-15.

Poppe, S., Schlage, M., Schneider, M. and Weisemuller, W. (1975).
    Field beans, a protein feed for growing pigs. Tierzucht.
    28, 359-361.
Presber, A.A.W. (1972). European experience with the small faba
    bean (Horse bean). Canada Grains Council., Winnipeg, Manitoba.
Sarwar, G. and Bowland, J.P. (1976). Protein quality evaluation of
    low glucosinolate-low erucic acid rapeseed meal and unpro-
    cessed faba beans in young pigs. J. Nutr., 106, 350-360.
Slinger, S.J. (1977). Improving the nutritional properties of
    rapeseed. J. Am. Oil Chemists' Soc., 54, 94A-99A.
Stringam, G.R., McGregor, D.I. and Pawlowski, S.H. (1974). Chemical
    and morphological characteristics associated with seedcoat
    color in rapeseed. In, 'Proceedings of the 4th International
    Rapeseed Congress' Giessen, West Germany.
Walz, O.P. (1974). Untersuchungen zum Einsatz von Ackerbohnen
    (Vicia faba) in der Schweinemast. Z. Tierophysiol. Tierer-
    naehr. Futtermittelkd, 33, 183-184.
Whittemore, C.T. and Taylor, A.G. (1973). Digestibility and
    nitrogen retention in pigs fed diets containing dried and
    undried field beans treated with propionic acid. J. Sci. Fd
    Agric., 24, 1133-1136.
Wilson, B.J. and McNab, J.M. (1972). The effect of autoclaving
    and methionine supplementation on the growth of chicks
    given diets containing field beans (Vicia baba L.). Br. Poult.
    Sci., 13, 67-73.
Wilson, B.J., McNab, J.M. and Bentley, H. (1972a). Trypsin
    inhibitor activity in the field bean (Vicia faba L.). J. Sci.
    Food Agric., 23, 679-684.
Wilson, B.J., McNab, J.M. and Bentley, H. (1972b). The effect on
    chick growth of a trypsin inhibitor isolate from the field
    bean (Vicia faba L.). Br. Poult. Sci., 13, 521-523.

25

PRODUCTION OF ANIMAL PROTEIN FROM NONPROTEIN NITROGEN CHEMICALS

William Chalupa

School of Veterinary Medicine, University of

Pennsylvania, Kennett Square PA 19348

Ruminants obtain amino acids (AA) from microbial protein synthesized in the rumen and from feed proteins that escape ruminal degradation. Synthesis of microbial protein provides a mechanism for
obtaining AA from NPN. Effectiveness of NPN utilization depends upon
production and utilization of ammonia by rumen microbes. Because
ammonia is produced from protein and NPN, feeding proteins resistant
to microbial degradation forces utilization of ammonia derived from
NPN. The quantity of microbial cells formed in the anaerobic rumen
fermentation system is primarily dependent upon energy supply but can
be modulated by types and supplies of other nutrients (i.e. amino-N,
minerals, growth factors) and by growth rate of rumen bacteria.
Potential quantities of NPN that can be utilized with different feed
ingredients can be estimated from amounts of feed protein degraded in
the rumen, and requiring transformation into protein via growth of
rumen microbes, and from amounts of energy provided by feed ingredients. High energy feed ingredients with low amounts of degradable
protein are most favorable for NPN utilization, but NPN has also been
used successfully with high-fibrous, low energy feed materials.
Growth, lactation and reproduction have been obtained on diets containing more than 97% of the nitrogen from NPN, but microbial protein
alone cannot provide quantities of AA needed for high levels of productivity. Regulating ruminal degradation of dietary protein and
utilizing NPN for rumen protein production is a highly desirable
strategy for producing human foods with ruminants.

INTRODUCTION

The metabolic machinery of ruminants, like that of other animals
must be supplied with the proper types and amounts of amino acids.

The mixture of amino acids available for absorption from the small intestine is supplied by microbial protein synthesized in the rumen, undegraded food proteins which bypass the rumen, and endogenous secretions. Probably little can be done to influence directly the amino acids provided by endogenous secretions. However, amino acids supplied by microbial protein and materials which bypass the rumen can be controlled. The desirable end result would logically be to optimize rumen protein production from NPN chemicals, minimize ruminal degradation of dietary amino nitrogen and supplement with rumen nondegradable amino acids if needed. This system takes advantage of the mechanism for NPN utilization provided by rumen microbes, minimizes losses incurred in the transformation of dietary protein to absorbable protein in the form of rumen microbes, and recognizes that at a given level of energy consumption, the amount of protein synthesized in the rumen is not always sufficient to meet requirements for maintenance plus production (Chalupa, 1973; 1975ab).

SYNTHESIS OF RUMEN MICROBIAL PROTEIN

The quantity of microbial cells formed in the rumen is a nutritional function of supplies of nitrogen, energy and other growth factors, and is modulated by growth rates of rumen bacteria.

Considerable attention has been focused on the quantitative relationship between rumen fermentation and microbial growth and it is recognized that cell yields in the anaerobic fermentation are lower than in aerobic systems (Hungate, 1966). A panel of experts (Anonymous, 1972) concluded that 90 to 230 g microbial protein per kg organic matter digested in the rumen could be produced and this wide range of cell yields is supported by summaries published in reviews by Henderickx (1976), McMemiman, Ben-Ghedalia and Armstrong (1976) and Preston (1976). Growth rate is an important determinant of yields and efficiency of microbial protein production because at high growth rates, more of the energy derived from fermentation is used for cell growth rather than for maintenance of the microbial population (Isaacson, Hinds, Bryant and Owens, 1975).

When energy is not limiting, rumen protein production may be regulated by the amounts and forms of nitrogenous nutrients. Protozoa can incorporate free exogenous amino acids, but it appears that nitrogen is usually incorporated into bacterial cells first and appears in protozoa cells following ingestion of bacteria by protozoa (Allison, 1969, 1970). Ammonia is the central intermediate in the degradation and assimilation of nitrogen in the rumen and is the preferred or required nitrogenous nutrient of many species of rumen bacteria (Bryant, 1970). Amination and transamination reactions appear to be the major mechanisms for assimilation of ammonia by rumen bacteria (Allison, 1969, 1970, Annison, 1975). Enzymes systems potentially important and Km's for ammonia of these enzymes in non-rumen microorganisms are presented in Table 1. Living cells, however, are able to concentrate ammonia (Buttery, 1976) and thus minimal ammonia concentrations required to maximize growth of rumen bacteria may deviate considerably from the listed Kms.

NPN chemicals are utilized by producing ammonia concentrations in the rumen which will satisfy bacterial requirements. When ammonia requirements are met, growth of ammonia- utilizing bacteria is not increased by additional supplies and ammonia accumulates. Thus a method of assessing the quantity of NPN which might be utilized with a particular diet would be to monitor rumen ammonia concentrations in relation to NPN additions (Satter and Roffler, 1975). Minimum ammonia concentrations needed to meet bacterial requirements and maximize rumen protein production are probably low but have not been completely defined (Mercer and Annison, 1976). In vitro growth of Bacteriodes amylophilus and the mixed rumen microbial population was limited at ammonia concentrations below 6-8 mg/dl (Henderson, Hobson and Summers, 1969; Allison, 1970; Satter and Slyter, 1974). Linear accumulations of rumen ammonia when concentrations exceeded 5 mg/dl indicated that the fractional amount of ammonia incorporated by microbes was not influenced by concentration (Roffler, Schwab and Satter, 1976). Hume, Moir and Somers (1970) showed that in sheep fed purified diets there was no increase in rumen tungstic acid precipi- table nitrogen above an ammonia level of 8.8 mg/dl. Miller (1973), however, found that the rumen ammonia concentration which maximized the flow of tungstic acid precipitable protein through the omasum was 13 mg/dl or higher.

Studies with ^{15}N (Al-Rabbat, Baldwin and Weir, 1971a,b; Mathison and Milligan, 1971; Nolan, 1975; Pilgram, Gray, Weller and Belling, 1970) demonstrated that not all the nitrogen used for microbial growth cycled through the rumen ammonia pool. Some species of rumen bacteria use peptides directly and some amino acids, notably methionine and cysteine are stimulatory to certain strains of rumen bacteria (Allison, 1970; Bryant, 1970, Buttery, 1976). Cell yields in vitro of washed suspensions of rumen bacteria were increased by replacement of a portion of the urea in the culture mixture with amino acids (Maeng, Van Nevel, Baldwin and Morris, 1976).

Because nutrients other than energy and nitrogen are needed for cell growth, (Bryant, 1970, Buttery, 1976) branched-chain volatile fatty acids, mineral elements or other growth factors may need to be supplied in the diet of ruminants given NPN to obtain maximum protein production in the rumen.

QUALITY OF MICROBIAL PROTEIN SYNTHESIZED IN THE RUMEN

Isolated preparations of rumen bacteria and protozoa have been reported to contain 35-80% and 17-55% crude protein respectively (Table 2). The wide range in crude protein contents is probably

TABLE 1

Ammonia fixing enzyme systems
(Buttery, 1976)

Enzyme	Source	Km	pH of determination
Alanine dehydrogenase	S. subtilis	3.8×10^{-2} M	8.0
Glutamate dehydrogenase (NADH)	Yeast	5.0×10^{-4} M	7.6
Aspartase	B. cadavaris	3.0×10^{-2} M	6.8
Asparagine synthetase	S. bovis	4.0×10^{-3} M	7.2
Glutamine synthetase	E. coli	1.8×10^{-3} M	7.0
Carbamoyl phosphate synthetase	E. coli	1.2×10^{-2} M	8.0

TABLE 2

Crude protein contents and nutritive value
of rumen bacteria and protozoa
(Chalupa, 1972)

	Crude Protein %		True Digest. %		Biolog. Value %		Net Protein Utiliz. %	
	B[b]	P[b]	B	P	B	P	B	P
Wheat hay chaff (0.89%N)	58	24						
Lucerne hay chaff (2.91%N)	69	41						
Wheat straw, oats, urea (0.92%N)	65	17						
Mixed green pasture	76	49						
Forage and concentrate	42	27	74	91	81	80	60	73
Alfalfa meal, ground corn, urea	35	50	75	87	85	82	63	71
Green feed			62		80		50	
Dry feed			65		78		50	
	45	55	55	86	66	68	36	58
Average	55	38	66	88	78	77	52	67

[a]Major dietary ingredients of animal from which bacteria and protozoa were obtained. [b]B = bacteria; P = protozoa.

mainly due to varying degrees of contamination of microbial preparations with digesta.

The nutritive value of rumen microbial protein has been determined by feeding isolated preparations of bacteria and protozoa
to rats. Generally, rumen protozoa are only slightly higher in
biological value than bacteria, but because of higher true
digestibilities, net utilization of protozoal protein is greater
(Table 2). However, digestibility of rumen microbial protein may
warrant further investigation because methods such as drying and
lypholization which were employed have been shown to increase
digestibility of non-rumen bacteria (Chalupa, 1975b). Recent
experiments suggest that the digestibility of rumen microbes in the
small intestine of sheep may vary from 30 to 70% (Smith, 1975).

Experiments reveiwed by Purser (1970) and Chalupa (1972) indicated that rumen micro-organisms contain substantial amounts of
nucleic acid N and the pattern of amino acids exhibits a remarkable
consistency which does not appear to be influenced by diets. There
are reports (reviewed by Chalupa, 1973) which indicate that the
nutritive value of rumen microbial protein may vary, but manipulation
of the quality of rumen microbial protein does not appear to be a
major point of control in the production of edible protein in
ruminant animals.

QUANTITY OF MICROBIAL PROTEIN SYNTHESIZED IN THE RUMEN

Both rumen microbes and ruminant tissues require energy for
protein synthesis, but the anaerobic rumen system has a lower
potential energy supply than the aerobic tissue system. Thus, at a
given level of energy consumption, ruminant tissues can potentially
utilize more absorbable amino acids than can be provided by
microbial protein (Chalupa, 1975a). Amino acid requirements of
ruminants are not constant, but vary in relation to changing
productive or physiological state (Figure 1). The dashed line
represents incorporation of microbial protein into tissue protein.
Provided energy is not limiting, rumen microorganisms appear to
provide sufficient protein for maintenance, slow growth and early
pregnancy, but not for fast growth, late pregnancy or early
lactation.

Protein requirements of ruminants cannot simply be stated as
crude or digestible protein (nitrogen X 6.25) in a given diet. It is
necessary to consider that the utilizable amino acids available to
the animal for maintenance plus production are functions of the
amount of rumen microbial protein produced from ammonia and amino
acids and the amount of dietary protein which is resistant to degradation and by-passes the rumen. Thus, except where low levels of
production are normal or can be tolerated, protein that escapes rumen
degradation is needed.

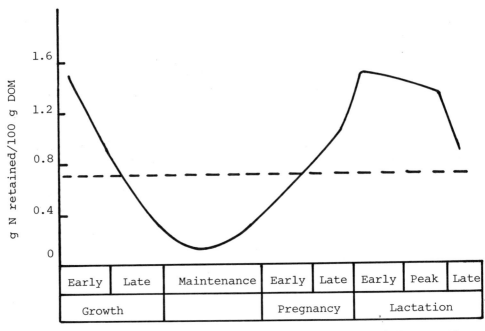

Figure 1.   Effect of physiological state on potential retention
            of nitrogen in relation to digestible organic matter
            intake (Orskov, 1970)

DIETARY PROTEINS RESISTANT TO RUMINAL DEGRADATION

     Potent rumen microbial proteases and deaminases degrade proteins
and amino acids which are soluble in the rumen liquid phase
(Chalupa, 1975b). Rumen bacterial proteases are cell bound, but are
located on the cell surface to provide free access to substrate and
are comprised of both exo- and endopeptidases. Proteolytic enzymes
enable rumen protozoa to digest bacterial protein which is a major
source of amino acids for growth of these microbes (Allison, 1970).
In vitro studies with mixed and pure cultures of rumen bacteria
demonstrated that total ruminal degradation of amino acids is the
result of intensive bacterial interaction and may vary greatly
depending upon the predominant types of microorganisms present
(Chalupa, 1976B; Scheifinger, Russell and Chalupa, 1976).

     Protein vary in solubility but the amount of protein which
escapes degradation and bypasses the rumen also depends upon rate
of passage because degradable fractions disappear from the rumen
by degradation or passage whereas undegradable fractions disappear
only by passage (Waldo, Smith and Cox, 1972). Thus, the

proportion of feed protein bypassing the rumen can be described by the ratio $k_r/(k_r + k_p)$ where k_r and k_p are rate constants for turnover of ruminal contents and ruminal proteolysis, respectively (Broderick, 1977).

Minimizing ruminal degradation of protein can improve the nitrogen economy of ruminants by (a) forcing rumen microbes to use ammonia derived from NPN rather than from dietary protein and (b) eliminating the unavoidable losses incurred when dietary protein is degraded to ammonia which then must be transformed into microbial protein to be of nutritional value. The efficiency of converting dietary crude protein into absorbable microbial protein has been estimated to be only about 50% (Black, 1971, Chalupa, 1975a). These estimates considered that not all the ammonia produced from ruminal degradation of dietary protein is assimilated by rumen microbes, rumen microbial cells contain 10 to 20% non-nutritious nucleic acid nitrogen and microbial protein is lower in digestibility than many plant proteins which bypass the rumen (Figure 2). On the other hand the only digestion losses incurred with dietary crude protein which resists ruminal degradation of bypasses the rumen is that fraction which is not digested and absorbed in the abomasum and small intestine (Figure 2).

Information in Table 3 illustrates that there can be wide differences between feed ingredients in the extent of ruminal degradation of the protein fraction. Additionally, degradation of protein in specific ingredients can vary greatly from the average values presented (Chalupa, 1975b). Methods to increase ruminal

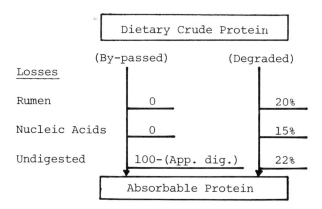

Figure 2. Losses incurred in obtaining absorbable protein from dietary crude protein which bypasses the rumen versus dietary crude protein which is degraded in the rumen and reformed into rumen microbial protein.

TABLE 3

Rumen degradation of protein in selected feed ingredients
(Chalupa, 1975b)

Ingredient	Ruminal Degradation (%)
Urea	100
Casein	90
Barley	80
Cottonseed meal	70
Peanut meal	65
Soybean meal	60
Alfalfa hay	60
Milo	40
Corn	40
Fish meal	30

bypass of protein and amino acids include (a) normal procedures used
in the manufacture of feed ingredients, especially those in which
heat is generated or applied, (b) chemical treatment of proteins,
(c) encapsulation of amino acids, (d) amino acid analogs, (e)
esophageal groove closure and (g) manipulation of rumen metabolism
(Broderick, 1975; Chalupa, 1975b; Ferguson, 1975). All methods offer
potential but probably require additional research before practical
use is widespread. It is important that procedures employed protect
against ruminal degradation but do not interfere with ruminal
metabolism or post ruminal digestion and absorption.

Although it is recognized that the quantity of protein which
escapes degradation and bypasses the rumen is a key factor determining the animal's nitrogen economy (Chalupa, 1975a,b; Clark, 1975b
Kempton, Nolan and Leng, 1977) obtaining definitive information is
complicated because of difficulties in distinguishing between
microbial and dietary proteins in ruminal, abomasal or intestinal
digesta. Because of the time and labor involved in in vivo
estimates of protein degradation, more convenient and rapid methods
are needed.

Solubility is an inherent characteristic which is largely
determined by the protein classes present in the feedstuff.
Albumins and globulins are the most soluble and prolamins and
glutelins are the more insoluble fractions of feedstuffs (Clark,
1975b). A primary factor regulating susceptibility to degradation
is solubility in the rumen liquid phase (Chalupa, 1975b).

The quantity of ammonia produced by rumen microbes is highly correlated with solubility in mineral buffer solutions (Satter, Whitlow and Beardsley, 1977; Chalupa, unpublished observations) but, review of the early literature (Satter, Whitlow and Beardsley, 1977) reveals no basis for directly equating soluble protein with rumen degradable protein and insoluble protein with undegradable protein. Buffer mineral solutions primarily extract nonprotein nitrogen (Chalupa, unpublished observations; Pichard and VanSoest, 1977) and regression of ammonia accumulation in energy deficient in vitro batch cultures of the mixed rumen microbial population versus protein solubility indicated that rumen microbes were degrading protein which was insoluble in a buffer mineral solution which simulated ruminant saliva (Chalupa, unpublished observations). Subjecting proteins to the action of a purified bacterial protease (Pichard and VanSoest, 1977) or to rumen microorganisms (Broderick, 1978) appears to provide better differentiation between quantities which will be degraded or resist ruminal degradation.

In spite of the deficiencies of in vitro protein solubility measurements, inverse relationships between protein solubility versus nitrogen retention (Sniffen, 1972; Wohlt, Sniffen, Hoover, Johnson and Walker, 1976; Evans and Nomani, 1972; Evans and Biddle, 1973) and versus the supply of essential amino acids to the mammary gland (Dingley, Sniffen, Johnson, Hoover and Walker, 1975) indicates that rations formulated to contain more insoluble protein provided increased quantities of absorbable amino acids. Evans and Nomani (1972) found that 26% more soluble than insoluble nitrogen was required to result in equal nitrogen retention in growing steers. Increased milk production resulted from feeding concentrate mixes formulated to contain regulated levels of soluble protein (Braund and Dolge, 1976). The foregoing responses are probably the result of providing a more optimum ratio of ammonia to energy in the rumen, but this may be a consequence of selecting feed ingredients which contain less NPN, rather than proteins which are resistant to ruminal degradation.

IMPORTANCE OF RUMEN TURNOVER RATE

The rumen approximates a continuous fermentation system (Hungate, 1966). Fresh feed and saliva mix with the fermenting mass, and fluids and particulate matter leave in quantities equivalent to those entering. Rumen liquids and solids have differential turnover rates (Hungate, 1966). The turnover rate of liquids in particular is a major factor influencing the function of the rumen ecosystem and outflow of nutrients (Chalupa, 1977; Leng, 1976; Leng and Preston, 1976; Owens and Isaacson, 1977; Sutherland, 1976). Substances which move with the liquid phase because they are soluble or microparticulate will bypass the rumen to greater extents at higher liquid turnover rates. Thus, as indicated earlier turnover rates will influence quantities of dietary protein which escape degradation and bypass the rumen. Increasing turnover rates encourages selection of rumen microbes with fast growth rates since slower growing microbes will be washed out of the system. Additionally maintenance energy requirement per unit of microbial mass becomes smaller as turnover rate is increased. Thus, changes in turnover rate can be expected to alter efficiency of microbial growth, microbial cell yields, and the types and quantities of fermentation products.

Selonomonads and bacteriodes predominated in the rumens of sheep with low liquid turnover rates, but increasing turnover rate by dietary inclusion of mineral salts resulted in microbial populations in which bacteriodes decreased and Gram-variable chain forming cocci became the predominant organism (Latham and Sharpe, 1975). Protozoa, because of their slow growth rates, should be especially vulnerable to changes in rumen turnover rates. For example, sheep fed molasses based diets have slow rumen turnover rates and large numbers of protozoa (Leng, 1976; Leng and Preston, 1976). Large numbers of rumen protozoa could decrease ruminal outflows of microbial protein since rumen microbial protein synthesis was 20 to 35% greater in defaunated animals (Sutherland, 1976).

The rate of rumen turnover is a function of the nature of the feed ingested, the level of feeding and the pattern of feeding (Sutherland, 1976). The rate of water removal from the rumen is faster in animals fed fresh versus dried forage (MacRae, 1976) and forage versus concentrate diets (Hodgson and Thomas, 1975; Bauman, Davis, Frobish and Sachan, 1971). The increased turnover rate observed with fresh forage is probably not due to water content since intraruminal infusion of water did not produce the effect (Harrison, Beever, Thomson and Osbourn, 1975). It may be an osmotic pressure phenomena since fresh forage contains large amounts of macro-elements, especially potassium, and there appears to be a relationship between the duodenal flow of non-ammonia nitrogen and the intake and duodenal flow of potassium in sheep given fresh forage (MacRae, 1976). When increasing levels of the same feed are ingested, rumen volume may show little change but outflow and therefore turnover rates are increased (Sutherland, 1976). Pattern of feeding may affect both rumen volume and outflow. A relatively high rumen liquid volume was observed in sheep fed cubed dried grass twice daily, but this was accompanied by low turnover rates (Sutherland, 1976). Supplying the same ration from a continuous feeding device gave much smaller rumen liquid volumes but increased turnover rates (Sutherland, 1976).

The turnover rate of the rumen liquid has been increased by
ruminal infusion of artificial saliva and sodium bicarbonate
(Harrison, Beever, Thomson and Osbourn, 1975), inclusion of the
mineral salts of artificial saliva into the diet (Thomson, Beever,
Murdell, Elderfield and Harrison, 1975), ingestion of saline (1.3%
w/v NaCl) drinking water (Potter, Walker and Forest, 1972) and
inclusion of high levels of salt (ca. 20%) into the diet (Hemsley,
1967). Ruminal infusion of water alone did not change rumen liquid
turnover rate (Harrison, Beever, Thomson and Osbourn, 1975).

NPN CHEMICALS AS COMPONENTS OF RUMINANT DIETS

Because of problems associated with feeding NPN, it is doubtful
whether NPN would be used as a component of ruminant diets unless
feed protein sources were limited in supply and/or the cost were in
favor of NPN. NPN chemicals cannot be used successfully and their
use should not be recommended in situations of questionable
management practices and capabilities. However, if problems of
feeding diets containing NPN are understood and the known biochemical and physiological aspects of NPN utilization are employed
to identify effective use situations, NPN chemicals can be a
viable component of ruminant diets.

Problems associated with feeding NPN chemicals. Replacement of
dietary protein with NPN is not without problems, but fears of many
animal feeders are often the result of exaggerations based upon
few facts. There is no doubt that acute ammonia toxicity and death
can occur from accidental overconsumption of NPN chemicals (Chalupa,
1972). However, if use situations are effectively identified and
accepted feeding methods are employed, it is doubtful that acute
toxicity will be encountered. There is no experimental evidence to
indicate urea and nitrate are additive in their toxic effects upon
ruminants (Huber, 1976a) nor has reproductive performance been
adversely affected as a consequence of feeding recommended levels of
urea (Ryder, Hillman and Huber, 1972).

Feed mixtures containing NPN are consumed in lesser amounts than
those supplemented with protein. The situation is more acute with
dairy cattle and the correlation between impaired feed intake of
urea containing diets and reduced milk yields has been demonstrated
in many experiments (Kertz and Everett, 1975). Generally, not more
than 1 to 2% urea is recommended in concentrated mixtures fed to
dairy cattle. However, even at levels of 1% , urea in high moisture
concentrates (14 to 16% moisture) can cause intake problems (Kertz
and Everett, 1975). Intake depressions in beef cattle are also
recognized and the low acceptability of urea currently limits its
use to 25 to 30% of total diet protein. Fonnesback, Kearly and Harris
(1975) reviewed experiments in which the "unpalatability" of NPN
supplements prevented animals from consuming sufficient nitrogen to
meet their protein requirements. In the experiments of Conrad and

Hibbs (1975), meal length was shorter with urea vs. protein feeds, but daily consumption was equivalent because animals fed urea had more meals.

Reasons for aversion towards urea containing diets are not completely understood. Cattle and other ruminants reject bitter tasting materials. Goatcher and Church (1970a) reported that sheep consistently rejected solutions containing 2.5 and 5% urea and these same workers (1970b) concluded that cattle generally respond to dietary chemicals at lower concentrations than sheep or goats. Huber and Cook (1972) concluded that intake depressions were due to the undesireable taste of urea and not ruminal or post-ruminal effects, but Martz, Wilson, Campbell and Hilderbrand (1973) suggested that intake of urea-containing rations may be regulated by non-taste factors.

Ammonia arising from hydrolysis of urea in feed has been implicated as a cause of decreased consumption of urea containing rations by cattle, but ammonia odor did not cause rejection of a non-urea ration (Kertz, Brockett, Davidson and Betz, 1977). Blood annomia concentration is a function of the rate of entry from the rumen and the rate of utilization by the liver for urea synthesis. Chalupa, Clark, Opliger and Lavker (1970) found that urea-fed animals had decreased activities of certain enzyme systems (i.e. carbamyl phosphate synthetase, ornithine transcarbymylase and arginase) needed to convert ammonia to urea and that ruminants were able to detoxify additional ammonia absorbed from the digestive tract by mechanisms which involved increasing the concentrations of liver ornithine, the key intermediate in the hepatic synthesis of urea. It was further suggested that liver ammonia detoxication systems could easily be exceeded when NPN is fed. Ruminants fed NPN do not normally exhibit acute toxicity characterized by symptoms such as restlessness, frequent urination, awkward locomotion and eventually convulsions, bloating and death (Chalupa, 1972). However biochemical derangements produced by ammonia in liver and other tissues implicate a subclinical ammonia toxicity in the decreased productivities of ruminants fed NPN. Blood ammonia may influence feed intake at two sites, the liver and brain, before the usually recognized symptoms become overt.

There are several reports which describe attempts to suppress aversions to diets supplemented with NPN. Holter, Colcvos and Urban (1968) suggested that grain mixes which contain several ingredients versus only two or three enhance the acceptability of urea. Better acceptance of urea-containing rations has been reported when urea was mixed with dehydrated alfalfa meal (Conrad and Hibbs, 1968) and when urea was provided in an intimate mixture with gelatanized starch (Helmer, Bartley and Deyoe, 1970). Dissolution of urea in molasses masked the undesireable taste of a concentrate containing 3.5% urea, but simply mixing urea and molasses into the

concentrate did not alleviate aversions (Huber and Cook, 1972).
Palatability studies with urea-treated silages have not given
consistent results (Helmer and Bartley, 1971). Some workers have
observed decreased intakes, others have observed increased intakes,
and several report similar intakes. The unpalatability of urea-
containing rations at 2% or higher has not been overcome in numerous
experiments using various flavors, odors, coatings, extusions and
other physical or processing methods (Kertz and Everett, 1975).

Effective use situations. NPN chemicals have been important
components of ruminant diets for 25 years. Unfortunately, most of
the 800,000 tons of urea per year used in livestock feeds in the
U.S. are incorporated into diets at levels dictated by rule of
thumb constants without adequate consideration given to the known
biochemical and physiological aspects of NPN utilization.
Consequently, unknown but probably substantial quantities of urea
are used in diets which are not suitable to effective utilization
of NPN and there are probably dietary situations that could support
greater utilization of NPN than we currently expect.

    Nature of the diet, especially protein content, quantity of
protein degraded in the rumen and energy availability are the primary
determinants of how effectively ammonia from NPN supplements will
be transformed into microbial protein.

    Although precise information is not currently available, it is
possible to estimate the quantities of urea that potentially can be
utilized with different feed ingredients (Chalupa, 1975a). The
urea utilization values for feed ingredients contained in Table 4
were calculated using potential rumen energy availability and the
estimated quantity of protein degraded in the rumen and requiring
transformation into protein via growth of ruminal microbes. Corn
grain and milo are excellent feed ingredients to use in diets
containing NPN because they provide ruminal energy in excess of
that needed to utilize ammonia produced by proteolysis and
deamination. Barley is a high energy feed ingredient, but the
quantity of barley protein estimated to be degraded in the rumen
and requiring transformation into microbial protein creates an
energy deficit and a negative urea utilization factor. Liquid
molasses contains energy for reutilization of its rumen degraded
protein (22 g/kg) plus 12 g of urea (38.8 g crude protein per kg),
with 18 g/kg of crude protein resisting ruminal degradation. Thus,
molasses contains sufficient energy to yield a liquid supplement
containing 78.8 g of crude protein per kg (7.99% crude protein).
If NPN is added to produce higher crude protein molasses based
supplement, other feed ingredients must supply energy for
ammonia utilization or the additional NPN cannot be utilized
efficiently. Forages and roughages vary considerably in protein
and energy contents and can be fair to poor ingredients to use with
NPN. The excellent quality alfalfa (20% crude protein) listed in

TABLE 4

Potential urea utilization with selected feed ingredients
(Chalupa and Davis, 1976)

Ingredient	Crude protein (g/kg)				Digestible energy (Mcal/kg)			Urea utilization[6] (g/kg)
	Content	Rumen degraded[1]	Rumen loss[2]	Microbial[3]	Microbial requirement[4]	Rumen supply[5]	Supply-required	
Corn	100	40	8	32	1.45	2.51	1.06	10
Milo	120	48	10	38	1.72	2.40	0.68	7
Barley	130	94	19	75	3.40	2.67	-.73	-7
Molasses	45	27	5	22	1.00	2.25	1.25	12
Alfalfa	200	120	24	96	4.36	2.02	-2.34	-23
Cottonseed hulls	45	23	5	18	0.82	1.71	0.89	8
Cottonseed meal	450	315	63	252	11.45	2.65	-8.80	-86
Soybean meal	520	260	52	208	9.45	2.42	-7.03	-69
Peanut meal	500	315	63	252	11.45	2.90	-8.55	-84
Fish meal	540	135	27	108	4.90	2.45	-2.45	-24

[1]See review by Chalupa (1975b)
[2]Assumes 20% of rumen degraded protein is lost from the rumen
[3]Quantity of rumen degraded protein not lost from the rumen and requiring transformation into microbial protein.
[4]22 g of microbial crude protein produced per Mcal of digestible energy in the rumen.
[5]Assumes 75% of dietary digestible energy is available in the rumen.
[6]Assumes 20% of the urea nitrogen is lost from the rumen with the remaining 80% used for microbial protein as a function of energy availability at the rate described in footnote 4.

Table 4 is energy deficient for NPN utilization, whereas cottonseed hulls provide energy for the utilization of 8 g of urea per kg. Cottonseed hulls are often considered to be a low quality roughage but, this feed ingredient contains sufficient digestible energy (2.28 Mcal/kg) for ammonia utilization. Cottonseed hull protein has a negative digestion coefficient but the recent experiment of Oltjen Dinius and Georing (1975) demonstrated effective NPN utilization. Cattle fed cottonseed hulls alone lost .19 kg/day, but animals receiving urea or biuret supplements gained .49 and .54 kg/day, respectively. The inability of rumen protein production to meet the animal's requirements was indicated by the increased gains obtained when either fish meal or soybean replaced 20% of the supplemental NPN. As might be expected, protein supplements all have negative urea utilization values.

The importance of dietary energy and the quantity of protein degraded in the rumen upon the quantities of NPN that can be effectively utilized is further illustrated in Table 5. The well known fact that NPN utilization is energy dependent is demonstrated.

TABLE 5

Effect of rumen bypass of diet protein and diet energy on maximum effective crude protein supplies (theoretical considerations)[1] (Chalupa and Davis, 1976)

Crude protein supplied by diet ingredients (g/kg)	Bypass Protein (%)					
	40			60		
	Diet digestible energy (Mcal/kg)					
	2.25	2.75	3.25	2.25	2.75	3.25
	Maximum effective crude protein (g/kg)					
80	79[b,2]	87[c]	95[c]	91[c]	100[c]	108[c]
100	89[a]	100[b]	106[c]	105[c]	113[c]	122[c]
120	99[a]	108[a]	116[b]	118[b]	127[c]	135[c]
140	109[a]	118[a]	126[a]	132[a]	141[b]	149[c]
160	120[a]	129[a]	137[a]	146[a]	154[a]	162[b]
180	131[a]	139[a]	147[a]	159[a]	168[a]	176[b]

[1]Calculations assumed 20% of degraded protein is lost from rumen, 75% of dietary DE is available in the rumen and 22 g of microbial crude protein are synthesized per Mcal of DE in the rumen.

[2]Using the 80 g/kg crude protein-2.25 Mcal diet as an example, 79 was calculated as follows:

$$80 + .75(2.25) - \frac{(80 \times .60) - 9.60}{22} \times 22$$

[a]Insufficient energy to utilize rumen degraded protein.
[b]Sufficient energy to utilize only rumen degraded protein.
[c]Sufficient energy to utilize rumen degraded protein plus NPN.

<u>Examples of successful utilization</u>. The potential for animal-protein
production from NPN was demonstrated in experiments of Virtanen
(1966) and Oltjen (1969). Growth, reproduction and lactation were
obtained on protein-free diets containing more than ninety-seven
per cent of the N from NPN. Animal productivity was lower than
is considered desirable but lesser reductions result when a smaller
quantity of NPN is used. In some instances, lowered rates of animal
productivity which might result from feeding NPN may be offset by
the economics and availability of NPN compared with plant protein.

NPN is used mainly as a replacement for oilseed meals and is
most commonly added to concentrate mixtures, to complete feeds, to
molasses-based liquid supplements, or to corn silage either at
ensiling or at feeding (Chalupa, 1970b). Usually the basal rations
supplemented with NPN are not especially low in protein and may
already supply approximately seventy per cent of the animal's total
protein requirement. Positive benefits are obtained primarily
because rations are high in energy content and are fed ad lib.
Experiments reviewed by Huber (1975, 1976b) indicated that if feed
ingredients used as components of NPN-supplemented diets are
selected with care, NPN is effectively utilized by lactating cows
and high producers do as well as low producers.

Grains are available for livestock feeding only when their
production exceeds the quantity needed for human consumption. The
absence of indigenous grain production has hindered the development
of a viable livestock industry in many areas. The tropics, with
their high yielding carbohydrate rich crops, offer many possibilities
for ruminant livestock production (Preston, 1976). Sugar cane, in
the form of by-products from normal sugar production such as
molasses and bagasse, or processing the entire sugar cane plant
without extraction, provides a basis for intensive animal production
systems (Leng and Preston, 1976). NPN can be used to alleviate a
portion of the nitrogen deficiency of low protein - high carbohydrate
crops, but because of the thermodynamic limits of the anaerobic
rumen fermentation system, some dietary protein which escapes
ruminal degradation appears to be needed to maximize productivity
(Preston, 1972, 1976, Leng and Preston, 1976).

Use of NPN with high-fibrous, low-energy feed materials cannot
be ignored. Sixty-four percent of the world's agricultural land is
suitable only for forage production. In addition, crop and
industrial by-products are a large reservoir of plant carbon which
can be converted into animal carbon by ruminants. Compatibility of
NPN with such feed ingredients may necessitate treatment(s) to
increase availability of rumen energy or may involve the use of
NPN compounds which give patterns of ammonia-release different from
that of urea. Oltjen, Williams, Slyter and Richardson (1969)

demonstrated that respectable animal performance could be obtained in fattening beef cattle fed forage-based NPN diets. Timothy-hay diets supplemented with urea and biuret yielded daily gains of 0.81 and 0.74 kg when fed ad lib. Biuret was clearly the superior NPN source when diets were fed twice daily.

Low-protein forages often available to grazing ruminants are usually consumed in adequate amounts and deficiencies of both protein and energy are encountered. In these situations, reduction of weight losses and future productivity of the animals rather than positive weight gains may be the primary objective. Ammerman, Verde, Moore, Burns and Chicco (1972) and Fick, Ammerman, McGowan, Loggins and Conell (1973) reported that urea biuret or natural protein supplementation increased intakes of low-quality forages and improved N retention in sheep. NPN chemicals increase consumption of diets low in protein by alleviating rumen ammonia deficiencies. However, in order to provide sufficient quantities of utilizable amino acids, protein supplements which escape ruminal degradation are also needed. The improvement in production obtained with supplements of by-pass protein are, in many instances, largely mediated through stimulation of feed intake (Kempton, Nolan and Leng, 1977).

The use of NPN sources other than urea as components of ruminant diets has been reviewed (Chalupa, 1970a). Unfortunately, most alternative NPN sources have not been adequately researched in animal trials.

SUPPLEMENTARY AMINO ACIDS AND PROTEIN

Although considerable proportions of dietary protein are resistant to ruminal degradation, quantities which bypass the rumen do not appear to be sufficient to supplement rumen-protein production completely. Post ruminal supplements of high quality proteins, such as casein and mixtures of amino acids have consistantly increased nitrogen retention in growing steers (Chalupa, 1975a, 1976a) and milk production and milk protein yields in dairy cows (Clark, 1975ab). Attempts to elucidate primary limiting amino acids have not been conclusive. Perhaps experimental techniques employed could not detect small responses from supplements of single amino acids or growing and lactating cattle, unlike sheep used for wool growth, may not be suffering from specific amino acid deficiencies (Chalupa, 1976a). In growing cattle, nitrogen retention usually was increased with post ruminal supplements of methionine plus lysine plus threonine (Chalupa, 1975a, 1976a). Methionine alone did not always significantly increase nitrogen retention, but methionine had to be present in order to obtain responses from other amino acids. In lactating cows, methionine and lysine plus possibly threonine, isoleucine and phenylalanine are the most limiting amino acids for milk and milk protein

production (Schwab, Satter and Clay, 1976; Baisdell, Clark, Wohlt
and Spires, 1977).

Whether to provide for rumen bypass of single amino acids will
depend upon whether shortages of a few or many amino acids are
limiting production.

REFERENCES

Allison, M. J. (1969). Biosynthesis of amino acids by ruminal
    mircoorganisms. J. Anim. Sci., 29, 797-807.
Allison, M. J. (1970). Nitrogen metabolism in ruminal microorganisms.
    Pages 456-473, In, 'Physiology of Digestion in the Ruminant',
    A. T. Phillipson (Editor). Oriel Press Ltd., New Castle upon
    Tyne, England.
Al-Rabbat, M. F., Baldwin, R. L. and Weir, W. C. (1971a). In vitro
    [15]nitrogen-tracer technique for some kinetic measures of ruminal
    ammonia. J. Diary Sci., 54, 1150-1161.
Al-Rabbat, M. F., Baldwin, R. L. and Weir, W. C. (1971b). Microbial
    growth dependence on ammonia nitrogen in the bovine rumen.
    J. Dairy Sci., 54, 1162-1172.
Ammerman, C. B., Verde, G. J., Moore, J. E., Burns, W. C. and Chicco,
    C. F. (1972). Biuret, urea and natural proteins as nitrogen
    supplements for low quality roughage for sheep. J. Anim. Sci.,
    35, 121-127.
Annison, E. F. (1975). Microbial protein synthesis in relation to
    amino acid requirements. Pages 141-152, In, ' Tracer Studies
    on Non-protein nitrogen for Ruminants II' Int. Atomic Energy
    Agency, Vienna.
Anonymous. (1972). Conclusions and recommendations. Pages 171-176,
    In, 'Tracer Studies on Non-protein Nitrogen for Ruminants'.
    Int. Atomic Energy Agency, Vienna.
Bauman, D. E., Davis, C. L., Frobish, R. A. and Sachan, D. S. (1971).
    Evaluation of polyethylene glycol method in determining rumen
    fluid volume in dairy cows fed different diets. J. Dairy Sci.,
    54, 928-930.
Black, J. L. (1971). A theoretical consideration of the effect of
    preventing ruminal fermentation on the efficiency of utiliza-
    tion of dietary energy and protein in lambs. Brit. J. Nutr.,
    25, 31-55.
Blaisdell, F. S., Clark, J. H., Wohlt, J. E. and Spires, H. R.
    (1977). Effects of postruminal infusions of casein or amino
    acids on milk and milk protein production. Amer. Soc. Anim.
    Sci. Abstracts, 221.
Braund, D. G. and Dolge, K. L. (1976). Pro:right feeds. A new
    approach to dairy nutrition and production. Agway Cooperator,
    Sept., 1-2.
Broderick, G. A. (1975). Factors affecting responses to protected
    amino acids and proteins. Pages 211 to 259, In, 'Protein

Nutritional Quality of Foods and Feeds', Vol. 1, Part 2. Mendel
Friedman (Editor). Marcell Dekker Inc., NY

Broderick, G. A. (1978). In vitro procedures for estimating rates
of ruminal protein degradation and proportions of dietary protein escaping the rumen undegraded. J. Nutr., 108, 181-190.

Bryant, M. P. (1970). Microbiology of the rumen. Pages 484-515,
In, 'Duke's Physiology of Domestic Animals', 8th ed. E. J.
Swenson (Editor). Cornell Univ. Press, Ithaca.

Buttery, P. J. (1976). Protein synthesis in the rumen: Its implication in the feeding of nonprotein nitrogen to ruminants. Pages
145-168, In, 'Principles of Cattle Production', H. Swan and
W. H. Broster (Editors). Butterworths, Boston.

Chalupa, W. (1970a). NPN sources other than urea as components of
ruminant diets. Clemson Univ. Dairy Sci. Res. Series, 54, 1-22.

Chalupa, W. (1970b). Urea as a component of ruminant diets. Proc.
Cornell Nutr. Conf., 64-76.

Chalupa, W. (1972). Metabolic aspects of nonprotein nitrogen utilization in ruminant animals. Fed. Proc., 31, 1152-1164.

Chalupa, W. (1973). Utilization of non-protein nitrogen in the
production of animal protein. Proc. Nutr. Soc., 32, 99-105.

Chalupa, W. (1975a). Amino acid nutrition of growing cattle. Pages
175-194, In, 'Tracer Studies on Non-protein Nitrogen for
Ruminants II'. Int. Atomic Energy Agency, Vienna.

Chalupa, W. (1975b). Rumen bypass and protection of protein and
amino acids. J. Dairy Sci., 58, 1198-1218.

Chalupa, W. (1976a). Approaches to determining amino acid require-
ments in producing ruminants. Pages 99-109, In, 'Reviews in
Rural Science II', T. M. Sutherland, J. R. McWilliam and R. A.
Leng (Editors). Univ. New England Publ. Unit, Armidale, NSW,
Australia.

Chalupa, W. (1976b). Degradation of amino acids by the mixed rumen
microbial population. J. Anim. Sci., 43, 828-834.

Chalupa, W. (1977). Manipulating rumen fermentation. J. Anim. Sci.,
45, 585-599.

Chalupa, W., Clark, J., Opliger, P. and Lavker, R. (1970). Detoxication of ammonia in sheep fed soy protein or urea. J. Nutr.,
100, 170-176.

Chalupa, W. and Davis, R. F. (1976). An update on the use of urea
in ruminant feeding. Proc. Maryland Nutr. Conf., 6-14.

Clark, J. H. (1975a). Lactational responses to postruminal administration of proteins and amino acids. J. Dairy Sci., 58, 1178-
1197.

Clark, J. H. (1975b). Pages 261-304, In, 'Protein Nutritional Quality
of Foods and Feeds', Vol. 1, Part 2. Mendel Friedman (Editor).
Marcell Dekker, Inc., NY.

Conrad, H. R. and Hibbs, J. W. (1968). Nitrogen utilization by the
ruminant. Appreciation of its nutritive value. J. Dairy Sci.,
51, 276-285.

Conrad, H. R. and Hibbs, J. W. (1975). Association of nonprotein
nitrogen with decreased meal size and eating intervals.

J. Dairy Sci., 58, 746.

Dingley, P. Y., Sniffen, C. J., Johnson, L. L., Hoover, W. H. and
      Walker, C. K. (1975). Protein solubility and amino acid supply
      to the udder. J. Dairy Sci., 58, 1240.

Evans, J. L. and Biddle, G. N. (1973). Utilization in growing cattle
      of N in sources that differ in soluble N. J. Anim. Sci., 37,
      367.

Evans, J. L. and Nomani, M. Z. A. (1972). Influence of level and
      source of diet nitrogen on its utilization. J. Anim. Sci., 35,
      284.

Ferguson, K. A. (1975). The protection of dietary proteins and amino
      acids against microbial fermentation in the rumen. Pages 448-
      463, In, 'Digestion and Metabolism in the Ruminant', I. W.
      McDonald and A. C. I. Warner (Editors). Univ. New England Publ.
      Unit, Armidale, NSW, Australia.

Fick, K. R., Ammerman, C. B., McGowan, C. H., Loggins, P. E. and
      Conell, J. A. (1973). Influence of supplemental energy and
      biuret nitrogen on the utilization of low quality roughage by
      sheep. J. Anim. Sci., 36, 137-143.

Fonnesbeck, P. V., Kearly, L. C. and Harris, L. E. (1975). Feed
      grade biuret as a protein replacement for ruminants. J. Anim.
      Sci., 40, 1150-1184.

Goatcher, W. D. and Church, D. C. (1970a). Taste responses in
      ruminants. II. Reactions of sheep to acids, quinine, urea, and
      sodium hydroxide. J. Anim. Sci., 30, 784-790.

Goatcher, W. D. and Church, D. C. (1970b). Taste responses in
      ruminants. IV. Reactions of pygmy goats, normal goats, sheep
      and cattle to acetic acid and quinine hydrochloride. J. Anim.
      Sci., 31, 373-382.

Harrison, D. G., Beever, D. E., Thomson, D. J. and Osbourn, D. F.
      (1975). Manipulation of rumen fermentation in sheep by in-
      creasing the rate of flow of water from the rumen. J. Agric.
      Sci., 85, 93-101.

Helmer, L. G., Bartley, E. E. and Deyoe, C. W. (1970). Feed process-
      ing. VI. Comparison of starea, urea and soybean meal as protein
      sources for lactating dairy cows. J. Dairy Sci., 53, 883-887.

Helmer, L. G. and Bartley, E. E. (1971). Progress in the utilization
      of urea as a protein replacement for ruminants. A Review.
      J. Dairy Sci., 54, 25-51.

Hemsley, J. A. (1967). Sodium chloride intake and flow through the
      rumen. Aust. J. Exp. Biol. Med. Sci., 45, 39.

Henderickx, H. K. (1976). Quantitative aspects of the use of non-
      protein nitrogen in ruminant feeding. Cuban J. Agric. Sci.,
      10, 1-18.

Henderson, C., Hobson, P. N. and Summers, R. (1969). Proc. IV Int.
      Symp. on the Continuous Culture of Microorganisms. P. 189.
      Czechoslovak Academy of Sciences, Prague.

Hodgson, J. C. and Thomas, P. C. (1975). A relationship between the
      molar proportion of propionic acid and the clearance rate of

the liquid phase in the rumen of the sheep. Brit. J. Nutr., 33, 447-456.

Holtor, J. B., Colovas, N. F. and Urban, W. E. (1968). Urea for lactating dairy cattle. IV. Effect of urea vs. no urea in the concentrate on production performance in a high producing herd. J. Dairy Sci., 51, 1403-1408.

Huber, J. T. (1975). Protein and nonprotein nitrogen utilization in practical dairy rations. J. Anim. Sci., 41, 954-961.

Huber, J. T. (1976a). NPN fears unfounded. Anim. Nutr. and Health, June/July, 12-13.

Huber, J. T. (1976b). Use of nonprotein nitrogen by lactating cows. Feedstuffs, Dec. 6, 13-14.

Huber, J. T. and Cook, R. M. (1972). Influence of site of administration of urea on voluntary intake of concentrate by lactating cows. J. Dairy Sci., 55, 1470-1473.

Hume, I. D., Muir, R. J. and Somers, M. (1970). Synthesis of microbial protein in the rumen. I. Influence of level of nitrogen intake. Aust. J. Agric. Res., 32, 283-296.

Hungate, R. E. (1966). The Rumen and its Microbes. Academic Press, NY.

Isaacson, H. R., Hinds, F. C., Bryant, M. P. and Owens, F. N. (1975). Efficiency of energy utilization by mixed rumen bacteria in continuous culture. J. Dairy Sci., 58, 1645-1659.

Kertz, A. F., Brockett, M. K., Davidson, L. E. and Betz, N. L. (1977). Influence of ambient ammonia odor on acceptance of a nonurea ration by lactating cows. J. Dairy Sci., 60, 788-790.

Kertz, A. F. and Everett, J. P. (1975). Utilization of urea by lactating cows — An industry viewpoint. J. Anim. Sci., 41, 945-953.

Latham, J. J. and Sharpe, M. E. (1975). Rumen microbial population changes of lambs given mineral-supplemented diets. Proc. Nutr. Soc., 34, 113A.

Leng, R. A. (1976). Factors influencing net protein production by rumen microbiota. Pages 85-91, In, 'Reviews in Rural Science II', T. M. Sutherland, J. R. McWilliam and R. A. Leng (Editors). Univ. New England Publ. Unit, Armidale, NSW, Australia.

Leng, R. A. and Preston, T. R. (1976). Sugar cane for cattle production: Present constraints, perspectives and research priorities. Trop. Anim. Prod., 1, 1-22.

Kempton, T. J., Nolan, J. V. and Leng, R. A. (1977). Principles for the use of non-protein nitrogen and by-pass proteins in diets of ruminants. World Anim. Rev., 22, 2-10.

MacRae, J. C. (1976). Utilization of the protein of green forage by ruminants at pasture. Pages 93-97, In, 'Reviews in Rural Science II', T. M. Sutherland, J. R. McWilliam and R. A. Leng (Editors). Univ. New England Publ. Unit, Armidale, NSW, Australia.

Maeng, W. J., Van Nevel, C. J., Baldwin, R. L. and Morris, J. G. (1976). Rumen microbial growth rates and yields: Effect of amino acids and protein. J. Dairy Sci., 59, 68-79.

Martz, F. A., Wilson, G., Campbell, J. R. and Hilderbrand, E. S. (1973) Voluntary intake of urea diets for ruminants.

J. Dairy Sci., 37, 351.

Mathison, G. W. and Milligan, L. P. (1971). Nitrogen metabolism in
   sheep. Brit. J. Nutr., 25, 351-366.

McMeniman, N. P., Ben-Ghedalia, D. and Armstrong, D. G. (1976).
   Nitrogen-energy interactions in rumen fermentation. Pages 217-
   229, In, 'Protein Metabolism and Nutrition', D. J. A. Cole,
   K. N. Boorman, P. J. Buttery, D. Lewis, R. J. Neale and H. Swan
   (Editors). Butterworths, Boston.

Mercer, J. R. and Annison, E. F. (1976). Utilization of nitrogen in
   ruminants. Pages 397-416, In, 'Protein Metabolism and Nutrition'
   D. J. A. Cole, K. N. Boorman, P. J. Buttery, D. Lewis, R. J.
   Neale and H. Swan (Editors). Butterworths, Boston.

Miller, E. L. (1973). Evaluation of foods as sources of nitrogen and
   amino acids. Proc. Nutr. Soc., 32, 79-84.

Nolan, J. V. (1975). Quantitative models of nitrogen metabolism in
   sheep. Pages 416-431, In, 'Digestion and Metabolism in the
   Ruminant', I. W. McDonald and A. C. I. Warner (Editors). Univ.
   New England Publ. Unit, Armidale, NSW, Australia.

Oltjen, R. R. (1969). Effects of feeding ruminants nonprotein nitrogen as the only nitrogen source. J. Anim. Sci., 28, 673-682.

Oltjen, R. R., Dinius, D. A. and Goering, H. K. (1975). Cottonseed
   hulls plus NPN-protein supplements for wintering calves.
   J. Anim. Sci., 41, 412.

Oltjen, R. R., Williams, E. E., Slyter, L. L. and Richardson, G. V.
   (1969). Urea versus biuret in a roughage diet for steers.
   J. Anim. Sci., 29, 816-822.

Orskov, E. R. (1970). Proceedings of the 4th Nutrition Conference
   for Feed Manufacturers. Univ. Nottingham, Churchill, London.

Owens, F. N. and Isaacson, H. R. (1977). Rumen microbial yields:
   Factors influencing synthesis and bypass. Fed. Proc., 36, 198-
   202.

Pichard, G. R. and Van Soest, P. J. (1977). Solubility of forage
   nitrogen fractions. Amer. Soc. Anim. Sci. Abstracts, 125.

Pilgram, A. F., Gray, F. V., Weller, R. A. and Belling, C. B. (1970).
   Synthesis of microbial protein in the sheep's rumen and the
   proportion of dietary nitrogen converted into microbial nitrogen.
   Brit. J. Nutr., 24, 589-598.

Potter, B. J., Walker, D. J. and Forrest, W. W. (1972). Changes in
   intraruminal function of sheep when drinking saline drinking
   water. Brit. J. Nutr., 27, 75-83.

Preston, T. R. (1972). Quantitative aspects of animal protein produc-
   tion from NPN in ruminants. Pages 1-10, In, 'Tracer Studies on
   Non-protein Nitrogen for Ruminants'. Int. Atomic Energy Agency,
   Vienna.

Preston, T. R. (1976). Protein supplementation in intensive feeding
   situations for growth and lactation. Pages 129-133, In, 'Reviews
   in Rural Science II', T. M. Sutherland, J. R. McWilliam and R. A.
   Leng (Editors). Univ. New England Publ. Unit., Armidale, NSW,
   Australia.

Purser, D. B. (1970). Nitrogen metabolism in the rumen. Microorganisms as a source of protein for the ruminant animal. J. Anim. Sci., 30, 988-1001.

Roffler, R. E., Schwab, C. G. and Satter, L. D. (1976). Relationship between ruminal ammonia concentration and nonprotein nitrogen utilization by ruminants. III. Influence of intraruminal urea infusion on ruminal ammonia concentration. J. Dairy Sci., 59, 80-84.

Ryder, W. L., Hillman, D., and Huber, J. T. (1972). Effect of feeding urea on reproductive efficiency in Michigan dairy herd improvement association herds. J. Dairy Sci., 55, 1290-1294.

Satter, L. D. and Roffler, R. E. (1975). Nitrogen requirement and utilization in dairy cattle. J. Dairy Sci., 58, 1219-1237.

Satter, L. D. and Slyter, L. L. (1974). Effect of ammonia concentration on rumen microbial protein production in vitro. Brit. J. Nutr., 32, 199-208.

Satter, L. D., Whitlow, L. W. and Beardsley, G. L. (1977). Resistance of protein to rumen degradation and its significance to the dairy cow. Proc. Dist. Feed. Res. Council, 63-72.

Scheifinger, C., Russel, N. and Chalupa, W. (1976). Degradation of amino acids by pure cultures of rumen bacteria. J. Anim. Sci., 43, 821-827.

Schwab, C. G., Satter, L. D. and Clay, A. B. (1976). Response of lactating dairy cows to abomasal infusion of amino acids. J. Dairy Sci., 59, 1254-1270.

Smith, R. H. (1975). Nitrogen metabolism in the rumen and the composition and nutritive value of nitrogen compounds entering the duodenum. Pages 399-415, In, 'Digestion and Metabolism in the Ruminant', I. W. McDonald and A. C. I. Warner (Editors). Univ. New England Publ. Unit, Armidale, NSW, Australia.

Sniffen, C. J. (1974). Nitrogen utilization as related to solubility of NPN and protein in feeds. Proc. Cornell Nutr. Conf., 12-18.

Sutherland, T. M. (1976). The overall metabolism of nitrogen in the rumen. Pages 65-72, In, 'Reviews in Rural Science II', T. M. Sutherland, J. R. McWilliam and R. A. Leng (Editors). Univ. New England Publ. Unit, Armidale, NSW, Australia.

Thomson, D. J., Beever, D. E., Mundell, D. C., Elderfield, M. L. and Harrison, D. G. (1975). The effect of altering dilution rate on the pattern of fermentation in the rumen. Proc. Nutr. Soc., 34, 111A.

Virtanen, A. I. (1966). Milk production of cows on protein-free feed. Science, 153, 1603-1607.

Waldo, D. R., Smith, L. W. and Cox, E. L. (1972). Model of cellulose disappearance from the rumen. J. Dairy Sci., 55, 125-129.

Wohlt, J. E., Sniffen, C. J., Hoover, W. H., Johnson, L. L. and Walker, C. K. (1976). Nitrogen metabolism in wethers as affected by dietary protein solubility and amino acid profile. J. Anim. Sci., 42, 1280-1289.

26

ANALYSIS FOR AVAILABILITY OF AMINO ACID SUPPLEMENTS IN FOODS AND
FEEDS: BIOCHEMICAL AND NUTRITIONAL IMPLICATIONS

Henry T. Ostrowski

Biochemistry Department, Bendigo College of Advanced

Education, Bendigo, Victoria 3550, Australia

ABSTRACT

In formulated diets based on cereal grains, lysine and/or methionine are usually deficient as well as often being the first amino
acids limiting the nutritional value of such diets. Deficiency of
these two amino acids in nutritional practice is compensated by synthetic L-lysine and DL-methionine supplementation or by the introduction of various protein sources - rich in lysine and methionine.
Among all essential amino acids lysine is most liable and subject
to damage during the processing of foods and feeds which can cause
the "deepening" of the lysine deficiency not on the total but on
the physiologically-available lysine basis. Hence, the simultaneous lysine deficiency and biological "sufficiency" problem is discussed using examples of practical diets in which a balance of biologically-active substances was achieved by the formulation and
optimalisation according to the needs of animals, taking into account physiological lysine "accessibility" - "availability".

Growth rate, nitrogen balance data and chemical composition of
the tissues in long term trials are the most valid indication just-
ifying the quantity of amino acid supplements to the practical
diets. Prediction of the practical results of dietary amino acid
balance from various short-term chemical and biological tests can
give misleading results. Their application in nutritional practice
is restricted to particular types of foods/feeds, and to specific
processing systems and test conditions. Observations of the appearances of most limiting, dietary amino acids in the blood after the
meal do not provide a complete nutritional characteristic of practical rations due to complex regulatory mechanisms in protein and
amino acid metabolism much of which are not yet fully understood.

INTRODUCTION

The degree to which dietary proteins are utilised for body metabolism and specific functions depends mainly on their amino acid composition particularly the concentration of limiting amino acids and their biological availability. Hence, in modern nutritional practice diets are so formulated to balance energy, essential amino acids and other dietary ingredients to obtain a final composition, as chemically determined, that would be the closest to the standards and requirements described as optimal for the particular type of organism. Optimalisation of diets in modern terms involving computerised formulation requires a knowledge of the chemical characteristics of the raw product, range of its application, cost, limitations and finally its eventual evaluation in biological terms. Such an overall and detailed quality control is a complex problem since the computerisation of our activities requires quality control in quantitative terms.

There is sufficient evidence to suggest that of all essential amino acids lysine and sulfur amino acids methionine and cystine, are the most indispensible in most foods, feeds and practical diets used in both human and animal nutrition. To formulate a well-balanced diet it is necessary to mix various dietary ingredients in such proportions to use the surplus of amino acids and other substances from one ingredient to cover the deficiencies in the others and reverse. With present low prices of synthetic amino-acids a few dollars per kilogram as compared to a few thousand dollars per kilogram some 15 years ago - a dietary essential amino acid balance can also be economically achieved by synthetic amino acid supplementations. The principal aim of dietary formulation in modern food and feed industries, and particularly important to animal production is to achieve a nutritionally-adequate balance by amino acid supplementation which in turn has to be justified by the economy of such a procedure. The ways, techniques and methods which can be used to measure the response of animals to dietary amino acid supplementation in protein and/or synthetic amino acid form will be discussed in this paper.

The present article will be limited to studies conducted by the author on two amino acids, lysine and methionine which are generally present in insufficient amounts in the practical diets for growing pigs and therefore they have to be supplemented to the appropriate requirement levels established as "optimal". Particular attention will be paid to chemical and biological tests which could be used as an indication of the dietary amino acids "sufficiency" and to methods which can be used for detecting biological availability of amino acids from the basal diets and from protein supplements to the practical rations. The following questions were put forward in this presentation: Which chemical or biological tests should be recommended for measuring limitations and the avail-

ability of amino acids in foods, feeds and various diets? Is
the amino acid availability test, particularly the availability of
lysine a reliable criterion for the evaluation and prediction
of the nutritive value of the practical rations? Which of the
analytical methods should be used to predict the effects of the
application of diets which were modified by amino acid supplementation at dietary formulation stage? - These questions however
cannot be answered definitely due to our incomplete knowledge of
the regulatory mechanisms in the protein and amino acid metabolism.
However, the experimental data presented in this paper should
encourage the reader to draw his own conclusions.

PRACTICAL DIETS FOR PIGS AND ESSENTIAL AMINO ACID BALANCE

Most of the common varieties of cereal grains and cereal-based
diets for monogastric farm animals are deficient in certain essential amino acids, lysine being most often the first limiting and
methionine the second. Figure 1 shows an aminogram of barley which
is still the main ingredient of the practical cereal-based diets
for meat-type pigs in many countries and indicates distinct lysine
and sulfur amino acids deficiency relative to the essential amino
acid requirements of young growing pigs listed by the NRC (1968)
and ARC (1967). The lysine and methionine deficiency in such diets
is compensated for by synthetic L-lysine and DL-methionine supple-

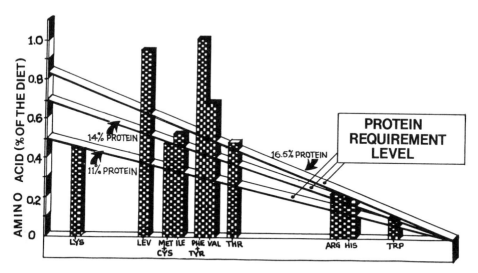

Figure 1. Essential amino acids in barley in relation to the
requirements of growing pigs (11 to 32 kg live weight) at recommended 16.5% dietary crude protein level and indication of protein
levels at which lysine (11.1%) and sulfur containing amino acids
(Methionine + cystine) (14%) would cover pigs requirements for
these amino acids (Ostrowski, 1972f).

ments or by other protein sources high in these amino acids, i.e.
proteins of animal origin such as milk, fish and meat, and/or food
legume proteins of plant origin such as soya bean. Although barley
is being used as a major ingredient in most of the practical rations
for growing meat-type pigs, the fact that high potato yields can be
achieved in various climatic zones, is encouraging the partial or
complete replacement of barley. Potatoes contain less but a high
quality protein as measured by essential amino acid composition
(Koreleski & Ostrowski, 1970) compared to barley in which lysine is
deficient, being the first limiting amino acid, with a methionine
level higher than that found in potatoes (Ostrowski & Koreleski,
1970).

Optimal diet for pigs with maximal predispositions to meet
tissue formation and minimum fat tissue deposition is that known
to be based on barley and skim milk (Clausen, 1965). When replacing milk in such a diet with other cheaper sources of protein such
as soya bean meal, ground nut meal, meat and bone meal, to

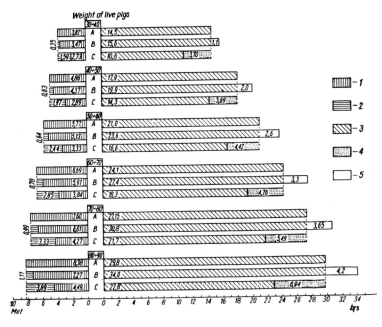

Figure 2. Lysine and methionine levels in barley and skimmed
milk diet (A) and quantity of synthetic forms of these two amino
acids added to high (B) and low (C) protein diets where barley was
replaced by dried potato flakes (1, dietary methionine; 2, DL-
methionine supplement; 3, dietary lysine; 4, L-lysine supplement;
5, excess of dietary lysine above the level in diet A) (Ostrowski
& Ryś, 1969).

TABLE 1

Effect of L-lysine and DL-methionine supplementation to the diets in which barley was replaced with potatoes at two dietary protein levels (Ostrowski & Ryś, 1969).

Diet	Daily gains (g/24 hr) (1)	Protein (N X 6.25) Conversion (g/kg gain)	Meat to Fat Relation
"OPTIMAL" - BARLEY & MILK	681	411	4.30
POTATO & MILK - HIGH PROTEIN:			
methionine deficient	576	514	3.75
methionine supplemented	643	487	3.83
POTATO & MILK - LOW PROTEIN:			
-lysine & methionine deficient	531	321	3.49
-methionine deficient (+ L-lysine only)	521	341	3.73
-lysine deficient (+ DL-methionine only)	583	322	3.73
+lysine & methionine together (as in "optimal" diet)	627	275	3.85

(1) Feeding period from 30 to 90 kg live weight.

achieve similar results as when barley and skimmed milk diet is used, a supplementation with synthetic amino acids L-lysine and DL-methionine is necessary.

Taking lysine and methionine concentrations in barley and skimmed milk diet as the "optimal" ones and then replacing barley by dried potato flakes at the same protein level, this results in a deficiency of methionine and an excess of dietary lysine. (Figure 2). Reduction of milk in potato-based diet, without changing the dietary energy content, decreases the protein concentration much below the established by ARC (1967) and NRC (1968) requirement levels: i.e. from 15 to 11% for young animals and from 13 to 8% for older ones. This results in both lysine and methionine being deficient in the diet causing low production effects as measured by growth rate, protein conversion efficiency and meat to fat relation as compared to "optimal" barley and milk diet (Table 1). Supplementation of the deficient potato and milk diets with either synthetic DL-methionine or L-lysine and DL-methionine to the "optimal" level, improves production effects close to, but still below those observed with "optimal" barley and milk diet.

TABLE 2

Performance and nitrogen metabolism of pigs fed with low protein, plant-origin diet either with or without synthetic amino acids supplementation (Ostrowski & Ryś,* - 1973a or; ** - 1973b).

Supplements & Measurement	Trial 1*		Trial 2**	
Lysine & methionine supplements[1]	-	+	-	+
PRODUCTION RESULTS:				
Average daily gains (g/24 hr)	516	594	616	640
Protein (N X 6.25) conversion efficiency (g/1 kg gain)	441	411	437	423
Meat/fat relation	3.4	3.7	4.1	4.0
NIGROGEN METABOLISM DATA:				
Apparent N-digestibility (%)	75	80	77	81
N-retention (g/24 hr)	16.0	20.9	16.7	23.8

(1) Diet composed of dried potatoes & dried sugar beet flakes (1:1) and protein concentrates mixture of plant origin.

The positive effects of amino acid supplementation to the practical diets for pigs shows the importance of proper dietary formulation in terms of an amino acid balance saving substantial amounts of valuable feedstuffs (milk, barley) which in turn can be used as a foodstuff in human nutrition. A saving of over 8 kg of crude protein on one animal, by means of reducing milk consumption with simultaneous synthetic L-lysine and DL-methionine supplementation, led to further trials in which milk was completely eliminated from the rations and replaced by proteins of plant origin. However, dietary lysine and methionine were kept on the "optimal" barley and milk diet level.

In two subsequent Trials, conducted in identical conditions using two different bulk feed supplies, it was shown that balancing diets based exclusively on plant-originated ingredients with methionine and lysine led only to a slight improvement in the performance and nitrogen digestibility despite a simultaneous notable increase in nitrogen retention (Table 2). Despite the L-Lysine and DL-methionine supplementation to diets containing plant protein mixtures instead of milk, achieved results were in each case worse than those obtained with the use of the "optimal"-barley and milk diet.

The question arises whether the diets used previously which were based on plant origin feedstuffs, were properly balanced and whether it is possible to formulate high nutritive value diet from low value plant ingredients by a proper balance of dietary substances according to presently known requirement standards.

DIETARY BALANCE AND CONSEQUENCES OF DEFICIENCIES IN PRACTICE

The prospects of a proper dietary balance by means of an appropriate formulation of the extremely low-protein, plant-originated diet and the importance of dietary supplementation with lysine, the first limiting amino acid in the ration are demonstrated in Figure 3. Diet was composed from 85% of barley and dried potato flakes mixture (1:1) and wheatings (15%). It contained 10% of crude (6.5% digestible) protein and as low as 0.37% of the total lysine and 0.23% chemically determined "available" as FDNB - reactive lysine. The growth and nitrogen balance of pigs fed with such a diet - even in short term balance trial, was very poor. When this diet was supplemented with synthetic amino acids, vitamins, macro-and microelements (in premix form) in the quantities equating concentrations of these substances in the diet according to the ARC (1967) requirements levels, then the nitrogen metabolism of the animals fed on such a balanced diet was notably improved (Figure 3, A & B diet 11).

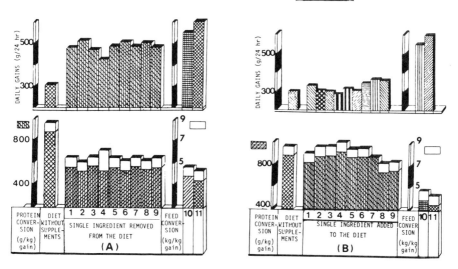

Figure 3. The long-term effect of the elimination of (A) or supplementation with (B) the single biologically active substance from the low protein of plant origin diet previously supplemented with the commercially manufactured premix (10) on daily gains, feed conversion and protein conversion efficiency and comparison of the results with the same diet balanced according to ARC (1967) requirement levels (11). Single ingredient removed from or added to the diet: 1, vit. B_{12}; 2, pantothenic acid; 3, choline; 4, lysine; 5, methionine; 6, oxyterracine; 7, phosphorus; 8, copper; 9, cobalt; (Ostrowski, 1972f).

Lysine deficiency which caused a simultaneous amino acid imbalance resulted in a consistant reduction in growth and nitrogen metabolism
data. Despite other biologically-active substances being present
in the diet the results were only slightly better than those observed in the imbalanced - unsupplemented diet.

     Of all supplements present in the properly formulated diet
(according to ARC, 1967), lysine showed itself to be the most
critical when excluded from the ration, causing greatest depression
in production effects expressed as daily live weight gains, protein
and feed conversion efficiency (Figure 3A). On the other hand
individual supplementation of the low-lysine and low-protein of
plant origin diet with the single ingredient, without balancing
others to the animal requirements standards,did not improve the
daily live weight gains in long term - productive type-trial as
compared to the basic diet without any supplements (Figure 3B).
Lysine supplementation to the imbalanced diet resulted in both
growth and feed conversion efficiency depression while with either
methionine (5), vitamin B12 (1), phosphorus (7), cobalt (9) and
copper (8) supplementation there resulted a slight growth rate
improvement. This may be an indication of lysine toxicity which
usually takes place in imbalanced diets with an excess of one amino
acid (Harper & Benevenga, 1970). Lowering in performance of animals
due to lack of lysine and/or other single dietary ingredient is due
to a dietary imbalance which affects their nitrogen metabolism.
Growth of pigs as recorded in short-term trial with lysine elimin-
ation/supplementation agree with nitrogen balance data (Figure 4).

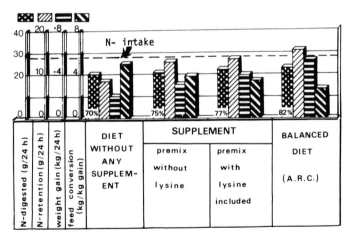

     Figure 4. The effect of L-lysine exclusion from the low pro-
tein of plant origin diet for growing pigs previously balanced in
biologically active substances either by supplementation with the
commercially manufactured premix or supplementation according to
the ARC (1967) requirement levels (Ostrowski, 1972e).

TABLE 3

A comparison of the results obtained in short- (S) and long- (L)
term Trials on pigs fed diets either imbalanced or balanced in some
biologically active substances (Ostrowski, 1972e).

DIET	N-digestibility (%)	N-retention (g/24 hr)	Daily Live Weight gains (g/24 hr)		Feed Conversion (kg/kg gain)	
	S	S	S	L	S	L
DIET WITHOUT SUPPLEMENTS	70	8.2	379	311	4.6	6.8
SINGLE INGREDIENT REMOVED FROM THE DIET:						
Vitamin B12	74	12.3	433	487	3.8	4.3
Pantothenic acid	72	12.0	510	516	4.3	4.1
Choline chloride	74	11.4	503	478	2.9	4.4
L-lysine	76	11.6	450	432	4.1	5.3
DL-methionine	75	12.9	553	491	4.0	4.3
Oxyterracine	78	14.6	611	509	4.9	4.1
Phosphorus	76	12.0	488	482	2.9	4.3
Copper	76	13.3	514	502	2.8	4.2
Cobalt	75	13.3	567	485	3.2	4.3
DIET WITH COMMERCIAL PREMIX	78	14.1	586	556	2.9	3.8
DIET BALANCED ACCORDING TO A.R.C. REQUIREMENTS	82	15.4	641	604	2.7	3.5
Significance	**	**	**	**	**	**
S.E. of mean	1.7	0.9	30	39	0.3	0.4

Also there was a general agreement in results obtained in short and
long-term Trials (Table 3) confirming lysine to be the first limiting amino acid in the diets of plant origin. Pigs showed a higher
sensitivity to lysine deficiency than to methionine deficiency
which is contrary to results obtained by Said, Hegsted & Hays
(1974) who observed slow rate of nitrogen depletion as a result of
feeding with a lysine-free diet as opposed to methionine. This may
be due to several factors other than lysine. When balancing practical diets with a number of ingredients one has to take into consideration various interactions, antagonisms, synergisms which can
drastically alter typical requirement levels and hence adding an
extra problem to food and/or feed formulation process (Ostrowski,
1972b, c). There are several interactions between protein and
essential amino acids, amongst the amino acids, between the essential

amino acids, vitamins and minerals discussion of which exceed the limit of this paper.

Since lysine appears to be the most limiting amino acid and therefore most important in the practical cereal type diets,followed by methionine, the effects of dietary supplementation with these two amino acids will be discussed further with particular emphasis being given to lysine. The first problem with amino acid supplementation is the knowledge of the levels of the requirements of animals for lysine and methionine so as to establish the validity of the norms used for calculation of the quantities of amino acid supplements.

LYSINE AND METHIONINE SUPPLEMENTATION AND REQUIREMENT LEVELS FOR PIGS

The requirement of pigs for lysine as determined by different workers has been shown to vary between 0.41% and 1.3% of the diet (Ostrowski, 1972d). Using a lysine deficient diet the requirements of pigs in various weight intervals has been established in relation to maximal nitrogen deposition at various dietary lysine levels (Figure 5A).

Requirement for methionine has also been determined in order to establish a level to which this amino acid should be supplemented together with lysine in diets for pigs. In nutritional practice it is convenient to use sum of methionine and cystine rather than methionine itself since cystine can cover up to 50% of the organism requirement for methionine. Requirement of growing pigs for the sum of methionine and cystine as determined by different workers vary between 0.23% and 0.8% of the diet (Ostrowski 1972f). Using methionine and cystine deficient diet the requirement for these two

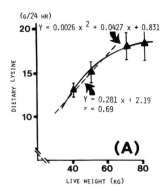
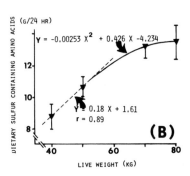

Figure 5.   Requirement of growing pigs for lysine (A) (Ostrowski, 1972d) and sulfur containing amino acids: methionine + cystine (B) at different live weight intervals.

sulfur containing amino acids was determined similarly as requirement for lysine from the maximum nitrogen deposition at various
dietary sulphur amino acid contents (Figure 5B).

The requirement levels of both lysine and sulphur containing
amino acids as presented on Figure 5 were similar or close to those
concentrations in barley and milk diet (Clausen, 1965). The next
question arose as to which of the measurements recorded in both
short- and long-term Trials appears to be the most reliable criterion of dietary lysine, sulfur-containing and other essential
amino acids "sufficiency" and how various measurements are related
to lysine absorption and deposition in the tissues as a consequence
of lysine and methionine balance in the diet.

NUTRITIONAL AND BIOCHEMICAL CONSEQUENCES OF DIETARY LYSINE AND
METHIONINE SUPPLEMENTATION

When a lysine and methionine deficient diet, composed of ingredients of plant origin, was supplemented with synthetic forms of
these two amino acids to the level present in barley and milk diet
- considered as "optimal" for growing meat type pigs (Figure 6) -
then, except for apparent nitrogen digestibility, both production

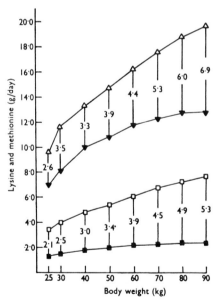

Figure 6. Total lysine (▼) and methionine (■) level in the
potato and plant protein mixture diet and quantity of synthetic L-
lysine and DL-methionine supplementation to the "optimal" - barley
and milk diet for growing pigs (Δ □) (Ostrowski, 1969).

TABLE 4

Effect of synthetic L-lysine and DL-methionine supplementation on production effects and nitrogen metabolism of pigs given diet either deficient (LLM) or "optimal" (OLM) in lysine and methionine (Ostrowski, 1969).

Measurement	Diet		S.E. of mean (+)	Signi- ficance
	LLM	OLM		
PRODUCTION EFFECTS:				
Average daily gain (g/24 hr)	504	576	18.8	*
Protein (N X 6.25) conversion (g/1 kg gain)	477	428	12.1	**
Meat/fat relation	3.26	3.58	0.10	*
NITROGEN METABOLISM DATA:				
Apparent N-digestibility (%)	66.84	71.26	1.99	NS
N-retention (g/24 hr)	11.16	15.89	1.032	**

effects and nitrogen retention results notably improved (Table 4). Higher nitrogen retention at the "optimal" dietary lysine and methionine level (OLM) led to an increase in weight of the longissimus dorsi muscle and its protein content with a simultaneous decrease in intramuscular fat (Table 5) as compared to the low protein of plant origin diet, deficient in lysine and methionine (LLM). Looking at lysine absorption from the diets and deposition in the tissues as presented in Table 6 there were significant differences in lysine concentrations in the blood, liver and muscle between the animals in LLM and OLM diets, which could be ascribed to a higher absorption of lysine from OLM diet and this could in turn lead to a greater lysine deposition.

The higher blood lysine level in the OLM group corresponds to a higher lysine content in the liver, and the liver to blood lysine ratio which is nearly equal for both LLM and OLM groups (6.1 and 6.0 respectively). This, despite the same ratio between liver and muscle lysine and muscle and blood lysine is significantly different on the two treatments. In other words, blood lysine concentration is closely associated with the concentration in the liver. Dalgliesh and Tabechian (1956) observed that after a labelled amino acid solution had been administered to rats by stomach tube, the activity of the "protein-bound" fraction and soluble amino acids in liver increased but most of the activity was in the muscle. Results of an investigation on dogs reported by Van Slyke and Meyer (1913a, b) also showed that musculature is the major reservoir of amino acids, although the percentage content of amino acids in muscle is less than in liver.

TABLE 5

Effect of synthetic L-lysine and DL-methionine supplementation on the weight and composition of m. longissimus dorsi (Ostrowski,1969).

Measurement	Diet		S.E. of mean (+)	Signi-ficance
	LLM	OLM		
COMPOSITION OF M. LONGISSIMUS DORSI:				
Weight of the muscle (kg)	1.31	1.86	0.10	**
Dry matter %	27.2	28.8	0.97	NS
Total dry matter (g)	356	499	31	**
Protein (N X 6.25) (%)	21.9	23.3	0.32	**
Total N X 6.25 in muscle (g)	287	454	31	**
Fat (%)	4.14	2.52	0.32	**
Total fat in muscle (g)	54.2	46.9	1.5	**
Ash (%)	1.14	1.00	0.10	NS
Total ash in muscle (g)	14.9	18.6	0.76	**

In the past years many reports have given attention to the controversial concept of labile body protein reserves contributing to the free amino acid pools in the organism (Ashley & Fisher, 1967; Fisher, 1967; Munro, 1964). In one of the first studies on amino acid accumulation in the animal body, Van Slyke & Meyer (1913c) reported that amino acid reserves in the tissues do not tend to be extensively depleted in fastings. On the other hand, it could be supposed that, following a period of starvation, administration of a higher level of amino acids in the diet should increase the amino acid content in muscle. The results obtained in many of the experiments are not in agreement, and as emphasised by Christensen (1964) in a review of tissue amino acids, our understanding of the function of tissue amino acid accumulation is very incomplete, despite this being a dominant aspect of amino acid nutrition.

According to Munro (1970) free amino acids of the body can follow three different pathways - protein synthesis, synthesis of a variety of low molecular compounds and degradation through the pathways of amino acid catabolism. In the new-born organisms intense protein synthesis is much greater than the degradation of circulating amino acids which results in an increase in tissue amino acid levels and augmented protein synthesis in the liver. Discussing the regulatory mechanism in protein metabolism, Munro (1970) explained that the mechanism of protein synthesis and its degradation was due to the engagement of ribosomes with the messenger RNA to form polysomes. Discussing results presented above it

TABLE 6

Effect of synthetic L-lysine and DL-methionine supplementation on lysine content of m. longissimus dorsi, liver and blood (Ostrowski, 1969).

Measurement	Diet		S.E. of mean (+)	Signi-ficance
	LLM	OLM		
Blood lysine: (mg/100 ml)	8.2	21.5	3.2	**
Liver lysine: (mg/100 g)[1]	50	129	19.5	**
Total liver lysine (g)	0.7	2.3	0.31	**
Muscle lysine: (mg/100 g)[1]	58.6	76.17	5.58	*
Total muscle lysine (g)	0.8	1.42	0.01	**
as % of crude protein	0.28	0.33	0.02	NS
Lysine in pressed muscle juice (mg/100 ml)	66	74	2.47	*
Ratio of:				
Liver : blood lysine [1]	6.1	6.0	0.28	NS
Liver : muscle lysine [1]	0.9	1.7	0.20	**
Muscle : blood lysine	7.1	3.5	0.54	**
(1) fresh weight.				

can be assumed, as did Munro (1970), that with ingestion of a diet supplemented in lysine and methionine an influx of amino acids after each meal is connected with more ribosoms being engaged with the messenger to form polysomes resulting in an acceleration of protein formation and consequently a more rapid increase in the protein content in the liver as compared to imbalanced amino acid mixture entering liver after ingestion of a meal deficient in these two amino acids. Omsted & Van der Decken (1974) found that animals given a synthetic diet deficient in lysine show a very distinctive reduction in lysine deposition in livers and muscles which was accompanied by the substantial decrease in ribosomal RNA in skelctal muscle and liver. Refeeding with a high lysine diet resulted in an increase of lysine and RNA concentrations, however to a lesser extent in the liver than in the muscle.

It was calculated that the degree of nitrogen deposition in the muscle was very closely related to the lysine level in the muscle since both LLM and OLM groups have virtually the same ratio of muscle lysine to % N retention, equal to 5.0 and 4.8 respectively. The relation of dietary lysine intake to nitrogen retention was also the same in each group (1.0). Table 7 demonstrates that all correlation coeficients in the OLM diet between lysine in the blood,

TABLE 7

Correlation coefficients between blood, liver and muscle lysine
level and their correlation with some other indices (Ostrowski,1969).

Measurement	Units	OLM Diet		
		Blood lysine	Liver lysine	Muscle lysine
Liver lysine	mg/100 g	0.956	-	-
Muscle lysine	mg/100 g	0.971	0.917	-
Total liver lysine	g	0.788	0.984	0.906
Total muscle lysine	g	0.918	0.871	0.992
Lysine in pressed m. juice	mg/100 ml	0.949	0.947	0.996
Protein in muscle	%	0.756	0.783	0.924
N-retention	%	0.928	0.932	0.943
Lysine intake	g	0.968	0.927	0.960

liver and muscle and lysine intake and nitrogen retention reached
a high level and were highly significant. Lysine in the blood
appears to be an accurate indication of lysine intake and nitrogen
retention; the correlation between these measurements being 0.968
and 0.928 respectively. Kelly & Scott (1968) also reported a
very high correlation (r = 0.95) between lysine intake and lysine
blood plasma level in the chick which is very similar to that given
in Table 7.

BLOOD PLASMA LYSINE AS AN INDICATION OF LYSINE "SUFFICIENCY" IN
DIETS

     In the OLM diet i.e. with lysine supplementation to LLM diet
there occurs a greater absorption of lysine from the intestine to
the blood which is accompanied by a higher blood lysine concentration. However, after starvation, when pigs are fed on diets containing unequal amounts of lysine, differences in the lysine content of
blood plasma are usually small (Krysciak, Ostrowski & Rys, 1966;
Rerat & Lougnone, 1965). Whatever may be the short term effect,
Table 6 shows that the blood lysine level, even after the 18 hour
starvation period, is higher on an optimal lysine regime than on
one which is deficient in lysine. It can be assumed that this is
the result of long term differences in lysine levels in the diet,
whereas the majority of previous experiments on lysine intake were
conducted during short growth periods of animals with observations
lasting for only a few days. Also, the lysine level was evaluated
in the whole blood while in the majority of other works lysine is

TABLE 8

Production effects and nitrogen metabolism of pigs as a result of
feeding with diet of different lysine content with either increasing
concentrations of sulfur containing and other essential amino acids
(casein supplement) or with essential amino acids other than lysine
remaining at the constant level (l-lysine supplement).

Supplement (Group)		Dietary Lysine (%)		Dietary Meth-ionine + Cys-tine(%)	Daily Live Weight Gains (g/24 hr)	Protein Digest-ibility (%)	Nitrogen Retention (g/24 hr)
		Total	Avail-able				
Casein	A	0.59	0.48	0.55	487	78	14.4
	B	0.80	0.67	0.58	524	81	17.2
	C	1.00	0.85	0.63	561	83	17.9
	D	1.20	1.02	0.72	603	85	18.0
L-lysine	A	0.59	0.48	0.55	516	75	15.5
	B	0.83	0.71	0.55	578	79	18.1
	C	1.08	0.94	0.56	612	80	18.5
	D	1.32	1.17	0.56	627	78	18.6

Meal composed of 550g barley; 125g ground nut meal and 34g vitamin-mineral mixture (two meals a day) with casein or L-lysine
supplements.

usually evaluated in the blood plasma. This may indicate that
whole blood analysis could be a more sensitive indication of dietary lysine content than lysine in plasma.

It has been observed that the limitations in dietary amino
acids can be detected from the appearance of these amino acids in
animals' blood plasma after the meal (Longenecker,1963). Consequently,there has been growing interest in measuring the quantity of
lysine and other amino acids in pigs' blood plasma after ingestion
of several types of formulated diets with various amino acid levels
as a useful biological test indicating the degree of amino acids
"sufficiency" in the diet (Rerat & Lougnone,1965; Pion et.al., 1966).

The high degree of correlation between lysine intake and blood
lysine level, as demonstrated in Table 7 invites one to query to
what extent do plasma lysine levels reflect dietary lysine concentrations and whether the relation between the dietary and plasma
lysine could be embraced in a formula suitable for analysis of

availability of amino acid supplements in foods and feeds. This
could give an indication of production and nitrogen balance results
or in synthetic form. Also, how much are plasma lysine levels dependent on the dietary essential amino acids balance, and whether
there is any interaction between dietary lysine, and lysine plasma
levels as a result of dietary sulfur containing and other essential
amino acids contents.

Lysine as the First Limiting Amino Acid : Response of Animals to
Amino Acid Supplementation

Increasing concentrations of dietary lysine with a simultaneous either increase or constant sulfur containing and other essential amino acids in the ration (Figure 7) produced gradually higher
live weight gains of pigs and an increase in nitrogen retention,
(Table 8); the relationship between dietary lysine (x) and N-ret-

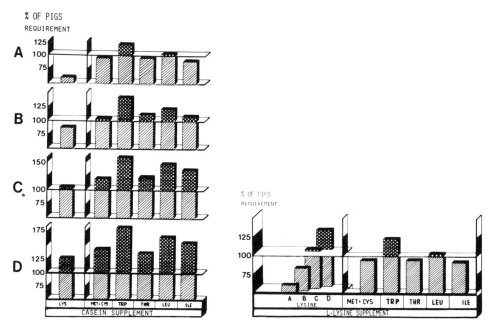

Figure 7. The effect of casein or synthetic L-lysine supplementation to the diet deficient in lysine (first limiting amino
acid) on the aminograms of the daily rations fed to pigs; essential
amino acids expressed as a percentage of pig requirements; the level
100% represents essential amino acid requirements according to
Clausen (1965) (Ostrowski, 1975).

ention (y) being expressed by the regression equation: $Y = 0.08 \; x^2$ + 2.32 X 1.05.   The highest dietary lysine concentration at constant sulfur containing other essential amino acids (with synthetic L-lysine supplement) showed slightly declining N-digestibility values as compared to the former level.   Increases in the dietary lysine level, despite the lysine source added, resulted in a characteristic sharpening of the lysine peak built up from relative lysine concentrations (percentages of the fast lysine content) measured within the first three reconrding points - 0, 1 and 2 hours after ingestion of the meal (Figure 8) Relative plasma concentrations in their maximums, despite the level of lysine in the diet, were higher when synthetic L-lysine was used as lysine supplement as compared to casein.   Accumulated relative plasma lysine concentrations after ingestion of meal showed an increase in overall recorded values.   These values corresponded with the increasing dietary lysine levels but only within the first three levels (A, B

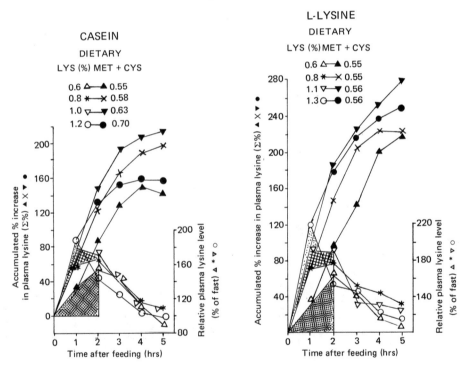

Figure 8. Changes in the relative lysine concentrations (mg/ 100 ml) expressed as percentages of the fast plasma lysine level (open asterisks) and accumulated increases in relative plasma levels (closed asterisks) summed up after ingestion of diet providing four lysine levels, both total and "available" (chemically determined as FDNB-reactive lysine), achieved by supplementation with casein or synthetic L-lysine.

and C) while the highest dietary lysine concentration (D) showed a deflating effect within both the lysine sources used.

Casein used as a source of lysine caused slightly lower plasma lysine concentrations and later maximums' appearance after the meal, as compared to synthetic L-lysine, providing pigs with similar dietary lysine levels. This is contrary to results presented by Longenecker & House (1959) who found a similar lysine absorption rate from both intact proteins and from L-lysine. When pigs were fed with diets containing different levels of lysine from two different sources, both with or without constant ratio between lysine and other amino acids, it was shown that changes in the plasma lysine were of similar function of dietary lysine with the only difference being the rate of lysine absorption. This may indicate that lysine from casein, as compared to synthetic L-lysine, was completely absorbed, but due to the digestion process, consequent lysine absorption from the intestines to the blood was slower and its subsequent appearance in the plasma was delayed.

The better response in performance an apparent protein diges-

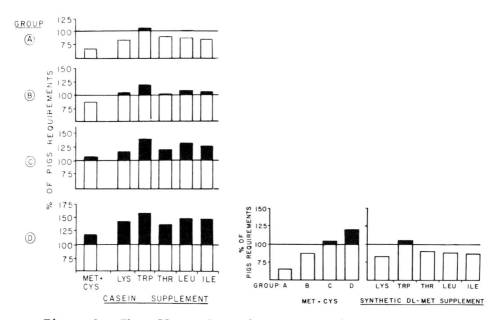

Figure 9. The effect of casein or synthetic DL-methionine supplementation to the diet deficient in methionine + cystine (first limiting amino acids) on the aminograms of the daily rations fed to pigs; essential amino acids expressed as a percentage of pig requirements; the level 100% represents requirements according to Clausen (1965).

tibility with L-lysine than with casein may be caused also by the
lower lysine availability in casein as compared with synthetic L-
lysine. Although it is assumed that casein should be completely
digested by pigs, however when it was analysed chemically for available lysine, only 92.7% of lysine in casein was available. Also
some microbial degradation of total lysine entering the small
intestine can occur before or after absorption causing a lowering
in the N-digestibility with the highest dietary lysine concentrations.
According to Harper (1968) and Rerat (1971) lower protein digestibility can be explained in terms of the lack of balance between
essential amino acids and interactions between lysine and other
amino acids.

Methionine + Cystine as the First Limiting Amino Acids in the Diet:
    Response of Animals to Amino Acid Supplementation

    Using casein supplementation to the basic diet with sulfur
containing first limiting amino acids methionine and cystine,
four diets were prepared (Figure 9): Diet A deficient in all essential amino acids; diet B deficient in sulfur containing amino acids
with sufficient lysine and other amino acids (according to animal
requirements); diet C, sulfur containing amino acids on the requirement level, and diet D, sulfur containing amino acids in excess of
pigs' requirement, with lysine and other amino acids in excess
in both C and D diets.

    With DL-methionine supplementation only the amounts of sulfur
containing amino acids increased with increasing levels of supplement, while lysine and other essential amino acids were within
the range of animal requirement levels with a slight excess of
tryptophan.

    When dietary lysine concentrations increased together with sul-
fur containing and other essential amino acids, as a result of casein
supplementation to sulfur amino acid deficient diet, then the production results and nitrogen metabolism of pigs were improved
notably. The degree of this improvement was similar to those observed as a result of increasing dietary sulfur containing amino
acids by DL-methionine supplement (Table 9). The relationship
between dietary sulfur containing amino acids (x) and nitrogen
retention of growing pigs (y) has been established as $Y = 0.52 \ X^2 +
10.9 \ X - 40.1$.

    Ingestion of a methionine and cystine deficient diet, simultan-
eously deficient in lysine and other essential amino acids, resulted
in only a slight blood plasma lysine rise after the meal. With
casein supplementation when all essential amino acids were balanced,
according to the requirements of animals, the blood plasma lysine
concentrations reached their maximums on the second hour after the
meal and maximas reflected rising dietary lysine levels at constant

TABLE 9.

Production effects and nitrogen metabolism of pigs as a result of feeding with diet deficient in sulfur containing amino acids in which sulfur containing amino acids were supplemented in casein form or with DL-methionine.

Supplement	Dietary Lysine (%)		Dietary Sulfur Amino Acids (methionine + cystine) (%)	Daily Live Weight Gains (g/24h)	Protein Digestibility (%)	Nitrogen Retention (g/24 hr)
	Total	Available				
Casein	0.78	0.62	0.39	150	73	4.1
	0.95	0.76	0.47	400	78	10.9
	1.10	0.90	0.54	529	81	14.4
	1.22	1.01	0.59	577	83	15.7
DL-methionine	0.78	0.62	0.39	202	74	5.5
	0.78	0.62	0.49	481	74	13.1
	0.78	0.62	0.58	599	73	16.3
	0.78	0.62	0.66	672	74	18.3

Meal composed of 375g barley; 135g soyabean meal; 135g corn starch 25g sugar and 35g of vitamin-mineral mixture (two meals a day) with casein or DL-methionine supplements.

ratios between lysine, sulfur containing and other essential amino acids (Figure 10). However, supplementation of the same diet with DL-methionine, keeping lysine and other essential amino acids in the diet at constant - deficient levels (except tryptophan) also resulted in a gradual increase in plasma lysine concentrations with increased methionine content. This shows that supplementation of

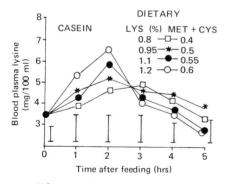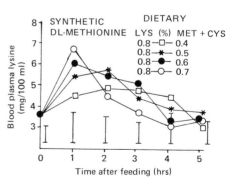

Figure 10. Lysine concentrations in peripheral blood plasma after ingestion of methionine and cystine deficient diet with various quantitities of either casein or DL-methionine. (Lines mark S.D.)

the diet, with the deficient amino acid being first limiting one
improves the absorption of the other dietary essential amino acids
as judged by the appearance of lysine in peripheral blood plasma.

In experiments with either L-lysine or simultaneous L-lysine
and DL-methionine supplementations to the diet deficient in these
two amino acids validity of the assumption was tested whether methionine added together with lysine to the diet increases the absorption of dietary lysine as measured by its appearance in the
peripheral blood, and whether the system of amino acid administration to the diet has an effect on pigs performance and blood plasma
levels in the long-term feeding trial.

Utilisation of Amino Acid Supplements by Pigs as a Result
of Administration Method

An excess of amino acids in blood after ingestion of food or
feed is usually metabolised and excreted with urine without being
utilised for tissues protein synthesis. To keep blood lysine and
methionine evenly distributed over a longer period of time after
feeding so that the animal would utilise better the lysine and
methionine ingested, synthetic L-lysine and DL-methionine were fed
to pigs in a drink form, two hours after feeding. Results summar-
ised in Table 10 show that by delaying the administration of lysine
and lysine with methionine to pigs till after the meal the growth
rate and protein conversion efficiency is greatly affected whereas
protein digestibility and nitrogen metabolism remains unaffected.
(Ostrowski et al. 1972b).

By administering L-lysine two hours after the meal, plasma

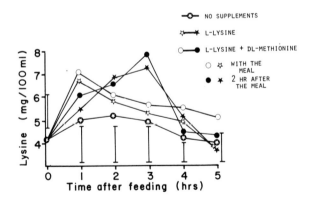

Figure 11. Blood plasma lysine as a result of dietary supplementations with L-lysine alone or together with DL-methionine and
effect of synthetic amino acid administration with the meal or 2
hours after the meal. (Vertical lines mark pooled S.D.)

TABLE 10

Supplementation of the low protein deficient in lysine and methionine diet with L-lysine alone or together with DL-methionine and
effect of their administration with the meal or 2 hours after the
meal on production results and nitrogen metabolism of pigs
(Ostrowski et al., 1972b).

Measurement	Meal without supp- lements	L-lysine supplement		L-lysine + DL-methionine	
		With Meal	2 hr after the meal	With Meal	2 hr after the meal
Daily live weight gains (g/24 hr)	382	534	514	578	525
Protein (N X 6.25) conversion effic- iency (g/1 Kg gain)	517	430	443	404	441
Nitrogen metabolism:					
N-digestibility (%)	87	86	86	87	88
N-retention (g/24 hr)	8.8	12.5	12.9	13.1	13.3

lysine concentrations gradually increased reaching the highest
level on the 3rd hour after the meal (Figure 11.). This however
had no effect on performance results and nitrogen metabolism of pigs
as compared to animals receiving lysine and/or methionine supplements together with the meal which were characterised by sharp
picks of plasma lysine in the first hour after the meal followed by
a gradual decrease up to the last sampling on the 5th hour after
the meal.

DIETARY AMINO ACIDS AND THEIR BIOLOGICAL "ACCESSIBILITY"

In studies presented earlier all diets were supplemented with
synthetic L-lysine and DL-methionine based on total amino acid content in the dietary ingredients. It is known however that while
synthetic DL-methionine and L-lysine is completely (or almost completely) absorbed and biologically available, thus these amino acids
from foods and feeds - particularly from those previously processed
- are only partially "available" for monogostric organisms
(Carpenter & Woodham 1974; Boyne et al., 1975). Hence it was
reasonable to suppose that despite lysine and methionine supplementation these two amino acids could be still in insufficient
amounts as compared to the "optimal" diet taken as an essential
amino acid standard. Hurrel & Carpenter (1977) demonstrated that
food and feed processing and/or storage is accompanied with a

decrease in amino acid "availability" of which basic amino acids, lysine in particular, are most subject to damage in biochemical and biological terms. In processed cereal foods or plant-originated diets a substantial reduction in nutritive value is observed due to combined action; lysine and other essential amino acid deficiency in unprocessed material ("by nature") which is followed by further depression by the destruction of part of the physiologically-active lysine during processing and/or storage. Therefore, there is, the problem of detecting the degree of lysine and other amino acids deficiency and their "unavailability" in foods and feeds so as to allow food technologists to control the nutritional quality of processed products and then to enable dieteticians and nutritionists to make the appropriate formulation of the high nutritional quality diets and sufficient supplementation with synthetic amino acids. All this to ensure for the organism a proper amino acid and other nutrients balance in the diet, and prevent lysine and/or other essential amino acids from becoming deficient due to partial unavailability (Carpenter, 1974).

DAMAGE TO AMINO ACIDS IN FOODS AND FEEDS DUE TO PROCESSING AND/OR STORAGE

Even under mild conditions of heating which occurred at food or feed processing stages or during storage, some essential amino acids in protein particles are significantly damaged and hence become partially unavailable. Such reactions can occur particularly between ε-amino groups of lysine incorporated in the protein chain and sugar aldehyde groups. Consequently the lysine unit, most sensitive to unfavourable processing or storage conditions, links with sugars becoming unavailable to the organism as a source of lysine (Early Maillard Reaction). As a result of severe heat treatment during food processing, even in the absence of carbohydrates, damage occurs not only to a large proportion of lysine but also to other amino acids, like arginine and to a lesser extent to tryptophan, methionine, cysteine and histidine (Advanced Maillard Reaction). The third type of reaction: protein - protein, occurs in slower rate than the previous two and takes place in the absence of reducing sugars. Nutritional consequences of such reactions have been reviewed by Hurrel & Carpenter (1977).

LYSINE "SUFFICIENCY" IN FEED FORMULATION - DILEMA: TOTAL OR "AVAILABLE" LYSINE?

To determine whether the growth of pigs, nitrogen retention and lysine absorption from the intestine to the blood can be ascribed to either total lysine or to the chemically determined "available" - dietary FDNB-reactive lysine, four diets were prepared, each providing approximately 0.65% available lysine and 71.6% total digestable nutrients (TDN) (Figure 12). They were based on barley meal with either meat and bone meal (MBM), white fish meal (WFM), soyabean meal (SBM) or groundnut meal (GNM). Cassava

TABLE 11

Amino Acid composition of the diets (%) (Ostrowski, Jones & Cadenhead, 1971).

	MBM	WFM	SBM	GNM
Crude Protein	16.7	11.1	15.1	19.8
Arginine	0.9	0.7	0.9	1.9
Histidine	0.4	0.3	0.4	0.4
Lysine	0.72	0.70	0.73	0.71
Tryptophan	0.1	0.1	0.2	0.2
Cystine	0.2	0.2	0.3	0.3
Methionine	0.5	0.5	0.5	0.5
Tyrosine	0.4	0.4	0.5	0.7
Phenylalanine	0.7	0.5	0.8	1.0
Threonine	0.5	0.5	0.5	0.6
Leucine	1.2	0.8	1.0	1.3
Iso-leucine	0.6	0.6	0.7	0.9
Valine	0.8	0.7	0.8	0.9

meal and maize starch were used to equate the available lysine and TDN concentrations between diets. Supplements of DL-methionine were added so that all diets provided adequate amounts of sulfur amino acids according to their requirements. The amino acid composition of the diets given in Table 11 shows that apart from those

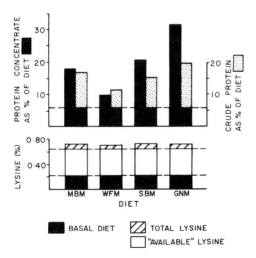

Figure 12. Characteristic of the barley-based diet supplemented with four protein concentrates providing different levels of both crude protein and total lysine but the same chemically determined "available" FDNB reactive lysine (Ostrowski, Jones & Cadenhead, 1971).

TABLE 12

Productive effects, nitrogen metabolism data and carcass quality of pigs fed with four protein concentrates at constant "available" FDNB reactive lysine level (Ostrowski, Jones & Cadenhead, 1971).

Measurement	Protein Concentrate				Significance of Difference
	MBM	WFM	SBM	GNM	
PRODUCTIVE RESULTS:					
Live weight gains (g/24 hr)	751	741	741	737	NS
Food conversion efficiency (g/1 kg gain)	2.61	2.63	2.68	2.64	NS
N-METABOLISM RESULTS:					
Apparent digestibility	83.9	82.0	81.6	83.1	NS
N-retention: (g/24 hr)	20.8	16.9	21.7	21.0	**
- (% of N-intake)	41.4	47.4	45.6	37.7	**
- (% of N-digested)	49.4	57.7	56.1	41.7	**
CARCASS QUALITY:					
Specific gravity of half carcass	1.050	1.038	1.054	1.048	*
Average weight of the psoas m. (g)	166	143	200	194	*
N X 6.25 in the muscle (%)	19.3	18.1	19.6	19.3	*
Fat in the muscle (%)	4.6	6.8	4.1	4.1	*

amino acids which were supplied in excess of the estimated require-ment, the fish meal diet was lower in valine and phenylalanine than the other rations, but these amino acids are unlikely to be the second or third limiting amino acids.

Growth, Nitrogen Balance and Carcass Quality as Affected by Lysine Availability

While there were no differences in the digestibility of nitro-gen between the diets and both growth rate and food conversion efficiency were similar in all treatments, the values for nitrogen retention (g/day) were identical on MBM, SBM and GNM with only about 20% lower N-retention on the diet containing white fish meal (Table 12). The total protein content of the fish meal diet was low hence, it is possible that the low nitrogen retention on the fish meal ration might have been due to an insufficient supply of protein or nitrogen in the form of the non-essential amino acids. When the dietary crude protein concentration was high, interactions were found between protein and lysine concentrations in the effects on the nitrogen retention of pigs. So at high concentration, dietary crude protein per se becomes important. The high fat contents of the psoas muscles and the low specific gravities of the carcasses of the pigs given fish meal, both of which are indication of high fat content in the carcass, reflect the lower nitrogen retention by these pigs. The low protein content of the fish meal diet would mean that the energy : protein ratio in this diet was increased relative to that of the other three and this could be expected to lead to a high rate of fat deposition in the carcass.

Lysine Apparent Digestibility and Lysine Availability

Apparent lysine digestibility coefficients were similar in all groups (Table 13), showing however, overall higher values than the apparent nitrogen digestibilities (see Table 12). It could be concluded that apparent lysine digestibility reflects lysine "availability" as chemically determined by FDNB reactive lysine since digestibility values obtained for different protein sources, fed on both varied protein and total lysine levels but with the same FDNB reactive lysine quantities, were similar. Older pigs showed slightly higher apparent lysine digestibility values which can be explained by the more intensive microbial fermentation in the large intestines. Despite the alteration in the absolute amounts of lysine excreated, which is the mixture of "unavailable" lysine and lysine produced by microflora in large intestines, the lysine digestibility was even higher in older pigs than those chemically determined, and was consistant reflecting the dietary lysine availability analysed as FDNB reactive lysine.

Digestibility of amino acids as a measurement of their absorption from the intestines to the blood is not the most favourable technique and is treated with reserve as a nutritional test. This is due to deamination by microorganisms in the coecum and colon of pigs yielding ammonia and various amines which in turn can be incorporated into amino acids to synthesise in the large intestines depending on the dietary composition, level and type of protein. Thus, the result of amino acid availability, as determined in digestibility and metabolism studies, can be subject to error resulting in reduced or increased digestibility values. It was found that amino acid fermentation in the large intestine obscures or reduces differences in digestibility values between different dietary proteins tested (Holmes et al 1974). Analysis of the ileal contents is considered to be both more convenient and meaningful technique for individual amino acids digestibility studies (Holmes et al., 1974; Varnish & Carpenter, 1975), requiring however, animals fitted with re-entrant cannulas which in practice can create some extra technical problems. In addition, lysine digestibility can also be altered and notably over-estimated due to the analytical procedure and technique used in digestibility studies. Up to 11% losses in feacal total lysine and up to 51% in

TABLE 13

Lysine digestibility coefficients (%)[1] as a result of feeding
with four diets of constant "available" lysine levels as chemically determined.

Weight of Pigs	Diet				Significance of Difference	SE of mean
	MBM	WFM	SBM	GWM		
41 kg.	89	91	90	88	NS	1.7
74 kg.	95	94	97	94	NS	3.1
"Availability" as FDNB reactive lysine	92	93	90	87	NS	2.8

[1] Calculated from true total dietary lysine intake minus total
lysine excreated in feaces expressed as percent of total
lysine intake.

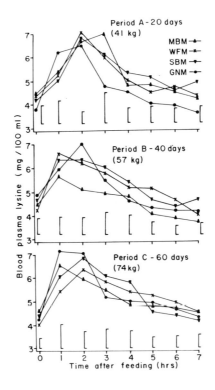

Figure 13. Changes in the plasma lysine concentrations (mg
/100 ml) after ingestion of four diets providing the same chemically determined "available" (FDNB reactive) lysine, on pigs of
average 41, 57 and 74 kg live weight (vertical lines mark S.D.).

"available" feacal lysine were recorded with different analytical procedures which indicates that the lysine "balance" and lysine digestibility values should be treated with reserve (Ostrowski, 1970a).

The experiments carried out so far suggest that, within certain limits, most of the variability in the performance and nitrogen metabolism of genetically similar pigs could be accounted for in terms of differences.in "available" lysine intake. The question arose however whether the dietary FDNB-reactive lysine, chemically determined as "available", and lysine digestibility correspond with the lysine which is actually absorbed and can be determined by the lysine appearance in the blood after the meal and also how these changes correlate with the growth assay, lysine digestibility and nitrogen retention of animals.

Plasma Lysine as an Indication of Lysine Avail-
bility from the Diet

Even though the diets containing the same amounts of "available" (FDNB-reactive) lysine, produced similar results as measured by growth rate, the appearance of lysine in systemic blood after ingestion of meal is dissimilar as measured by the area or the height of the lysine peaks (Figure 13). In all cases free lysine concentration in pigs' plasma, reached the maximum between the first and third hour after ingestion of feed. The fasting lysine level was similar despite the diet used. When lysine values were expressed as percent of the 18 hr fast level (time 0) and then

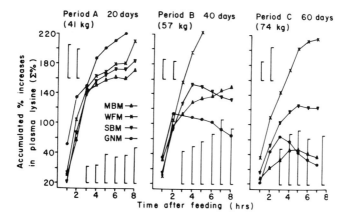

Figure 14.   Changes in relative plasma lysine concentrations and expressed as accumulated increases in plasma levels given as percentages of fast lysine contents after ingestion of the meal containing four protein concentrates(vertical lines mark S.D.).

TABLE 14

Pooled within groups correlation coefficients[1] between plasma
lysine picture after ingestion of feed and body weight gains, N-
retention and dietary total and "available" lysine.

Measurement	Blood Sampling Time After Meal (hr)	Live Weight Gains (g/24 hr)	Nitrogen Retention (g/24 hr)	Dietary Lysine (% DM)	
				Total	FDNB-reactive ("available")
Plasma Lysine	0	0.593**	0.584**	-0.023	-0.015
(mg/100 ml)	1	0.490*	0.499*	0.747**	0.726**
	2	-0.252	-0.233	-0.182	-0.181
Accumulative	1	0.230	0.258	0.001	0.619**
Relative Plasma	2	-0.111	-0.062	0.077	0.412
Level (%)	3	-0.242	-0.176	0.212	0.275

[1] Based on 20 animals (17 d.f.)

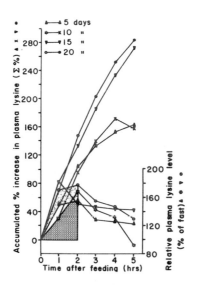

Figure 15. Changes in the relative plasma lysine concentrations expressed as percent of plasma fast level (open asterisks),
and/or accumulated increases in relative plasma levels (closed
asterisks) summed up after ingestion of meal consumed by pigs over
5, 10, 15 or 20 days.

when the percentage increases were accumulated over the blood collection period, similar values were obtained in the third hour after the meal in young pigs (41 kg) despite the protein concentrate used as a protein source (Figure 14). This would suggest the use of such a "3 hour plasma lysine test" as an indication of lysine absorption, and lysine availability of pigs. However, despite the same pigs and diets being used on two other occasions, when the pigs were older (57 or 74 kg), big variations in accumulated lysine percentages were observed after the meal. This indicates that the age of pigs, used as test animals, had a pronounced effect on the lysine picture in the blood plasma after ingestion of feed. Davey et al. (1973) reported a similar tendency. This suggests the use of rather younger animals for lysine absorption studies so as to obtain clear and/or a more consistent response to dietary lysine. Figure 15 also demonstrates the affect of the length of the introductory feeding period before blood sampling on the lysine concentration in the blood plasma after the meal. The longer the period of feeding with the test diet before blood sampling, the earlier the appearance of the peak after the meal.

When the nitrogen balance results from the series of balance periods which ended with consecutive blood sampling were then used to determine the degree of correlation with plasma lysine after the meal and with production results on a pooled, within group basis (Table 14), then live weight gains and nitrogen retention (g/24 hr) were highly correlated with fasting lysine level and plasma lysine level at one hour after the meal was significantly correlated with feed conversion efficiency, nitrogen retention and both dietary total and available lysine levels. Accumulative relative plasma lysine values were significantly correlated with protein conversion efficiency from (r=-0.620 to -0.793) and also in the first hour after the meal with dietary "available" lysine (r=0.619). There were however no significant correlations between the plasma lysine picture expressed as change in relative values over 3 hours after the meal, and the dietary both total and "available" lysine in protein concentrates used as a lysine source. It appears from the correlation coefficients that dietary lysine can be related to plasma lysine concentration as determined in the first hour after the meal. However, in another experiment (see Table 10 and Figure 11), while L-lysine, administered together with DL-methionine, increased plasma lysine levels after the meal (despite the mode of amino acids administration to pigs) there was no significant correlation between the blood plasma lysine profiles and both growth rate and/or nitrogen metabolism data.

Pigs responded to DL-methionine supplementation to a much higher extent than they did to L-lysine supplementation (see Tables 8 & 9). This indicates that the deficiency of sulfur containing amino acids has much more destructive effects on production results and nitrogen metabolism of pigs than does the deficiency of lysine, a fact which has also been observed by Said, Hegstead &

Hays (1974). They demonstrated that an animal given a lysine-free
diet does not lose body nitrogen at the rate comparable to other
essential amino acids. Looking at lysine appearances in the systemic blood plasma after meals containing different quantities of
sulfur amino acids at constant lysine level (Figure 10) one could
conclude that methionine stimulates lysine absorption from the diet.

The plasma lysine picture observed in the first 3 hours after
ingestion of the meal can give useful complementary information on
the rate and degree of lysine absorption from the diet which can
characterise dietary lysine sufficiency or imbalance with other
amino acids on a relative-qualitative rather than on a quantitative
basis.

The question arises whether systemic venous blood can characterise the extent of dietary lysine absorption and utilisation
from feeds. The majority of experiments on amino acids absorption
were based on analyses of portal blood. Christensen (1964) showed
that sampling of the venous plasma of the systemic blood circulation produced similar changes in the amino acid levels to those
occuring in the portal blood plasma but to a lesser extent. Rolls,
Porter & Westgarth (1972) found even higher systemic and lower portal lysine concentrations in rats with a particularly sharp rise
in systemic plasma lysine in the first hour after ingestion of
lysine supplemented protein with portal lysine showing less distinctive changes after the ingestion of a similar meal.

Correlations between both the dietary lysine and "available"
lysine and the extent to which lysine concentrations in peripheral
plasma increased after the administration of various diets in different modes is rather conflicting and difficult to explain. It is
believed that the pattern of appearance for amino acids in peripheral plasma is unrelated to the dietary amino acids as digested
(Nasset, 1963) since the influence of liver and tissue uptake and
release of amino acids makes for the ingested protein to be mixed
with several times its mass of endogenous protein so that an amino
acid mixture as absorbed from the intestines to the portal blood is
of relatively constant composition. Nasset's (196) postulation
was questioned by number of workers (Marrs, et al., 1975; Varnish
& Carpenter, 1975b) and the results presented so far do not
support Nasset's theory either.

Analyses of the amino acids in blood plasma are laborious and
time consuming so that in order to find some simpler method to
observe the degree of lysine absorption from the ingested diet a
physico-chemical method, chemiluminescence was applied for lysine
balance studies. Blood lysine levels after ingestion of the meal
(Figure 16B) were related to dietary lysine and nitrogen balance
results (Figure 16A). Chemiluminescence of the peripheral blood
gives profiles of overall enzyme activity changes similar to those
as observed with blood lysine after the meal (Figure 17). When

the chemiluminsecence activity was correlated with dietary lysine
and then with chemically determined dietary "available" lysine then
correlation coefficients were 0.735 and 0.942 respectively. On the
other hand chemiluminescence values of the whole blood and nitrogen
retention of pigs were also highly correlated : 0.771 for blood
sampled after starvation and 0.924 for blood sampled 1 hour after
the meal. Despite a number of factors which can affect biolumin-
escence activity other than lysine it appears that this technique,
after proper standardisation for a definite purpose (e.g. for lysine or other amino acids absorption studies) could be a valuable
fast screening procedure to predict nutritional value of diets,
foods and feeds(Ostrowski, 1972a).

Rolls, Porter & Westgarth (1972) and Davey et al. (1973) emphasised that because of the many factors influencing the plasma
amino acid picture, its utility as an indication of lysine absorption from the diet remains in doubt. This is mainly due to the
incomplete knowledge of factors responsible for the variation in
the availability of individual amino acids. Some of the factors
are discussed further using lysine as an example.

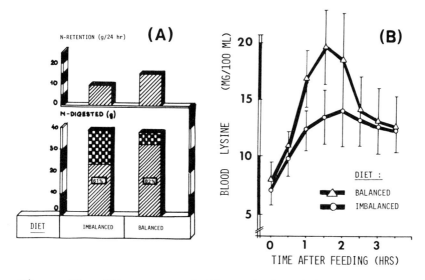

Figure 16. Nitrogen metabolism of pigs (A) consuming low
protein of plant origin diet either without (imbalanced diet) or
with supplements providing macro- and micro-nutrients according to
ARC (1967) requirement levels (balanced diet) as well as corresponding lysine concentrations in the whole blood (B) after feeding
with these two diets (Ostrowski, 1972a).

SOME FACTORS AFFECTING LYSINE ABSORPTION AND APPEARANCE IN
THE BLOOD PLASMA - RELIABILITY OF PLASMA LYSINE TEST

Explanation of the relationship between the dietary amino acid
composition and appearances of free amino acids in systemic blood
is not an easy task since in addition to all the controversial
issues mentioned earlier, Elwyn (1969) demonstrated on a cannulated
dog that after feeding a meal the greater part of amino acid load
absorbed from intestine does not pass through the liver but about
60% is transformed within the liver into urea, about 20% into liver
protein and about 10% into plasma proteins leaving only some 10%
for distribution to other tissues by way of systemic circulation.

Interpretation of the plasma aminograms can be even more complicated by the fact that when pigs were fed semipurified diet composed of starch, glucose and celulose without any source of protein or amino acids then plasma lysine concentrations in systemic
blood after the meal increased showing a similar profile as observed with pigs fed with the same diet in which 20% of wheat starch
was replaced by casein (Figure 18). The most confused results
however were obtained with starved pigs (without the meal) which
were allocated in metabolic cages next to animals fed semipurified
diet either protein free or with casein supplement. Despite the
fact that the other animals were fed while these starved pigs were
not, a sharp peak of lysine appeared in their systemic blood plasma
1 hour after the time when the starved pigs were usually fed a

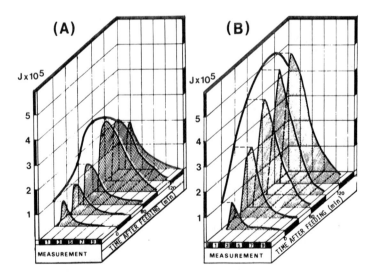

Figure 17. Photon emission (J) of blood as measured by chemiluminescence technique after ingestion of either lysine deficient
(A) or lysine balanced diet (B).

morning meal. This last result demonstrates our incomplete knowledge of amino acid metabolism in the organism supporting the concept of diurnal cycles in polysome aggregation and disaggregation
as mentioned by Munro (1970), and also giving some additional
evidence to the supporters of the labile amino acids reserves in
the tissues (Christensen, 1964).

Diurnal cycles however can be completely dissynchronised by
physical and/or climatic stressors. Figure 19 demonstrates the
example of pigs which were immediately after the meal exposed to
pain stress, by applying pressure to a wire loop through a pig's
nose for a two minute period. After the stressor application, the
lysine plasma concentration level fell notably only to be followed
by an increase with maximum lysine concentration much below that
as observed without stress application. A similar effect was
observed when with the end of the meal pigs were exposed for next
1 hour to cold at 4°C climatic stressor. The immediate decrease
in lysine concentration was followed by the return to the level
before the food intake, (Figure 19B), however, without the characteristic "peak" formation as observed in all previously presented
studies. The first major metabolic response to short-term stress
appears to be a lowering in apparent digestibility of dietary
protein (Ostrowski, 1975a) with a simultaneous but slight increase
in fat digestion (Figure 19A).

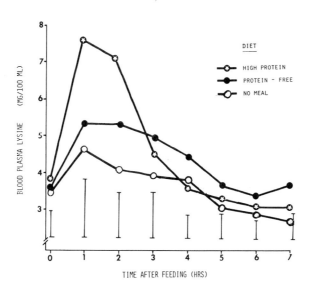

Figure 18. Lysine concentrations in peripheral blood plasma
after ingestion of semi-purified diet either: high in protein (20%)
(✪) and protein free (●), or by animals deprived of the regular
meal while other animals were fed (○).

In reference to results presented in <u>Figure 17</u> it is reasonable to suppose that the depressions in plasma amino acid concentrations immediately after ingestion of feed as reported by
Longenecker & House (1961) on dogs and Krysciak, Ostrowski & Rys
(1966) could be due to the stress factor connected with the particular techniques applied for blood sampling after the meal.

All the above results demonstrate the difficulties connected
with the standardisation of the plasma lysine test as an indication
of quantitative lysine absorption from the practical diets.   While
Said, Hegsted & Hays (1974) pointed out that lysine is the most
abberant essential amino acid the question remains why does lysine
in the blood plasma not reflect the quantity of lysine in the ingested diet - in biologically accessible - "available" form - and
why the lack of protein and lysine in the meal results in an increase in plasma lysine concentrations which would be ascribed to
the digestion of the lysine containing diet.

DIETARY FORMULATION AND AMINO ACID SUPPLEMENTATION

The question arises whether we have sufficient knowledge of
the regulatory mechanism of plasma and tissue free amino acid concentrations to explain animals' responses to dietary lysine and
methionine deficiency and amino acid supplementation and the possible disproportions between them? Harper and Benevenga (1970)

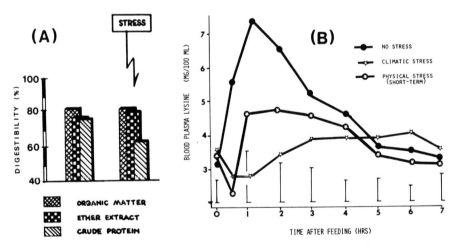

Figure 19.   Changes in apparent digestibility coefficients as
a result of application of short term physical stress (A) and lysine concentrations in peripheral blood plasma after the meal (B)
followed by the application of etiher short-term physical stress
(●) or longer-term, climatic stress (4°C for 1 hr) (✡).

discussed three possible types of organism responses to disproportionate amounts of amino acids in the diet. Alternatively an
organism may (1) tolerate a measure of disproportion among the
dietary amino acids without showing evidence of adverse effects,
(2) depending upon physiological and nutritional state tolerance
of the organism as mentioned in (1) can vary and (3) depending upon the degree of disproportion of dietary amino acids there is a
continuous gradation of disproportion effects on organism from
innocuous to toxic. The data presented and discussed in this
paper can generally fall into all these three categories. However,
the knowledge of the general trend in amino acid homeostatic
regulation and wisdom on the processes that contribute to regulation of free amino acid concentrations including tissue protein
synthesis and degradation and amino acid degradation and excretion
do not help to provide the practical measure of availability of
the amino acids from the diet and dietary supplements. As was
shown in Figure 18 a protein meal is not necessary to produce
evidence of amino acid "absorption" from the hypothetical protein
which does not exist. The effect of the digestion of protein-
free diet can be measured as an increase in plasma lysine concentrations similar to those observed with the normal high protein
and high lysine diet. On the other hand, a high dietary lysine
level cannot produce any evidence of lysine presence in the diet
when animals are subject to stress after being fed (Figure 19).
In a way this supports the theory about homeostatic regulation,
in a slightly different form as that presented by Harper and
Benevenga (1970), and again opens discussion on amino acids accumulation in the body and labile amino acid reserves in the tissues
which "do not tend to be extensively depleted even in fasting" -
an observation made by Van Slyke and Mayer in 1913. Discussion of
this problem however exceeds the limit of this presentation. One
fact remains obvious and that is that the proper dietary formulation can increase the nutritional value of low quality feeds of
plant origin to be similar or even higher than those of high quality - animal origin feedstuffs. In Table 15 a result of such a
formulation is demonstrated when by supplementing synthetic amino
acids and synthetic fatty acids to a low protein plant origin diet,
with a simultaneous balancing of other biologically active substances to the recommended requirement levels, the production
effects and nitrogen balance of pigs were even better than those
obtained on high protein of animal origin diet.

The results demonstrated in this paper indicate that the
quantities of amino acids supplementation should be calculated
from the quantities necessary to cover animals' needs, as determined by the appropriate requirement tables and from actual concentrations of amino acids in the dietary components. This taking
into consideration, the biological availability of amino acids in
basic formulated diets and in the products used as sources of
amino acids supplement. Hence the problem of choice of the most
appropriate assay to determine concentrations of nutritionally -

TABLE 15

Performance and nitrogen metabolism of pigs fed either animal-origin, high protein diet or low protein, plant-origin diet without or with synthetic amino acids (AA) and synthetic fatty acids (FA) supplementation (Ostrowski, Ryś & Morstin, 1972).

Supplements & Measurement	High Protein, Animal Origin Diet		Low Protein, Plant Origin Diet		
Supplements	–	FA	–	AA	AA+FA
PRODUCTION RESULTS:					
Average daily gains (g/24 hr)	640	651	506	604	724
Protein (N X 6.25) conversion efficiency (g/1 kg gain)	488	401	529	494	413
Meat/fat relation	2.95	2.71	2.91	2.73	2.79
NITROGEN METABOLISM DATA:					
Apparent N-digestibility (%)	81	80	64	78	92
N-retention (g/24 hr)	16.4	19.2	13.1	16.3	18.6

biologically active essential amino acids in foods, feeds and diets. This is particularly important when foods and feeds are heat treated during processing which causes damage to protein and reduction in contents of amino acid "accessible" to organism.

ANALYSIS OF SUPPLEMENTED AMINO ACIDS IN FOODS AND FEEDS
- CHOICE OF METHOD

At present the choice of method for amino acid balance study and/or technique for measuring physiological "sufficiency" of limiting amino acid in the consumed diet and the effect of amino acid supplementation to the diet in nutritional practice is the matter of compromise between less or more inaccurate chemical or biological methods, their simplicity and efficiency in labor and economy terms.

In recent years a number of different methods have been proposed for the control of protein damage in processed foods and feedstuffs. A large proportion of these methods, particularly in reference to processed high protein foods and feedstuffs, is based on the determination of availability of the amino acids most limiting in foods and practical diets, i.e. sulfur amino acids - methionine and cystine, lysine, tryptophan and isoleucine (Carpenter and Woodham, 1974; Boyne et al., 1975).

Combs & Nott (1967) attempted to tabulate the amino acid availability of all the main sources of protein in poultry diets in the U.S.A. The values are approximate "guestimetes" and were designed for average quality foodstuffs, i.e. typical products used commercially. According to the classification given originally by Combs & Nott (1967) and slightly modified later (Allen, 1973) average amino acid availabilities of typical feedstuffs for use in formulation of the diets for poultry ranged from 100 - 95% in milk through to 65% in blood meal and feather meal. According to Carpenter (1974) tabulated availability figures give reasonable estimates of available amino acid content under condition that the foodstuffs are of average quality - an assumption which again needs to be tested. The only means by which quality of processed foods or feeds can be proved in terms of amino acids "sufficiency" is chemical and/or biological test.

Chemical Procedures for Amino Acid "Availability" Determination

In general practice the damage to proteins as a result of technological processing and/or storage are measured by the changes in "available" lysine content, as this amino acid is easy to determine both chemically and biologically, (Carpenter & Booth, 1973). Also for "available" methionine and cystine determination both chemical and biological assays are used (Pieniazek et al. 1975) however to a lesser extent. "Available" isoleucine and tryptophan can be determined in biological assay only which is not recommended for general use due to lack of accuracy in the procedure.

The major problem associated with analysis of amino acid availability in various processed foods and feeds is the most convenient and accurate method which should be used for availability determination. Table 16 demonstrates on lysine example that different chemical procedures are giving different indications of "availability" in standard protein due to various type of heat treatment. A distinctive discrepancy between the various methods is rather confusing for the feed formulator who would like to know the correct analytical result rather than methodological problem which is of no value for the computer operator who is programming and formulating practical diets and who has to use absolute results in terms of definite values. Validity of the analytical determinations for practical use can be checked in biological assays. (Erbersdobler, 1976).

Biological Assays for Amino Acid "Availability" Determination

A number of biological assays for determining amino acid availability have been proposed which can be grouped as microbiological, enzymic and those biological tests based on digestibility

TABLE 16

Variation in lysine "availability" results determined using different chemical techniques as a result of various types of heat treatment and/or storage of bovine plasma albumin.

Procedure	Unprocessed & unstored bovine plasma albumin	TYPE OF REACTION[1]			
		Maillard		Protein:Protein	
		Early (2)	Advanced(3)	without heating (4)	heated (5)
REACTIVE LYSINE	(g/16g N)				
FDNB-reactive: "direct" (Carpenter, 1960)	12.6	93	30	47	19
FDNB-reactive:"by differen ce (Ostrowski et al.,1970)	12.8	91	33	76	28
TNBS-reactive: "direct" (Kakade & Liener, 1969)	11.5	95	29	79	25
DYE-BINDING CAPACITY	(mM/16g N)				
Acid Orange G 12 (Hurrel & Carpenter, 1974)	133	84	15	105	96
Remazol Brilliant Blue (Pruss & Ney, 1972)	257	89	18	60	8
Cresol Red (Fröhlich, 1954)	1.05	11	92	179	214

[1] All values expressed as percentages of the corresponding value for unstored and unheated bovine plasma albumin.

[2] Storage in plastic containers at $22^{\circ}C$ at 8.2% moisture content for 4 weeks.

[3] Heating at $135^{\circ}C$ for 24 hr.

[4] Storage of the mixture of bovine plasma albumin and glucose at $22^{\circ}C$ at 8.2% moisture for 4 weeks.

[5] As (4) followed by heat treatment at $135^{\circ}C$ for 30 minutes.

in vivo and in vitro, animal growth assays and plasma amino acid
levels (Carpenter & Booth, 1973).

From microorganisms used for amino acid availability studies
those commonly used are : Leuconostoc mesenteroides and Strepto-
coccus faecalis - for percentage lysine availability and/or digestible lysine evaluation ; Streptoccus zymogenes - proteolytic
microorganism; for most of the essential amino acids availability
except for lysine (it does not require lysine for growth) and
Tetrahymena pyriformis - the protozoon with proteolytic power; for
available lysine estimation. (Boyne et al., 1975; Shorrock, 1976).

Enzymic digestion of protein in vitro followed by amino acid
activity estimation using several micro organisms is a short and
convenient method for determining biological "accessibility" of
amino acids from processed foods or feeds. However, despite the
advantages of using microbiological assays there is a general re-
luctance among quality-control laboratories to apply them in
practice. This is probably due to a strong chemical orientation in
some centres while other centres dealing with test animals in terms
of both classification and reasonable size to be handled "mis-treat"
this type of test organism.

Amino acid digestibility in vivo is based on the measurement
of amino acid intake and the amounts of amino acids excreted in
the faeces. The interpretation of the amino acid digestibility
values for estimating digestibility and biological value of proteins is complicated by the existence of a micro-flora in the large
intestines which can cause, by uncontrolled fermentation, a modification to undigested protein residues and which can make for
misleading digestibility values. However, this technique does
give a good indication of changes in nutritional value of processed
foods resulting from dietary amino acid composition and their
biological "availability". (Dammers,1964; Varnish and Carpenter,
1975).

Despite amino acid levels in blood plasma reflecting changes
in dietary amino acid concentrations this assay is subject to great
biological variation and to difficulties in its standardisation.
Hence, its effective usefulness as a criterion in food and feed
formulation is in doubt. The complex aspect of this problem has
already been shown earlier on the lysine example.

Animal growth assays despite the fact they are expensive, slow
and "inprecise" (in chemical terms), due to great variational
response between individual animals, are according to Carpenter
(1973) the only measure and practical check-up of chemical and
microbiological tests. By observation of growth in various more or
less complicated tests on laboratory or farm animals as a result of

TABLE 17

Correlation of the results from production experiment on pigs with those obtained in the test with rats (Ostrowski, Morstin & Kościńska, 1972).[1]

Total lysine	0.67	0.68	0.68	0.69	0.69
Lysine availability (%)	81	79	75	72	67

	Correlation Coefficients (r)	
	P I G S :	
R A T S :	Live Weight g.	Protein Conversion
Live weight gains	0.026	-0.171
Protein conversion	-0.171	0.504
NPU	-0.236	-0.268
PER	-0.018	-0.540

[1] Productive experiment on pigs from 30 to 96 kg and on rats 14 days; feeding system ad libitum; Diet:Barley (30%), Rye (15%), Maize (15%), Oat (7%) & Potato Flakes (40%) mixed in various proportions with wheatings, soyabean meal, fish meal and cotton seed meal to obtain constant dietary 9.7% of digestible protein concentration.

practical application of the tested food, feed or complete diet we can claim for the nutritive relevance of values. The final result of the growth test can be taken as an absolute measure of the nutritional value of the tested material - a value which is measured in productive results showing the degree to which the nutritional value of the diet or proteinaceous material could be improved. The biological test, most commonly used in nutritional practice, is the biological value test with rats in which additional information could be obtained regarding protein efficiency ration (PER) and net protein utilization (NPU). The biological value of proteins (BV) is regarded as dependent upon amino acid composition. This supposition assumes that all proteins are completely hydrolysed in the digestive tract to free amino acids and that amino acids are absorbed by the organism. The results obtained by the three biological measurements, BV, PER and NPU, usually differ and hence in nutritional practice the validity of the tests mentioned above is questioned in terms of their application to amino acid supplementation and availability studies (Woodham & Clarke, 1977).

There is also a number of predictive biochemical methods for
BV evaluation, the most common being the Amino Acid Score known
also as "chemical score" and Essential Amino Acid Index (EAAI).
The amino acid score is based on the analysis of the limiting amino
acids, without taking into account their availability and their excessive amounts in relation to the requirement of the organism - a
factor contributing to the inaccuracy of this particular test. In
the other test, Essential Amino Acid Index (EAAI), in which all
essential amino acids are incorporated in the calculations, the
same objections apply as to "Chemical Score". It was shown by
Said, Hegsted & Hayes (1974) that in conventional tests on rats BV
or NPU over-estimate the nutritive value of low quality ,lysine-
deficient nutrients and hence rats are not recommended for lysine
deficiency and/or lysine availability studies. When rats were used
for a prediction of nutritive value of formulated diets for pigs
there arose a noticeable discrepancy between predicted and actually
achieved values in practical experiment which caused a lack of
correlation in responses of pigs and rats to the same dietary factor - both in the lysine level and its availability (Table 17).
Another complication with using rats for lysince balance is the
different response of different breeds of rats and sexes to the
same dietary factor. This makes the prediction of results for
pigs in tests on rats far from the expected accuracy for nutritionists and feed formulators (Ostrowski, Morstin & Kościńska,1972).
While tests on rats and their reponse to dietary lysine and its
availability is different depending on breed and sex, the reactions
of pigs to the same factors is definite, even in short term metabolism trials. This is reflected by the high correlation coefficients between dietary lysine, both total and "available", as chemically determined and nitrogen metabolism of pigs ($r = 0.846$ and
0.883 respectively) (Ostrowski 1971b).

It is difficult to decide which of the biological assays is
the more favourable one to use for the detecting the degree of
"availability" of the amino acid added to the protein concentrate
in which content of the biologically-active amino acid was notably
decreased due to heat damage. As shown in Table 18 the degree of
the amino acid damage due to heat treatment and lysine supplementation determined by different biological methods varied and
depended on the test used. This can cause serious controversy
between chemical and biological or nutritional laboratories
confusing the feed formulator. Hence, the growth test with the
use of diets and animals for which the diet is formulated and
supplemented with the appropriate quantity of amino acids remains
the most valuable and practical biological test. Various factors
however, which can influence the growth of the test animal (change
in amino acid balance of the whole diet, system of supplément's
administration etc.), cannot be eliminated in the single test and
hence growth tests are usually carried out in several alternative,
long-term experiments before the more or less definite and undoubtful answers can be known.

TABLE 18

"Sensitivity" of various biological assays in measuring the degree
of different types of heat damage to milk protein and the response
to L-lysine supplementation.[1]

Measurement	Not heated	SPRAY-DRIED MILK Heated[1]	
		unsup-plemented	supplement-ed with L-lysine[2]
CRUDE PROTEIN (N x 6.25)(%DM)	32.5	99	124
LYSINE (g/16gN):			
Total	6.7	94	123
"Available" (FDNB-reactive)	4.9	61	100
ENZYMIC in vitro DIGESTION (%):			
Nitrogen	95	91	90
Lysine	97	87	83
In vivo DIGESTION (%):			
Rats	88	82	81
Pigs	93	89	87
BLOOD LYSINE(mg/100ml):			
Fast Level: rats	4.7	87	91
pigs	7.3	63	94
1 hr after meal: rats	14.5	71	90
pigs	19.8	66	97
PLASMA LYSINE(mg/100ml):			
Fast Level: rats	3.8	103	98
pigs	4.6	99	102
1 hr after meal: rats	7.3	86	97
pigs	6.1	90	109
GROWTH ASSAY (RATS):			
BV	0.83	69	91
NPU	0.61	53	70
PER	2.72	76	93
Slope-Ratio	86	81	97
N-digestibility (%)	79	87	95
Lysine digestibility (%)	88	86	78
GROWTH ASSAY (PIGS):			
Growth rate (g/24hr)	647	84	97
Protein conversion(kg/kg gain)	393	146	112
N-retention (g/24h)	17.3	62	93

[1] Values of heated milk expressed as percentage of the corresponding value for unheated milk.

[2] L-lysine was supplemented to balance loss of lysine in spray-
dried milk due to heating as chemically determined.

Nevertheless,it appears from the data presented in this paper that biological and nutritional consequences of amino acid "disorders" in the diet as well as the consequences of dietary amino acid modification by proper amino acid and other biological active substances supplementation should be studied on organisms for which prediction is made about consequential benefits of such modification as measured by metabolic indices and/or in productive terms. One can question, whether there is any point in continuing to analyse the reduction in nutritional value of proteinaceous products due to processing and storage by application of more or less accurate chemical or short-term biological tests. If so, to do this with full knowledge of the methodological inaccuracies, imperfections and restrictions in practical application of the chosen method.

Simple chemical methods (e.g. _in vitro_ or dye binding methods) can give as valid prediction as do complicated biological tests once restrictions in application of the chosen method to measure particular type of effects are clearly known and specified. In other words, each of the methods discussed in this presentation could be used in food science and nutritional practice, but with certain limitations in its application to specific processes and to various types of processed or raw products and type of ration or diet.

SUMMARY

Analysing data with lysine deposition in the muscles and liver, absorption of lysine from the diet, as measured by lysine digestibility and lysine plasma profiles after ingestion of meal as a result of dietary lysine concentration and its chemically determined availability, one can conclude that none of the measures as discussed in this paper gives undoubtful indication of lysine physiological sufficiency, and "accessibility" for the metabolic functions and production effects of growing animals. Despite a number of significant correlations between various measurements characterising nutritional _status quo_ in both diet and organism as due to deficiency or supplementation with deficient amino acid, further explanations for a number of conflicting results cannot be given without further studies. It is reasonable to suppose however that the organism has a well developed adaptation mechanism allowing him to conserve lysine and other amino acids for the period of time when ingested diet is completely deficient or contains insufficient amounts of amino acid. This natural "protective" and "defensive" side of amino acid metabolism in living organism suggests we turn our attention to the controversial labile amino acid pool and amino acid storage problem in the tissues in order to explain several conflicting findings in the amino acid metabolism area.

It appears also from the results presented that despite the method used for lysine deficiency and/or lysine availability determination, it is more appropriate to formulate diets for pigs taking into account the concentration of limiting amino acids (lysine and sulfur containing amino acids) and lysine "availability" rather than the dietary protein level. Once the essential amino acids, other biologically-active substances and energy in the practical diet are well balanced and supplied in amounts covering the physiological and productive demands, the dietary protein level can be substanitally decreased far below the traditionally established levels. Together with a decrease in absolute amounts of protein fed to pigs, protein of animal origin can be completely eliminated and replaced by feeds of lower nutritional value without deteriorating the productive effects. This can be achieved by a proper formulation process of diets with a physiological balance of nutrients (supplementation, fortification, processing, etc.). As was demonstrated in this paper, using all available technical, biochemical and nutritional knowledge it is possible to modify foods and feeds of low nutritional value to be of high quality and nutritionally "optimal" and hence fully productive and highly efficient in both biological and economic terms.

ACKNOWLEDGEMENTS

The work was initiated at the Rowett Research Institute, Bucksburn, Aberdeen, Scotland, when the author was in receipt of a grant from the Food and Agriculture Organisation of the United Nations, and continued at the Nutritional Biochemistry Department, Division of Animal Nutrition, Institute of Zootechnics in Cracow, Poland, then when the author was in receipt of a grant from the New Zealand National Research Advisory Council at the Nutrition Centre, Ruakura Research Station, Hamilton, New Zealand and finally in Biochemistry Department, Bendigo College of Advanced Education, Bendigo, Victoria, Australia. Thanks are due to Dr. A. S. Jones and Professor D. R. Ryś for giving the use of facilities to conduct the experiments and also to Dr. J. B. Hutton and Mr. R. McKenzie for opportunity to work on the problem in their Departments.

REFERENCES

Agricultural Research Council (1967). Nutrient Requirement of Farm Livestock. No. 3, Pigs, London.

Allen, R. D. (1973). Ingredient Analysis Table, Feedstuffs Yearbook. Miller Publ. Co. Minneapolis. 24.

Ashley, J. H. and Fisher, H. (1967). Protein reserves and muscle constituents of protein-depleted and repleted cocks. Br. J. Nutr., 21, 661-670.

Boyne, A. W., Ford, J. E., Hewitt, D. and Schrimpton, D. H. (1975).
    Protein quality of feeding-stuffs. 7. Collaborative studies
    on the microbiological assay of available amino acids. Br. J.
    Nutr., 34, 153-162.
Carpenter, K. J. (1960). The estimation of available lysine in
    animal-protein foods. J. Biochem., 77, 604-10.
Carpenter, K. J. (1974). Problems of amino-acid availability. In,
    'Nutrition Conference for Feed Manufacturers', H. Swan and
    D. Lewis (editors). University of Nottingham, London, Butter-
    worths, 71-89.
Carpenter, K. J. and Booth, V. H. (1973). Damage to lysine in food
    processing : its measurement and its significance. Nutr.
    Abstr. Rev., 43, 6, 423-447.
Carpenter, K. J. and Woodham, A. A. (1974). Protein quality of
    feeding-stuffs. 6. Comparison of the results of collaborative
    biological assays for amino acids with those of other methods.
    Br. J. Nutr., 32, 647-660.
Clausen, H. (1965). The protein requirements of growing meat-type
    pigs. World Rev. Anim. Prod., 1, 1-28.
Combs, . F. and Nott, H. (1967). Amino acid availability of the
    protein sources used in poultry diets. Feedstuffs, 39, Oct. 21,
    36.
Christensen, H. W. (1964). Free amino acids and peptides in
    tissues. In, 'Mammalian Protein Metabolism' Vol.I, Chapter 4.
    H. N. Munro and J. B. Allison, (Editors). Academic Press, New
    York and London, 105-124.
Dagliesh, C. E. and Tabechian, J. (1956). Comparison of the meta-
    bolism of uniformly 14C Labelled L-Phenyloalenine, L-Tyrosine
    and L-Tryptophan in the rat. Biochem. J. 62, 625.
Dammers, J. (1964). Digestibility in the pig. Factors influencing
    the digestion of the components of the feed and the digest-
    ibility of the amino acids. Inst. Veevoedingsonderzoek,
    'Hoorn', 1-152.
Davey, R. J., Phelps, J. W. and Thomas, C. H. (1973). Plasma free
    amino acids of swine as influenced by diet protein level,
    animal age and time of sampling. J. Anim. Sci., 37, 1, 81.
Elwyn, D. (1969). In, 'Mammalian Protein Metabolism', H. N. Munro
    (Editor). Academic Press, New York.
Erbersdobler,H.F.(1976). Amino acid availability. In, 'Protein
    Metabolism and Nutrition', D. J. A. Cole, K. N. Borrman, P. J.
    Buttery, D. Lewis, R. J. Neale and H. Swan (Editors). Butter-
    worths, London.
Fisher, H. (1967). Nutritional aspects of protein reserves. In,
    'Newer Methods of Nutritional Biochemistry'. A. A. Albanese,
    (Editor) Vol. 3, Chapter 2. New York and London: Academic
    Press, 101-124.
Fröhlich, A. (1954). Reaction between Phthalein Dyes and heated
    foodstudffs. Nature, 174, 879.

Harper, A. E. (1968). Diet and plasma amino acids. Am. J. Clin. Nutr. 21, 5, 358-366.

Harper, A. E. and Benevenga, N. J. (1970). Effects of disproportionate amounts of amino acids. In, 'Proteins as Human Food', R. A. Lawrie (Editor). Academic Press, Cambridge, 417-447.

Holmes, J. H. G., Bayley, H. S., Leadbeater, P. A., Horney, F. D. (1974). Digestion of protein in small intestine of the pig. Br. J. Nutr., 32, 479-489.

Hurrell, R. F. and Carpenter, K. J. (1974). Mechanism of heat damage in proteins. 4. The reactive lysine content of heat-damaged material as measured in different ways. Br. J. Nutr., 32, 589-604.

Hurrell R. F. and Carpenter, K. J. (1977). Nutritional significance of cross-link formation during food processing. In, 'Protein crosslinking : Nutritional and medical consequences', M.Friedman (Editor). Plenum Publishing Company, New York. 231-244.

Kakade, M. L. and Liener, I. E. (1969). Determination of available lysine in proteins. Anal. Biochem., 27. 273-280.

Kelly, M. and Scott, H. M. (1968). Plasma lysine titers in the chick in relation to source of lysine and mode of administration. J. Nutr., 94, 326-330.

Koreleski, J. and Ostrowski, H. T. (1970). The effect of nitrogen fertilisers on nutritional value of potatoes proteins. Bull. Inst. Zootech., 3/58, 57-69.

Krysciak, J., Ostrowski, H. T. and Rys, R. (1966). Changes in the content of free amino acids in pig blood plasma after ingestion of food. Acta biochem. pol., 13, 229-235.

Longenecker, J. B., House, N. L. (1959). Relationship between plasma amino acids and composition of the ingested protein. Arch. Biochem. Biophys., 84, 46-52.

Longenecker, J. B. and House, N. L. (1961). Relationship between plasma amino acids and composition of ingested protein. II. A shortened procedure to determine plasma amino acid ratios. Am. J. Clin. Nutr., 4, 356-364.

Longenecker, J. B. (1963). Utilisation of Dietary Proteins. In, 'Never Methods Nutritional Biochemistry', A. A. Albanese (Editor), Vol. 1, Academic Press, New York and London, 113-144.

Marrs, T. C., Addison, J. M., Burston, D. and Matthews, D. M. (1975). Changes in plasma amino acid concentrations in man after ingestion of an amino acid mixture simulating casein, and tryptic hydrolysate of casein. Br. J. Nutr., 34, 259-265.

Munro, H. N. (1964). General aspects of the regulation of protein metabolism by diet and by hormones. In, 'Mammalian Protein Metabolism'. Vol.I, Chapter 10. H. N. Munro and J. B. Allison (Editors), New York and London: Academic Press.

Munro, H. N. (1970). Regulatory mechanisms in mammalian protein metabolism. In, 'Proteins as human food', R. A. Lawrie (Editor). Academic Press, Cambridge. 403-415.

Nasset, E. S., Ganapathy, S. N. and Goldsmith, D. P. S. (1963). Amino acids in dog blood and gut contents after feeding zein. J. Nutr., 81, 343-347.

NRC, (1968). 'Nutrient requirements of swine'. National Academy of Sciences, Research Council, Washington, D.C.

Omstedt, P. T. and Von der Decken, A. (1974). Dietary amino acids: effect of depletion and recovery on protein synthesis in vitro in rat skeletal muscle and liver. Br. J. Nutr., 31, 67-76.

Ostrowski, H. T. (1969). The effects of dietary supplementation with lysine and methionine on body and tissue composition in the pig. Anim. Prod., 11, 4, 521-532.

Ostrowski, H. T. (1970). Some problems concerning errors in the nitrogen and lysine balance studies on animals. Bull. de L Academia Polonaise des Science, Serie des Sciences biologiques. C1. II, XVIII, 11-12, 727-729.

Ostrowski, H. T. (1971). Available lysine as an indication of nutritional evaluation of feedstuffs. IV. An attempt of the application of lysine availability test in feed mixtures as an indication of their nutritional quality in pig nutrition. Bull. Przem. Pasz., 3, 1-8.

Ostrowski, H. T. (1972a). Chemiluminescence as a method for malabsorption syndrome detection. Proc. XIVth Congress Gastroenterology, Praque, p.268.

Ostrowski, H. T. (1972b). Nutritional and physiological role of biostimulators used in "premix" form in feed mixtures. Sci. Publ. Centr. Lab. Feed Ind. Lublin, 1, 12-25, 1972.

Ostrowski, H. T. (1972c). Problem of synergism and antagonism between biostimulators using as component of the feed mixtures for farm animals. Sci. Publ. Centr. Lab. Feed Ind., 1, 26-36.

Ostrowski, H. T. (1972d). Requirements of growing meat type pigs for lysine. Rocz. Nauk rol., 94-B-3, 75-87.

Ostrowski, H. T. (1972e). The studies on premix composition for growing pigs and comparison of the production results with nitrogen balance studies. Scient. Public. Central Lab. Feed Ind., Lublin, 1, 37-80.

Ostrowski, H. T. (1972f). Premixes for growing pigs fed with diets of plant origin with low protein level. Sci. Public. Central Lab. Feed Ind., CLPP, Lublin, 1-139.

Ostrowski, H. T. (1975a). Effect of dietary lysine imbalance on the apparent digestibility of protein, organic matter, and ether extract for pigs. N.Z. J. Agric. Res., 18, 13-18.

Ostrowski, H. T. and Rys, R. (1969). Attempt of total replacement of barley by potato flakes in bacon fattening with simultaneous completion of the diet with synthetic amino acids L-lysine & DL-methionine. Rocz, Nauk Roln., 92-B-1, 71-92.

Ostrowski, H. T., Jones, A. S. and Cadenhead, A. (1970). Availability of lysine in protein concentrates and diets using Carpenter's method & a modified Silcock method. J. Sci. Fd. Agric., 21, 103-107.

Ostrowski, H. T. and Koreleski, J. (1970). The effect of nitrogen fertilisers on nutritional value of cereal protein. Bull. Inst. Zootech., 3/58, 39-56.

Ostrowski, H. T., Jones, A. S. and Cadenhead, A. (1971). Nitrogen Metabolism of the Pig. III. Utilisation of protein from different sources. J. Sci. Fd Agri., 22, 34-37.

Ostrowski, H. T., Ryś, R. and Morstin, E. (1972). The applying synthetic fatty acids & their sodium salts & amino acids in growing pigs nutrition. Rocz. Nauk rol., 94-B-2, 45-52.

Ostrowski, H. T., Ryś, R., Morstin, E. and Kościńska, A. (1972). Studies on the effect of synthetic L-lysine & DL-methionine supplements given to pigs after being mixed with feed or separately two hours after the meal. Bull. Przem. Pasz., 3-4, 75-80.

Ostrowski, H. T., Morstin, E. and Kościńska, A. (1972). A comparison of nutritional value of feed mixtures for pigs in experiments on rats & pigs. Zesz. Probl. Post. Nauk roln., 126, 143-149.

Ostrowski, H. T. and Ryś, R. (1973a). Rapeseed oil meal as a protein component of diets for fattening pigs. I. Rocz. Nauk roln., 94-B-4, 83-103.

Ostrowski, H. T. and Ryś, R. (1973b). Rapeseed oil meal as a protein component of diets for fattening pigs. II. Rocz. Nauk roln., 94-B-4, 105-122.

Pieniążek, D., Rakowska, M., Szkiłłądziowa, W. and Grabarek, Z. (1975). Estimation of available methionine and cysteine in proteins of food products by in vivo and in vitro methods. Br. J. Nutr., 34, 175-190.

Pion, R., Fauconneau, G. and Rerat, A. (1966). Etude de la digestion des proteines chez le proc par la mesure de L'aminoacidemie porte. Cachier No. 6. (Amino acids, peptides, proteins), 326-339.

Pruss, H. D. and Ney, K. H. (1972). Determination of the "available" lysine in whey powder, whey protein and rannet-precipitated casein by the Remazolbrillantblue-R-method. Z. Lebensmitt. - Untersuch. 148. 347-351.

Rerat, A. (1971). La valeur biologique des proteines : quelques acquisitions recentes. Ann. de Zootech., 20, 2, 193-246.

Rerat, A. and Lougnon, J. (1965). Les besoins en amino acides pore en croissance. Cachier A.E.C. No. 6. (Amino acids, peptides, proteins), 342-421.

Richardson, L. R., Hale, F. and Ritchey, S. J. (1965). Effect of fasting and level of dietary protein on free amino acids in pig plasma. J. Anim. Sci., 24, 368-372.

Rolls, B. A., Porter, J. W. G. and Westgarth, D. R. (1972). The course of digestion of different food proteins in rat. III. The absorption of proteins given alone and with supplements of their limiting amino acids. Br. J. Nutr., 28, 283-293.

Said, A. K., Hegsted, D. M. and Hayes, K. C. (1974). Response of adult rats to deficiencies of different essential amino acids. Br. J. Nutr., 31, 47-57.

Schorrock, C. (1976). An improved procedure for the assay of available lysine and methionine in feedstuffs using Tetrahymene pyriformis W. Br. J. Nutr., 35, 333-341.

Van Slyke, D. D. and Meyer, G. M. (1913a). The absorption of amino acids from the blood by the tissues. J. Biol. Chem., 16, 197-212.

Van Slyke, D. D. and Meyer, G. M. (1913b). The locus of chemical transformation of absorbed amino acids. J. Biol. Chem., 16, 213-229.

Van Slyke, D. D. and Meyer, G. M. (1913c). The effect of feeding and fasting on the amino acid content of the tissues. J. Biol. Chem., 16, 231-233.

Varnish, S. A. and Carpenter, K. J. (1975). Mechanism of heat damage in proteins. VI. The digestibility of individual amino acids in heated and propionyleted proteins. Br. J. Nutr., 34, 339-349.

Woodham, A. A. and Clarke, E. M. W. (1977). Nutritive value of mixed proteins. II. As determined by net protein utilisation and protein efficiency ratio tests. Br. J. Nutr., 37, 309-319.

27

N-SUBSTITUTED LYSINES AS SOURCES OF LYSINE IN NUTRITION

Paul-André Finot, Françoise Mottu, Eliane Bujard and

Jean Mauron

Nestlé Products Technical Assistance Co. Ltd.

CH-1814 La Tour-de-Peilz - Switzerland

ABSTRACT

Twenty seven α-N- and ϵ-N-substituted derivatives of lysine belonging to eight different classes: (1)natural dipeptides, (2) α-N-acyl-, (3)ϵ-N-acyl-, (4)ϵ-N-(α-amino acyl)-, (5)ϵ-N-(ω-amino acyl)-, (6)α-N-ϵ-N-di-amino acyl-, (7)ϵ-N-acylglycyl- and (8) Schiff's bases were synthesized. The "in vitro" utilization of some of them was tested by a rat growth assay. Only the derivatives which provided biologically available lysine were hydrolysed by one or more of the intestinal mucosa, liver or kidney homogenates. It is argued that derivatives which can be split by any of the above homogenates are potential sources of lysine. The derivatives of classes (1),(4),(6) and (8) are nearly as efficient as free lysine while lysine in classes (2) and (7) is not utilized at all. From the classes (3) and (5) only some are utilized: ϵ-formyl- and ϵ-acetyl- partially and ϵ-(γ-glutamyl)- totally. The biologically available derivatives were 4 to 7 times less reactive than free lysine in the Maillard reaction and could therefore be used to fortify foods which have to be submitted to severe heat-treatments. A cheap method of synthesis of ϵ-(γ-glutamyl)-lysine is proposed and its metabolic transit described.

INTRODUCTION

Lysine is the limiting essential amino acid in many vegetable proteins, especially cereals. To improve the biological value of

these proteins, particularly for the nutrition of children, whose
lysine requirements are considerable, it is necessary to add this
amino acid in the form of lysine-rich protein or as free lysine
(lysine monohydrochloride). Lysine has on its side chain, however,
a free amino group which is susceptible to reaction with the
surrounding medium, and so it takes part in various chemical
reactions in the course of technological treatments which result
in the formation of biologically non-available derivatives:
reaction with reducing sugars (non-enzymic browning), reaction
with glutaminyl and asparaginyl residues to give isopeptides
(Bjarnason and Carpenter, 1970) formation of lysinoalanine (Bohak,
1964; Patchornick and Sokolovsky, 1964).

A deeper knowledge of the biological availability of lysine
derivatives is thus of particular interest, for two reasons:
firstly, to show to what extent protein-linked lysine whose ε-
amino group has been substituted, either unintentionally during
industrial processing, or deliberately (to give particular functional properties to the proteins), is still biologically available; and secondly to indicate, with a view to enriching lysine
deficient proteins, the biologically available lysine substitutes
having the best efficiency and functional properties better than
that of free lysine.

The biological availability of a certain number of N-substituted lysines has already been described by various authors.
Availability zero for α-N-acetyl-L-lysine (Neuberger and Sanger,
1943; Bjarnason and Carpenter, 1969; Mauron, 1970), for ε-N-
propionyl-L-lysine (Bjarnason and Carpenter, 1969) and for ε-N-
acetylglycyl-L-lysine (Mauron, 1970). Availability of about 50 %
for ε-N-acetyl-L-lysine (Neuberger and Sanger, 1943; Bjarnason and
Carpenter, 1969; Mauron, 1970). Availability of about 80 to 100 %
for ε-N-(γ-L-glutamyl)-L-lysine (Mauron, 1970; Waibel and
Carpenter, 1972), for ε-N-(α-L-glutamyl)-L-lysine and ε-N-glycyl-
L-lysine (Mauron, 1970).

From these fragmentary studies, it is impossible to make
general rules on the relation between the structure of these
lysine derivatives and their utilization as lysine sources in
nutrition. On the other hand, none of these derivatives has been
the object of research on the possible advantages which it could
have over free lysine in nutrition and food technology. This study
bears on 8 classes of lysine derivatives for which the biological
utilization has been determined either directly by growth tests on
rats, or indirectly by studying their "hydrolyzability" by the
homogenates of intestinal mucosa, liver and kidney.

SYNTHESIS OF N-SUBSTITUTED LYSINES

The N-substituted lysines were synthesized by the conventional methods of peptide synthesis (Greenstein and Winitz, 1961; Schröder and Lubke, 1965). All reagents and intermediates necessary for the different syntheses were obtained from Fluka AG, Buchs SG, Switzerland. The natural peptides were supplied by Bachem, Basel, Switzerland. The purity of the derivatives was verified by paper electrophoresis and the lysine content estimated by ion exchange chromatography after acid hydrolysis; this last value was used as a basis for the biological evaluation.

Copper complex of L-lysine : ($C_6H_{14}O_2N_2$, Cu/2, HCl, H_2O according to Greenstein and Winitz, 1961) was used as an intermediate in the synthesis of the ε-N-substituted lysines. It was synthesized as follows : L-lysine monohydrochloride (100 g) was dissolved in 700 ml water; 50 g copper hydroxy-carbonate ($CuCO_3 \cdot Cu(OH)_2$) were added gradually until all CO_2 was released. The solution was then heated for 1 hr at 60°C, filtered and concentrated to 200 ml. The copper complex of lysine was crystallized by adding 1 litre of ethanol to the stirred solution. After keeping the suspension overnight at 4°C, the complex was filtered off and dried at room temperature (m.p. 229-230°C). Elementary analysis gave the following results (with the expected values in parentheses) : C 31.42 (31.00), H 7.28 (7.32), N 12.00 (12.06).

A) Natural peptides

L-alanyl-L-lysine monohydrochloride was purchased from Bachem (m.p. 147 - 150°C). Elementary analysis : C 42.96 (42.60), H 7.76 (7.89), N 16.29 (16.57); % lysine 47.51 (57.59). According to these analyses, this preparation was not pure. It was, however, free from any other ninhydrin positive substance; the purity of the peptide was caculated on the basis of its lysine content.

L-glutamyl-L-lysine was purchased from Bachem, (m.p. 160 - 165°C). Elementary analysis : C 46.86 (48.00), H 7.77 (7.66), N 14.24 (15.27); % lysine 39.71 (53.09). As for the previous peptide, the purity of this preparation free from any other ninhydrin positive substance, was calculated on the basis of its lysine content.

L-lysyl-L-alanyl dihydrobromide was purchased from Bachem. Before utilization, HBr was removed on ion-exchange resin Dowex-2 (form OH⁻). (m.p. 90 - 92°C). Elementary analysis : C 29.07 (28.50), H 5.99 (5.54), N 10.92 (11.08); % lysine 34.55 (38.52).

α-N-glycyl-L-lysine monoacetate was synthesized by the mixed carboxylic-carbonic acid anhydride method (or the mixed anhydride method) according to Erlander and Brand (1951). N-carbobenzoxy-glycine (2.09 g) and triethylamine (1 g) dissolved in 50 ml tetrahydrofuran and cooled at -10°C was treated with isobutyl chloroformiate (1.5 g). After 30 min, ε-N-carbobenzoxy-lysine benzyl ester (3.3 g) dissolved in tetrahydrofurane (80 ml), dimethyl formamide (80 ml) and triethylamine (1.25 g) was added slowly. After several hours, the mixture was added to a large volume of water and the condensation product was crystallized. After hydrogenation on palladium in an acetic acid - ethanol solution (1/1) (Greenstein and Winitz, 1961) the peptide was obtained as monoacetate. Elementary analysis : C 45.65 (45.60), H 8.31 (8.00), N 16.08 (16.00), % lysine 46.18 (55.51).

B) α-N-acyl-L-lysines

α-N-formyl-L-lysine was synthesized according to Hofmann et al. (1960) (m.p. 200 - 201°C). Elementary analysis : C 48.40 (48.27), H 8.22 (8.04), N 16.06 (16.09).

α-N-acetyl-L-lysine was synthesized according to Neuberger and Sanger (1943) (m.p. 225- 226°C with decomposition). Elementary analysis : C 51.20 (51.06), H 8.59 (8.51), N 14.84 (14.89).

C) ε-N-acyl-L-lysines

ε-N-formyl-L-lysine was synthesized according to Hofmann et al. (1960) (m.p. 205°C). Elementary analysis : C 48.33 (48.27), H 8.16 (8.04), N 16.10 (16.09).

ε-N-acetyl-L-lysine was prepared according to Neuberger and Sanger (1943) (m.p. 218 - 219°C). Elementary analysis : C 51.05 (51.06), H 8.72 (8.51), N 14.83 (14.89).

ε-N-lauryl-L-lysine was synthesized by coupling lauric acid chloride (8 g in 150 ml of dimethylformamide) with the copper complex of lysine (12.5 g in 150 ml H_2O treated with 10 g of triethylamine dissolved in 50 ml of dimethylformamide). The blue precipitate obtained, i.e. ε-N-lauryl-L-lysine (copper complex), was filtered off and the copper was removed in N HCl (stirring at 40°C until complete decoloration of the product). The white precipitate of ε-N-lauryl-L-lysine was dissolved in acetic acid and then reprecipitated by dilution with water. Elementary analysis : C 66.05 (65.90), H 11.17 (10.96), N 8.49 (8.53).

ε-N-palmityl-L-lysine was obtained by a similar technique to

that for ε-N-lauryl-L-lysine. Elementary analysis : C 68.96
(68.75), H 11.70 (11.45), N 7.45 (7.29).

ε-N-linoleyl-L-lysine was obtained by the mixed anhydride
method. Linoleic acid (13 g) and triethylamine (5 g) dissolved in
tetrahydrofurane (250 ml) and cooled at -10°C was treated with
isobutyl chloroformiate (7.5 g). After stirring for 30 min, the
solution of the copper complex of lysine (18 g in 100 ml of H_2O,
15 ml of triethylamine and 50 ml of tetrahydrofurane) was added
slowly. After one hour, the mixture was added to a large volume
of water and the blue derivative filtered off. The copper was
removed as for the two previous derivatives. Elementary analysis :
C 64.15 (70.50), H 10.14 (10.70), N 6.65 (6.85).

ε-N-L-pyroglutamyl-L-lysine was synthesized by reaction of
L-pyrrolidone carboxylic acid with the copper complex of lysine
in the presence of N-N'-dicyclohexyl-carbodiimide in a homogeneous
mixture of dimethylformamide, ethanol, tetrahydrofuran and water.
The copper was removed by treatment with a cation-exchange resin
(Dowex-50, NH_4^+ form) and the peptide purified by chromatography
on Dowex-50, (H+ form) eluted with 0.5 N HCl. After treatment
with Amberlite IR-4B (OH⁻ form) to remove HCl, the peptide was
crystallized from water (m.p. 235°C with decomposition). Elementary analysis : C 51.45 (51.36), H 7.67 (7.39), N 16.21 (16.34).

D) ε-N-(α-aminoacyl)-L-lysines

ε-N-glycyl-L-lysine monoacetate was synthesized by the mixed
anhydride method, according to Theodoropoulos (1958). N-carbobenzoxy-glycine (10.5 g) and triethylamine (5.05 g)dissolved in
200 ml tetrahydrofurane and cooled at -10°C was treated with
isobutyl-chloroformiate (7,5 g). After 30 min, the copper complex
of lysine (17.5 g) dissolved in a mixture of water (100 ml),
tetrahydrofurane (60 ml) and triethylamine (12.6 g) was added
slowly. After two hours, the condensation product was precipitated
in a large volume of water(1.2 litre), filtered off, suspended
in 20 % acetic acid solution (80 ml) and treated with 10 %
potassium cyanide (50 ml). After 12 hrs the white precipitate was
washed with water, dissolved in 33 % acetic acid and precipitated
at pH 4.5 with NaOH. The last step was done twice more. The
carbobenzoxy group was removed by hydrogenation on palladium as
described for the α-N-glycyl-L-lysine. The derivative was
crystallized as monoacetate (m.p. 178 - 182°C). Elementary
analysis : C 45.60 (45.60), H 7.95 (8.00), N 15.95 (16.00), %
lysine 53.40 (55.51).

ε-N-L-phenylalanine-L-lysine monohydrochloride was synthesi-

zed by the mixed anhydride method from N-carbobenzoxy-L-phenyl-
alanine and α-N-carbobenzoxy-lysine benzyl ester (benzenesulpho-
nate) (Bezas and Zervas, 1961). After hydrogenation on palladium
in 1 $\underline{N}$ hydrochloric acid the peptide was purified by crystallization from ethanol (m.p. 210 - 211°C). Elementary analysis :
C 54.87 (54.63), H 7.54 (7.28), N 12.71 (12.75).

ε-N-L-arginyl-L-lysine trihydrochloride was synthesized by
reacting α-N-carbobenzoxy-L-lysine benzyl-ester prepared according
to Bezas and Zervas (1961) with N-carbobenzoxy-L-arginine in the
presence of N-N'-dicyclohexyl-carbodiimide. After treatment with
HBr in acetic acid, then with Dowex-2 (OH$^-$ form) to remove
excess HBr, the peptide was purified by chromatography on Dowex-50
(NH$_4^+$ form) with 1 $\underline{N}$ NH$_4$OH as eluting solution. After evaporation
the peptide was acidified by HCl, then crystallized (m.p. 155°C
with decomposition). Elementary analysis : C 35.82 (34.99),
H 7.94 (7.05), N 21.07 (20.41).

ε-N-(α-L-glutamyl)-L-lysine was prepared by coupling
N-carbobenzoxy-γ-benzyl-L-glutamic acid (Hanby et al. 1950) with
the copper complex of lysine according to the mixed anhydride
method. γ-benzyl-N-carbobenzoxy glutamic (9.5 g) and triethylamine
(3.5 ml) were dissolved in tetrahydrofurane (80 ml), cooled at
-10°C and treated with isobutylchloroformiate (3.42 g). After
30 min, the copper complex of lysine (9.0 g) dissolved in water
(50 ml), tetrahydrofurane (30 ml) and triethylamine (7 ml) was
added slowly. The condensation product was precipitated in a
large volume of water. After removal of copper with potassium
cyanide, as for ε-N-glycyl-L-lysine and hydrogenation on
palladium in ethanol/water (50:50), the peptide was crystallized
in absolute ethanol. Elementary analysis : C 48.22 (48.00),
H 7.79 (7.64), N 15.42 (15.25), % lysine 48.15 (53.09).

E) ε-N-(ω-aminoacyl)-L-lysines

ε-N-(γ-L-glutamyl)-L-lysine was synthesized by coupling the
copper complex of lysine with N-carbobenzoxy-α-t.butyl-γ-glutamyl
azide freshly prepared from the corresponding hydrazide derivative
(Taschner et al, 1961). N-carbobenzoxy-α-t.butyl-γ-glutamyl
hydrazide (6 g) dissolved in acetic acid (200 ml) and 1 $\underline{N}$ HCl
(80 ml) was cooled at -5°, and treated with 1 $\underline{N}$ sodium nitrite
(25 ml) during 10 min then diluted with cold water (500 ml). The
azide formed was extracted with ether and the organic phase
washed with a solution of sodium bicarbonate until complete
neutralization. This solution was then treated with the copper
complex of lysine (6 g) dissolved in water (65 ml), dimethyl-

formamide (35 ml) and triethylamine (9.5 ml). After stirring for
3 hrs at 0°C the condensation product was precipitated in a large
volume of water (600 ml), dissolved with 5 $\underline{N}$ NH$_4$OH, passed through
a column of Dowex-50 (NH$_4^+$ form) and eluted with 5 $\underline{N}$ NH$_4$OH to remove the copper. The fractions containing ε-(N-carbobenzoxy-α-t.
butyl-γ-L-glutamyl)-L-lysine were evaporated, dissolved in acetic
acid and treated with the same volume of acetic acid saturated
with HBr. After 15 min the solution was precipitated in a large
volume of ether. After washing with ether and drying, the precipitate was dissolved in water and passed through a column of
Dowex-2 (OH⁻ form) to remove HBr. The isopeptide was then eluted
with 1 $\underline{N}$ acetic acid and crystallized in water (m.p. 245 - 250°C).
Elementary analysis : C 47.62 (48.00), H 7.78 (7.64), N 15.19
(15.25); % lysine 42.42 (53.09).

   ε-N-(γ-L-glutamyl)-[U-^{14}C]-L-lysine. This radioactive isopeptide was synthesized by reacting N-carbobenzoxy-α-t.butyl-γ-L-
glutamyl-azide prepared from 200 mg N-carbobenzoxy-α-t.butyl-γ-L-
glutamyl-hydrazide with the copper complex of [U-^{14}C]-L-lysine
prepared from 30.3 mg L-lysine(HCl),diluted with 160 μci [U-^{14}C]-
L-lysine purchased from Amersham (England). All the steps of
condensation, removal of protective groups and purification were
performed as described previously for the synthesis of the
unlabelled isopeptide.(specific activity : 0.89 μci/μ mole).

   ε-N-(β-L-aspartyl)-L-lysine dihydrochloride was synthesized
by the mixed anhydride method using the procedure published by
Swallow et al., (1958) and modified as follows : reaction of
N-carbobenzoxy-L-aspartic-α-benzyl-ester with α-N-carbobenzoxy-L-
lysine-benzyl-ester prepared according to Bezas & Zervas (1961).
After hydrogenation on palladium to remove the blocking groups,
the peptide was purified by crystallization (m.p. 250°C with
decomposition). Elementary analysis : C 36.40 (35.93), H 6.51
(6.29), N 12.10 (12.57).

   ε-N-(β-alanyl)-L-lysine was synthesized by the acid chloride
method: N-carbobenzoxy-β-alanine (10.3 g) dissolved in ether was
transformed by addition of PCl$_5$ (9.6 g) into N-carbobenzoxy-β-
alanyl-chloride which was then after separation added slowly to
a solution of α-N-carbobenzoxy-L-lysine (12.25 g) dissolved in
50 ml 1 $\underline{N}$ NaOH cooled at 0°C. After reaction, the condensation
product was extracted with ether in acidic medium, and reduced
by hydrogen in the presence of palladium in ethanol/acetic
acid (50:50). The isopeptide was then purified by chromatography
on Dowex-50 by elution with 3 $\underline{N}$ NH$_4$OH.

F) ε-N-acylglycyl-L-lysines

ε-N-acetylglycyl-L-lysine was obtained by the mixed anhydride
method :   ε-N-acetylglycine was coupled with the copper complex
of lysine and copper removed on a cation exchange   resin (Dowex-
50, NH_4^+ form). Elementary analysis : C 48.82 (48.97), H 8.02
(7.75), N 17.23 (17.14).

ε-N-laurylglycyl-L-lysine was synthesized in two steps : a)
synthesis of laurylglycylmethyl ester by coupling the methyl
ester of lysine with lauric acid chloride, b) synthesis of ε-N-
laurylglycyl-L-lysine, by coupling the copper complex of lysine
with the laurylglycyl azide prepared from the laurylglycyl methyl
ester and followed by removal of the copper in the same way as
for ε-N-lauryl-L-lysine. Elementary analysis : C 62.34 (62.33),
H 10.08 (10.12), N 10.91 (10.91).

ε-N-palmitylglycyl-L-lysine was obtained by a technique
similar to that for ε-N-laurylglycyl-L-lysine. Elementary
analysis : C 65.49 (65.30), H 10.60 (10.65), N 9.48 (9.52).

ε-N-linoleylglycyl-L-lysine was synthesized in two steps :
a) synthesis of linoleylglycyl methyl ester by the mixed
anhydride method, b) synthesis of ε-N-linoleylglycyl-L-lysine by
coupling linoleylglycine with the copper complex of lysine by the
mixed anhydride method followed by the removal of copper by the
same technique as for ε-N-lauryl-L-lysine. Elementary analysis :
C 65.94 (67.09), H 9.89 (10.10), N 9.43 (9.00).

G) α-N-ε-N-diaminoacyl-L-lysines

α-N-ε-N-diglycyl-L-lysine was prepared by reacting an excess
of the mixed anhydride of N-carbobenzoxyglycine with lysine
ethyl ester. After saponification and reaction with HBr in
acetic acid to remove the carbobenzoxyl group, the peptide was
freed of HBr by treatment with anion-exchange resin (Amberlite
IR-4B, OH⁻ form) and purified by chromatography with 1 N NH_4OH on
a Dowex-50 (NH_4^+ form) column (m.p. 155°C with decomposition).
Elementary analysis : C 48.05 (46.15), H 7.51 (7.69), N 18.54
(21.54); % lysine 34.2 (49.3); % glycine 33.5 (50.7) (ratio
glycine/lysine = 1.9). This preparation contained only one
ninhydrin positive substance.

α-N-ε-N-di-L-alanyl-L-lysine was synthesized by the carbodiimide method : reaction of L-lysine ethyl ester with twice as
much N-carbobenzoxy-L-alanine (Fluka AG) in dichloromethane.
After reaction, dicyclohexyl-urea was filtered off and the solu-

tion washed, dried with Na_2SO_4 and then evaporated. After removal
of the blocking group using HBr in acetic acid, the peptide was
precipitated in diethyl-ether, treated with Dowex-2 (acetate form)
to eliminate HBr, saponified in a solution of 4 $\underline{N}$ NaOH in acetone
and purified by ion-exchange chromatography on Dowex-50 (NH_4^+ form)
using 1 $\underline{N}$ NH_4OH as eluting solution. The peptide was isolated
in a pure form and separated from ε-N-L-alanyl-L-lysine synthesized as the same time as the tripeptide. (m.p. 180 - 184°C with
decomposition). Elementary analysis : C 50.15 (50.00), H 8.38
(8.33), N 19.16 (19.44);% lysine 40 (45), % alanine 44 (55).

H) Schiff's bases of lysine

ε-N-benzylidene-L-lysine was synthesized according to Bezas
and Zervas (1961). Elementary analysis : C 66.50 (66.67), H 7.71
(7.69), N 11.90 (11.96). (m.p. 182°C) % lysine 55.9 (62.39).

ε-N-salicylidene-L-lysine was synthesized following the
procedure of Bezas and Zervas (1926) with minor modifications;
0.1 mole of L-lysine monohydrochloride was dissolved in 150 ml of
water containing 0.1 mole of NaOH. 0.1 mole of salicylaldehyde
was then slowly added to the stirred solution. The yellow crystals
which appeared were filtered after keeping overnight at 4°C.
Elementary analysis : C 62.53 (62.40), H 7.37 (7.2), N 11.14
(11.20) (m.p. 199 - 200°C) % lysine 55.7 (58.40).

BIOLOGICAL AVAILABILITY OF N-SUBSTITUTED
LYSINES AND HYDROLYSIS BY THE TISSUES

The biological availability of N-substituted lysines was
determined by growth trials on rats, by comparison of the
responses of the animals receiving a diet poor in lysine enriched
with lysine derivatives, with those of the animals receiving the
same diet but enriched with free lysine. In addition, the lysine
derivatives were incubated with homogenates of the intestinal
mucosa, liver and kidneys of rats, in order to find the organ (or
organs) responsible for their hydrolysis and the resulting
release of lysine.

A) Growth trials on rats

The method used was that of Mottu and Mauron (1967) with
some modifications. The basal diet was composed of wheat gluten
(10 %), zeine (10 %), potato starch (42.8%), sucrose (25.0 %),
peanut oil (5.0 %), salts according to Hawk-Oser (4.0%),
histidine (0.10 %), tryptophan (0.12 %), threonine (0.30 %),
methionine (0.35 %), valine (0.35 %) and vitamins. The protein

level (N x 6.25) was 18.2 % and the available lysine was evaluated at 0.12 g/100 g of diet.

Each trial was carried out with several groups of 6 rats, one receiving the basal diet with 0 % added lysine, a second one receiving the basal diet enriched by a quantity of lysine varying between 0.12 % and 0.24 % of lysine monohydrochloride (for which the added lysine is considered as being 100 % utilized) and several groups of 6 rats each receiving the basal diet enriched with a lysine derivative at the same level as that of free lysine. In these conditions, the weight gain of the animals per 100 g of ingested food is proportional to the amount of added lysine (Mottu and Mauron, 1967). The response of the animals receiving diets enriched with a lysine derivative can be expressed as a percentage (% utilization) of the response of the animals receiving the diet enriched with lysine monohydrochloride.

B) Hydrolysis by the homogenates of the intestinal mucosa, liver and kidney of the rat

The N-substituted lysines were incubated for 4 hours at 37°C at a concentration of 1 mg equivalent of lysine per ml (3.5 mg equivalent of lysine dissolved in 2.5 ml buffer, plus 1 ml homogenate prepared in the same buffer). The homogenates of liver and kidney were prepared at a concentration of 20 % in a 0.01 M phosphate buffer of pH 7.4, and the intestinal mucosa homogenates were obtained from the scrapings of the small intestine of one rat, homogenized in 10 ml of 0.2 M Tris buffer of pH 7.6. Under these conditions, the natural dipeptides of lysine were 100 % hydrolyzed. The released lysine was determined manometrically by lysine decarboxylase or by paper electrophoresis and expressed as a percentage of the lysine content of the derivative.

C) Results

The results given by the "in vivo" rat trials and the "in vitro" hydrolyses permit the classification of N-substituted lysines into three groups: those derivatives which are very well utilized as lysine source, those which are partially utilized, and those which are not utilized.

1. The derivatives which are very well utilized as lysine source belong to five different classes. (Table 1).

a) The natural dipeptides : they are utilized with the same efficiency as free lysine and are completely hydrolyzed under our experimental conditions by the homogenates of

Table 1

Derivatives of which the lysine is readily biologically available.
Hydrolytic action of the homogenates of the intestinal mucosa,
liver and kidneys of the rat.

Derivative	% utilization	% hydrolysis by homogenate of		
		intestinal mucosa	liver	kidney
Natural dipeptides				
glycyl-lysine	86-97	100	100	100
alanyl-lysine	106	100	100	100
glutamyl-lysine	107	100	100	100
lysyl-alanine	92	100	100	100
ε-N-(α-aminoacyl)-lysines				
ε-N-glycyl-	93-57 84-63	15-28	11-16	70-100
ε-N-phenylalanyl-	82	7	38	90-100
ε-N-(α-glutamyl)-	82-81	49-50	37-40	78-93
ε-N-arginyl-		50	100	100
ε-N-(α-aspartyl)-				+
ε-N-alanyl-				+
ε-N-leucyl-				+
Schiff's bases of lysine				
ε-N-benzylidene-	113-91			
ε-N-salicylidene-	102			
ε-N-(ω-aminoacyl)-lysines				
ε-N-(γ-glutamyl)-	102-98	5-6	0	86-86
α-N-ε-N-diaminoacyl-lysines				
α-N-ε-N-dialanyl-		100	30	100

+ Hydrolysis by ε-lysine acylase (Padayatti and Van Kley, 1966)

intestinal mucosa, liver and kidney.

b) The ε-N-(α-aminoacyl)-lysines : they are hydrolyzed at
    different rates by the homogenates of the three tissues
    tested. It appears that, for the three derivatives tested on
    rats, even if the intestinal mucosa has only weak hydrolytic
    action, the derivatives are still used as lysine source if
    the liver or kidneys can hydrolyze them. This observation
    suggests that these derivatives can be absorbed by the
    intestine and eventually hydrolyzed in the interior of the
    organism, mainly by the kidneys which possess an ε-lysine
    acylase (Paik and Benoiton, 1963; Leclerc and Benoiton, 1968)
    active on these derivatives just as on ε-N-(α-aspartyl)-
    lysine, ε-N-alanyl-lysine and ε-N-leucyl-lysine, as has been
    shown by Padayatti and Van Kley (1966). These latter
    derivatives are thus probably used as lysine source.

c) The Schiff's bases of lysine : these result from a reversible
    reaction between the ε-amino group of lysine and an aromatic
    aldehyde. They are hydrolyzed in acid medium and it is
    probable that "in vivo" they release lysine at the level of
    the stomach.

d) ε-N-(γ-glutamyl)-lysine : this isopeptide belongs to the
    class of ε-N-(ω-aminoacyl)-lysines of which certain derivati-
    ves are not biologically available (Table 3). It is hydro-
    lyzed only by the kidneys. It is thus absorbed by the
    intestine unmodified and its hydrolysis occurs in the
    kidney, which releases lysine. It has been confirmed on
    perfused rat liver that the radioactive isopeptide was not
    at all hydrolyzed by the liver.

e) The α-N-ε-N-diaminoacyl-lysines : only one derivative of this
    class was tested, α-N-ε-N-dialanyl-lysine. It is completely
    hydrolyzed by the intestinal mucosa and the kidney, and
    partially so by the liver. It is thus certainly biologically
    available.

2. The derivatives which are partially utilized as lysine source
    are ε-N-formyl- and ε-N-acetyl-lysines. They belong to the
    group of ε-N-acyl-lysines, the other members of which are
    not biologically available (Table 2). They are negligibly
    hydrolyzed by intestinal mucosa and liver, and only slightly
    so by the kidneys. According to Paik and Benoiton (1963)
    and Leclerc and Benoiton (1968) it is renal ε-lysine
    acylase which is responsible for their hydrolysis.

Table 2

Derivatives of which the lysine is partially available. Hydrolytic action of the homogenates of intestinal mucosa, liver and kidney of the rat.

Derivative	% utiliza- tion	% hydrolysis by homogenate of		
		intestinal mucosa	liver	kidney
ε-N-acyl-lysines				
ε-N-formyl-	58	0-5	0-7	20-21
ε-N-acetyl-	51-52	0-5	0-5	18-43
	79			

3.   The derivatives which are not used as lysine source belong to four different classes (Table 3).

a)   The α-N-acyl-lysines. They are not hydrolyzed by any of the tested tissues and are not used as lysine source. Here again is found the relation between the inability of the tissues to hydrolyze the lysine derivatives and their non-availability.

b)   The ε-N-acyl-lysines. The first two derivatives of this class, ε-N-formyl- and ε-N-acetyl-, have been found to be partially utilized. On the other hand, ε-N-lauryl- and ε-N-palmityl- are not utilized and would even have an inhibiting effect on growth as they have negative utilization rates. Elsewhere it has been shown that ε-N-propionyl-lysine was not utilized (Bjarnason and Carpenter, 1969) and was not hydrolyzed by ε-lysine acylase (Paik and Benoiton, 1963; Leclerc and Benoiton, 1968). Of this class of derivatives, only the first two of the series are utilized (partially) as lysine source (Table 2).

c)   The ε-N-acylglycyl-lysines. None of the four derivatives of this class is used as lysine source; moreover none is

Table 3

Derivatives of which the lysine is not biologically available.
Hydrolytic action of the homogenates of intestinal mucosa, liver
and kidney of the rat.

Derivative	% utiliza-tion	% hydrolysis of the homo-genates of		
		intestinal mucosa	liver	kidney
α-N-acyl-lysines				
α-N-formyl-	(-3) 24	0-5	0	0
α-N-acetyl-	(-15)11	0	0	0
ε-N-acyl-lysines				
ε-N-propionyl-	0*			0**
ε-N-lauryl-	(-3)(-23)	0	0	0
ε-N-palmityl-	(-36)	0	0	0
ε-N-acylglycyl-lysines				
ε-N-acetylglycyl-	(-2) 29			
ε-N-laurylglycyl-	(-35)			
ε-N-palmitylglycyl-	(-34)			
ε-N-linoleylglycyl-	22			
ε-N-(ω-aminoacyl)-lysines				
ε-N-(β-alanyl)-		0	0	6-8
ε-N-(β-aspartyl)-	12	0	0	4

*   according to Bjarnason and Carpenter (1969)
**   according to Paik and Benoiton (1963) and Leclerc and Benoiton
     (1968), the renal ε-lysine acylase does not hydrolyze it.

hydrolyzed by the homogenates of the three tested tissues.
According to Paik and Benoiton (1963), the first derivative
of this series, ε-N-acetylglycyl-lysine, is not hydrolyzed by
renal ε-lysine acylase.

d)   The ε-N-(ω-aminoacyl)-lysines. Of this class, only ε-N-(γ-
     glutamyl)-lysine was found to be very well utilized as lysine
     source (Table 1). Its homologue, ε-N-(β-aspartyl)-lysine, on
     the contrary, is not utilized at all. Furthermore, like ε-N-
     (β-alanyl)-lysine, it is not hydrolyzed "in vitro".

We suggest the trivial name PROLYSINE for the biologically
available derivatives of lysine.

STABILITY TOWARDS THE MAILLARD REACTION

Biologically available lysine derivatives (prolysines) could
be used instead of free lysine if they offered actual physiological or technological advantages. From a technological point of
view, the addition of free lysine to food has the disadvantage of
the high reactivity of lysine with respect to the reducing sugars.
Substitution of an amino group of lysine, especially the more
reactive ε-amino group, should reduce its reactivity.

With the aim of quantifying this phenomenon, some lysine
derivatives were heated in the presence of glucose, in the same
conditions, and a comparison was made of the evolution of browning
as a function of time. (0.1 M lysine, 0.1 M glucose in 0.1 M
phosphate buffer of pH 6.5, heated at 100°C in a sealed tube;
readings at 500 nm). Under these conditions, Lento et al. (1958)
observed differences in the rate of browning of the α- and ω-amino
acids. All the lysine derivatives were found to be much less
reactive than free lysine. In the class of natural peptides, lysyl-
alanine, alanyl-lysine and glycyl-lysine were about two times less
reactive than lysine, whereas glutamyl-lysine was four times less
reactive. (Fig. 1). In the class of acyl-lysines, the α-acyl derivatives were two times less reactive than lysine and the ε-acyl
derivatives were four times less so (Fig. 2). Among the isopeptides, the ε-aminoacyl-lysines behaved like the ε-acyl derivatives,
except for ε-N-glycyl-lysine which behaved like an α-acyl derivative and ε-N-(α-glutamyl)-lysine which was seven times less reactive than free lysine (Fig. 3).

Thus it appears that the natural peptides, the ε-acyl-,ε-pep-
tides and the α-ε-diaminoacyl-lysines, which are partially or well
utilized biologically, are less susceptible to reaction with
reducing sugars than free lysine, and have a certain technological
advantage when they must be incorporated in foods containing
reducing sugars.

Elsewhere, these "prolysines" could have an application in
at least parenteral nutrition with the following two advantages:

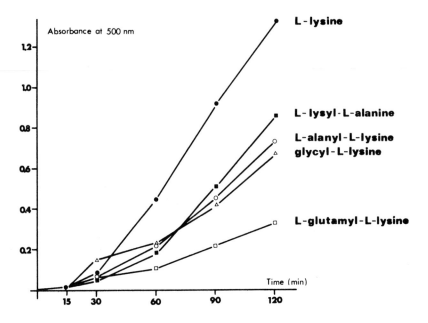

Fig. 1   Browning of natural dipeptides of lysine

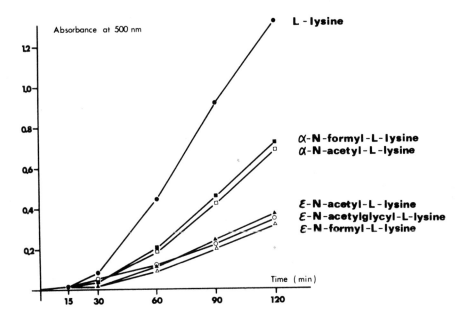

Fig. 2   Browning of α-N- and ε-N-acyl lysines

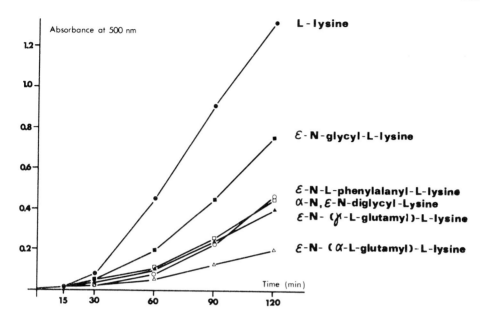

Fig. 3   Browning of ε-N-aminoacyl- and α-N-ε-N-diaminoacyl-
lysines

a)   during heat sterilization of the perfusate containing a
mixture of amino acids and glucose, the Maillard reaction
would take place to a much less extent than with free lysine.
The presence of such derivatives in the perfusate will not
cause any problems since they are rapidly hydrolyzed in the
kidney.

b)   the use of isopeptides may give a certain reduction of the
osmolarity of the perfusate.

ε-N-(γ-GLUTAMYL)-LYSINE AS A POTENTIAL PROLYSINE

In spite of the interest of these "prolysines" from a technological point of view, their use is greatly limited in practice
because of their prohibitive cost. Their synthesis often requires
several reaction stages for the blocking and unblocking of groups
to be protected, in addition to the condensation reaction, and
the yield is never optimum. For example, the synthesis of ε-(γ-

glutamyl)-lysine requires 9 reaction stages and the final yield is below 10 %. At the current market price of about $100 per gramme, it is evidently impossible to imagine its use, or the use of similar derivatives, as source of supplementary lysine in staple foods. We have attempted to overcome this problem by introducing the method of thermal condensation, usually used industrially to prepare amides. The salt lysine glutamate, resulting from the neutralization of the γ-carboxyl group of glutamic acid and of the ε-amino group of lysine, can easily be obtained from an aqueous solution of monosodium glutamate and lysine monohydrochloride. By addition of methanol this salt can be isolated from sodium chloride and crystallized with a yield of 100 %.

$$\text{Na glutamate + lysine HCl} \rightarrow \text{NaCl + lysine glutamate}$$

When this salt is heated under optimum conditions, it loses one molecule of water and is transformed into the expected isopeptide ε-N-(γ-glutamyl)-lysine with a yield of 50 % (Finot et al., 1975).

$$\text{lysine glutamate} \rightarrow H_2O + \varepsilon\text{-}(\gamma\text{-glutamyl})\text{-lysine}$$

Under these conditions, 50 % of glutamic acid is transformed into pyrrolidone carboxylic acid and other non-identified condensation products containing lysine. Lysine which has not reacted can be recovered and recycled in the process.

METABOLISM OF $[U\text{-}^{14}C]$-L-LYSINE AND ε-(γ-GLUTAMYL)-$[U\text{-}^{14}C]$-L-LYSINE

The problem which now arises is to know whether there are observable differences between the metabolism of free lysine and that of the isopeptides. The case of ε-N-(γ-glutamyl)-lysine has been studied. Rats of 100 - 120 g, starved for 24 h, received by stomach tube both $[U\text{-}^{14}C]$-L-lysine and ε-N-(γ-L-glutamyl)-$[U\text{-}^{14}C]$-L-lysine. 24 hours after oral ingestion, the incorporation in the different tissues was the same for lysine and for the isopeptide. However, the $^{14}CO_2$ peak appeared 165 to 195 min. after administration of the isopeptide and 30 min. after administration of lysine, a difference of more than 2 hours (Fig. 4).

When the two radioactive molecules were administered intravenously, the $^{14}CO_2$ peak occurred at the same time for each, that is to say 30 min. after injection (Fig. 4).

This observation shows that the isopeptide is available to the organism with a delay of 2 hours relative to free lysine, that the delay is due to the fact that the isopeptide is absorbed

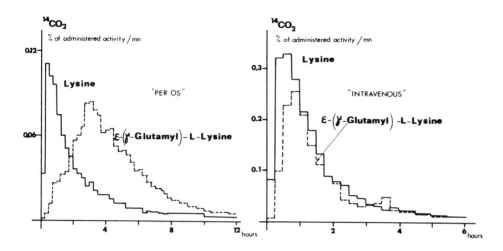

Fig. 4 $^{14}CO_2$ expiration after "per os" and intravenous administration of $[U-^{14}C]$-L-lysine and ε-(γ-L-glutamyl)-$[U-^{14}C]$-L-lysine

in the distal part of the small intestine, and that it is completely hydrolyzed by a different organ, in the event the kidneys, which confirms the trials carried out on the tissue homogenates.

Little information exists on the speed of appearance in the blood of free lysine and protein-linked lysine. However, it seems likely that the speed of appearance in the blood of linked lysine is closer to that of the isopeptide than that of free lysine.

CONCLUSION

The study of the biological availability, measured in trials with rats, of 8 classes of N-substituted lysines and of their hydrolysis by homogenates of intestinal mucosa, liver and kidney, permits their classification into 3 groups.

a)   The biologically non-available derivatives : the α-N-acyl-, ε-N-acyl- (whose radical possesses more than 2 carbon atoms), ε-N-acylglycyl- and ε-N-(ω-aminoacyl)-lysines (except ε-N-(γ-glutamyl)-lysine).

b)   The biologically partially available derivatives : the ε-N-
     formyl- and ε-N-acetyl-lysines.

c)   The derivatives which are available with an efficiency
     comparable to that of free lysine : the natural dipeptides,
     the ε-N-aminoacyl-, α-N-ε-N-diaminoacyl-, ε-N-(γ-glutamyl)-
     lysines and the Schiff's bases.

The latter are hydrolyzed by intestinal mucosa and liver
with variable efficiency according to their structure, but always
hydrolyzed readily by the kidney. This confers on them the
property of releasing lysine into the blood stream with a certain
delay with respect to free lysine, as has been shown for ε-N-(γ-
glutamyl)-lysine. They are more stable with respect to the reducing sugars than is free lysine, and have thus a certain technological advantage over free lysine as additives to foods rich in
reducing sugars. They can also be utilized advantageously in
parenteral nutrition. Their synthesis can be improved in order to
reduce their cost, as has been shown for ε-N-(γ-glutamyl)-lysine,
for which we have developed the method of thermal condensation.

We suggest for these derivatives the term PROLYSINES.

ACKNOWLEDGEMENTS

The authors wish to thank all the collaborators who contributed to this work : Miss S. Schupbach, Miss E. Magnenat,
Mrs C. Constantin, Mr J.P. Corbaz, Mr M. Studer, Mr S. Heyland,
Dr G. Spohr and Dr M. Arnaud for the syntheses, Miss I. Verkleij
and Mr R. Deutsch for the "in vitro" evaluations, Mrs I. Bougeon,
Mr Ch. Dormond for the biological evaluations, Miss E. Magnenat
and Mrs R. Madelaine for the metabolic studies, Dr P. Hirsbrunner
and Mr R. Bertholet for preparing ε-(γ-glutamyl)-lysine by
thermal condensation and Dr K. Eder (School of Medecine, Geneva)
for the elementary analyses.

REFERENCES

Bezas, B. and Zervas, L. (1961). On the peptides of L-lysine.
     J. Am. Chem. Soc. 83, 719-722

Bjarnason, J. and Carpenter, U.K. (1969). Mechanism of heat
     damage in proteins. I. Models with acylated lysine units.
     Br. J. Nutr. 23, 859-868

Bjarnason, J. and Carpenter, U.K. (1970). Mechanism of heat
    damage in protein. 2. Chemical changes in pure proteins. Br.
    J. Nutr. 24, 313-329

Bohak, Z. (1964). N-Epsilon-(DL-2-amino-2-carboxy-ethyl)-L-lysine.
    A new amino acid formed on alkaline treatments of proteins.
    J. Biol. Chem. 239, 2878-2887

Erlander, B.F. and Brand, E. (1951). Optical rotation of peptides.
    III. Lysine dipeptides. J. Am. Chem. Soc. 73, 4025-4027

Finot, P.A., Hirsbrunner, P. and Bertholet, R. (1975). Verfahren
    zur Herstellung von epsilon-(gamma-glutamyl)-lysin. German
    Patent 25 12 583. Preparation of ε-(γ-glutamyl)-lysine. 1976.
    British patent 1 471 850
Greenstein, J.P. and Winitz, M. (1961). Chemistry of the amino
    acids; J. Wiley and Son Inc.

Hanby, W.E., Waley, S.G. and Watson, J. (1950). Synthetic poly-
    peptides. Part II. Polyglutamic acid. J. Chem. Soc. 3239-3249

Hofmann, K., Stutz, E., Spühler, G., Yajima, H. and Schwartz, E.T.
    (1960). Studies on polypeptides. XVI. The preparation of ε-
    N-formyl-L-lysine and its application to the synthesis of
    peptides. J. Am. Chem. Soc. 82, 3727-3732

Leclerc, J. and Benoiton, L. (1968). Further studies on ε-lysine
    acylase. The ω-N-acyl-diamino acid hydrolase activity of
    avian kidney. Can.J. Biochem. 46, 471-475

Lento, H.G., Underwood, J.C. and Willits, C.O. (1958). Browning
    of sugar solutions. II. Effect of the position of amino group
    in the acid molecule in dilute glucose solutions. Food
    Research, 23, 68-71

Mauron, J. (1970). Comportement chimique des protéines lors de la
    préparation des aliments et ses incidences biologiques.
    J. Internat. Vitaminol. 40, 209-227

Mottu, F. and Mauron, J. (1967). The differential determination of
    lysine in heated milk. II. Comparison of the "in vitro"
    methods with the biological evaluation. J. Sci. Fd. Agric.
    18, 57-62

Neuberger, A. and Sanger, F. (1943). The availability of the acetyl
    derivatives of lysine for growth. Biochem. J. 37, 515-518

Padayatti, J.D. and Van Kley, H. (1966). Studies on ε-peptidase.
    Biochemistry, 5, 1394-1399

Paik, W.K. and Benoiton, L. (1963). Purification and properties
    of hog kidney ε-lysine acylase. Can. J. Biochem. Physiol.
    41, 1643-1654

Patchornick, A. and Sokolovsky, M. (1964). Chemical interactions
    between lysine and dehydroalanine in modified bovine
    pancreatic ribonuclease. J. Am. Chem. Soc. 86, 1860-1861

Schröder, E. and Lübke, K. (1965). Methods of peptides synthesis.
    Vol. I, Acad. Press

Swallow, D.L., Lockhart, I.M. and Abraham, E.P. (1958). Synthesis
    of ε-aspartyl-lysines and isohexylamides of aspartic acid.
    Biochem. J. 70, 359-364

Taschner, E. Wasielewski, C. Sokolowska, T. and Biernat, J.F.
    (1961). Neue Veresterungsmethoden in der Peptidchemie, VII.
    Darstellung von tosyl- und carbobenzoxy-glutaminsäure-α-tert.
    -butylestern und ihre Verwendung zur Synthese von γ-glutamyl-
    peptiden. Ann. Chem. Liebigs 646, 127-134

Theodoropoulos, D. (1958). Synthesis of ε-peptides of lysine.
    J. Org. Chem. 23, 140

Waibel, P.E. and Carpenter, K.J. (1972). Mechanism of heat damage
    in protein. 3. Studies with ε-(γ-L-glutamyl)-L-lysine. Br.
    J. Nutr. 27, 509-515

28

BIOAVAILABILITY OF ACETYLATED DERIVATIVES OF METHIONINE, THREONINE, AND LYSINE

R. W. Boggs

The Procter & Gamble Company, Miami Valley Laboratories

P.O. Box 39175, Cincinnati, OH 45247

ABSTRACT

Supplementation of vegetable proteins with various essential amino acids is an effective means of improving protein quality. Unfortunately, simple amino acid additions to foods which must be heat processed and cooked is not without consequences. Under these conditions, methionine interacts with reducing sugars yielding methional through the Strecker degradation reaction. This generation of methional during heat treatment imparts undesirable sulfur odors and flavors to the food rendering it organoleptically unacceptable. Similarly, threonine and lysine are also susceptible to interaction with reducing sugars rendering them nutritionally unavailable.

Acetylated derivatives of methionine, threonine and lysine have been studied to determine their utility in overcoming the inherent problems associated with each amino acid. To this end, N-acetyl-L-methionine and N-acetyl-L-threonine were found to be fully available to promote growth of rats. To the contrary, neither the α nor the ϵ, monoacetylated derivative of L-Lysine nor the α, ϵ diacetyl derivative of L-Lysine were effective in significantly promoting the growth of rats.

Utilization of N-acetyl-L-methionine by humans has also been studied and shown to be as effective as methionine in improving the quality of vegetable proteins deficient in sulfur amino acids.

INTRODUCTION

Supplementation of vegetable proteins with the limiting essential amino acid is an effective means of improving the biological quality. As such the quality of soybean protein can be improved by adding methionine, wheat protein by adding lysine and peanut protein by adding threonine. Unfortunately, in food products that must be heat processed and cooked, amino acid additions are not without consequences; methionine develops objectionable odors and flavors while lysine becomes unavailable. Since these undesirable side effects result from the interaction of the amino acids with the reducing sugars present in the food, protection of the amine of the amino acid by acetylation offers a practical solution to the problem. The utilization and metabolism of acetylated derivatives of methionine and lysine is important to the food processor and thus the subject of this presentation.

Furthermore acetylated amino acids occur naturally and the metabolism of threonine appears to be highly specific, thus the utilization of acetyl-threonine is of interest to further our understanding of acetylated amino acids.

BIOAVAILABILITY OF ACETYL-METHIONINE

Ballance (1961) showed that methionine produces methional by means of the Strecker reaction and it is this methional which results in the objectionable odors and flavors in methionine supplemented foods. Damico (1975) has shown that replacing methionine with acetyl-methionine prevents the production of methional (Figure 1).

Since acetyl-methionine offers a solution to the inherent odor and flavor problems associated with methionine supplementation of foods, an understanding of the bioavailability and metabolism of acetyl-methionine is necessary if it is to be considered as a potential food constituent. To this end, considerable confusion is found in the literature regarding the matabolism of acyl-methionine derivatives. Jackson and Block (1933, 1937) found that

$$\text{Methionine + Sugar + Water} \xrightarrow[\text{2 hours}]{100\%} \text{Methional + Methionine}$$

$$\text{Acetylmethionine + Sugar + Water} \xrightarrow[\text{2 hours}]{100\%} \text{Acetylmethionine}$$

Figure 1. Reaction of methionine and acetylmethionine with reducing sugars.

N-formyl-L-methionine supported growth of rats but N-formyl-D-methionine was ineffective. To the contrary, Rahm (1954), Beneditti et. al. (1968), Jenkins et. al. (1974), and Amos et. al. (1975) have all suggested both the D and L isomers of acetyl-methionine are available and utilized by experimental animals.

Due to the confusion in the literature, it seemed appropriate to conduct an experiment to resolve the confusion. N-acetyl-L-methionine and N-acetyl-D-methionine were fed to rats under conditions of limiting total dietary sulfur amino acids. The results of this study clearly showed that N-acetyl-L-methionine was fully available to the rat for growth, and that N-acetyl-D-methionine was not utilized by the rat for growth (Table 1). In addition, this study also allowed us to determine the source of confusion related to previous studies; namely, those who fed DL-isomers of acetyl-methionine. Those authors who reported apparent utilization of N-acetyl-DL-methionine fed the compound to rats at levels which was more than two times the rats' dietary requirement for total sulfur amino acids.

In order to further understand the metabolism of N-acetyl-L-methionine, two metabolic studies were conducted; one involving ^{14}C-N-acetyl-L-methionine and the other ^{35}S-N-acetyl-L-methionine. N-(1-^{14}C)-acetyl-L-methionine was administered to rats both orally and intraperitonally to study the hydrolysis and metabolic fate of the acetyl portion of the molecule. Equimolar sodium (1-C^{14})-acetate was used as a control to determine the degree of hydrolysis of the acetyl group from N-acetyl-L-methionine. Either route of

TABLE 1

Weight gains measured in rats fed diets supplemented with DL-methionine, L-methionine, D-methionine, N-acetyl-DL-methionine N-acetyl-L-methionine, or N-acetyl-D-methionine

Level of Methionine Equivalents Added to Diet	Body Weight Gain
	g
0.0	26.6 ± 8.3
0.4% DL-methionine	64.0 ± 16.3
0.4% L-methionine	64.8 ± 14.0
0.4% D-methionine	53.9 ± 10.5
0.4% N-acetyl-DL-methionine	54.3 ± 10.4
0.4% N-acetyl-L-methionine	62.7 ± 9.5
0.4% N-acetyl-D-methionine	23.9 ± 0.6

administration resulted in quantitative hydrolysis of the acetyl group from N-acetyl-L-methionine (Figures 2 and 3). Studies utilizing ^{35}S labelled N-acetyl-L-methionine and comparison to ^{35}S labelled L-methionine also showed that the rate of incorporation of the methionine moiety from N-acetyl-L-methionine was equivalent to L-methionine (Table 2).

Since these experiments provide compelling evidence that N-acetyl-L-methionine was metabolized, it seemed important to understand its enzymatic hydrolysis. Greenstein (1961) extensively studied the enzyme acylase, which hydrolyzes N-acetyl-L-methionine to acetate and methionine, and showed the kidney to be the organ of predominant enzymatic activity (Table 3).

Based on observations from in vitro intestinal studies suggesting an apparent hydrolysis of N-acetyl-L-methionine, we extended Greenstein's earlier organ studies to include the digestive tract. Table 4 shows the results of a study where the entire small intestine of the rat, chick and monkey was divided into 8 equal segments and assayed for acylase activity. Note that the entire small intestine of the rat, chick and monkey possessed acylase activity.

TABLE 2

Distribution of ^{35}S from L-methionine - ^{35}S

or N-acetyl-L-methionine - ^{35}S

24 Hours After Dosing

% of Dose

Source	L-Met-^{35}S	NAL-Met-^{35}S
G.I. tract	9.3 ± 0.7	9.0 ± 0.2
G.I. wash	2.1 ± 0.3	1.0
Carcass	38.3 ± 2.3	38.2 ± 0.9
Liver	12.3 ± 0.9	11.9 ± 1.1
Kidneys	2.3 ± 0.3	2.1 ± 0.1
Testes	1.1 ± 0.1	1.1 ± 0.1
Skin-hair	19.4 ± 3.1	18.3 ± 3.4
Urine	7.7 ± 7.9	6.9 ± 1.7
Feces	1.5 ± 1.0	1.6 ± 0.5
Recovery	93.8 ± 4.5	90.5 ± 1.9

% of the Dose/Gram of Tissue

Muscle	0.18 ± 0.09	0.17 ± .04

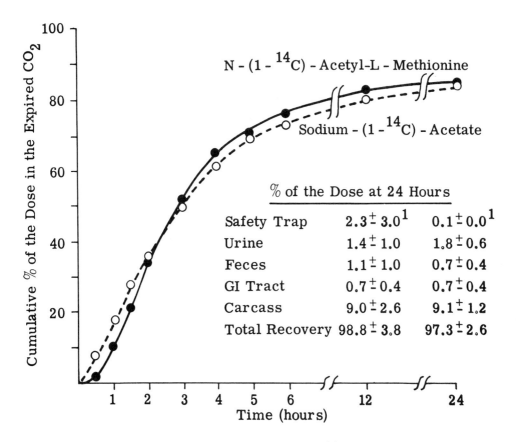

Figure 2. Metabolism of orally dosed N-(1-^{14}C)-acetyl-L-methionine and sodium-(1-^{14}C)-acetate.

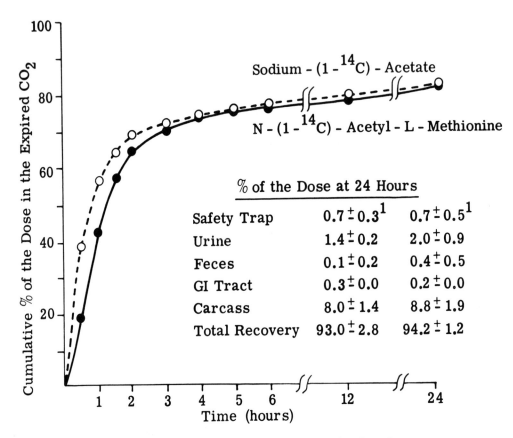

Figure 3. Metabolism of intraperitoneally dosed
N-(1-^{14}C)-acetyl-L-methionine and sodium-(1-^{14}C)-acetate.

TABLE 3

Rate of hydrolysis of N-acetyl-L-methionine
by Rat Tissues

Tissue	Rate μ moles NALM hydrolyzed/mg prot/hr
Kidney	44.0
Liver	5.4
Brain	4.8
Heart	1.2
Lungs	1.2
Muscle	0.6
Spleen	0
Pancreas	0

Greenstein et. al., Chemistry of Amino Acids, Vol. 2,
Chapter 20, pg. 1758. Greenstein-Winitz (1961).

TABLE 4

Acylase activity of rat, chick, and monkey
small intestine as a function of intestinal location

Segment No.	Species		
	Rat	Chick	Monkey
1	0.100	0.096	0.196
2	0.051	0.088	0.180
3	0.040	0.099	0.173
4	0.050	0.098	0.198
5	0.048	0.090	0.228
6	0.047	0.067	0.220
7	0.043	0.059	0.250
8	0.023	0.050	0.269

Activity expressed as μ g N-acetyl-L-methionine hydrolyzed/mg
tissue protein/hour.

Furthermore, if the total organ, in this case the intestine, is considered as a metabolic entity, Table 5 shows that the small intestine of the rat contains as much acylase activity as the kidney, whereas the stomach and large intestine contain very little enzymatic activity. Enzymatic activity in the human intestine at two locations, the jejunum and the ileum, exceeds that of the rat and chick but is less than that of the monkey (Table 6).

The effect of age on acylase activity is shown in Table 7. Both the kidney and the small intestine showed an increase in activity from day 28 to day 42 after which no further increase was noted. The presence or absence of N-acetyl-L-methionine in the diet had no effect on enzymatic activity.

The availability of various acyl chain lengths added to L-methionine is shown in Table 8. We have concluded that addition of the acyl chains longer than propionyl (C-3) results in a significant reduction in bioavailability. Enzymatic studies reported by Damico (1975) suggests that the decreased solubility of the long chain acyl methionine derivatives is the cause for the reduced availability.

The specificity of the acylase enzyme with regard to bio-availability was further studied by modifying the chemical constituent attached to the methionine-amino group. If the group is an acyl group, availability is reduced but not diminished. To the contrary, if succinic acid is substituted for butyric acid, availability is abolished (Table 9). These results suggest that enzymatic specificity is a function of the group attached to the amine of the methionine.

TABLE 6

A comparison of acylase activity in the small
intestine of various species

	Acylase Activity	
	μg N-Acetyl-L-Methionine Hydrolyzed/ mg Tissue Protein/Hour	
	Jejunum	Ileum
Rat	0.0482 ± 0.0126	0.0230 ± 0.0243
Chick	0.0940 ± 0.024	0.0590 ± 0.0170
Human	0.1060 ± 0.0300	0.0230 ± 0.0060
Monkey	0.1726 ± 0.1053	0.2119 ± 0.0868

TABLE 7

Organ acylase activity as a function of age
and size of rat

	Acylase Activity	
	μg NALM Hydrolyzed/Total Organ	
Weight of Animal	Kidney	Small Intestine
68 g (28 days)	29.3 ± 0.5	10.8 ± 3.1
170 g (42 days)	54.8 ± 0.2	56.9 ± 4.1
270 g (90 days)	52.2 ± 1.9	59.9 ± 5.2

TABLE 8

Availability of N-acyl derivatives of
Methionine

Derivative	Relative Availability
L-methionine	100
N-formyl-L-methionine (C_1)	105
N-acetyl-L-methionine (C_2)	98
N-propionyl-L-methionine (C_3)	93
N-butyl-L-methionine (C_4)	82
N-hexyl-L-methionine (C_6)	52
N-octyl-L-methionine (C_8)	66
N-decyl-L-methionine (C_{10})	70
N-oleoyl-L-methionine (C_{18})	34

Relative availability:

$$\frac{\text{gain of exptal} - \text{gain of control}}{\text{gain of methionine} - \text{gain of control}} \times 100 =$$

TABLE 9

Specificity of acylated derivates of methionine

Compound	Structure	Availability
Methionine	$CH_3-S-CH_2-CH_2-CH-COOH$ $\quad\quad\quad\quad\quad\quad H_2N(R)$	100
N-acetyl-L-methionine	$R = -\overset{O}{\overset{\|}{C}}-CH_3$	100
N-butyl-L-methionine	$R = \overset{O}{\overset{\|}{C}}-CH_2-CH_2-CH_3$	82
N-succinyl-L-methionine	$R = -\overset{O}{\overset{\|}{C}}-CH_2-CH_2-\overset{O}{\overset{\|}{C}}-OH$	0
N-hexyl-L-methionine	$R = -\overset{O}{\overset{\|}{C}}-CH_2CH_2-CH_2CH_2-CH_3$	52

Finally, specificity, as measured by bioavailability, directed at modification of the methionine carboxyl group was studied. Data in Table 10 show that addition of a methyl or ethyl ester to N-acetyl-L-methionine does not affect its availability. Both compounds were fully available to the rat. These data suggest that enzymatic hydrolysis of the esters and the acetyl groups occurs simultaneously or independently without interference from the counter constituent.

Finally, utilization of N-acetyl-L-methionine has been assessed in humans and shown to be complete. Experiments similar to those done in rats using N-(1-^{14}C)-acetyl-L-methionine were conducted and showed a similar response. Figure 4 shows that after 6 hours of exposure the N-acetyl-L-methionine was hydrolyzed and the 1-^{14}C-acetate appeared in the respired breath as $^{14}CO_2$ at a rate equivalent to equimolar sodium-1-^{14}C-acetate.

TABLE 10

Bioavailability of N-acetyl-L-methionine esters

Compound	B.W. Gain (grams)	Bioavailability
Soybean protein isolate	47 ± 4	–
L-methionine	99 ± 11	100
N-acetyl-L-methionine	103 ± 12	104
N-acetyl-L-methionine-methyl ester	95 ± 7	96
N-acetyl-L-methionine-ethyl ester	102 ± 8	103

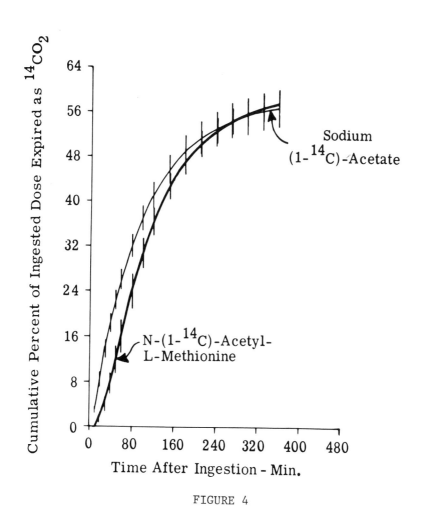

FIGURE 4

Metabolism of N-(1-^{14}C) Acetyl-L-Methionine
and Sodium (1-^{14}C)-Acetate by Human Subjects

BIOAVAILABILITY OF N-ACETYL-L-THREONINE

Since threonine and lysine deficient proteins are more difficult
to formulate, we chose to use an amino acid diet for these two
studies. The composition of the diet is shown in Table 11, while
the amino acid composition is shown in Table 12. These diets were
duplicated from those published by Rogers and Harper (1965) with a
slight modification which included feeding the diet as a dry mix
rather than as an agar and using the modified Barnhart and Tomarrilli
salt mix.

Using these amino acid diets, the availability of N-acetyl-
L-threonine was considered. We were interested in acetyl-threonine
because Greenstein had suggested that the amino acid constituent
significantly affected the specificity of the acylase to hydrolyze
the attached acyl group. The availability of N-acetyl-L-threonine
was shown to be at least 90% of L-threonine when fed to young
growing rats for 16 days (Table 13). Some adaptation to the
supplement may be apparent as indicated by the increase in apparent
availability from day 6 to 16.

These studies are of even greater interest when it is noted that
most analogs of threonine are not available (Table 14). Only N-
acetyl-L-threonine was available to any extent.

TABLE 11

Amino acid diet

Diet Ingredient	g/100 g
Corn starch	33.48
Sucrose	33.48
Salt mix (Barnhardt & Tomarelli)	5.0
Vitamin mix	0.5
Corn oil	10.0
Choline chloride	0.2
Amino acid mix	17.35
Total	100.00

TABLE 12

Amino acid mix

Amino Acid	% of Mix	Amino Acid	% of Mix
His·HCl·H$_2$O	3.46	Valine	5.19
Isoleucine	5.19	Na acetate	4.96
Leucine	6.92	Arg·HCl	5.76
Lysine·HCl	8.07	Asparagine	5.76
Methionine	3.17	Serine	2.88
Cystine	2.31	Proline	5.76
Phenylalanine	4.32	Glycine	5.76
Tyrosine	2.88	Glutamic acid	17.29
Threonine	4.03	Alanine	2.88
Tryptophan	1.15	Na acetate	2.25

Rogers & Harper, J. Nutr., 1965

TABLE 13

Bioavailability of N-acetyl-L-threonine

Amino Acid	Body Weight Gain (Grams) 6 Days	16 Days
−Threonine	−11 ± 3	−14 ± 4
+Threonine (control)	35 ± 5 (100)	113 ± 10 (100)
+N-acetyl-L-threonine	28 ± 5 (80)	101 ± 13 (90)

TABLE 14

Bioavailability of threonine analogs

Amino Acid		Relative Bioavailability
Threonine (control)	$CH_3-\overset{\overset{OH}{\mid}}{C}-\overset{\overset{H}{}}{C}-COOH$ $\overset{}{H}\ \overset{}{NH_2}$	100
α Hydroxy analog threonine	$CH_3-\overset{\overset{OH}{\mid}}{C}-\overset{\overset{H}{}}{C}-COOH$ $\overset{}{H}\ \overset{}{OH}$	0
α Keto analog threonine	$CH_3-\overset{\overset{OH}{}}{C}-\overset{}{C}-COOH$ $\overset{}{H}\ \overset{}{O}$	0
L-homoserine	$\overset{\overset{}{CH_2}}{\underset{OH}{}}-CH_2-\overset{\overset{H}{}}{C}-COOH$ $\overset{}{NH_2}$	0
α Acetamido β keto methyl butyrate	$CH_3-\overset{\overset{O}{}}{C}-\overset{\overset{H}{}}{C}-\overset{\overset{O}{}}{C}OCH_3$ $\overset{\overset{}{O}}{HN-\overset{}{C}-CH_3}$	0
N-acetyl-L-threonine	$CH_3-\overset{\overset{OH}{\mid}}{C}-\overset{\overset{H}{}}{C}-COOH$ $\overset{}{H}\ \overset{\overset{O}{}}{HN-C-CH_3}$	90

BIOAVAILABILITY OF α AND ε ACETYL LYSINE

The bioavailability of acetyl-derivatives of lysine is also confusing. Neuberger and Sanger (1943) suggested that ε-acetyl-L-lysine was available to the rat but that α-acetyl-L-lysine was not metabolized. Paquet (1977) has published data showing that α-palmityl-L-lysine is not metabolized by the rat. Gordon (1939) published results suggesting that α-N-methyl lysine did not support growth of rats.

None of these previously cited workers have tested the α, ε-diacetyl derivative of L-lysine. To this end, we have evaluated α-acetyl-L-lysine, ε-acetyl-L-lysine and α, ε-diacetyl-L-lysine. When these compounds were added individually to amino acid diets devoid of lysine, we found α-acetyl- and α, ε-diacetyl-L-lysine were unavailable to the rat. ε-N-acetyl-L-lysine was partially available (30%) to the rat (Table 14).

TABLE 15

Bioavailability of α and ε Acetylated
Derivatives of L-Lysine

	6 Days	16 Days
+Lysine (control)	35 + 5	113 + 10
-Lysine	-7 + 3	-7 + 3
+α-N-Acetyl-L-Lysine	-4 + 5	-6 + 4
+ε-N-Acetyl-L-Lysine	12 + 3	38 + 7
+α,ε-N-Diacetyl-L-Lysine	1 + 2	-

These data seem to clarify some of the confusion regarding the availability of acetyl-lysine derivatives. Since the enzyme which hydrolyzes α-acetyl is different from that which hydrolyzes ε-acetyl-L-lysine, the bioavailability results may be explained by an enzymatic rationale.

SUMMARY

The utilization and metabolism of N-acetyl-L-methionine has been well characterized in experimental animals and humans.

Utilization of acetylated derivatives of amino acids is dependent upon the enzyme acylase. These studies have shown the N-acetyl-L-methionine is as effectively utilized as L-methionine by animals and humans. In addition, these studies have shown that increasing the chain length of the acyl derivative on the L-methionine reduces the availability of the N-acyl-L-methionine. To the contrary, addition of methyl or ethyl esters to N-acetyl-L-methionine does not reduce the availability of the derivative compared to L-methionine.

The bioavailability of threonine analogs and derivatives have also been studied. Of those studied, only N-acetyl-L-threonine showed nutritive value to the rat. These results suggest that the acylase activity of rat tissues is sufficient to meet the threonine requirements of the rat when N-acetyl-L-threonine is added to a threonine-free diet.

The utilization of acetylated derivatives of lysine is much less effective than for either N-acetyl-L-methionine or N-acetyl-L-threonine. The ε-acetyl-L-lysine showed a partial availability (30%) when compared to L-lysine. To the contrary, neither α-N-acetyl-L-lysine nor α,ε-N-diacetyl-L-lysine promoted the growth of rats.

REFERENCES

1. Amos, H.E., Schelling, G.T., Digenis, G.A. Swintosky, J.V., Little, C.O., and Mitchell, Jr., G.E. (1975) Methionine replacement value of N-acetylmethionine and homocysteine-thiolactone hydrochloride for growing rats, J. Nutr. 105, 577-580.

2. Ballance, P.E. (1961) Production of volatile compounds related to the flavor of foods from Strecker degradation of DL-methionine, J. Sci. Food Agr. 12, 532-536.

3. Beneditti, P.C., Mariani, A., Spadoni, M.A. and Tagliamonte, B. (1968) Use of acetyl-methionine as supplementing factor of diets low in sulfurated amino acids. Quad. Nutr. 28, 209-224.

4. Damico, R. (1975) An investigation of N-substituted methionine derivatives for food supplementation. J. Agr. Food Chem. 23, 221-224.

5. Gordon, W.G. (1939) The metabolism of N-methylated amino acids I. The availability of α-N-monomethyl lysine and α-N-dimethyl lysine for growth. J. Biol. Chem. 127, 487-494.

6. Greenstein, J.P., Winitz, M. (1961) Chemistry of Amino Acids, Vol. 2, Chapter 20, John Wiley and Sons, Inc.

7. Jackson, R. W. and Block, R. J. (1933) Metabolism of d- and l-methionine. Proc. Soc. Exp. Biol. Med. 30, 587-588.

8. Jackson, R. W. and Block, R. J. (1937) The metabolism of cystine and methionine. J. Biol. Chem. 122, 425-432.

9. Jenkins, M. Y., Mitchell, G.V. and Adkins, J.S. (1974) Evaluation of the biological potency of various methionine isomers and derivatives. Fed. Proc. 33, 681.

10. Neuberger, A., and Sauger, F. (1943) The availability of the acetyl derivatives of lysine for growth. Biochem. J. 37, 515-518.

11. Rahm. L.D.W. (1954) A study of the utilization of acetyl-methionine and ethionine by animal organisms. Diss. Abstr. 14, 598-599.

12. Stephens, C.A., Veen-Baigent, M.J., Paquet, A., and Anderson, G.H. (1977) Digestibility and nutrient value of palmitoyl-L-lysine derivatives in weanling rats. Can. J. Physiol. Pharmacol 55, 434-438.

29

A METHOD FOR IMPROVING THE NUTRITIONAL VALUE OF FOOD PROTEINS: COVALENT ATTACHMENT OF AMINO ACIDS

Antoine J. Puigserver*, Lourminia C. Sen, Andrew J. Clifford**, Robert E. Feeney and John R. Whitaker

Department of Food Science and Technology and Department of Nutrition
University of California, Davis, California 95616

I. ABSTRACT

Casein was modified by use of a series of active N-hydroxy-succinimide esters of amino acids in order to study the effects of new covalently linked hydrophobic or hydrophilic groups on its physical and nutritional properties. Tryptophan was used to determine the best conditions for the chemical reaction and to study the stability of the newly formed amide linkage (isopeptide bond). Casein was also modified with glycine, alanine, methionine, N-acetyl-methionine and aspartic acid. In vitro hydrolysis studies using bovine chymotrypsin, pancreatin and rat bile-pancreatic juice indicated that digestibility of the modified casein derivatives was lower than that of the untreated protein. Since solubility was not significantly changed (except for tryptophyl-casein), the decreased in vitro digestibility is probably due to other factors such as steric hindrance as well as to decrease in lysine residues available to trypsin in pancreatin and rat pancreatic juice. Plasma amino acid patterns for rats fed a 10% protein diet of highly modified glycyl-casein or methionyl-casein suggest that the ε-aminolysyl derivatives are readily hydrolyzed in vivo. This was confirmed by the growth response of rats fed the following isonitrogenous diets (protein source listed only): casein, casein + free methionine, methionyl-casein, casein + free

---

*Present address: Centre de Biochimie et de Biologie Moléculaire (C.N.R.S.), 31, Chemin Joseph-Aiguier. 13009 Marseille - France.

**Department of Nutrition, University of California, Davis.

N-acetyl-methionine, N-acetyl-methionyl-casein. Covalently
attached methionine appeared to be as readily available as the
free amino acid; bound N-acetyl-methionine was also available but
to a slightly lower extent. Although this study is preliminary,
the covalent attachment of amino acids to proteins appears to be
a promising method for improving the biological value of food proteins.

II. INTRODUCTION

While it is becoming increasingly clear that more of the
world's requirement for proteins must be met by use of proteins
from plants, single cells and other less conventional sources, it
is also evident that most of these proteins must have their biological quality improved. In addition to specific problems characterizing each class of food protein, such as naturally occurring
toxicants in plant proteins or high levels of nucleic acids in
protein from microbial sources, it is well known that these proteins are often deficient in one or more essential amino acids.
Because of the economical, political and nutritional importance of
this problem, a number of important studies have been done on food
proteins, either to improve their functional properties or nutritional values.

Chemical and enzymatic modification of proteins have been
widely used to study their structure-function relationships alone
and in biological systems (Spande et al., 1970; Means and Feeney,
1971; Hoelzl Wallach, 1972; Heinrikson and Kramer, 1974; Knowles,
1974; Horecker et al., 1975; Louvard et al., 1975; Mobley et al.,
1976). More recently, a variety of chemical and enzymatic methods have been applied to food proteins, or suggested for use, by
biochemists and enzymologists working in food-related areas.
Up-to-date information on these topics is available in a recently
published book (Feeney and Whitaker, 1977) as well as in separate
studies (Kinsella, 1976; Galembeck et al., 1977). It has been
possible, for example, to improve the functional properties of
leaf and fish protein isolates by acylation (Franzen and Kinsella,
1976; Miller and Groninger, 1976). These chemical modifications
may be useful in increasing the acceptability of unconventional
protein sources and may offer new possibilities for food
scientists and technologists interested in new products.

Since many plant proteins have limited nutritional value because of their low content of one or more essential amino acids,
it is important to investigate the feasibility of covalently
attaching amino acids to proteins. It is equally important to
determine the biological availability of the newly bound amino
acid. Fortunately there are chemical and enzymatic methods al-

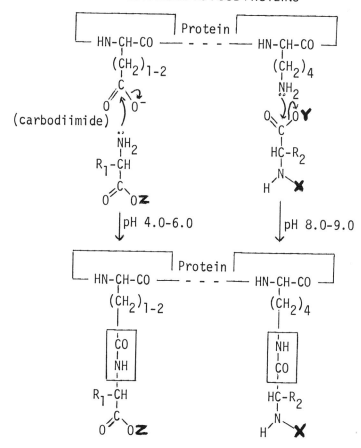

Fig. 1. General scheme for isopeptide bond formation between amino acyl side chains of proteins and additional amino acids. **X** and **Z** are amino and carboxyl protecting groups, respectively; **Y** is a carboxyl activating group.

ready available for the covalent attachment of amino acids to proteins in aqueous medium.

III.   CHEMICAL ATTACHMENT OF AMINO ACIDS TO PROTEINS

Chemical methods for attaching amino acids to proteins are directly derived from procedures for peptide synthesis. The synthesis of peptides in homogeneous solution and by solid phase peptide synthesis are well documented (Merrifield, 1969; Fridkin and Patchornik, 1974; Katsoyannis and Schwartz, 1977; Doscher,

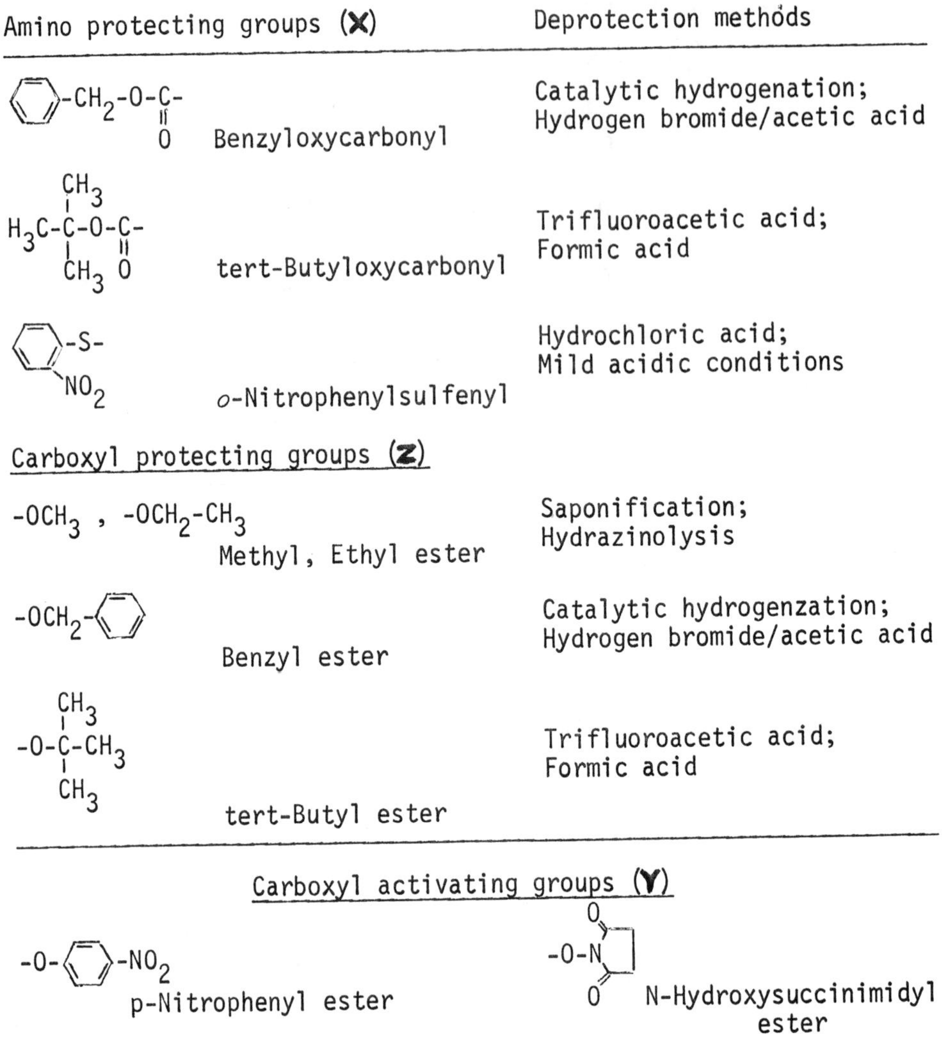

Amino protecting groups (**X**)	Deprotection methods
Benzyloxycarbonyl	Catalytic hydrogenation; Hydrogen bromide/acetic acid
tert-Butyloxycarbonyl	Trifluoroacetic acid; Formic acid
o-Nitrophenylsulfenyl	Hydrochloric acid; Mild acidic conditions

Carboxyl protecting groups (**Z**)

$-OCH_3$, $-OCH_2-CH_3$ Methyl, Ethyl ester	Saponification; Hydrazinolysis
$-OCH_2-$ Benzyl ester	Catalytic hydrogenzation; Hydrogen bromide/acetic acid
tert-Butyl ester	Trifluoroacetic acid; Formic acid

Carboxyl activating groups (**Y**)

$-O-$ $-NO_2$ p-Nitrophenyl ester $-O-N$ N-Hydroxysuccinimidyl ester

Fig. 2. Protecting and activating groups used in peptide synthesis and covalent attachment of amino acids to proteins. More detailed information is available in articles by Merrifield (1969), Stewart and Young (1969), and Katsoyannis and Schwartz (1977).

1977). The usefulness of such techniques for studies of the relationship of structure to activity or for verification of structures of natural peptides is well documented in the above references and will not be discussed further here.

Two different approaches are possible in peptide synthesis, that of fragment condensation and stepwise synthesis. Both strategies require that one amino acid have its amino group protected and its carboxyl group activated and that the second amino acid have its amino group free and its carboxyl group protected. As shown in Figure 1, the amino group responsible for the nucleophilic attack of an activated carboxyl group may be either the ε-amino group of a lysyl residue of a protein or the free amino group of an added amino acid. In both cases involving proteins, the resulting amide linkage is known as an isopeptide bond. The most important amino and carboxyl group protectors and the deprotection methods generally used in peptide synthesis are listed in Figure 2.

A major requirement of an amino protecting group is that it preclude racemization which may occur during activation of carboxyl groups. Racemization proceeds generally through the formation of an oxazolone intermediate (Katsoyannis and Ginas, 1969) as depicted in Figure 3. Protection of the α-amino group by an acyl moiety (acetyl, benzoyl) allows formation of an oxazolone followed by some degree of racemization. By contrast, urethan-type protecting groups (benzyloxycarbonyl, tert-butyloxycarbonyl), or the o-nitrophenylsulfenyl group which is carbonyl-free, do not permit racemization because formation of an oxazolone is not possible.

At the end of a peptide synthesis, amino or carboxyl protecting groups may be removed. Conditions used for deprotection are listed in Figure 2. Although catalytic hydrogenation is the most elegant way to remove carbobenzoxy groups, this procedure cannot be used for peptides or proteins containing sulfur amino acids. All the other conditions listed are somewhat drastic for proteins; therefore, development of more easily removable groups would be useful for the covalent attachment of amino acids to proteins. If deblocking is not a required step, acetyl and amide groups are the best amino and carboxyl protectors as they occur naturally in biological systems.

Activation of carboxyl groups of proteins or free amino acids, followed by coupling with free amino groups of a second compound, leads to peptide bond formation (Fig. 1). The carbodiimide method (Sheehan and Hess, 1955; Carraway and Koshland, 1972) has been used to activate protein carboxyl groups in aqueous medium. Use of a water-soluble carbodiimide (1-ethyl-3-(3-dimethylaminopropyl)carbodiimide) allowed the attachment on chymotrypsinogen of glycinamide (Carraway et al., 1969; Abita et al., 1969) and 1-aminoglucose (Wriston, 1973). Limitations of this chemical modification are the large excess of both nucleophilic reagent and carbodiimide needed to drive the reaction to com-

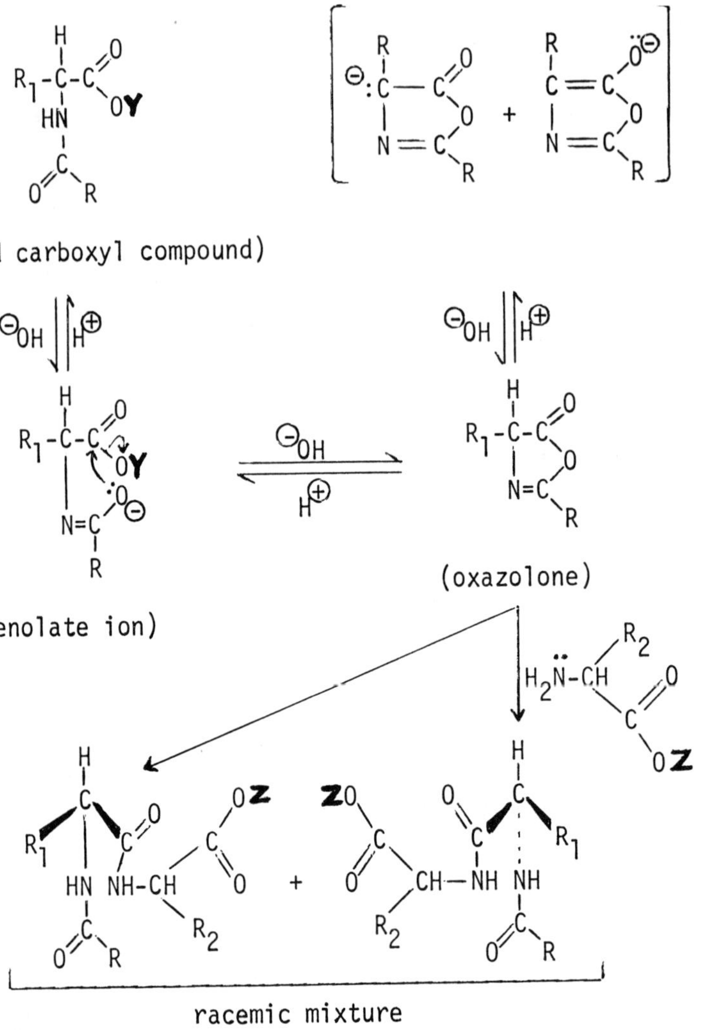

(activated carboxyl compound)

(enolate ion)   (oxazolone)

racemic mixture

Fig. 3. Interpretation of racemization process which may occur
during peptide bond formation (adapted from Katsoyannis and
Ginos, 1969).

pletion on the one hand and side reactions with tyrosines and
sulfhydryls on the other hand (Carraway and Koshland, 1968;
Carraway and Triplett, 1970).

Two active esters of amino-protected amino acids, p-nitro-
phenyl (Bodansky and du Vigneaud, 1959) and N-hydroxysuccinimidyl
(Anderson et al., 1964) are widely used in peptide synthesis
(Fig. 2).

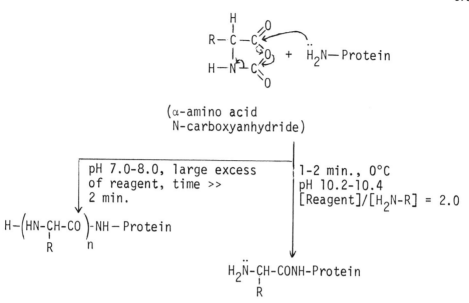

(α-amino acid
N-carboxyanhydride)

| pH 7.0-8.0, large excess of reagent, time >> 2 min. | 1-2 min., 0°C pH 10.2-10.4 [Reagent]/[H_2N-R] = 2.0 |

$$H-\left(HN-\underset{R}{CH}-CO\right)_n-NH-Protein$$

$$H_2\ddot{N}-\underset{R}{CH}-CONH-Protein$$

Fig. 4. Single or multiple addition of α-amino acid N-carboxy-anhydride to protein amino groups.

After chemical removal of amino terminal residues of small proteins, tert-methyloxycarbonyl-L-amino acid-N-hydroxysuccinimide esters (Boc-amino acid-O-Su) allowed replacement reactions in organic solvents (Borrás and Offord, 1970; Lode et al., 1974). This reagent has been used also in aqueous media to investigate the effect of polypeptide chain elongation on biological activity of various proteins such as ε-guanidinated trypsin (Robinson et al., 1973), thermolysin (Blumberg and Vallee, 1975), pancreatic phospholipase A_2 (Slotboom and de Haas, 1975), soybean trypsin inhibitor (Kowalski and Laskowski, Jr., 1976b) and subunit III of bovine procarboxypeptidase A (Puigserver, unpublished results). Moreover, the use of BOC-amino acid-O-Su may permit introduction of isotopically labeled amino acids at selected sites in proteins (Garner and Gurd, 1975).

Another method used in the controlled and sequential synthesis of peptides in aqueous medium involves α-amino acid N-carboxy anhydrides (Leuchs' anhydrides). These reagents are prepared by direct treatment of the unprotected amino acid with phosgene (Hirschmann et al., 1971); however, protection of the additional functional group was required with lysine, histidine, serine,

cysteine and threonine. N-Carboxy-α-amino acid anhydrides have
been primarily used for the synthesis of poly-α-amino acids. The
physicochemical and biological properties, as well as the usefulness of these synthetic polymers, are summarized in two review
articles (Katchalski and Sela, 1958; Sela and Katchalski, 1959).

Proteins react under mild conditions with α-amino acid-N-
carboxyanhydrides to yield either peptidyl- or polypeptidylpro-
teins (Fig. 4). Reaction proceeds at alkaline pH without detectable racemization (Denkewalter et al., 1966; Manning and Moore,
1968) but, with large excess of reagent or with prolonged reaction time, multiple addition of the added amino acid on the same
protein amino group may occur (Hirschmann et al., 1967). The
reaction is usually stopped by addition of a nucleophile or by
lowering the pH. A number of proteins have been chemically modified with N-carboxy-amino acid anhydrides and their properties
investigated. A partial list includes ribonuclease (Anfinsen
et al., 1962), trypsin (Glazer et al., 1962), insulin (Virupakska
and Tarver, 1964) and soybean trypsin inhibitor (Kowalski and
Laskowski, Jr., 1976a). This chemical modification was used to
increase the water solubility of gliadins (Sela et al., 1962) and
edestin (St. Angelo et al., 1966).

IV. COVALENT ATTACHMENT OF AMINO ACIDS TO PROTEINS BY ENZYMATIC METHODS

Enzymatic methods may also be used to link amino acids to
proteins. Since the pioneering investigations using papain
(Bergmann and Fraenkel-Conrat, 1937) and chymotrypsin (Bergmann
and Fruton, 1938) to demonstrate enzyme-catalyzed amide or peptide
bond synthesis, many investigators have reported use of the same
or other proteolytic enzymes (Blau and Waley, 1954; Kimmel and
Smith, 1957; Goldberg and Fruton, 1969). Proteolytic enzymes have
been used to increase the content of essential amino acids of food
proteins and to decrease the amount of an amino acid for specific
purposes (Yamashita et al., 1971, 1976). This technique has been
called the plastein reaction. Recently, carboxypeptidase B
(Sealock and Laskowski, Jr., 1969) and trypsin (Kowalski and
Laskowski, Jr., 1976b) were used to replace the arginyl residue in
the reactive site of soybean trypsin inhibitor by a lysyl residue
and to catalyze a peptide bond formation in the modified inhibitor, respectively. Using a more alkaline pH and much more enzyme
than usually required for peptide hydrolysis, chymotrypsin was
found to be useful for peptide synthesis (Morihara and Oka, 1977).
However, as shown in Figure 5, concentrations of amino acid or
peptide derivatives used as nucleophiles must be high enough to
compete with water and lead to peptide formation in a good yield.
Extent of synthesis is also dependent on the solubility of the
newly synthesized peptides.

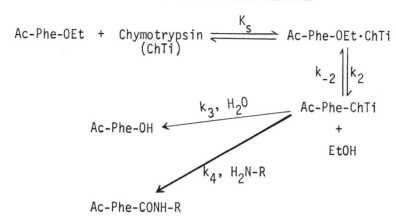

Fig. 5. Chymotrypsin-catalyzed peptide synthesis (from Fastrez and Fersht, 1973).

Although enzymatic synthesis of peptides is attractive because of its stereospecificity, mild conditions of reaction and elimination of need to protect amino acid side chains, this method probably has limited commercial application for modifying food proteins.

V. CHEMICAL MODIFICATION OF CASEIN WITH ACTIVE ESTERS OF AMINO ACIDS

The initial objective of this research was to investigate a method for covalent introduction of a limiting essential amino acid into a protein in aqueous solution. Casein was chosen as a model for a food protein because it is highly digestible, it has a limiting amount of methionine and it is commercially available at low cost. Moreover, since this protein has been widely used in feeding experiments with rats, it was considered ideal for studying the biological availability of amino acids covalently bound to the lysyl residues via isopeptide bonds.

N-Hydroxysuccinimide esters of tert-butyloxycarbonyl amino acids (Boc-amino acid-O-Su), described already for chemical modification of proteins in aqueous solution (Blumberg and Vallee, 1975; Slotboom and de Haas, 1975), was used for attaching amino acids to amino groups of casein. The tryptophan derivative was used to determine the best conditions for the reaction. In a typical experiment performed at room temperature, casein dissolved

in 0.1 M N-2-hydroxyethylpiperazine-N'-2-ethanesulfonate (HEPES)
buffer (pH 8.0) was incubated with a 10% (v/v) aqueous dimethyl
formamide solution containing the active ester. After 2 hr incubation, the modified casein was separated from reaction by-products by gel filtration on a Bio-Gel P-6 column (1.3 X 17 cm)
equilibrated with 0.05 M Tris-HCl buffer (pH 8.0) at room temperature. The column was quite effective for purification of 1.0 ml
of reaction mixture containing about 5 mg of protein.

     Under the above-described conditions, BOC-tryptophan
added to functional groups other than amino groups, namely the
hydroxyl group of tyrosyl residues. There was a linear relationship between the extent of modification and protein concentration
up to 10-12 mg casein/ml buffer. Then, the extent of reaction
reached a plateau, because of limitation on available active ester
as a result of base-catalyzed hydrolysis of the reagent and incomplete solubility of the active ester in the aqueous medium at
higher protein concentrations. Most of the amino groups of
casein (80-85% of the total) were covalently modified. Increasing
the reagent solubility with higher concentrations of dimethylformamide sharply increased ester formation and to a lesser extent
amide formation. Under conditions where most of the reagent was
soluble, ester bond formation was greater suggesting that increasing the concentration of soluble reagent via increasing concentration of dimethylformamide is not the method of choice for driving
the modification of amino groups to completion. By contrast, the
total amount (soluble and insoluble) of reagent used is very important. Complete modification of the ε-amino groups was achieved
with about 3-fold molar excess of reagent over the amount of amino
groups.

     Stability of the tryptophyl residues presumably linked to
tyrosines via ester linkages was studied (Fig. 6). Tryptophyl
ester bonds were quite stable at pH 7.0 and 25°C but were readily
removed in the presence of 1.0 M hydroxylamine. The extent of
formation and stability of ester bonds may be different with
different amino acids (Blumberg and Vallee, 1975).

     When reactions were performed in the following buffers:
sodium citrate pH 6.0, potassium phosphate pH 7.0, HEPES pH 8.0,
sodium borate pH 9.0 and sodium bicarbonate pH 10.0, maximum
modification occurred at pH 9.0. The reaction was 15% more
efficient at pH 9.0 than at pH 8.0. Therefore, the following
conditions were used for the large scale modification of casein.
A 5% suspension of vitamin-free casein in 0.1 M sodium borate
buffer (pH 9.0) was stirred for 30 min at room temperature, incubated for 1 hr at 45°C in order to increase solubility and then
cooled to 25°C. The active ester dissolved in 15% (v/v) aqueous
dimethylformamide was added slowly and the solution incubated for

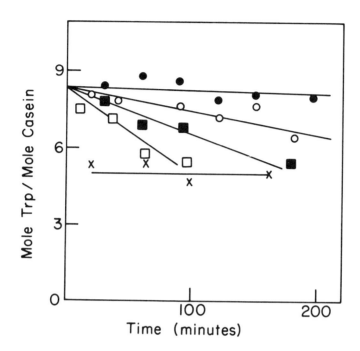

Fig. 6. Stability at 25°C of tryptophyl residues linked to casein by ester bonds. After casein was modified with a 1.0 molar ratio of BOC-Trp-OSu to amino groups as described in the text, pH of the reaction mixture was lowered to 7.0 and the modified protein separated from reagents and products by gel filtration. A Sephadex G-25 column (1.1 X 56 cm) equilibrated with 0.025 $\underline{M}$ Tris-HCl buffer (pH 7.0) was used for 2.0 ml reaction mixtures at room temperature. Concentration of pooled fractions was adjusted to 5 mg protein/ml with Tris-HCl buffer of the appropriate pH. For the stability study at pH 9.0, 25 m$\underline{M}$ sodium borate buffer was used. Stability of tryptophyl ester bonds was studied at pH 7.0 (●), 8.0 (○), 9.0 (■), 8.0 in the presence of a final concentration of 0.4 $\underline{M}$ hydroxylamine (□) and in the presence of a final concentration of 1.0 $\underline{M}$ hydroxylamine (X). After incubation for varying times, free BOC-Try was removed on Bio-Gel columns and bound Try estimated as described by Edelhoch (1967).

4 hr at room temperature. During the reaction, the pH was maintained at pH 9.0 with addition of NaOH solution. After hydroxylamine treatment at pH 8.0, as described before, the reaction mixture was dialyzed at 4°C for 3 days and lyophilized.

Removal of BOC groups was readily achieved by treatment of
proteins with anhydrous trifluoroacetic acid under conditions
where peptide and isopeptide bonds are expected to be stable.
BOC-group removal occurred very rapidly (less than 5 min) when 50
mg of lyophilized BOC-glycyl-casein were dissolved in 1.0 ml of
anhydrous TFA and incubated at room temperature. No additional
amino groups could be detected on further incubation of the protein up to 2 hr. A 30-fold molar excess of TFA over BOC groups
(300 mg protein/ml TFA) was generally used for complete removal
of amino protecting groups. The protein was then slowly dispersed
with stirring in 0.5 $\underline{M}$ Tris-HCl buffer (pH 8.0-9.0) with continuous adjustment of pH with 10 $\underline{N}$ NaOH. Precipitation always occurred when the protein was changed from TFA to an aqueous medium;
on further stirring, it dissolved. Following dialysis against
water, protein solutions were either lyophilized or precipitated
by adjusting the pH to 4.5 with 3 $\underline{N}$ HCl, freeze-dried and ground
into a powder for feeding experiments.

VI. PROPERTIES OF MODIFIED CASEINS

Viscosity of 2% solutions of modified casein was not changed
when a large number of hydrophobic groups (for example, 10 BOC-
alanyl residues/mole protein corresponding to an 8% weight increase in hydrophobic residues) was linked to the ε-amino groups
of the protein (Puigserver et al., unpublished data). This was
true even with bulky groups (BOC-Try) or negatively charged hydrophobic groups (BOC-Asp). When the amino group of the newly
attached amino acid was freed of the BOC group, the aspartyl-
casein derivative was the only modified protein with a significantly increased viscosity. This increase could be the result of
a conformational change through electrostatic repulsions. Changes
in solubility were not appreciable except for tryptophyl-casein;
tryptophan is known for its poor solubility in aqueous medium.
Casein has very little tertiary structure which may help explain
the viscosity and solubility results. It has been generally
assumed that hydrophobic residues are in the interior of a globular protein (one with tertiary structure) whereas the hydrophilic
side chains are on the outside. Therefore, a conformational
change might be expected when hydrophobic groups are attached to
the side chain of lysyl residues because they would tend to move
into the hydrophobic interior of the molecule. However, it is now
known that several globular proteins have accessible hydrophobic
groups (Klotz, 1970; Hofstee, 1975). With proteins lacking

ordered tertiary structure such as casein (Taborsky, 1974), the attachment of hydrophobic groups may have little effect on inducing tertiary structure.

In vitro enzyme digestion of casein modified through covalent attachment of hydrophobic and hydrophilic amino acids is reported in Table 1. Liberated amino groups, determined by trinitrobenzene sulfonic acid (TNBS) analysis (Fields, 1972), were used as a measure of the rate and extent of enzymatic digestion. When the amino protecting group was still present, the decrease in initial rates of digestion of α-chymotrypsin may be correlated with the extent of modification. There is a direct relationship between the increase in size of modifying amino acids (BOC-Gly < BOC-Ala < BOC-Met < BOC-Asp) and the decrease in initial rates of hydrolysis as determined with pancreatic enzymes mixtures. Removal of the BOC group increased the initial rates of digestion indicating the importance of steric hindrance (and/or substrate inhibition) in chymotrypsin-catalyzed hydrolysis of peptide bonds in modified caseins. The higher extent of digestion of alanyl-casein by chymotrypsin compared to aspartyl-casein, despite their almost identical solubility, confirmed this. Using reductive alkylation of protein amino groups (Means and Feeney, 1968; Means, 1977), several investigators have established that in vitro digestibility of various alkylated proteins is significantly lowered (Lin et al., 1969; Galembeck et al., 1977; Lee et al., 1978; Sen et al., unpublished data).

VII. BIOAVAILABILITY OF METHIONINE AND N-ACETYL-METHIONINE COVALENTLY LINKED TO CASEIN

Levels of free amino acids in plasma from rats fed casein modified by covalent attachment of glycine and methionine were determined in order to establish whether the isopeptide bond, formed between the ε-amino group of lysine and the carboxyl group of the newly added amino acid, was cleaved in vivo or not. For this purpose, four groups of 5 rats each (weanling Sprague-Dawley males) with approximately equal mean initial weights (63 ± 4 g) were fed a 10% protein diet containing either unmodified casein, glycyl-casein, methionyl-casein or isopropyl-casein for 3 days. The alkylated casein (a gift of H. S. Lee) was selected as a control since it has already been established that ε-N-isopropyl-lysine is unavailable as a lysine source for rats (Lee et al., 1978). Plasma levels of some important amino acids, in regard to this experiment, are reported in Table 2. The plasma amino acid patterns of rats fed glycyl- or methionyl-casein were normal compared to the pattern of those fed isopropyl-casein. This latter behavior with isopropyl-casein is typical of lysine deficiency

TABLE 1

In vitro Digestion Studies of Modified Caseins

Protein	Modification[a] (%)	Relative initial rate[b] (%)		Relative extent of digestion[c] (%)	
		- TFA	+ TFA	- TFA	+ TFA
Control casein	0	100	100	100	100
Alanyl- casein	44	49	43	64	92
	79	18	43	44	85
	88	10(34)	43(68)	55	84
Tryptophyl- casein	54	0	0	57	80
	87	0	0	36	68
	95	0	0	35	67
	97	0	0	32	77
Aspartyl- casein	36	18	65	69	77
	65	2	39	51	73
	83	2(15)	18(57)	38	60
Glycyl- casein	91	[50]	[73]		
Methionyl- casein	89	[32]	[46]		

[a]Determined by amino group estimation with TNBS (Fields, 1972) and by amino acid analysis following hydrolysis of proteins in 6 N HCl at 110°C for 24 hr.

[b]Performed with bovine α-chymotrypsin, bovine pancreatin ( ) and rat bile-pancreatic juice [ ]. Bovine enzymes were from Sigma Chemical Co., St. Louis, Mo. while rat pancreatic juice was a gift of B. Schneeman, UCD Dept. of Nutrition. Reaction mixtures containing 0.1% protein in 0.1 M phosphate buffer, pH 7.0, for pancreatin and pancreatic juice assays or in 0.02 M borate buffer, pH 8.2, for α-chymotrypsin assays, were incubated at 38°C with 1:60 (w/w; enzyme to protein) pancreatin, 1:3000 (v/v) pancreatic juice and 1:3,000 (w/w) α-chymotrypsin.

[c]Determined as above with 1:300 (w/w) α-chymotrypsin to protein after a 48 hr incubation period.

TABLE 2

Plasma Concentration of Some Free Amino Acids in Rats
Fed 10% Protein Diets[a]

Proteins	μmoles/100 ml plasma[b]				
	Lys	Thr	Ser	Gly	Met
Control casein	101	19	34	32	5
Met-casein[c]	96	17	33	27	39
Gly-casein[c]	72	19	34	30	8
iPro-casein[c]	17	46	44	40	6

[a]Average of 5 blood samples collected after a 3 day-test period by decapitation.

[b]Blood samples were collected at room temperature in centrifuge tubes containing 1.2% EDTA in 0.9% NaCl. After centrifugation, plasma samples were deproteinized with equal volumes of 6% sulfo-salicylic acid and kept frozen until analysis.

[c]Casein derivatives (methionyl-, glycyl- and isopropyl-) were highly modified (>90%) as determined by TNBS assay (Fields, 1972) and by amino acid analysis following hydrolysis of protein at 110°C for 24 hr in 6 N HCl.

(Gray et al., 1960; Morrison et al., 1961; Muramatsu et al., 1973; Lee et al., 1978).

The high level of methionine in the plasma of rats fed methionyl-casein might be related to an efficient cleavage of the corresponding isopeptide bond and a subsequent normal absorption through the intestinal wall. By contrast, the level of glycine in the plasma is not changed suggesting that hydrolysis of the ε-glycyllysine bond is less efficient than with the methionyl derivative. This may have some relationship with the diarrhea observed for the group of rats fed glycyl-casein and with the quite different physical aspect of this casein derivative compared to unmodified or methionyl-casein. Diarrhea was also observed when rats were fed isopropyl-casein (Lee et al., 1978). Diarrhea may also be the result of digestibility problems since it was shown that ε-N-glycyllysine was able to almost completely replace lysine (Mauron, 1970). However, results obtained with the dipeptide may be completely different from those arising from a protein because it is now well known that there are close relationships between peptide transport and hydrolysis (Ugolev, 1972; Matthews, 1975; Silk, 1977; Kim, 1977).

Another way to examine efficiency of hydrolysis of the isopeptide bond is to compare growth response of rats fed diets containing the same amount of an individual amino acid, either free or covalently linked. Since casein is slightly deficient in methionine and since methionine is one of the more limiting essential amino acids in several plant proteins (Henry and Ford, 1965; Miladi et al., 1972), it was decided to use methionyl-casein for this study. The effect of adding this amino acid would be higher with a protein even more deficient in methionine, such as a plant protein, but digestibility problems may also lower the response. As the nutritional similarities of methionine and N-acetyl-L-methionine have been demonstrated (Boggs et al., 1975), it was important to know whether this similarity is preserved when they are covalently attached to the ε-amino groups of a protein. Conversion of N-acetyl-L-methionine to its N-hydroxysuccinimide ester was performed essentially according to an already described method (Blumberg and Vallee, 1975). Its attachment to casein was achieved using the same experimental conditions as with methionine.

The protein composition of the isonitrogenous diets used in this feeding trial is listed in Table 3. As shown in Figure 7, the growth response of rats fed methionyl-casein was similar to that of rats fed a diet supplemented with free methionine. By contrast, N-acetyl-methionine linked to lysyl residues through an isopeptide bond was not as available as the free derivative. This may be the result of a less efficient hydrolysis of the isopeptide bond or of decreased absorption because of the protected amino group. Since the site of cleavage of the acyl moiety has not been clearly located in vivo (Rotruck and Boggs, 1975) an explanation of the difference cannot be given.

The nutritive value (PER) of methionyl-casein was comparable to that of the corresponding control (D_4) (Table 4) but was somewhat lower than commercial casein supplemented with free methionine (D_2). This is probably the result of effect of treatment of the protein with trifluoroacetic acid. Therefore, covalently bound methionine appears to be as readily available as the free amino acid while covalently bound N-acetyl-methionine is somewhat less available than when added in free form (compare D_5 and D_6).

TABLE 3

Protein Composition of Isonitrogenous Diets Used
in Growth Response Studies of Rats[a]

Diet	Proteins and amino acids		Methionine in the diet (% by weight)[b]
D_1	10%	commercial casein	0.26
D_2	10%	commercial casein	0.26
	0.2%	free methionine[c]	0.20
D_3	5%	commercial casein	0.13
	5%	methionyl-casein	0.34
D_4	5%	commercial casein	0.13
	5%	control casein[d]	0.13
	0.2%	free methionine	0.20
D_5	3%	commercial casein	0.08
	7%	N-acetyl-methionyl-casein	0.39
D_6	3%	commercial casein	0.08
	7%	control casein	0.18
	0.26%	N-acetyl-methionine	0.21

[a]Methionyl-casein and N-acetyl-methionyl-casein used in these
studies were 59 and 42% modified, respectively. The remainder of
the diet was of standard composition (Lee et al., 1978).

[b]Calculated by amino acid analysis as methionine and methionine
sulfone after performic acid oxidation.

[c]L-Methionine and N-acetyl-L-methionine were from Sigma Chemical
Co., St. Louis, Mo.

[d]Control casein was carried through all the steps used in preparing modified casein but without the addition of the methionine
derivatives.

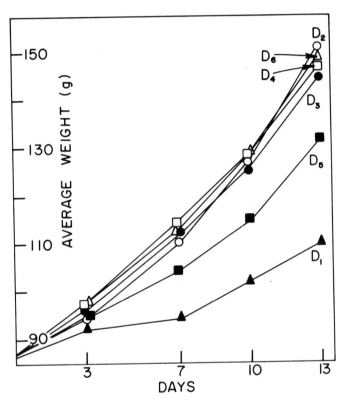

Fig. 7. Growth response of rats fed casein or casein derivatives as the sole protein source. Groups of 9 rats each with about the same mean initial weights were fed ad libitum 10% protein diets (see Table 3 for composition).

TABLE 4

Nutritive Values of Methionyl- and N-Acetyl-
methionyl-caseins for Rats[a]

Diet	Weight gain	Protein intake	PER[b]
D_1	72.6 ± 10.5	29.7 ± 3.6	2.46 ± 0.29
D_2	106.8 ± 9.7	33.7 ± 2.9	3.15 ± 0.23
D_3	60.5 ± 8.6	21.2 ± 1.5	2.92 ± 0.22
D_4	66.7 ± 10.6	22.2 ± 3.4	2.97 ± 0.30
D_5	89.8 ± 10.9	30.5 ± 4.0	2.95 ± 0.28
D_6	107.0 ± 9.9	33.6 ± 3.9	3.18 ± 0.29

[a]Groups of 9 rats each with about the same mean initial weights
were fed ad libitum 10% casein diets (see Table 3 for composition). All values are Mean ± SEM.

[b]Determined after a test period of 20 days. For groups fed
diets D_3 and D_4 the period was 14 days.

VIII. POTENTIAL COMMERCIAL APPLICATION OF COVALENTLY LINKED AMINO ACIDS TO PROTEINS

Fortification of foods with amino acids (Altschul, 1974) is
widely used in formulating animal feeds and must be considered as
an easy and relatively efficient way to improve the nutritional
value of food proteins. However many disadvantages, such as
flavor problems, loss of the added amino acids during processing
as well as side reactions occurring during processing or storage
are generally associated with this method. Reactions occurring
during processing generally result in a decrease of the nutritional value of the food. Moreover, it is becoming more and more
evident that, although the metabolism of amino acids free or
covalently attached in proteins is similar, it is not exactly the
same, primarily at the absorption level (Crampton, 1972; Matthews,
1972).

The quite efficient hydrolysis of the isopeptide bond of
ε-(methionyl)lysine _in vivo_ is important. The site-location of

the enzymatic activity responsible for this hydrolysis is of interest. To a certain extent, the isodipeptide ε-(methionyl)-lysine may be compared to the peptide ε-(γ-glutamyl)lysine. This latter peptide has been found in several tissues, namely body fluids, epithelial tissue and various proteins of wool and hair. The ε-(γ-glutamyl)lysine isopeptide bond, known to be formed enzymatically in blood clot formation or nonenzymatically during the heating of wool keratin, is very resistant to proteolysis (Kornguth et al., 1963). However, the peptide was able to replace lysine in rats and chicks fed lysine-deficient diets (Mauron, 1970; Waibel and Carpenter, 1972). As blood levels of the dipeptide in rats were lower when it was fed rather than intravenously infused, it has been postulated that an intestinal wall peptidase might be responsible for its hydrolysis (Folk and Finlayson, 1977). Such a situation may also be true for an ε-(amino acyl)lysine isodipeptide.

The covalent attachment of limiting essential amino acids to proteins is an attractive approach for improving the nutritional value of food proteins. The amino acid is biologically available as we have demonstrated in this work. It cannot be lost during processing. Moreover, the physical properties of proteins may be improved via the modification. The odor developed by addition of free methionine to foods, resulting from methional formation (Ballance, 1961), appears to be essentially eliminated when the amino acid is covalently bound to casein. By use of amino acids with protected amino groups, deteriorative reactions involving lysyl residues of protein (Carpenter and Booth, 1973; Feeney et al., 1975; Feeney, 1977; Cheftel, 1977) may be essentially eliminated during processing and storage.

Although biological activity of a number of enzymes are restored after TFA treatment when they are returned to aqueous solutions, this treatment cannot be applied to food proteins because of the toxicity of TFA. Thus, it is important to determine the usefulness of existing more labile amino-protecting groups such as diacid anhydrides (Dixon and Perham, 1968; Puigserver and Desnuelle, 1975) and other more complex compounds (Tesser and Balvert-Geers, 1975) and to design new reagents for use in modifying food proteins.

ACKNOWLEDGMENTS

The authors appreciate advice from Q. R. Rogers and H. S. Lee in conduct of the research, technical assistance from E. Gonzales-Flores and V. Crampton, and assistance of C. Robison in preparation of the manuscript. Financial support was received from grant FD 00568 from the Food and Drug Administration, from the University of California, Davis and from the Centre National de la Recherche Scientifique, Marseille, France.

REFERENCES

Abita, J. P., Maroux, S., Delaage, M. and Lazdunski, M. (1969). The reactivity of carboxyl groups in chymotrypsinogen. _FEBS Letters_, 4, 203.

Altschul, A. M. (1974). Fortification of foods with amino acids. _Nature_, 248, 643.

Anderson, G. W., Zimmerman, J. E. and Callahan, F. M. (1964). The use of esters of N-hydroxysuccinimide in peptide synthesis. _J. Am. Chem. Soc._, 86, 1839.

Anfinsen, C. B., Sela, M. and Cooke, J. P. (1962). The reversible reduction of disulfide bonds in polyalanyl ribonuclease. _J. Biol. Chem._, 237, 1825.

Ballance, P. E. (1961). Production of volatile compounds related to the flavor of foods from the Strecker degradation of DL-methionine. _J. Sc. Food Agr._, 12, 532.

Bergmann, M. and Fraenkel-Conrat, H. (1937). The role of specificity in the enzymatic synthesis of proteins. _J. Biol. Chem._, 119, 707.

Bergmann, M. and Fruton, J. S. (1938). Some synthetic and hydrolytic experiments with chymotrypsin. _J. Biol. Chem._, 124, 321.

Blau, K. and Waley, S. G. (1954). Chymotrypsin-catalyzed transpeptidations. _Biochem. J._, 57, 538.

Blumberg, S. and Vallee, B. L. (1975). Superactivation of thermolysin by acylation with amino acid N-hydroxysuccinimide esters. _Biochemistry_ 14, 2410.

Bodansky, M. and du Vigneaud, V. (1959). A method of synthesis of long peptide chains using a synthesis of oxytocin as an example. _J. Am. Chem. Soc._, 81, 5688.

Boggs, R. W., Rotruck, J. T. and Damico, R. A. (1975). Acetylmethionine as a source of methionine for the rat. _J. Nutr._, 105, 326.

Borrás, F. and Offord, R. E. (1970). Protected intermediate for the preparation of semisynthetic insulins. _Nature_, 227, 716.

Carpenter, K. J. and Booth, V. H. (1973). Damage to lysine in food processing: Its measurement and its significance. _Nutr. Abstr. Rev._, 43, 424.

Carraway, K. L. and Koshland, D. E., Jr. (1968). Reaction of tyrosine residues in proteins with carbodiimide reagents. _Biochim. Biophys. Acta_, 160, 272.

Carraway, K. L. and Koshland, D. E., Jr. (1972). Carbodiimide modification of proteins. _Meth. Enzym._, 25, 616.

Carraway, K. L., Spoerl, P. and Koshland, D. E., Jr. (1969). Carboxyl group modification in chymotrypsin and chymotryp-

sinogen. J. Mol. Biol., 42, 133.
Carraway, K. L. and Triplett, R. B. (1970). Reaction of carbo-
    diimides with protein sulfhydryl groups. Biochim. Biophys.
    Acta, 200, 564.
Cheftel, J. C. (1977). Chemical and nutritional modifications of
    food proteins due to processing and storage. In "Food Pro-
    teins," J. R. Whitaker and S. R. Tannenbaum, eds., Avi
    Publishing Co., Westport, Conn. p. 401.
Crampton, R. F. (1972). Nutritional and metabolic aspects of
    peptide transport. Peptide Transp. Bact. Mammalian Gut Symp.
    1971. Associated Scientific Publishers, Amsterdam.
Denkewalter, R. G., Schwam, H., Strachan, R. G., Beesley, T. E.,
    Veber, D. F., Schoenewaldt, E. F., Barkemeyer, H., Paleveda,
    W. J., Jr., Jacob, T. A. and Hirschmann, R. (1966). The
    controlled synthesis of peptides in aqueous medium. I. The
    use of α-amino acid N-carboxyanhydrides. J. Am. Chem. Soc.,
    88, 3163.
Dixon, H. B. F. and Perham, R. N. (1968). Reversible blocking of
    amino groups with citraconic anhydride. Biochem. J., 109,
    312.
Doscher, M. S. (1977). Solid phase peptide synthesis. Meth.
    Enzym., 47, 578.
Edelhoch, H. (1967). Spectroscopic determination of tryptophan
    and tyrosine in proteins. Biochemistry, 6, 1948.
Fastrez, Jacques and Fersht, A. R. (1973). Demonstration of the
    acyl-enzyme mechanism for the hydrolysis of peptides and
    anilides by chymotrypsin. Biochemistry, 12, 2025.
Feeney, R. E., Blankenhorn, G. and Dixon, H. B. F. (1975). Car-
    bonyl-amine reactions in protein chemistry. Adv. Prot.
    Chem., 29, 135.
Feeney, R. E. (1977). Chemical changes in food proteins. In
    "Evaluation of Proteins for Humans," C. E. Bodwell, ed., Avi
    Publishing Co., Westport, Conn. p. 233.
Feeney, R. E. and Whitaker, J. R., eds. (1977). "Food Proteins:
    Improvement Through Chemical and Enzymatic Modification."
    Adv. Chem. Series, 160, Am. Chem. Soc., Washington, D. C.
Fields, R. (1972). The rapid determination of amino groups with
    TNBS. Meth. Enzym. 25B, 464.
Folk, J. E. and Finlayson, J. S. (1977). The ε-(γ-glutamyl)-
    lysine crosslink and the catalytic role of transglutaminases.
    Adv. Prot. Chem., 31, 1.
Franzen, K. L. and Kinsella, J. E. (1976). Functional properties
    of succinylated and acetylated leaf protein. J. Agric. Food
    Chem., 24, 914.
Fridkin, M. and Patchornik, A. (1974). Peptide synthesis. Ann.
    Rev. Biochem., 43, 419.
Galembeck, F., Ryan, D. S., Whitaker, J. R. and Feeney, R. E.
    (1977). Reaction of proteins with formaldehyde in the pres-

ence and absence of sodium borohydride. _J. Agric. Food. Chem._, _25_, 238.

Garner, W. H. and Gurd, F. R. N. (1975). Semisynthesis of a specific NH_2-terminal [1-^{13}C] glycine adduct to sperm whale myoglobin: Intermediate protection of ε-amino groups with methyl acetimidate. _Biochem. Biophys. Res. Comm._, _63_, 262.

Glazer, A. N., Bar-Eli, A. and Katchalski, E. (1962). Preparation and characterization of polytyrosyl trypsin. _J. Biol. Chem._, _237_, 1832.

Goldberg, M. I. and Fruton, J. S. (1969). Beef liver esterase as a catalyst of acyl transfer to amino acid esters. _Biochemistry_, _8_, 86.

Gray, J. A., Olsen, E. M., Hill, D. C. and Branion, H. D. (1960). Effect of a dietary lysine deficiency on the concentration of amino acids in the deproteinized blood plasma of chicks. _Can. J. Biochem._, _38_, 435.

Heinrikson, R. L. and Kramer, K. J. (1974). Recent advances in the chemical modification and covalent structural analysis of proteins. In "Progress in Bioorganic Chemistry," _3_, E. T. Kaiser and F. J. Kezdy, eds., J. Wiley and Sons, N. Y.

Henry, K. M. and Ford, J. E. (1965). Nutritive value of leaf protein concentrates determined in biological tests with rats and by microbiological methods. _J. Sci. Food Agric._ 16, 425.

Hirschmann, R., Strachan, R. G., Schwam, H., Schoenewaldt, E. F., Joshua, H., Barkemeyer, B., Veber, D. F., Paleveda, W. J., Jr., Jacob, T. A., Beesley, T. E. and Denkewalter, R. G. (1967). The controlled synthesis of peptides in aqueous medium. III. Use of Leuchs' anhydrides in the synthesis of dipeptides. Mechanism and control of side reactions. _J. Organic Chem._, _32_, 3415.

Hirschmann, R., Schwam, H., Strachan, R. G., Schoenewaldt, E. F., Barkemeyer, H., Miller, S. M., Conn, J. B., Garsky, V., Veber, D. F. and Denkewalter, R. G. (1971). The controlled synthesis of peptides in aqueous medium. VIII. The preparation and use of novel α-amino acid N-carboxyanhydrides. _J. Am. Chem. Soc._, _93_, 2746.

Hoelzl Wallach, D. F. (1972). The dispositions of proteins in the plasma membranes of animal cells: Analytical approaches using controlled peptidolysis and protein labels. _Biochim. Biophys. Acta_, _265_, 61.

Hofstee, B. H. J. (1975). Accessible hydrophobic groups of native proteins. _Biochem. Biophys. Res. Comm._, _63_, 618.

Horecker, B. L., Melloni, E. and Pontremoli, S. (1975). Fructose 1,6-biphosphatase: Properties of the neutral enzyme and its modification by proteolytic enzymes. _Adv. Enzym._, _42_, 193.

Katchalski, E. and Sela, M. (1958). Synthesis and chemical properties of poly-α-amino acids. _Adv. Prot. Chem._, _13_, 243.

Katsoyannis, P. G. and Ginos, J. Z. (1969). Chemical synthesis

of peptides. Ann. Rev. Biochem., 38, 881.
Katsoyannis, P. G. and Schwartz, G. P. (1977). The synthesis of
     peptides by homogeneous solution procedures. Meth. Enzym.,
     47, 501.
Kim, Y. S. (1977). Intestinal mucosal hydrolysis of proteins and
     peptides. In "Peptide Transport and Hydrolysis." Ciba
     Found. Symp., 50, 151, Associated Scientific Publishers,
     Amsterdam.
Kimmel, J. R. and Smith, E. L. (1957). The properties of papain.
     Adv. Enzym., 19, 267.
Kinsella, J. E. (1976). Functional properties of proteins in
     foods: A survey. CRC Critical Rev. Food Sc. Nutr., 7, 219.
Klotz, I. M. (1970). Comparison of molecular structures of pro-
     teins: Helix content, distribution of apolar residues.
     Arch. Biochem. Biophys., 138, 704.
Knowles, J. R. (1974). Chemical modification and the reactivity
     of amino acids in proteins. In "Chemistry of Macromole-
     cules," 1, Gutfreund, H., ed., University Park Press,
     Baltimore. p. 149.
Kornguth, M. L., Neidle, A. and Waelsch, H. (1963). The stabil-
     ity and rearrangement of ε-N-glutamyl-lysines. Biochem-
     istry, 2, 740.
Kowalski, D. and Laskowski, M., Jr. (1976a). Chemical-enzymatic
     replacement of Ile[64] in the reactive site of soybean trypsin
     inhibitor (Kunitz). Biochemistry, 15, 1300.
Kowalski, D. and Laskowski, M., Jr. (1976b). Chemical-enzymatic
     insertion of an amino acid residue in the reactive site of
     soybean trypsin inhibitor (Kunitz). Biochemistry, 15, 1309.
Lee, H. S., Sen, L. C., Clifford, A. J., Whitaker, J. R. and
     Feeney, R. E. (1978). Effect of reductive alkylation of the
     ε-amino group of lysyl residues of casein on its nutritive
     value in rats. J. Nutr. In Press.
Lin, Y., Means, G. E. and Feeney, R. E. (1969). The action of
     proteolytic enzymes on N,N-dimethyl proteins. J. Biol.
     Chem., 244, 789.
Lode, E. T., Murray, C. L., Sweeney, W. V. and Rabinowitz, J. C.
     (1974). Synthesis and properties of Clostridium acidi-urici
     [Leu²]-ferredoxin: A function of the peptide chain and evi-
     dence against the direct role of the aromatic residues in
     electron transfer. Proc. Nat. Acad. Sci. USA, 71, 1361.
Louvard, D., Maroux, S., Vannier, C. and Desnuelle, P. (1975).
     Topological studies on the hydrolases bound to the intestinal
     brush border membrane. I. Solubilization by papain and
     Triton X-100. Biochim. Biophys. Acta, 375, 236.
Manning, J. M. and Moore, S. (1968). Determination of D- and L-
     amino acids by ion exchange chromatography as L-D and L-L
     dipeptides. J. Biol. Chem., 243, 5591.
Matthews, D. M. (1972). Rates of peptide uptake by small in-
     testine. Peptide Transp. Bact. Mammalian Gut Symp. 1971, 71.

Associated Scientific Publishers, Amsterdam.

Matthews, D. M. (1975). Intestinal absorption of peptides. Physiol. Rev., 55, 537.

Mauron, S. (1970). The chemical behavior of proteins during food preparation and its biological consequences. Int. Z. Vitaminforsch., 40, 209.

Means, G. E. and Feeney, R. E. (1968). Reductive alkylation of amino groups in proteins. Biochemistry, 7, 2192.

Means, G. E. and Feeney, R. E. (1971). "Chemical Modification of Proteins," Holden-Day, San Francisco.

Means, G. E. (1977). Reductive alkylation of amino groups. Meth. Enzym., 47, 469.

Merrifield, R. B. (1969). Solid-phase peptide synthesis. Adv. Enzym., 32, 221.

Milade, S., Hegsted, D. M., Saunders, R. M. and Kohler, G. O. 1972. The relative nutritive values, amino acid content and digestibility of the proteins of wheat mill fractions. Cereal Chem., 49, 119.

Miller, R. and Groninger, H. S., Jr. (1976). Functional properties of enzyme-modified acylated fish protein derivatives. J. Food Sci., 41, 268.

Mobley, W. C., Schenker, A. and Shooter, E. M. (1976). Characterization and isolation of proteolytically modified nerve growth factor. Biochemistry, 15, 5543.

Morihara, K. and Oka, T. (1977). α-Chymotrypsin as the catalyst for peptide synthesis. Biochem. J., 163, 531.

Morrison, A. B., Middleton, E. J. and McLaughlan, J. M. (1961). Blood amino acid studies. II. Effects of dietary lysine concentration, sex and growth rate on plasma free lysine and threonine levels in the rat. Can. J. Biochem., 39, 1675.

Muramatsu, K., Takeuchi, M. and Sakurai, K. (1973). The relationship between weight gain and free amino acid concentration of plasma and liver in rats fed a diet supplemented with various amounts of lysine. J. Nutr. Sci. Vitaminol., 19, 277.

Puigserver, A. and Desnuelle, P. (1975). Dissociation of bovine 6S procarboxypeptidase A by reversible condensation with 2,3-dimethyl maleic anhydride: Application to the partial characterization of subunit III. Proc. Nat. Acad. Sc. USA, 72, 2442.

Robinson, N. C., Neurath, H. and Walsh, K. A. (1973). The relation of the α-amino group of trypsin to enzyme function and zymogen activation. Biochemistry, 12, 420.

Rotruck, J. T. and Boggs, R. W. (1975). Comparative metabolism of L-methionine and N-acetylated derivatives of methionine. J. Nutr., 105, 331.

Sealock, R. W. and Laskowski, M., Jr. (1969). Enzymatic replacement of the arginyl by a lysyl residue in the reactive site of soybean trypsin inhibitor. Biochemistry, 8, 3703.

Sela, M. and Katchalski, E. (1959). Biological properties of poly-α-amino acids. Adv. Prot. Chem., 14, 391.

Sela, M., Lupu, N., Yaron, A. and Berger, A. (1962). Water-soluble polypeptidyl gliadins. Biochim. Biophys. Acta, 62, 594.

Sheehan, J. C. and Hess, G. P. (1955). A new method of forming peptide bonds. J. Am. Chem. Soc., 77, 1067.

Silk, D. B. A. (1977). Amino acid and peptide absorption in man. In "Peptide Transport and Hydrolysis," Ciba Found. Symp., 50, 15, Associated Scientific Publishers, Amsterdam.

Slotboom, A. J. and de Haas, G. M. (1975). Specific transformations at the N-terminal region of phospholipase A_2. Biochemistry, 14, 5394.

Spande, T. F., Witkop, B., Degani, Y. and Patchornik, A. (1970). Selective cleavage and modification of peptides and proteins. Adv. Prot. Chem., 24, 97.

St. Angelo, A. J., Conkerton, E. J., Dechary, J. M. and Altschul, A. M. (1966). Modification of edestin with N-carboxy-D,L-alanine anhydride. Biochim. Biophys. Acta, 121, 181.

Stewart, J. M. and Young, J. D. (1969). "Solid Phase Peptide Synthesis," W. H. Freeman and Company, San Francisco.

Taborsky, G. (1974). Phosphoproteins. Adv. Prot. Chem., 28, 1.

Tesser, G. I. and Balvert-Geers, I. C. (1975). The methyl-sulfonylethyloxycarbonyl group, a new and versatile amino protective function. Int. J. Peptide Protein Res., 7, 295.

Ugolev, A. M. (1972). Membrane digestion and peptide transport. Peptide Transp. Bact. Mammalian Gut Symp. 1971, 123, Associated Scientific Publishers, Amsterdam.

Virupaksha, T. K. and Tarver, M. (1964). The reaction of insulin with N-acetyl-DL-homocysteine thiolactone: Some chemical and biological properties of the products. Biochemistry, 3, 1507.

Waibel, P. E. and Carpenter, K. J. (1972). Mechanisms of heat damage in proteins. 3. Studies with ε-(γ-L-glutamyl)-L-lysine. Br. J. Nutr., 27, 509.

Wriston, J. C., Jr. (1973). Modification of chymotrypsinogen with 1-aminoglucose. FEBS Letters, 33, 93.

Yamashita, M., Arai, S., Tsai, S. J. and Fujimaki, M. (1971). Plastein reaction as a method for enhancing the sulfur-containing amino acid level of soybean protein. J. Agric. Food Chem., 19, 1151.

Yamashita, M., Arai, S. and Fujimaki, M. (1976). A low-phenylalanine, high-tyrosine plastein as an acceptable dietetic food. Method of preparation by use of enzymatic protein hydrolysis and resynthesis. J. Food Sci., 41, 1029.

30

INHIBITION OF LYSINOALANINE SYNTHESIS BY PROTEIN ACYLATION

Mendel Friedman

Western Regional Research Laboratory, U.S. Department of
Agriculture, Berkeley, California 94710

ABSTRACT

Treating wheat gluten, soy protein, and lactalbumin under
alkaline conditions at 65°C for various times destroys part of the
threonine, cystine, lysine, tyrosine, and arginine residues in these
proteins. The losses were accompanied by the appearance of lysinoalanine and unidentified ninhydrin-positive substances. Treating
wool under somewhat milder alkaline conditions destroys part of the
cystine and lysine residues, but not the other amino acids cited.
In this case, loss of cystine and lysine was accompanied by the
appearance of lanthionine and lysinoalanine. Amino acid analysis
of alkali-treated acylated proteins revealed that acylation by
acetic and succinic anhydrides prevents or minimizes destruction
of lysine residues and the formation of lysinoalanine in wheat
gluten and soy protein and, in wool, minimizes destruction of
cystine and lysine residues and the formation of lanthionine
lysinoalanine. Mechanisms are proposed to explain the observed
inhibiting effects of protein acylation and certain additives
on lysinoalanine formation.

INTRODUCTION

Alkali treatment of food proteins has been used for many
purposes including preparing meat analogues from vegetable (soy)
protein (Hamdy, 1974; Sternberg et al., 1977), destroying aflatoxin

(Goldblatt, 1969), peeling fruits and vegetables (Gee et al., 1974;
Schultz et al., 1977), and preparing protein concentrates, (e.g.,
Saunders et al., 1974; Wu et al., 1977).

Crosslinked amino acids have been found in hydrolysates of both
alkali-treated and heat-treated proteins (Provansal et al., 1975;
Friedman, 1977a; Hurrell and Carpenter, 1977). One of these crosslinked derivatives, lysinoalanine, has been found to cause histologi-
cal changes in the descending portion (pars recta) of the proximal
tubules of rat kidneys (Woodard et al., 1975; Gould and MacGregor,
1977; Friedman, 1977a); Cf. also, Finot et al., 1977). These
observations cause concern about the nutritional quality and
safety of alkali-treated proteins. The chemical changes that
produce unnatural amino acids such as lysino-alanine and
lanthionine during alkali treatment need to be explained and
strategies to minimize or prevent these reactions need to be
developed.

In previous papers we have (1) analyzed factors that are
expected to operate during alkali-induced crosslinking of amino
acid residues in proteins (Friedman, 1977a); (2) demonstrated inhibitory effects of mercaptoamino acids on lysinoalanine formation
during alkali treatment of casein and soy protein (Finley et al.,
1977); (3) observed alkali-induced changes in the amino acid composition of soy protein (Finley and Friedman, 1977); (4) studied the
transformation of lysine to lysinoalanine, and of cystine to
lanthionine residues in proteins and polyamino acids (Friedman,
1977a, Friedman et al., 1977); and (5) critically reviewed effects
of lysine modification on nutritional, chemical, and functional
properties of proteins (Friedman, 1977b). Related chemical and
photochemical transformations of wheat gluten, including reactions
in nonaqueous solvents such as dimethyl sulfoxide in the presence
of strong bases such as sodium hydride and metallic sodium are
described elsewhere (Cavins and Friedman, 1967, 1968; Krull, 1969;
Eskins and Friedman, 1970a, 1970b; Eskins et al., 1971; Friedman
et al., 1971; Wu et al., 1971; and Friedman, 1973). In this paper
the effect of alkali on amino acid profiles of wheat gluten, soy
protein, lactalbumin and wool is discussed.

MATERIALS AND METHODS

Commercial wheat gluten and lactalbumin were obtained from
Nutritional Biochemical Corporation, Cleveland, Ohio; Promine-D (soy
protein) was donated by Central Soya, Chicago, Illinois; acylated
wool derivatives were a gift of N. H. Koenig of this laboratory, and
the other derivatives were prepared as follows (Riordan and Vallee,
1972; Klapper and Klotz, 1972).

Acetylated Wheat Gluten. Gluten (12 g) was suspended in 100cc
of saturated sodium acetate solution to which was added 100cc of

water. The beaker was placed in an ice-bath. The suspension was
maintained at 0°C. Acetic anhydride (20 cc) was added with stirring
from a dropping funnel over a period of about ninety minutes (about
40 drops every ten minutes). The suspension was stirred for another
two hours, dialyzed against distilled water, and lyophilized.
Succinylated Wheat Gluten. Gluten (10 g) was suspended in 300cc of
water at 0°C. A 0.01 N NaOH solution was added to the gluten suspension until the pH reached 7.0. Succinic anhydride (Eastman)
(7 g) was added in seven portions over a period of about 70 minutes.
The pH was maintained at 7 by adding 1 N NaOH. The reaction mixture
was stirred for another hour, dialyzed against 0.01 N acetic acid,
and lyophilized.
Acetylated Soy Protein (Promine-D). Promine-D (12 g) suspended in
100cc saturated sodium acetate solution to which 100cc of water had
been added, was placed in an ice bath. The suspension was maintained at 0°C. Acetic anhydride (20cc) was added dropwise with
stirring over a period of 90 minutes. The reaction mixture was
stirred for another ninety minutes, dialyzed against water, and
lyophilized.
Succinylated Promine-D. Promine-D (10 g) was suspended in 200cc of
water and treated with 10 grams of solid succinic anhydride in ten
portions over a period of about one hour. The pH of the reaction
mixture was adjusted to 7.0 with 1N NaOH after each addition. The
mixture was stirred for another hour, dialyzed against water, and
lyophilized.

Examination of acylated wheat gluten and soy protein by the
manual ninhydrin reaction (Friedman and Williams, 1973; 1974;
Friedman and Broderick, 1977) revealed that 70 to 80% of the amino
groups had been modified.

Acylated Wool Derivatives. Wool was treated with the various
anhydrides in dimethylformamide for 30 minutes at 105°C as described
by Koenig (1965). Van Slyke analyses of modified wool swatches
indicated that this treatment modified about 80% of the free amino
groups.
Alkali Treatments. The following procedure, illustrated with wheat
gluten, was also used with the other food proteins. A solution or
suspension of gluten (for a 1% solution, 0.5 gram of protein per
50cc of solvent; for a 10% solution, 5.0 grams per 50cc) in a glass-
stoppered Erlenmeyer flask was placed a 65°C water bath. After the
indicated time, the solution was dialyzed against 0.01N acetic acid
for about 2 days and then lyophilized.
Amino Acid Analyses. A weighed sample (about 5 mg) of protein was
hydrolyzed in 15cc of 6N HCl in a commercial hydrolysis tube. The
tube was evacuated, placed in an acetone-dry ice bath, evacuated
and refilled with nitrogen twice before being placed in an oven at
110°C for 24 hrs. The cooled hydrolysate was filtered through a
sintered disc funnel, evaporated to dryness at 40°C, with the aid
of an aspirator, and the residue was twice suspended in water and

evaporated to dryness. Amino acid analysis of an aliquot of the
soluble hydrolysate was carried out on a Durrum Amino Acid Analyzer,
Model D-500 under the following conditions: single column Moore-
Stein ion-exchange chromatography method; Resin, Durrum DC-4A;
buffer pH, 3.25, 4,25, 7.90; photometer, 440 nm, 590 nm; column,
1.75 mm X 48 cm; analysis time, 105 mn. Norleucine was used as an
internal standard.

In this system, lysinoalanine (LAL) is eluted just before histidine. The color constant of LAL was determined with an authentic
sample purchased from Miles Laboratories. The results are summarized in Tables 1-12 and Figures 1-12.

RESULTS AND DISCUSSION

Effects of pH and Protein Concentration.

The results in Tables 1-12 are reported in terms of mole percent of amino acids accounted for and ratio to alanine rather than
as weights of moles of each amino acid per unit weight of sample.
(Alanine or any other amino acid that is presumed to be unaffected
by the treatment acts as an internal standard). The mole per cent
or ratio method are more consistent measures of amino acid composition of processed, commercial, or modified proteins because they
avoid errors due to moisture content (acylated proteins are highly
hygroscopic), protein content (the commercial wheat gluten, soy
protein, and lactalbumin contain carbohydrates, lipids, etc.),
molecular weights changes, and errors occurring in all operations
during amino acid analysis (Cf. Cavins and Friedman, 1968a).

The data (Tables 1-4; Figures 8-9 show that the following amino
acids are degraded or destroyed during the alkaline treatment of
gluten: Threonine, serine, cystine, tyrosine, lysine, and arginine.
Thus, treating 1% (w/v) gluten in a N NaOH (Tables 1-3) at 65°C
decreases the threonine content to about 70% of the original value
after one hour, 39% after three hours, and 25% after eight hours.

The corresponding values for serine are 63, 36, and 24%; for tyrosine, 84, 76, and 68%; for lysine, 67, 76, and 87%, and for
arginine, 82, 69, and 42%, respectively. The treatment also induces
the disappearance of cystine and the appearance of lysinoalanine
(LAL) residues. Examination of the Tables also shows that the
relative concentrations of both proline and glutamic acid appear
to be increasing and that of glycine seems to decrease with
increasing exposure time of wheat gluten to alkali. No obvious
explanations can be offered to explain these results.

Table 1

Effect of pH on amino acid composition of wheat gluten.
Conditions: 1% wheat gluten; 65°C; 3 hours.
Numbers are mole (residue) per cent[a] for each amino acid.

Amino Acid	Control	9.6	10.6	11.2	12.5	13.9
ASP	3.20	3.26	3.26	3.15	3.57	2.96
THR	3.19	3.10	3.05	3.01	2.67	1.20
SER	6.81	6.75	6.64	6.55	5.30	2.24
GLU	27.90	32.57	32.53	33.36	33.09	39.28
PRO	18.33	14.25	14.80	14.82	13.56	16.55
GLY	6.01	6.30	5.78	6.10	5.76	3.94
ALA	3.91	3.95	4.07	3.86	4.40	3.78
CYS	0.976	0.691	0.00	0.00	0.00	0.00
VAL	4.36	4.32	4.40	4.26	4.80	4.20
MET	1.35	1.25	1.18	1.33	1.68	1.17
ILEU	3.68	3.52	3.68	3.62	4.37	3.97
LEU	7.48	7.28	7.49	7.31	8.00	8.58
TYR	2.49	2.55	2.43	2.49	2.43	1.85
PHE	4.35	4.29	4.52	4.35	4.29	4.93
LAL	0.00	0.00	0.262	0.420	0.762	0.884
HIS	1.87	1.80	1.83	1.78	1.74	1.71
LYS	1.33	1.40	1.16	0.963	0.945	0.948
ARG	2.75	2.70	2.66	2.68	2.61	1.79

[a]Mole per cent is defined as moles of each amino acid recovered from the ion-exchange column divided by the sum for all amino acids listed times 100.

Table 2. Effect of alkali treatment on amino acid composition of
          gluten.
          Conditions: 1% wheat gluten in 1N NaOH; 65°C.
          A columns show mole per cent of residues accounted for
          and B columns, mole ratios to alanine.

Amino Acid	Gluten Control (untreated) A	B	Time of Treatment 1 HR A	B	3 HR A	B	8 HR A	B
ASP	3.20	0.819	3.28	0.801	2.96	0.810	2.77	0.825
THR	3.19	0.816	2.34	0.573	1.18	0.322	0.685	0.205
SER	6.81	1.74	4.49	1.10	2.29	0.627	1.39	0.414
GLU	27.90	7.13	25.00	6.11	31.24	8.56	31.32	9.35
PRO	18.33	4.68	23.31	5.69	25.09	6.87	28.10	8.38
GLY	6.01	1.54	4.83	1.18	3.55	0.745	3.08	0.916
ALA	3.91	1.00	4.09	1.00	3.65	1.00	3.35	1.00
CYS	0.976	0.250	0.00	0.00	0.00	0.00	0.00	0.00
VAL	4.36	1.11	4.70	1.14	4.06	1.11	4.27	1.27
MET	1.35	0.346	1.48	0.362	1.23	0.336	0.912	0.272
ILEU	3.68	0.939	4.37	1.06	3.94	1.08	3.96	1.18
LEU	7.48	1.91	8.84	2.16	8.80	2.41	9.21	2.74
TYR	2.49	0.638	2.19	0.535	1.78	0.486	1.49	0.436
PHE	4.35	1.11	5.24	1.28	5.40	1.48	5.46	1.62
LAL	0.00	0.00	0.654	0.160	0.634	0.174	0.611	0.188
HIS	1.87	0.477	1.88	0.459	1.63	0.446	1.80	0.450
LYS	1.33	0.340	0.943	0.230	0.857	0.234	0.900	0.269
ARG	2.75	0.703	2.35	0.574	1.72	0.470	0.990	0.295

Table 3. Effect of alkali-treatment on amino acid composition of wheat gluten. Conditions: <u>10% wheat gluten</u> in 1N NaOH; 65°C. A columns show mole per cent of residues accounted for and B columns, mole ratios to alanine.

Amino Acid	Gluten Control		Time of Treatment					
			1 HR		3 HR		8 HR	
	A	B	A	B	A	B	A	B
ASP	3.20	0.819	2.69	0.796	3.02	0.805	2.84	0.807
THRE	3.19	0.816	2.09	0.619	1.65	0.440	0.983	0.279
SER	6.18	1.74	3.80	1.13	2.52	0.671	1.53	0.500
GLU	27.90	7.13	37.10	10.9	35.70	9.52	39.47	1.1
PRO	18.33	4.68	19.65	5.82	19.75	5.26	21.14	5.99
GLY	6.01	1.54	4.52	1.34	3.94	1.10	3.59	1.02
ALA	3.91	1.00	3.38	1.00	3.75	1.00	3.52	1.00
CYS	0.976	0.00	0.00	0.00	0.00	0.00	0.00	0.00
VAL	4.36	1.11	3.93	1.16	4.24	1.13	4.02	1.14
MET	1.35	0.346	1.10	0.326	1.16	0.309	1.14	0.323
ILEU	3.68	0.939	3.42	1.01	4.11	1.09	3.40	0.965
LEU	7.48	1.91	7.19	2.13	8.30	2.21	8.29	2.35
TYR	2.49	0.638	1.94	0.574	2.06	0.550	1.58	0.450
PHE	4.35	1.11	4.41	1.30	4.64	1.23	4.50	1.27
LAL	0.00	0.00	<u>0.493</u>	0.146	<u>0.835</u>	0.222	<u>0.610</u>	0.173
HIS	1.87	0.477	1.68	0.498	1.61	0.428	1.45	0.410
LYS	1.33	0.340	0.774	0.195	0.846	0.225	0.846	0.240
ARG	2.75	0.703	1.83	0.541	1.85	0.495	1.06	0.300

Table 4. Effect of alkali-treatment on amino acid composition of soybean (Promine-D) protein. Conditions: 1% Promine-D in 1N NaOH; 65°C; A columns show mole per cent of residues accounted for and B columns, mole ratios to alanine.

Amino Acid	Promine-D Control		1 HR		3 HR		8 HR	
	A	B	A	B	A	B	A	B
ASP	11.62	1.77	12.82	1.98	3.39	2.15	14.78	2.39
THRE	4.49	0.684	2.75	0.425	1.97	0.317	1.58	0.256
SER	6.89	1.05	4.05	0.626	2.67	0.429	1.76	0.284
GLU	16.74	2.55	20.52	3.17	22.74	3.65	24.74	4.00
PRO	6.37	0.970	6.47	1.00	6.23	1.00	6.19	1.00
GLY	7.42	1.13	7.31	1.13	6.85	1.10	5.96	0.964
ALA	6.56	1.00	6.47	1.00	6.23	1.00	6.19	1.00
VAL	5.39	0.822	5.62	0.859	5.91	0.949	6.31	1.02
MET	1.07	0.163	1.09	0.168	0.75	4.121	1.04	0.168
ILEU	4.57	0.697	4.36	0.673	4.20	0.675	3.87	0.626
LEU	8.53	1.30	8.94	1.38	8.91	1.43	9.46	1.53
TYR	2.91	0.443	2.57	0.397	2.22	0.356	2.38	0.385
PHE	4.46	0.679	4.18	0.645	4.86	0.781	4.05	0.654
LAL	0.00	0.00	1.19	0.183	1.37	0.220	1.31	0.212
HIS	2.07	0.316	2.27	0.350	2.16	0.347	2.13	0.345
LYS	5.32	0.811	4.63	0.715	4.67	0.749	4.99	0.792
ARG	5.59	0.852	4.80	0.742	4.92	0.789	2.42	0.392

Time of treatment

Table 5. Effect of alkali-treatment on amino acid composition of
soybean (Promine-D) protein. Conditions: 10% Promine-D in 1N NaOH;
65°C, A columns show mole per cent of residues accounted for and
B columns, mole ratios to alanine.

Amino Acid	Promine-D Control		Time of treatment					
			1 HR		3 HR		8 HR	
	A	B	A	B	A	B	A	B
ASP	11.62	1.77	12.42	1.91	12.99	1.98	13.93	2.14
THRE	4.49	0.684	2.88	0.443	2.15	0.328	2.30	0.199
SER	6.89	1.05	4.20	0.647	2.92	0.446	1.80	0.276
GLU	16.73	2.55	20.62	3.17	21.84	3.33	24.29	3.73
PRO	6.37	0.970	6.51	1.00	6.48	0.988	7.49	1.15
GLY	7.42	1.13	7.29	1.12	7.28	1.11	6.77	1.04
ALA	6.56	1.00	6.51	1.00	6.56	1.00	6.51	1.00
VAL	5.39	0.822	5.30	0.814	5.81	0.886	5.89	0.904
MET	1.07	0.163	0.995	0.153	1.07	0.164	0.827	0.127
ILEU	4.57	0.697	4.32	0.664	4.29	0.654	3.80	0.583
LEU	8.53	1.30	8.91	1.37	9.12	1.39	9.57	1.47
TYR	2.91	0.443	2.62	0.403	2.37	0.361	2.17	0.333
PHE	4.45	0.679	4.30	0.662	4.25	0.648	4.16	0.638
LAL	0.00	0.00	1.29	0.198	1.52	0.232	1.64	0.252
HIS	2.07	0.316	2.18	0.335	2.22	0.339	2.18	0.335
LYS	5.32	0.811	4.60	0.707	4.64	0.708	4.83	0.742
ARG	5.59	0.852	5.04	0.774	4.45	0.679	2.82	0.433

Table 6. Effect of pH on amino acid composition of lactalbumin.
Conditions: 1% lactalbumin: 65°C; 3 hours. Numbers are mole
(residue) percent values of the total accounted for.

Amino Acid	Control	pH				
		9.60	10.60	11.20	12.50	13.90
ASP	12.02	11.68	11.34	12.31	12.14	15.55
THR	6.01	6.04	6.00	5.95	5.33	2.75
SER	6.18	6.11	6.17	6.08	5.44	2.26
GLU	14.35	14.82	14.96	14.14	14.96	14.10
PRO	5.13	5.20	5.52	4.83	5.35	4.52
GLY	3.65	3.70	3.76	3.71	4.02	4.51
ALA	7.40	7.78	7.74	7.50	7.97	8.22
CYS	0.952	0.558	0.190	0.00	0.00	0.00
VAL	5.94	5.94	5.96	5.84	6.12	6.40
MET	1.84	1.96	2.12	2.06	1.92	2.14
ILEU	5.08	5.06	5.21	5.18	5.21	5.15
LEU	13.08	13.04	12.92	13.49	13.20	15.67
TYR	2.59	2.56	2.75	2.70	2.90	2.42
PHE	2.93	2.91	3.04	3.00	3.21	2.72
LAL	0.00	0.255	1.04	1.52	2.62	3.87
HIS	1.66	1.60	1.67	1.64	1.51	1.20
LYS	8.94	8.57	7.47	7.45	6.48	7.19
ARG	2.14	2.22	2.15	2.12	1.61	1.32

Table 7

Effect of alkali-treatment on amino acid composition of
lactalbumin. Conditions: 1% lactalbumin in 1N NaOH; 65° C.
A columns show mole per cent of the residues accounted for
and B columns, mole ratios to alanine.

Amino Acid	Lactalbumin Control		1 Hr		3 Hrs		8 Hrs	
	A	B	A	B	A	B	A	B
ASP	12.09	1.46	13.07	1.51	13.93	1.60	14.97	1.71
THRE	6.43	0.776	4.59	0.530	1.92	0.221	1.85	0.211
SER	6.58	0.794	4.32	0.499	2.85	0.327	1.51	0.172
GLU	15.58	1.88	17.58	2.03	19.06	2.19	20.00	2.28
ALA	8.29	1.00	8.66	1.00	8.70	1.00	8.75	1.00
VAL	6.40	0.773	6.48	0.749	6.80	0.781	6.98	0.796
MET	2.10	0.254	2.14	0.247	1.75	0.201	2.10	0.240
ILEU	5.38	0.649	5.20	0.600	5.39	0.619	4.75	0.542
LEU	13.67	1.65	14.20	1.64	15.14	1.74	15.85	1.81
TYR	2.92	0.352	2.78	0.323	2.65	0.304	2.34	0.267
PHE	3.17	0.382	3.09	0.357	3.06	0.351	2.78	0.318
LAL	0.00	0.00	2.60	0.300	3.20	0.367	3.14	0.358
HIS	1.80	0.217	1.57	0.181	1.48	0.170	1.33	0.152
LYS	9.20	1.11	7.10	0.820	7.17	0.824	7.97	0.910
ARG	2.33	0.281	1.72	0.198	1.44	0.165	0.850	0.097

Table 8. Effect of alkali-treatment on amino acid composition of
lactalbumin. Conditions: 10% lactalbumin in 1N NaOH; 65°C.
A columns show mole per cent of residues accounted for and
B columns, mole ratios to alanine.

Amino	Lactalbumin		Time of Treatment					
Acid	Control		1 HR		3 HR		8 HR	
	A	B	A	B	A	B	A	B
ASP	12.09	1.46	13.04	1.51	13.65	1.53	14.48	1.63
THR	6.43	0.776	4.90	0.567	3.50	0.392	2.02	0.227
SER	6.58	0.794	4.61	0.534	3.26	0.365	1.79	0.202
GLU	15.58	1.88	17.62	2.04	18.38	2.06	19.19	2.16
GLY	4.06	0.490	4.77	0.552	5.49	0.615	5.49	0.618
ALA	8.29	1.00	8.64	1.00	8.92	1.00	8.89	1.00
VAL	6.40	0.773	6.50	0.753	5.30	0.594	7.06	0.795
MET	2.10	0.254	2.32	0.269	2.37	0.266	2.05	0.231
ILEU	5.38	0.649	5.23	0.606	5.43	0.609	5.13	0.578
LEU	13.67	1.65	14.25	1.65	15.17	1.70	15.81	1.78
TYR	2.92	0.545	2.73	0.316	2.72	0.305	2.41	0.272
PHE	3.17	0.382	3.06	0.354	3.03	0.340	2.84	0.320
LAL	0.00	0.00	2.74	0.271	3.22	0.361	3.43	0.386
HIS	1.80	0.217	1.39	0.161	1.42	0.160	1.22	0.138
LYS	9.20	1.11	7.25	0.840	6.95	0.779	7.36	0.828
ARG	2.33	0.281	1.31	0.152	1.16	0.130	0.773	0.087

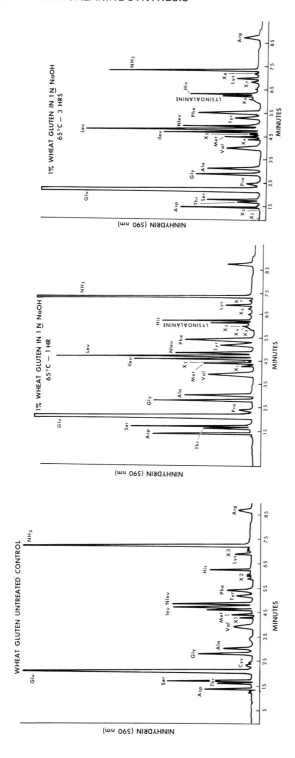

Figure 1. Amino acid analyses of hydrolysates of commercial wheat gluten and alkali-treated wheat glutens.

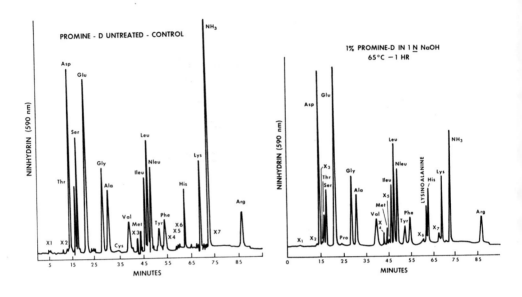

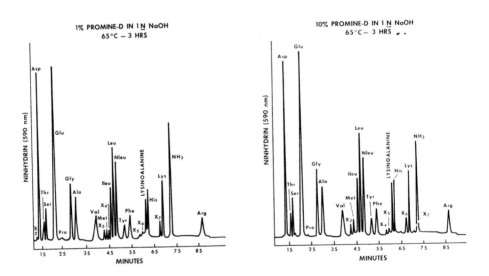

Figure 2.   Amino acid analyses of hydrolysates of commercial
            soy protein (promine-D) and alkali-treated promine-D.

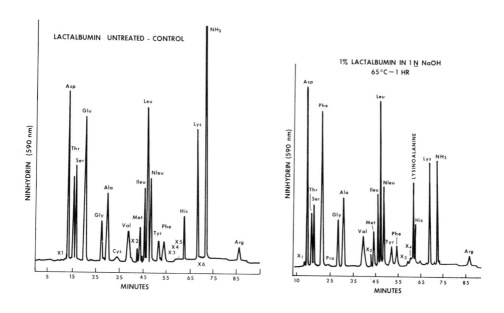

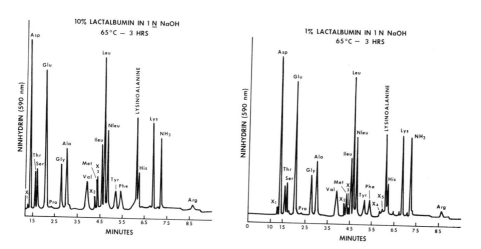

Figure 3. Amino acid analyses of hydrolysates of commercial lactal-bumins and alkali-treated lactalbumins.

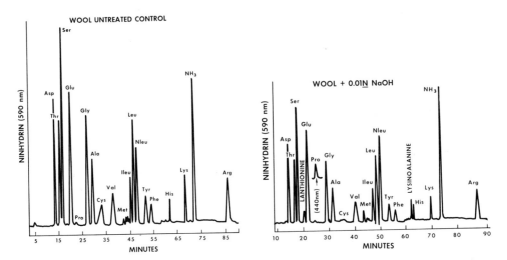

Figure 4.   Amino acid analyses of native and alkali-treated wools.

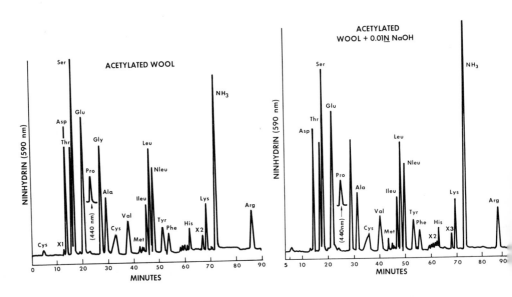

Figure 5.   Amino acid analyses of hydrolysates of acetylated and
alkali-treated-acetylated wools.

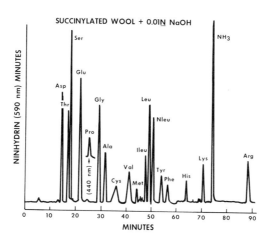

Figure 6.   Amino acid analysis of a hydrolysate of alkali-treated
            succinylated wools.

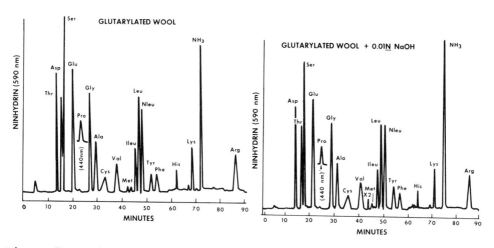

Figure 7.   Amino acid analyses of glutarylated and alkali-treated
            glutarylated wools.

The lysine content appears to go through a minimum. This unexpected result is consistent with the lysine peak being composite of lysine and ornithine, the latter derived from arginine by alkali-degradation (Friedman, 1977a). Another possibility is that lysinoalanine is destroyed (besides being formed) during alkaline treatment, regenerating lysine. An analogous reaction has been shown to occur when ε-cyanoethyl derivatives of lysine are subjected to alkaline conditions (Cavins and Friedman, 1967). The data suggest that after about one hour, the rate of lysinoalanine destruction may be as fast as its rate of formation. This conclusion is supported by the observed leveling off of lysinoalanine content after about one hour in all of the food proteins studied.

The destruction of alkali-labile amino acids appears to proceed at similar, although not identical, rates in soy protein and lactalbumin (Table 4-8; Figures 10-12). The amino acid composition sequence, conformation, and molecular weight of a specific protein, may all influence its reactivity with alkali. Therefore, differences in rates of destruction of alkali-labile amino acids in different proteins are not surprising. What is surprising is that the concentration of the substrate protein (e.g., wheat gluten) does not affect the extent of alkali-induced change in amino acid composition nor the rate of formation of lysinoalanine at high pH (cf. Sternberg and Kim, 1977). Thus, data in Tables 1-3 show that alkali-induced changes are about the same when 1% and 10% solutions of gluten, are treated in 1N NaOH at 65°C.

The observed apparent absence of a concentration effect can probably be explained as follows with the aid of Figures 13-15. Since elimination reactions of serine, threonine, and cystine to form dehydroalanine side chains are second-order reactions that depend on the concentration of both hydroxide ion and the susceptible amino acid, the extent of crosslinking should be a direct function of the hydroxide ion concentration. This is indeed the case (Whitaker and Feeney, 1977). Moreover, because reaction of the ε-amino group of lysine with a vinyl-type compound such as dehydroalanine to form a lysinoalanine side chain is also a second-order reaction (Friedman and Wall, 1964; Snow et al., 1976), an increase in protein concentration would be expected to increase the rate of lysinoalanine formation. Since this apparently does not occur, the major factor controlling lysinoalanine formation once the rate-determining precursor dehydroalanine is formed, may be the location of required partners for crosslink formation. Only dehydroalanine and lysine residues situated on the same or closely adjacent protein chains are favorably placed to form crosslinks. When the convenient sites have been used up, additional lysinoalanine or other crosslinks form less readily. Each protein, therefore, may have a limited fraction of potential sites for productive formation of crosslinked residues. The other sites are unproductive in the sense discussed. The number of productive sites may vary and

is presumably dictated by the protein's size, composition, conformation, chain mobility, and steric factors.

As already mentioned, the rates of both formation and
destruction of lysinoalanine may be greater in more concentrated
protein solutions, accounting for a limiting observed lysinoalanine
content that appears to be essentially independent of initial
protein concentration for wheat gluten, soy protein, and lactalbumin
at high pH.

Crosslinking reaction rates in concentrated protein solutions
or suspensions may also be influenced by protein-protein interactions that hinder accessability of reactants to one another.
Finally, because the rate of dehydroalanine formation depends
directly on hydroxide ion concentration, the rate of lysinoalanine
formation may depend on initial protein concentration when the reaction is carried out below at pH of about 11, where the slower
addition of ionized amino groups of lysine side chains (pK≈10) to
dehydroalanine residues to form lysinoalanine side chains rather
than hydroxide ion-catalyzed elimination of serine and cystine residues to form dehydroalanine side chains, is rate-controlling. This
statement implies that the rate of lysinoalanine formation at high
pH (above 12) may be governed mainly by the hydroxide ion concentration, while the corresponding rate at lower pH (below 11) is
controlled mainly by the amino group (protein) concentration. At
intermediate pH's, both the elimination and addition reactions
would then contribute to the rate determination.

The situation is even more complicated. Figures 8 and 11
show that cystine residues decompose at lower pH's than serine and
threonine residues. Consequently, the rate of formation of lysinoalanine as a function of pH in different proteins will also depend
on their relative contents of cystine, serine, and threonine.

Milder conditions (0.01 N NaOH instead of 1.0 N NaOH) were used
for wool because the more concentrated base completely dissolves
wool. Results in Table 11 show that this alkali treatment of wool
appears not to affect the threonine, serine, tyrosine, and arginine
content significantly. In contrast, the treatment did decrease the
cystine and lysine content. These decreases were accompanied by
the appearance of two new amino acids: lanthionine and lysinoalanine
(cf. Asquith and Otterburn, 1977).

Effect of Acylation. Since lysinoalanine formation from lysine
requires participation of an ε-amino group, protection of the amino
groups by acylation (acetylation, succinylation, etc.) as illustrated in Figures 16-17 should minimize or prevent lysinoalanine
formation under alkaline conditions if the protective group survives
the treatment. This expectation was, indeed, realized. Results in

Tables 9-11 demonstrate that acylations of wheat gluten, soy protein, and wool prevented or minimized lysinoalanine formation.
        In the case of wheat gluten and promine-D, either acetylation
or succinylation prevented both lysine destruction and lysinoalanine
formation. However, the other amino acid residues (cystine, serine,
threonine, arginine, and, to a lesser extent, tyrosine) were
modified.

        Exposure of native, acetylated, succinylated, or glutarylated
wool to (0.01 $\underline{N}$ NaOH, 65°C for one hr) gave unchanged amino acid
profiles. Thus, in the case of wool, acylation not only prevents
lysinoalanine and lanthionine formation but also loss of cystine
under the conditions examined. In contrast to wool, lanthionine was
absent in hydrolysates of alkali-treated native and acylated food
proteins.

        As previously noted (Friedman, 1977b), modifying proteins with
acetic anhydride is a widely used reaction to alter their functionality for various applications. Acetic anhydride transforms basic
amino groups to neutral amide side chains. In contrast, succinylation introduces a four-carbon side chain with a potentially
negatively-charged carboxyl group. Since such negatively charged
carboxyl groups electrostatically repel negatively charged hydroxyl
groups of the alkaline medium, succinylation was expected not only
to prevent lysinoalanine formation but also to minimize elimination
reactions leading to the destruction of serine, threonine, and
cystine. The data in Tables 10-12 do not support this expectation.
Possibly the repulsion of carboxylate ions causes unfolding of side
chains making the protein more accessible to attack by alkali.
(Cf. Habeeb et al., 1958 and Koenig and Friedman, 1977). In addition, the ionic strength of the medium may be high enough that the
local charges are screened from one another by the ion atmosphere.

        If acylated proteins turn out to be as nutritionally available
and safe as unmodified proteins (Cf. Friedman, 1977b), then acylation may be of practical value to protect proteins against formation
of lysinoalanine. It should be noted, however, that conditions
described in this paper are more severe than generally used in food
processing. Since commercial alkali treatment of proteins is
generally carried out above pH 10 at room temperature for short
periods, the actual lysinoalanine content of most alkali-treated
foods is probably small, although examination of the effect of pH
on the extent of lysinoalanine formation of wheat gluten,
and lactalbumin (Tables 1,6) reveals that after one hour
measurable amounts of the unnatural amino acids are formed at pH
10.6 and 65°C.

Mechanisms of Inhibiting Lysinoalanine Formation. As noted above,
lysinoalanine and related crosslinked amino acids may be derived
from reaction of lysine with dehydroalanine residues formed by

Table 9

Effect of acetylation and succinylation on amino acid composition of alkali-treated wheat gluten. Numbers for each amino acid are mole percentages of the total accounted for.

Amino Acid	Gluten Control untreated)	1% gluten + NaOH 3 Hrs	1% Acetylated gluten + NaOH 3 Hrs	10% Acetylated gluten + NaOH 1 Hr	10% Acetylated gluten + NaOH 3 Hrs	1% Succinylated gluten + NaOH 1 Hr
ASP	3.20	2.96	3.37	3.16	3.38	3.13
THRE	3.19	1.18	1.32	2.18	1.55	2.17
SER	6.81	2.29	2.64	4.31	2.85	4.19
GLU	27.90	31.24	30.58	35.42	35.77	35.45
PRO	18.33	25.09	20.43	16.42	16.94	16.46
GLY	6.01	3.55	4.79	5.30	4.89	5.37
ALA	3.91	3.65	4.02	3.96	4.21	3.92
VAL	4.36	4.06	4.74	4.27	4.59	4.43
MET	1.35	1.23	1.39	1.35	1.36	0.737
ILEU	3.68	3.94	4.26	3.59	3.83	3.92
LEU	7.48	8.80	9.41	7.68	8.38	8.11
TYR	2.49	1.78	2.14	2.23	2.03	2.44
PHE	4.35	5.40	5.75	4.59	4.63	4.98
LAL	0.00	0.634	0.00	0.00	0.126	0.00
HIS	1.87	1.63	1.76	1.75	1.79	1.77
LYS	1.33	0.857	1.54	1.39	1.59	1.14
ARG	2.75	1.72	1.82	2.37	2.02	1.77

Table 10

Effect of acetylation and succinylation on amino acid composition of acetylated and succinylated Promine-D.
Conditions: $\underline{1}$N NaOH; 65°C; 3 hrs. Numbers show, for each amino acid, the mole percentage of the total accounted for.

Amino Acid	Promine-D Control	Promine-D + NaOH	1% Acetylated Promine-D + NaOH	10% Acetylated Promine-D + NaOH	10% Succinylated Promine-D + NaOH
ASP	11.62	14.24	14.58	13.42	13.53
THRE	4.49	2.10	2.07	2.52	2.18
SER	6.89	2.84	2.34	3.67	2.71
GLU	16.74	17.55	17.60	16.60	17.39
PRO	6.37	6.82	6.77	7.06	6.85
GLY	7.42	7.29	7.73	8.12	8.00
ALA	6.56	6.62	7.36	7.07	7.27
VAL	5.39	6.29	6.62	5.94	6.54
MET	1.07	0.802	1.13	1.26	0.232
ILEU	4.57	4.47	4.64	4.28	5.02
LEU	8.53	9.47	10.16	9.16	10.62
TYR	2.91	2.36	2.35	2.44	2.92
PHE	4.46	5.17	4.15	4.00	5.09
LAL	0.00	1.46	0.412	0.416	0.138
HIS	2.07	2.30	1.97	2.44	2.15
LYS	5.32	4.96	6.13	6.50	4.93
ARG	5.59	5.23	3.92	5.12	4.34

Table 11

Effect of alkali on amino acid composition of wool and acylated wool wool derivatives.
Conditions: 400 mg of wool in 50 cc 0.01N NaOH -n-propanol (4:1); 65°C; 4 hours.
Numers are mole (residue) percentages of residues accounted for.

Amino Acid	Native wool No. 1	Native wool No. 2	Wool + NaOH	Acylated wool	Acylated wool + NaOH	Succinylated wool	Succinylated wool + NaOH	Glutarylated wool + wool	Glutarylated wool + NaOH
ASP	6.24	6.60	6.76	6.62	6.42	6.83	6.42	6.68	6.78
THR	6.52	6.77	6.65	6.96	6.71	6.88	6.47	6.62	6.73
SER	10.75	11.63	10.84	11.42	11.85	11.81	10.77	10.43	11.36
LAN	0.00	0.00	3.50	0.00	0.00	0.00	0.00	0.00	0.00
GLU	11.84	12.31	13.97	12.33	12.27	12.15	12.22	12.56	12.35
PRO	7.82	6.78	7.04	7.24	7.40	6.94	6.80	7.06	6.90
GLY	8.43	8.98	8.10	9.05	9.12	9.17	8.76	8.75	9.22
ALA	5.43	5.65	5.59	5.66	5.74	5.73	5.78	5.61	5.80
CYS	9.99	9.03	3.24	9.16	9.69	8.48	10.26	9.53	8.06
VAL	5.59	5.65	5.81	5.71	5.96	5.81	5.74	5.61	5.80
MET	0.434	0.451	0.374	0.362	0.419	0.459	0.407	0.432	0.348
ILEU	3.12	2.83	3.29	2.92	3.18	2.81	3.14	3.06	3.15
LEU	7.55	7.68	8.05	7.75	7.92	7.98	7.81	7.80	8.18
TYR	3.57	3.25	3.34	3.03	3.50	3.10	3.52	3.29	2.57
PHE	2.48	2.39	2.51	2.48	2.52	2.33	2.58	2.52	2.85
LAL	0.00	0.00	0.973	0.00	0.00	0.00	0.00	0.00	0.00
HIS	0.798	0.779	0.810	0.684	0.338	0.791	0.803	0.729	0.765
LYS	2.81	2.72	2.13	2.62	2.73	2.13	2.24	2.73	2.57
ARG	6.73	6.95	6.99	5.94	5.91	6.76	6.47	6.56	6.55

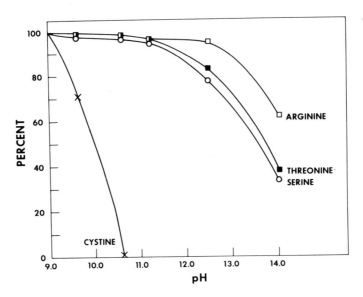

Figure 8. Effect of pH on degradation of susceptible amino acid
           residues in wheat gluten. Conditions: 1% wheat gluten;
           65°C; 3 hours.

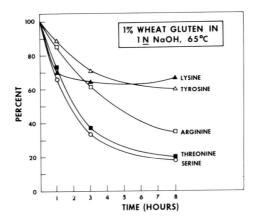

Figure 9. Effect of time on the extent of alkali-induced degrada-
           tion of susceptible amino acid residues in wheat gluten.

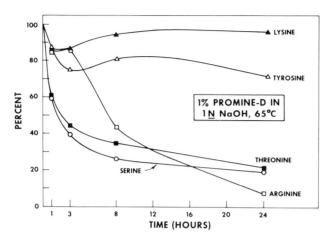

Figure 10.   Effect of time on the extent of alkali-induced degradation of susceptible amino acid residues in soy protein.

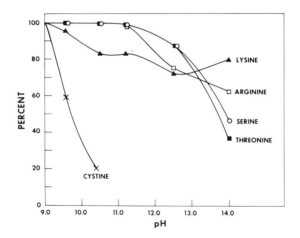

Figure 11.   Effect of pH on the extent of alkali-induced degradation of susceptible amino acid residues in lactalbumin. Conditions: 1% lactalbumin; 65°C; 3 hours.

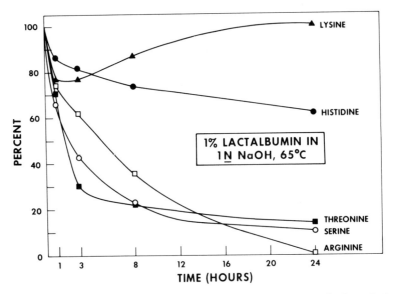

Figure 12. Effect of time on the extent of alkali-induced degradation of susceptible amino acid residues in lactalbumin.

elimination reactions of serine, cystine, and possibly cysteine
residues in proteins. Threonine residues may react similarly to
form methyl homologues. The double bond of dehydroalanine, which
is part of conjugated system, reacts readily with SH and NH_2 groups
of cysteine and lysine to form lanthionine and lysinoalanine,
respectively (Friedman, 1977a). The relative rates of these reactions and the accessability of reactive sites to one another appear
to determine the nature of heated or alkali-treated food proteins.

Inhibition of lysinoalanine formation by added thiols or other
nucleophiles such as sulfite ions can occur by at least three
distinct mechanisms (Friedman, 1977a; 1977b). First, by direct competition, the added nucleophile (mercaptide, sulfite, bisulfite,
thiocyanide, etc.) can trap dehydroalanine residues derived from
protein amino acid side chains to form their respective adducts.
In particular, lanthionine side chains, illustrated in Figures 18-20
are formed from added cysteine and N-acetyl-cysteine (direct competition mechanism). Second, the added nucleophile can cleave protein
disulfide bonds and thus generate free SH groups, which may, in
turn, combine with dehydroalanine residues, as illustrated in Figure
14 (indirect competition mechanism). Third, the added nucleophile,
by cleaving disulfide bonds, can diminish a potential source of
dehydroalanine, since the resulting cysteine residues would be
expected to undergo elimination reactions to form dehydroalanine
much less readily than the original cystine (disulfide) residues
(suppression of dehydroalanine formation mechanism, Figure 21).
Generally, it can be predicted that negatively charged protein side
chains such as sulfite (P-S$^-$), persulfide (P-S-S$^-$), sulfite
(P-SO$_3{}^-$), thiosulfate (P-S-SO$_3{}^-$), etc., will undergo base-catalyzed
elimination more slowly than neutral disulfide bonds because the
negative charge would repel the negatively-charged OH$^-$ ions. Thiol
derivatives, such as cysteine (Sternberg and Kim, 1977; Finley
et al., 1977), and sulfite ions (Friedman, 1977a) have been shown
to decrease the amount of lysinoalanine formed during alkali-
treatment of wool and several food proteins.

To gain further insight into the protective effect of such
external additives and to evaluate the relative effectiveness of
structurally different organic and inorganic nucleophiles, the
effects of several organic and inorganic compounds on the lysinoalanine and lysine contents of alkali-treated wheat gluten were
compared. Preliminary results in Table 12 show that all the compounds shown partly inhibit lysinoalanine formation. The extent of
inhibition may vary from protein to protein and should be related
to both the content and reducibility of the disulfide bonds. With
wheat gluten, acylation, rather than adding external nucleophiles,
appears more effective for preventing lysinoalanine formation.
Moreover, disulfide bond cleavage by added sulfite, sulfide, bisulfite, etc. destroys the original structural integrity of the
protein. Furthermore, Shapiro and Gazit (1977) have shown that

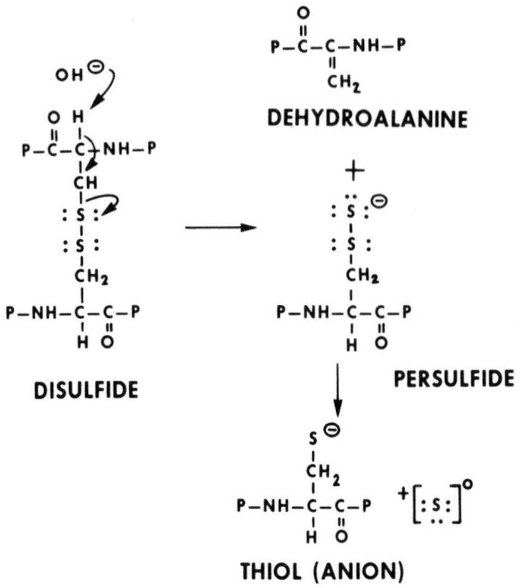

Figure 13. Possible mechanism for base catalyzed formation of one
            dehydroalanine side chain and one persulfide ion from a
            disulfide bond. The persulfide ion can decompose to a
            cysteine residue and elemental sulfur or combine with a
            dehydroalanine residue to reform a (different) disulfide
            bond.

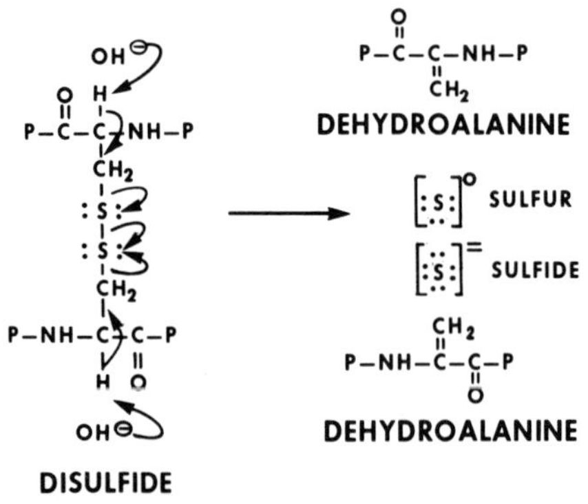

Figure 14. Possible mechanism of base-catalyzed transformation of a
            protein-disulfide bond to two dehydroalanine side chains,
            a sulfide ion, and elemental sulfur.

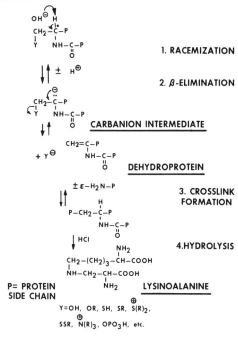

Figure 15.   Transformation of reactive protein side chains to lysino-
            alanine side chains via elimination and crosslink forma-
            tion. Note that the intermediate carbanion has lost the
            original asymmetry of the reactive amino acid side chain.
            The carbanion can either combine with a proton to regener-
            ate a racemized residue in the original amino acid side
            chain or undergo elimination to form dehydroalanine.

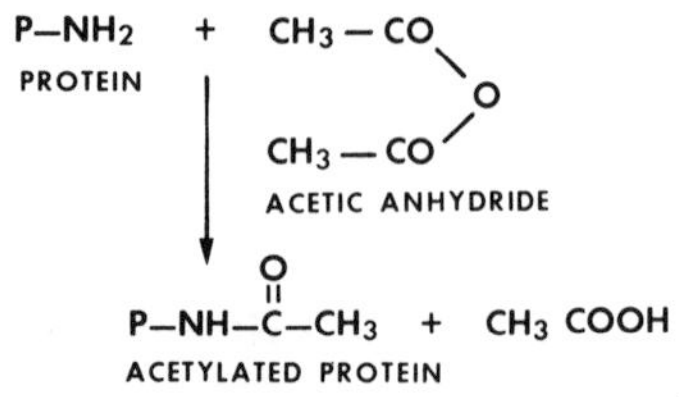

P—NH$_2$ +   CH$_3$—CO
PROTEIN   \   O
                 CH$_3$—CO /
                 ACETIC ANHYDRIDE

          O
          ‖
P—NH—C—CH$_3$ +   CH$_3$COOH
ACETYLATED PROTEIN

Figure 16. Acetylation of protein amino groups by acetic anhydride.

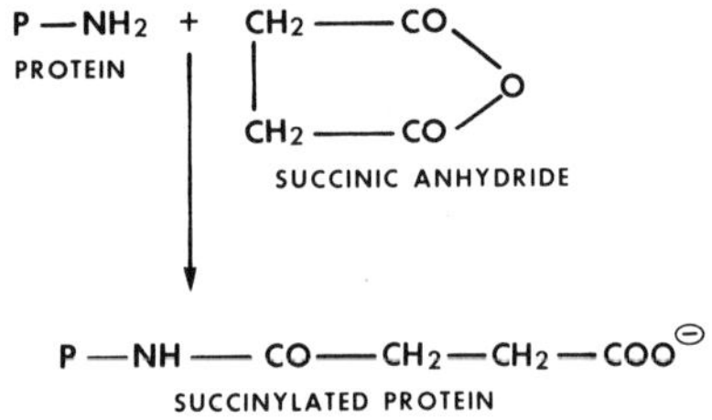

P —NH$_2$ +   CH$_2$ ——— CO
PROTEIN | \   O
                 CH$_2$ ——— CO /
                 SUCCINIC ANHYDRIDE

P —NH —— CO —— CH$_2$—CH$_2$ —COO$^{\ominus}$
SUCCINYLATED PROTEIN

Figure 17. Succinylation of protein amino groups by succinic anhydride.

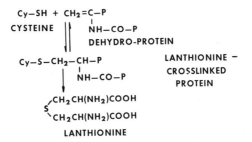

Cy—SH + CH$_2$=C—P
CYSTEINE ‖ NH—CO—P
             DEHYDRO-PROTEIN

Cy—S—CH$_2$—CH—P   LANTHIONINE –
              | CROSSLINKED
              NH—CO—P   PROTEIN

     /CH$_2$CH(NH$_2$)COOH
  S
     \CH$_2$CH(NH$_2$)COOH
   LANTHIONINE

Figure 18. Inhibition of lysinoalanine (crosslink) formation by added cysteine, which combines at a faster rate with the double bond of a dehydro-protein to form a lanthionine crosslink than does a lysine residue to form a lysino-alanine crosslink.

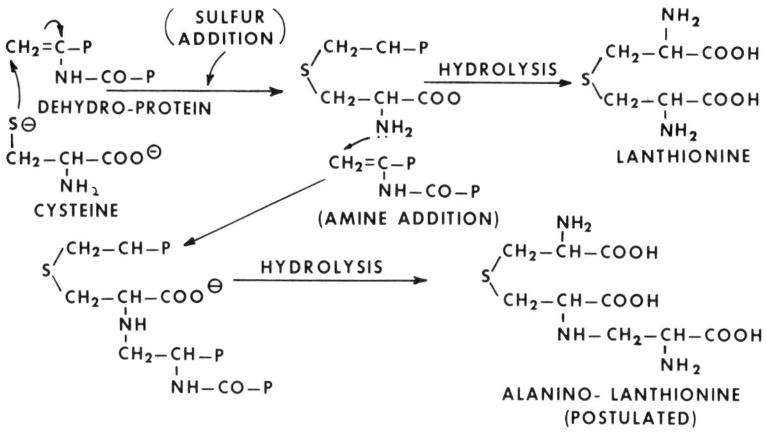

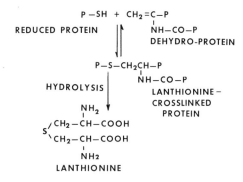

Figure 19. Competitive reactions of the ionized sulfhydryl and amino groups of cysteine with the double bond of a dehydro-protein.

Figure 20. Inhibition of lysinoalanine formation by indirect competition for a dehydro-protein, where the SH group of a reduced protein combines with the double bond of the dehydro-protein, thus preventing it from reacting with the ε-amino group of lysine to form lysinoalanine.

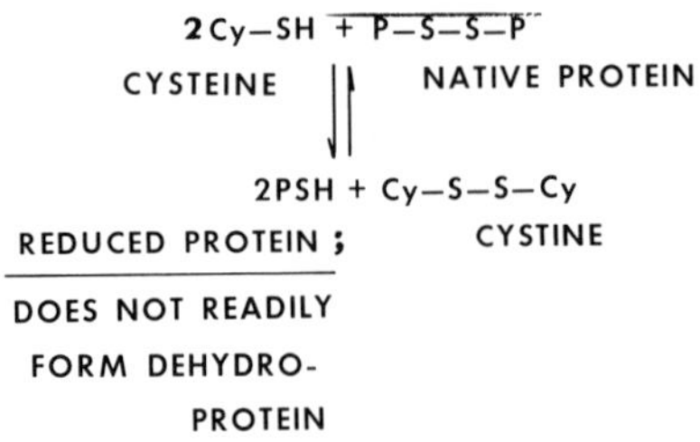

$$2\,Cy\!-\!SH + \overline{P\!-\!S\!-\!S\!-\!P}$$

CYSTEINE $\quad\Vert$ NATIVE PROTEIN

$$2PSH + Cy\!-\!S\!-\!S\!-\!Cy$$

REDUCED PROTEIN ; CYSTINE

DOES NOT READILY

FORM DEHYDRO-

PROTEIN

Figure 21. Inhibition of lysinoalanine formation by "suppression" of dehydro-protein formation, where added cysteine reduces the protein disulfide bond to two sulfhydryl groups. Note that the cysteine can prevent lysino-alanine formation by two mechanisms: it can combine with the double bond of a dehydro-protein, as shown in Figure 18 and/or reduce the disulfide bond of a protein, thus eliminating potential dehydro-protein precursor.

Table 12

Effect of additives on lysine and lysinoalanine content of wheat gluten. Conditions: 1% wheat gluten (1g/100cc) in 1N NaOH; 1 hour; 65°C. A columns show mole per cent of residues accounted for and B columns, mole ratios to alanine.

Compound added	A		B	
	Lysine	Lysinoalanine	Lysine	Lysinoalanine
Untreated gluten control	1.33	0.00	0.340	0.00
None	0.913	0.654	0.230	0.160
Sodium sulfite (200 mg)	1.23	0.552	0.273	0.123
Sodium bisulfite (200 mg)	0.733	0.253	0.210	0.072
L-Cysteine (50 mg)	0.987	0.263	0.272	0.073
N-Acetyl-L-cysteine (50 mg)	0.933	0.304	0.258	0.084
Thiourea (200 mg)	0.979	0.363	0.261	0.097

bisulfite ions can crosslink nucleic acids and proteins and may, therefore, be mutagenic. Furquharson and Adams (1977) have shown that vitamin B_{12} can react with bisulfite ions to form sulfitocobalamin. Consequently, use of such additives in foods and feeds is inadvisable without detailed nutritional and toxicological studies (Cf. also, Til et al., 1972).

ACKNOWLEDGMENTS

It is a pleasure to thank L. C. Lloyd and E. C. Marshall for excellent technical assistance, A. T. Noma for the amino acid analyses, and N. H. Koenig for preparing the acylated wool derivatives.

Reference to a company and/or product named by the Department is only for purposes of information and does not imply approval or recommendation of the product to the exclusion of others which may also be suitable.

Presented at the 10th National Conference on Wheat Utilization Research, Tucson, Arizona, November 14-16, 1977 and at the 175th National Meeting of the American Chemical Society, Anaheim, California, March 13-17, 1978. Abstracts: AGFD 4.

REFERENCES

Cavins, J. F., and Friedman, M. (1968a). Automatic integration and computation of amino acid analyses. Cereal Chem., 45, 172-176.
Cavins, J. F., and Friedman, M. (1968b). Specific modification of protein sulfhydryl groups with α,β-unsaturated compounds. J. Biol. Chem. 243: 3357-3360.
Cavins, J. F. and Friedman, M. (1967). New amino acids derived from reaction of ϵ-amino groups in proteins with α,β-unsaturated compounds. Biochemistry, 6, 3766-3770.
Eskins, K., and Friedman, M. (1970a). Graft photopolymerization of styrene to wheat gluten proteins in dimethyl sulfoxide. J. Macromol. Sci. A4, 947-956.
Eskins, K., and Friedman, M. (1970b). Photoaddition of dimethyl sulfoxide to polypeptides. Photochem. Photobiol. 12, 245-247.
Eskins, K., Dintzis, F., and Friedman, M. (1971). Photopolymerization of methyl acrylate in dimethyl sulfoxide. J. Macromol. Sci. A5 (3) 543-548.

Farquharson, J. and Adams, J. F. (1977). Conversion of hydroxo
    (aquo)- cobalamin to sulfitocobalamin in the absence of light:
    a reaction of importance in the identification of the forms of
    vitamin B$_{12}$, with possible clinical significance. Am. J. Clin.
    Nutri., 30, 1617-1622.
Finley, J. W. and Friedman, M. (1977). New amino acid derivatives
    formed by alkaline treatment of proteins. In "Protein Crosslink-
    ing: Nutritional and Medical Consequences," M. Friedman, Ed.,
    Plenum Press, New York, pp. 123-130.
Finley, J. W., Snow, J. T., Johnston, P. H., and Friedman, M.
    (1977). Inhibitory effect of mercaptoamino acids on lysino-
    alanine formation during alkali treatment of proteins. In
    "Protein Crosslinking: Nutritional and Medical Consequences,"
    M. Friedman, Ed., Plenum Press, New York, pp. 85-92.
Finot, P. A., Bujard, E., and Arnaud, M. (1977). Metabolic transit
    of lysinoalanine bound to protein and free radioactive ^{14}C-
    lysinoalanine. In "Protein Crosslinking: Nutritional and Medical
    Consequences", M. Friedman, Ed., Plenum Press, New York, pp. 51-
    71.
Friedman, M. (1977a). Crosslinking amino acids — stereochemistry
    and nomenclature. In "Protein Crosslinking: Nutritional and
    Medical Consequences," M. Friedman, Ed., Plenum Press, New York,
    pp. 1-27.
Friedman, M. (1977b). Effects of lysine modification on chemical,
    physical, nutritive, and functional properties of proteins. In
    "Food Proteins", J. R. Whitaker and S. R. Tannenbaum, Eds.,
    Avi, Westport, Connecticut, pp. 446-483.
Friedman, M. (1973). Reactions of cereal proteins with vinyl com-
    pounds. In "Industrial Uses of Cereal Grains", Y. Pomeranz, Ed.,
    American Association of Cereal Chemists, Minneapolis, Minnesota,
    pp. 237-251.
Friedman, M., and Broderick, G. A. (1977). Protected proteins in
    ruminant nutrition. In vitro evaluation of casein derivatives.
    In "Protein Crosslinking: Nutritional and Medical Consequences",
    M. Friedman, Ed., Plenum Press, New York, pp. 545-558.
Friedman, M., Krull, L. H. (1969). A novel spectrophotometric
    procedure for the determination of half-cystine residues in
    proteins. Biochem. Biophys. Res. Commun. 37, 630-633.
Friedman, M. and Wall, J. S. (1964). Application of a Hammett-Taft
    relation to kinetics of alkylation of amino acids and peptide
    model compounds with acrylonitrile. J. Am. Chem. Soc., 86, 3735-
    3741.
Friedman, M., and Williams, L. D. (1973). The reaction of ninhy-
    drin with keratin proteins. Analyt. Biochem., 54, 333-345.
Friedman, M., and Williams, L. D. (1974). Stoichiometry of
    formation of Ruhemann's purple in the ninhydrin reaction.
    Bioorganic Chemistry, 3, 267-280.
Friedman, M., Finley, J. W. and Yeh, Lai-Sue. (1977). Reactions
    of proteins with dehydrolanines. In "Protein Crosslinking:
    Nutritional and Medical Consequences", M. Friedman, Ed., Plenum
    Press, New York, pp. 213-224.

Gee, M., Huxsoll, C. C., and Graham, R. P. (1974). Acidification of dry caustic peeling was by lactic acid fermentation. American Potato J., 51, 126-131. .

Goldblatt, L. A. (1969). "Aflatoxin; Scientific Background, Control, and Implications", Academic Press, New York.

Gould, D. H., and MacGregor, J. T. (1977). Biological effects of alkali-treated protein and lysinoalanine: an overview. In "Protein Crosslinking: Nutritional and Medical Consequences", M. Friedman, Ed., Plenum Press, New York, pp. 29-48.

Habeeb, A. F. S. A., Cassidy, H. G., and Singer, S. J. (1958). Molecular structural effects produced in proteins by reaction with succinic anhydride. Biochim. Biophys. Acta, 29, 587-593.

Hamdy, M. (1974). The nutritional value of vegetable protein. Chem. Technol., 616-622.

Hurrell, F. R. and Carpenter, K. J. (1977). Nutritional significance of crosslink formation during food processing. In "Protein Crosslinking: Nutritional and Medical Consequences", M. Friedman, Ed., Plenum Press, New York, pp. 225-238.

Klapper, M. H. and Klotz, I. M. (1972). Acylation with dicarboxylic acid anhydrides. In "Methods in Enzymology", C.H.W. Hirs and S. N. Timascheff, Ed., Academic Press, New York, Vol. XXV, pp. 531-536.

Koenig, N. H. (1965). Wool modification with acid anhydrides in dimethylformamide. Text. Res. J., 35, 708-715.

Koenig, N. H. and Friedman, M. (1977). Comparison of wool reactions with selected mono- and bifunctional reagents. In "Protein Crosslinking: Biochemical and Molecular Aspects", M. Friedman, Ed., Plenum Press, New York, pp. 355-382.

Krull, L. H. and Friedman, M. (1967a). Anionic polymerization of methyl acrylate to protein functional groups. J. Polym. Sci., A-1, 5, 2535-2546.

Krull, L. H. and Friedman, M. (1967b). Reduction of protein disulfide bonds by sodium hydride in dimethyl sulfoxide. Biochem. Biophys. Res. Commun., 29, 373-377.

Provanasal, M.M.P., Cuq, J. L. A. and Cheftel, J. C. (1975). Chemical and nutritional modifications of sunflower proteins due to alkaline processing. Formation of amino acid cross-links and isomerization of lysine residues. J. Ag. Food Chem. 23, 938-943.

Riordan, J. F. and Vallee, B. L. (1972). Acetylation. In "Methods in Enzymology", C.H.W. Hirs and S. N. Timasheff, Eds., Academic Press, New York, Vol. XXV, pp. 494-499.

Saunders, R. M., Connor, M. A., Edwards, R. H., and Kohler, G. O. (1975). Preparation of protein concentrates from wheat shorts and wheat millrun by a wet alkaline process. Cereal Chem., 52, 93-101.

Schultz, W. G., Neuman, J. J., Schade, J. E., Morgan, J. P., Katsuyama, A. M., and Maagdengerg, H. J. (1977). Commercial feasibility of recovering tomato peeling residuals. Proc. 8th Nat'l. Symp. on Food Processing Wastes. Seattle WA, Industrial Environmental Research Laboratory, Office of Res. and Dev., U.S. Environmental Protection Agency, Cincinnati, pp 119-136.

Shapiro, R., and Gazit, A. (1977). Crosslinking of nucleic acids and proteins by bisulfite. In "Protein Crosslinking: Nutritional and Medical Consequences", M. Friedman, Ed., Plenum Press, New York, 633-640.

Snow, J. T., Finley, J. W., and Friedman, M. (1976). Relative reactivities of sulfhydryl groups with N-acetyl dehydroalanine and N-acetyldehydroalanine methyl ester. Int. J. Peptide Protein Res., 5, 177-186.

Sternberg, M., and Kim, C. Y. (1977). Lysinoalanine formation in protein food ingredients. In "Protein Crosslinking: Nutritional and Medical Consequences", M. Friedman, Ed., Plenum Press, New York, pp. 73-84.

Til, H. P., Feron, V. J., and DeGroot, A. P. (1972). Toxicity of sulfite. I. Long-term feeding and multigeneration studies in rats. Food Cosmet. Toxcol., 10, (3), 291-310.

Whitaker, J. R. and Feeney, R. E. (1977). Behaviour of O-glycosyl and O-phosphoryl proteins in alkaline solution. In "Protein Crosslinking: Nutritional and Medical Consequences", M. Friedman, Ed., Plenum Press, New York, pp. 155-175.

Woodard, C. J., Short, D. D., Alvarez, M. R. and Reyniers, J. (1975). Biologic effects of Nε-(DL-2-amino-2-carboxyethyl)-L-lysine, lysinoalanine. In "Protein Nutritional Quality of Foods and Feeds", M. Friedman, Ed., Marcel Dekker, New York, pp. 595-616.

Wu, Y. V., Sexson, K. R., Cluskey, J. E. and Inglett, G. E. (1977). Protein isolates from high protein oats preparation. Composition and properties. J. Food Sci., 42, (5), 1383-1386.

Wu, Y. V., Cluskey, J. E., Krull, L. H., and Friedman, M. (1971). Some optical properties of S-β-(4-pyridylethyl)-L-cysteine and its wheat gluten and serum albumin derivatives, Canad. J. Biochem., 49, 1042-1049.

31

MICROBIAL PRODUCTION OF ESSENTIAL AMINO ACIDS WITH CORYNEBACTERIUM GLUTAMICUM MUTANTS

Kiyoshi Nakayama, Kazumi Araki and Hiroshi Kase
Tokyo Research Laboratory, Kyowa Hakko Kogyo Co. Ltd.
Machida-shi, Tokyo

ABSTRACT

Amino acids produced by microbial process are generally L-forms. The stereospecificity of the amino acids produced by fermentation makes the process advantageous compared with synthetic process. Microorganisms employed in microbial process for amino acid production are divided into 4 classes; wild-type strain, auxotrophic mutant, regulatory mutant and auxotrophic regulatory mutant. Using such mutants of Corynebacterium glutamicum, all the essential amino acids but L-methionine are now being produced by "direct fermentation" from cheap carbon sources such as carbohydrate materials or acetic acid.

INTRODUCTION

Fermentative production of amino acids started with the discovery of an efficient glutamic acid producer, Corynebacterium glutamicum (synonym Micrococcus glutamicus), by Kinoshita et al. (1957). The bacterium was found during a time of increasing demand for monosodium glutamate as a flavoring agent. Following this, much research activity has been focused on microbial amino acid production. The primary reason for these efforts was the hope to improve the nutritional value of low-cost vegetable proteins by enrichment with essential amino acids. Once C. glutamicum was discovered by screening isolates from nature, similar efforts led to the isolation of bacteria producing L-valine. However, these wild-type strains could not accumulate other essential amino acids. Microbial production of these essential amino acids has become an industrial reality since the utilization of auxotrophic mutants of C. glutamicum in 1950s. At present, all the essential amino acids but L-methionine can be supplied by "direct fermentation" using the auxotrophic mutant and regulatory mutants. Most big production is L-lysine and total world production of it is probably in excess of 15,000 tons per year. In the present paper, we describe processes using C. glutamicum mutants.

RESULTS AND DISCUSSION

L-Lysine

Excretion and accumulation of L-lysine within or outside the microbial cells has long been studied (see review, Nakayama, 1972). The first prominent result for L-lysine production was obtained by a combination of diaminopimelate production by a lysine auxotroph of Escherichia coli and decarboxylation of the compound by Aerobacter aerogenes or wild-type E. coli. Soon afterwards, a more direct and economical process was developed by Kinoshita and Nakayama (Kinoshita et al., 1958). This process depends on the finding that a homoserine- (or methionine plus threonine) auxotrophic mutant of C. glutamicum accumulates a large amount of L-lysine in a culture medium. Molasses is generally used as a carbon source in the industrial production of L-lysine. Other carbohydrate materials, acetic acid and ethanol can also be used. The pH value of the medium is automatically maintained near neutrality during the fermentation by feeding ammonia or urea. Ammonia and ammonium salts are generally good nitrogen sources. Figure 1 exemplifies a fermentation using C. glutamicum No. 901 (a homoserine auxotroph) in a 2KL fermentor. Forty-four grams of L-lysine per liter was produced in 69 hr. Foaming in the aerated culture can be repressed by addition of proper antifoaming agents. Growth factors (homoserine or threonine and methionine) is supplied with acid-hydrolyzate of protein, and their amount should be appropriate for the production of L-lysine, i.e. the amounts suboptimal for the growth. Fermentation with acetic acid as substrate is carried out with feeding of acetic acid solution. The feeding is controlled automatically till the end of the fermentation, keeping the pH-value of the medium at near 7.0. The increase in lysine yield (more than 10% of yield in control culture) was obtained using a mutant of C. glutamicum, which requires homoserine and leucine and is resistant to S-(β-aminoethyl)-L-cysteine (AEC), a lysine analogue. It produced 39.5g of L-lysine in a medium containing 10% reducing sugars expressed as invert (as cane molasses), while the homoserine plus leucine auxotroph produced 34.5g of L-lysine per liter (Nakayama and Araki, 1973).

Regulation of lysine biosynthesis in C. glutamicum is represented in Figure 2. The blocking of homoserine synthesis at homoserine dehydrogenase(2) results in the release of the concerted feedback

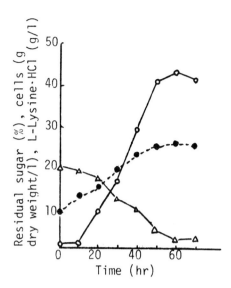

Figure 1. Time Course of L-Lysine Fermentation Using
          C. glutamicum No. 901 (homoserine)
                  (Nakayama, 1972)
Fermentation medium contains 20 % reduced sugars as invert
(as cane molasses) and 1.8 % soybean meal hydrolyzate (as
weight of meal before hydrolysis with H_2SO_4 and neutralization
with ammonia water).
—○— , L-Lysine;—△— , Residual sugar;···●···,Dry cell weight

inhibition by threonine and lysine on aspartokinase (1), and the
aspartic semialdehyde produced proceeds to lysine through the lysine
synthetic pathway on which no feedback inhibition is found.
Resistance to AEC brought by the desensitization of aspartokinase
also releases the concerted feedback inhibition. The conversion of
aspartic semialdehyde to threonine is feedback inhibited by L-
threonine. Thus the overproduced aspartic semialdehyde is channeled
into L-lysine production.

                           L-Threonine

     First efficient process for L-threonine production has been
developed by present authors (Kase et al., 1971) with an auxotrophic mutant Escherichia coli. Similar auxotrophic mutants of C.
glutamicum were unable to produce a large amount of L-threonine

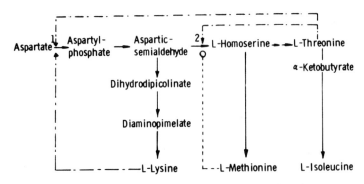

Figure 2. Regulation of Lysine Biosynthesis.
in C. glutamicum
(Nakayama, 1972)

◄·——·, Feedback inhibition; o········ , Repression.
1, Aspartokinase; 2, Homoserine dehydrogenase.

owing to feedback inhibition by L-threonine on homoserine dehydrogenase (Figure 2, enzyme 2). A mutant strain resistant to a
threonine analogue, α-amino-β-hydroxyvaleric acid (AHV), produced
L-threonine. A combination of polyauxotrophy and analogue-resistance
increased the ability to produce L-threonine (Kase and Nakayama,
1972). Thus strain KY 10440 which was obtained by stepwise mutagenic
improvement and is a methionine auxotroph resistant to AHV and AEC
produced 9.5g per liter of L-threonine in a medium containing 10%
glucose (Figure 3). The activities of homoserine dehydrogenase in
the mutants which produced L-threonine were slightly less susceptible
to inhibition by L-threonine than the activity in the original
strain, KY 9159. Thus genetical alteration of the enzyme may be a
cause of L-threonine production in these mutants.

L-Isoleucine

An L-isoleucine-producing mutant (ASAT 372) of Corynebacterium
glutamicum was isolated as a thiaisoleucine-resistant mutant from a
threonine-producing strain having three markers: methionine-less,
AHV-resistance, and AEC-resistance by mutation (Figure 4). A strain
ASAT 372 produced 5g of L-isoleucine and 5g of L-threonine per liter.
This strain was further improved by adding as markers: ethionine-
resistance, 4-azaleucine-resistance, and α-AB-resistance. RAM-83
thus obtained produced 9.7g of L-isoleucine per liter (Kase and
Nakayama, 1977).

Corynebacterium glutamicum	L-Threonine produced (g/l)
KY 9159 (Met$^-$)	
↓ AHV^r	
KY 10290	0.6
↓ AHV^{hr}	
KY 10484	2.3
↓ AEC^r	
KY 10440	9.5

Figure 3. Genealogy of L-Threonine-producing Mutants
(Kase and Nakayama, 1972)

Abbreviations: AHV, α-Amino-β-hydroxyvaleric acid; AEC,
S-(β-aminoethyl)-L-cysteine; AHV^{hr}, high resistance to AHV.

L-Leucine

An L-leucine production process using an auxotrophic mutant of
Corynebacterium glutamicum has been developed (Araki et al., 1974).
Mutant No. 190 was found to produce a large amount of L-leucine in
a culture medium. The nutritional requirements of the mutant are
rather complex but its growth was remarkably stimulated by L-
phenylalanine. Acetate (1.5-3.0%) or pyruvate (3%) stimulated
L-leucine production. A histidine auxotrophic derivative, Pα-219,
produced twice as much L-leucine as the parent strain, i. e.
L-leucine production by the strain reached 16g per liter in the
medium containing 12% glucose, 2.5% CH$_3$COONH$_4$ and other ingredients.
Figure 5 shows the time course of L-leucine production by this
mutant in a 5l jar fermentor. L-Tyrosine and L-valine accumulated
as by-products.

L-Valine

L-Valine-producing bacteria are often found in nature (see
review, Uemura et al., 1972). Processes using auxotrophic or
regulatory mutants have also been developed. Isoleucine and leucine
auxotrophic mutants of C. glutamicum produce a large amount of L-
valine in culture broths. L-Valine production by an isoleucine
auxotroph reached 11g or more per liter in a medium containing 7.5%
glucose (Nakayama et al., 1960). Limitation of growth factor
(isoleucine) is necessary for the valine production.

L-Tryptophan

Figure 6 shows the genealogy of L-tryptophan-producing mutants

Corynebacterium glutamicum	L-Isoleucine produced (g/l)
KY 10501 (Met$^-$, AHV^r, AEC^r)	1.3
$\downarrow$ S-Ile^r	
ASAT-372	5.0
$\downarrow$ Eth^r	
6E-211	5.0
$\downarrow$ Eth^{hr}	
ES-249	5.5
$\downarrow$ Monocolony	
F-84	6.0
$\downarrow$ AZL^r	
AZ-131	6.8
$\downarrow$ α-AB	
RAB-39-27	8.5
$\downarrow$ Monocolony	
RAM-83	9.7

Figure 4. Genealogy of L-Isoleucine-producers
(Kase and Nakayama, 1977)
Abbreviations: S-Ile, thiaisoleucine; AZL, 4-Azaleucine;
α-AB, α-Aminobutyric acid. Other abbreviations are the
same as those in Figure 3.

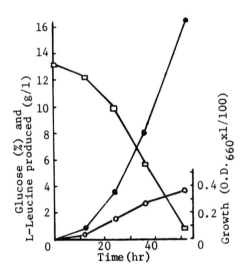

Figure 5. Time Course of L-Leucine Fermentation Using
C. glutamicum Pα-219
(Araki et al., 1974)

—●— , L-Leucine; —○— , Growth; —□— , Glucose.

of C. glutamicum. Mutants producing a large amount of L-tryptophan were derived from a phenylalanine and tyrosine double auxotroph, C. glutamicum KY 9456 which produced only a trace amount of L-tryptophan and anthranilate (Nakayama et al., 1976). A mutant Px-115-97, which stepwise acquired resistance to tryptophan-, phenylalanine, and tyrosine-analogues, produced 12g per liter of L-tryptophan in the medium containing 10% reducing sugars as invert (as cane molasses) and 2% $(NH_4)_2SO_4$.

Regulatory properties of the enzyme involved in aromatic amino acid biosynthesis in C. glutamicum wild and mutant strains were investigated (Nakayama et al., 1976). The overall control pattern (Figure 7) is a new addition to the list of control patterns in aromatic amino acid biosynthesis in microorganisms. A phenylalanine and tyrosine double auxotrophic L-tryptophan producer, Px-115-97, has anthranilate synthetase partially released from the inhibition by L-tryptophan and DAHP synthetase of a wild-type. The L-tryptophan production by the mutant appeared to be caused by the release from the feedback inhibition of anthranilate synthetase by L-tryptophan and blockage of chorismate mutase.

L-Phenylalanine

A tyrosine auxotrophic mutant, resistant to p-fluorophenylalanine and p-aminophenylalanine, produced 9.5g of L-phenylalanine

Corynebacterium glutamicum	L-Tryptophan produced (g/l)
KY 9456 (Phe⁻, Tyr⁻) ↓ 5MT^r, TrpHx^r, 6FT^r, 4MT^r 4MT-11	0.15
↓ PFP^r PFP-2-32	4.9
↓ PAP^r PAP-126-50	5.7
↓ TyrHx^r Tx-49	7.1
↓ PheHx^r Px-115-97	10.0
	12.0

Figure 6. Genealogy of L-Tryptophan-Producing Mutants
(Nakayama et al., 1976)

Abbreviations: 5MT, 5-Methyltryptophan; TypHx, Tryptophan hydroxamate; 6FT, 6-Fluorotryptophan; 4MT, 4-Methyltryptophan ; PFP, p-Fluorophenylalanine; PAP, p-Aminophenylalanine; TyrHx, Tyrosine hydroxamate; PheHx, Phenylalanine hydroxamate.

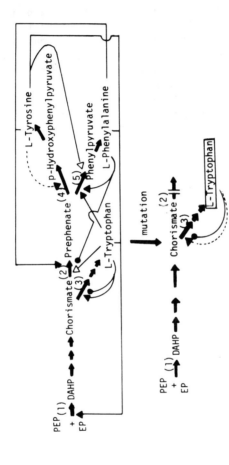

Figure 7. Regulation of Aromatic Amino Acid Biosynthesis in C. glutamicum and
Deregulation in Tryptophan-producing Mutants.
(Nakayama et al., 1976)

1, DAHP Synthetase; 2, Chorismate mutase; 3, Anthranilate synthetase; 4, Prephenate dehydrogenase;
5, Prephenate dehydratase. ━━→ , Feedback inhibition; ┈┈→ , Prtial inhibition; ◁━━ , Activation;
━━→ , Repression; ⊤ , Blocked reaction.
Abbreviations: PEP, Phosphoenolpyruvate; EP, Erythrose 4-phosphate; DAHP, 3-Deoxy-D-arabinose
heptulosonic acid 7-phosphate.

Corynebacterium glutamicum		L-Phenylalanine produced (g/1)
ATCC 13032 (Wild-type)		0
TL-3	Tyr⁻	1.0
	PFP (25 µg/ml)ʳ	
PFP-19		4.6
	PFP (50 µg/ml)ʳ	
PFP-19-31		6.7
	PAPʳ	
31-PAP-20-22		9.5

Figure 8. Genealogy of L-Phenylalanine-producing Mutants
(Hagino and Nakayama, 1974)
Abbreviations: See the legends of Figure 6.

per liter in the medium containing 10% reducing sugars as invert
(as cane molasses) (Figure 8, Hagino and Nakayama, 1974).

L-Methionine

L-Methionine production of C. glutamicum KY 9276 (Thr⁻) was
improved by sequential addition of resistance to five methionine-
analogues. The finally selected strain produced 2g of L-methionine
per liter of a medium containing 10% glucose (Kase and Nakayama,
1975). Methionine is now supplied with DL-form by chemical synthesis.

L-Arginine

A wild-type strain of C. glutamicum was found to be highly
resistant to the arginine analogues, canavanine, D-arginine and
arginine hydroxamate. A D-serine-sensitive mutant DSS-8 derived
from an isoleucine auxotroph was found to be sensitive to the
arginine-analogues and to produce a small amount of L-arginine.
The productivity of L-arginine in this mutant was improved stepwise
by mutation and selection (Figure 9, Nakayama and Yoshida, 1972).
Strain KY10576, a mutant derived from the D-serine-sensitive mutant,
and resistant to both D-arginine and arginine hydroxamate, produced
25 mg/ml of L-arginine in the cane molasses medium containing 15%
reducing sugars as invert. Strain DSS-8 may be a mutant with
increased permeability to D- and L-arginine, and has 3 to 11-fold
derepressed levels of at least three arginine enzymes: acetylonithine
aminotransferase (Figure 10, 4), transacetylase (5), ornithine
carbamoyltransferase (6). D-Arginine-resistant mutant KY 10479
has the acetylglutamate kinase which was altered to be resistant to
feedback inhibition by arginine and derepressed in arginine-synthetic

Corynebacterium glutamicum	L-Arginine produced (g/1)
KY 10025 (Wild-type)	
↓ Ile$^-$	
KY 10150	
↓ D-Ser^s	
DSS-8	1.5
↓ D-Arg^r	
KY 10479	6.8
↓ ArgHx^r	
KY 10480	16.6
↓ Ile$^+$	
KY 10508	19.6
↓ ArgHx^{hr}	
KY 10576	25.0

Figure 9. Genealogy of L-Arginine-producers
(Nakayama and Yoshida, 1972)

Abbreviation: ArgHx, Arginine hydroxamate.

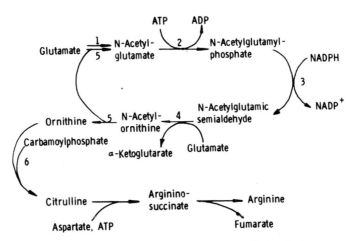

Figure 10. Biosynthetic Pathway of Arginine
in C. glutamicum
(Udaka and Kinoshita, 1958)

1, N-Acetylglutamate synthetase; 2, Acetylglutamate
kinase; 5, Transacetylase; 6, Ornithine carbamoyltransferase.

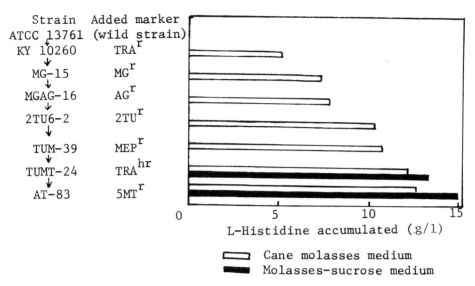

Figure 11. Increase in L-Histidine Productivity in C. glutamicum
        Mutants. (Araki and Nakayama, 1974a)
   Abbreviations: TRA, 1,2,4-Triazole-3-alanine; MG, 6-Mercapto-
guanine; AG, 8-Azaguanine; 2TU, 2-Thiouracil; MEP, 6-Methylpurine;
5MT, 5-Methyltryptophan.

enzymes. The deregulation of arginine biosynthesic pathway may be
a cause for the overproduction of L-arginine (Yoshida et al., 1977).

L-Histidine

     A 1,2,4-triazole-3-alanine(TRA)-resistant mutant, strain
KY10260, derived from the wild-type strain of C. glutamicum,
ATCC 13761, produced several grams per liter of L-histidine in a
cane molasses medium. The histidine productivity of KY10260
could be improved stepwise by successively introducing such
characters as purine analogue-resistance, pyrimidine analogue-
resistance and tryptophan analogue-resistance as shown in Figure
11 (Araki and Nakayama, 1974a). The improvement of L-histidine
productivity in each step was rather minor, but the mutant strain
finally selected, AT-83, produced approximately twice as much L-
histidine as the original strain KY10260. Feedback-resistance of
the first enzyme of the histidine pathway and the derepressed
formation of histidine enzymes explain the overproduction of L-
histidine in these L-histidine producers (Araki and Nakayama, 1974b).

Table 1   Production of Essential Amino Acids Using
C. glutamicum Mutants

Amino acids produced (g/1)	Type of strain	Main contributors to production
L-Valine (11)	Auxotrophic mutant	Ile^-; Leu^-.
L-Leucine (16)	"	Phe^-.
L-Lysine (>40)	"	$Homoserine^-$; Thr^-.
L-Lysine (>40)	Auxotrophic regulatory mutant	$Homoserine^-$, Leu^-, $Lys\text{-}analogue^r$.
L-Threonine(12)	"	Met^-, $Thr\text{-}analogue^r$.
L-Isoleucine(9.7)	"	Met^-, $Thr\text{-}analogue^r$, $Lys\text{-}analogue^r$, $Ile\text{-}analogue^r$.
L-Tryptophan(12)	"	Phe^-, Tyr^-, $Phe\text{-}analog^r$, $Tyr\text{-}analogue^r$, $Trp\text{-}analogue^r$.
L-Phenylalanine (9.5)	"	Tyr^-, $Phe\text{-}analogue^r$, $Tyr\text{-}analogue^r$.
L-Methionine(2.0)	"	Thr^-, $Met\text{-}analogue^r$.
L-Arginine (25)	Regulatory mutant	$Arg\text{-}analogue^r$.
L-Histidine(15)	"	$His\text{-}analogue^r$.

CONCLUSION

Using genetic techniques to avoid biosynthetic regulation, processes for the production of essential amino acids are established except for L-methionine which is supplied in DL-form by chemical synthesis. The laboratory data obtained are summarized in Table 1. Industrial productions are now being carried out by improved processes developed on the basis of these results.

REFERENCES

Araki, K., Nakayama, K. (1974a). Histidine production by Corynebacterium glutamicum mutants multiresistant to analogs of
histidine, tryptophan, purine and pyrimidine. Agric. Biol.
Chem., 38, 837-846.

Araki, K., Nakayama, K. (1974b). Feedback-resistant phosphoribosyl-ATP pyrophosphorylase in L-histidine-producing mutants of Corynebacterium glutamicum. Agric. Biol. Chem., 38, 2209-2218.

Araki, K., Ueda, H., Saigusa, S. (1974). Fermentative production of L-leucine with auxotrophic mutants of Corynebacterium glutamicum. Agric. Biol. Chem., 38, 565-572.

Hagino, H. Nakayama, K. (1974). L-Phenylalanine production by analog-resistant mutants of Corynebacterium glutamicum. Agric. Biol. Chem., 38, 157-161.

Kase, H., Tanaka, H., Nakayama, K. (1971). Studies on L-threonine fermentation. I. Production of L-threonine by auxotrophic mutants. Agric. Biol. Chem., 35, 2089-2096.

Kase, H., Nakayama, K. (1972). Production of L-threonine by analog-resistant mutants. Agric. Biol. Chem., 36, 1611-1621.

Kase, H., Nakayama, K. (1975). L-Methionine production by methionine analog-resistant mutants of Corynebacterium glutamicum. Agric. Biol. Chem., 39, 153-160.

Kase, H., Nakayama, K. (1977). L-Isoleucine produciton by analog-resistant mutants derived from threonine-producing strain of Corynebacterium glutamicum. Agric. Biol. Chem., 41, 109-116.

Kinoshita, S., Tanaka, K., Udaka, S., Akita, S. (1957). Glutamic acid fermentation. Proceedings of International Symposium on Enzyme Chemistry 2, 464-468.

Kinoshita, S., Nakayama, K., Kitada, S. (1958). L-Lysine production using microbial auxotroph. J. Gen Appl. Microbiol., 4, 128-129.

Nakayama, K., Kitada, S., Kinoshita, S. (1960). Valine fermentation using microbial auxotroph. Amino Acids, 2, 77-85 (Japanese).

Nakayama, K. (1972). Lysine and diaminopimelic acid, In The Microbial Production of Amino Acids. K. Yamada, S. Kinoshita, T. Tsunoda, K. Aida (Editors). Kodansha, Ltd., Tokyo, P.369.

Nakayama, K., Yoshida, H. (1972). Fermentative production of L-arginine. Agric. Biol. Chem., 36, 1675-1684.

Nakayama, K., Araki, K. (1973). Process for producing L-lysine. U. S. Patent 3,708,395, Jan. 2.

Nakayama, K., Araki, K., Hagino, H., Kase, H., Yoshida, H. (1976). Amino acid fermentations using regulatory mutants of Corynebacterium glutamicum. In Genetics of Industrial Microorganisms. K. D. MacDonald (Editor), Academic Press, London and New York, P.437.

Udaka, S., Kinoshita, S. (1958). Studies on L-ornithine fermentation. II. The change of fermentation product by feedback type mechanism. J. Gen. Appl. Microbiol., 4, 283-288.

Uemura, T., Sugisaki, Z., Takamura, T. (1972). Valine. In The Microbial Production of Amino Acids. K. Yamada, S. Kinoshita, T. Tsunoda, K. Aida (Editors). Kodansha Ltd., Tokyo.

Yoshida, H., Araki, K., Nakayama, K. (1977). Mechanism of arginine production in Corynebacterium glutamicum mutants. Agric. Biol. Chem. (manuscript in preparation).

32

NUTRITIONAL IMPROVEMENT OF FOOD PROTEINS BY MEANS OF THE PLASTEIN

REACTION AND ITS NOVEL MODIFICATION

Soichi Arai, Michiko Yamashita, and Masao Fujimaki

Department of Agricultural Chemistry, University of Tokyo

Bunkyo-ku, Tokyo 113, Japan

ABSTRACT

The paper reviews recent studies in the application of the plastein reaction for the improvement of amino acid compositions of food proteins; it describes in a large measure the specific incorporation of amino acid esters into protein hydrolysate during the plastein reaction with papain. The information obtained from this specificity study has been found useful in the improvement of several unconventional as well as conventional proteins by incorporating controlled amounts of essential amino acids through the plastein reaction. Prior to carrying out this reaction, however, it is necessary to prepare a protein hydrolysate as its substrate. The entire process thus requires two independent steps: enzymatic protein hydrolysis and resynthesis. In very recent work we have found it possible to incorporate amino acid esters directly into protein by one step when a proper reaction condition has been adopted. This novel "one-step process" is also discussed in comparison with the conventional plastein reaction.

INTRODUCTION

It is well known that in earlier days the plastein reaction was studied in some measure with the aim of elucidating a mechanism of protein biosynthesis (Tauber, 1951; Virtanen, 1951; Horowitz and Haurowitz, 1959). These were followed by work on the plastein reaction from the aspect of peptide chemistry (Determann, 1966). In recent years this reaction has been reinvestigated in more detail, especially from the standpoint of its application to improving food protein quality (Arai et al., 1975; Eriksen and

Protein —— at a very low concentration

↓   Hydrolysis with a protease at a specific pH

Hydrolysate —— at a very high concentration

↓   ← Amino acid ester

      Resynthesis with papain at pH 6

↓

Plastein enriched with the amino acid

Figure 1. Simplified scheme of amino acid incorporation
by means of the conventional process.

Fagerson, 1976; Hofsten and Lalasidis, 1976; Yamashita et al.,
(1976a). From a nutritional point of view it is interesting to
apply the plastein reaction as a tool for incorporating essential
amino acids used in ester form and thus make up plastein products
whose amino acid compositions have been improved from those of the
original proteins (Figure 1). In this regard Yamashita et al.
(1971) were the first to succeed in incorporating L-methionine and
enhancing a sulfur-containing amino acid level of soy protein.
Subsequently, similar trials have been made to improve conventional food proteins (Arai et al., 1974; Aso et al., 1974; Yamashita et al., 1976b) and, as discussed later to a greater extent,
some unconventional proteins of photosynthetic origin (Arai et al.,
1976). All these studies have used papain [EC 3·4·4·10] not only
because of its high ability to incorporate amino acids used in
ester form (Yamashita et al., 1976a) but also because this enzyme
has been well-defined for the catalytic function involved in the
hydrolysis of peptides, amides and esters (Glazer and Smith, 1971)
and in several kinds of unusual transfer reactions (Mycek and
Fruton, 1957; Glazer, 1966; Sluyterman and Wijdnes, 1972; Alecio
et al., 1974). Up to the present, however, no comprehensive
information has been obtained concerning a papain-catalyzed
reaction between peptide and amino acid ester to form a new bond,
especially reactions that proceed under the same conditions as
that of the plastein reaction which requires an exceptionally high
substrate concentration (Yamashita et al., 1970). Recently, Aso
et al. (1977) have attempted to find out how, during the plastein
reaction, different amino acid esters can react with specifically
different initial velocities which depend on their amino acid
side-chain and alcohol-chain structures, in order to obtain
general information that will be useful for the controlled alteration of amino acid compositions of food proteins.

SPECIFICITY FOR AMINO ACID INCORPORATION
DURING THE PLASTEIN REACTION WITH PAPAIN

The following experiments have been made and recently reported by Aso et al. (1977). A twice-crystallized preparation of papain, 27.0 BAEE units/mg/min (25°C), was used both for the protein hydrolysis and for the plastein synthesis (Figure 1). As the original protein, a reagent grade ovalbumin was used after denaturation with 0.01 N NaOH at room temperature. This protein was hydrolyzed with the papain preparation under the following conditions: ovalbumin concentration in reaction medium, 1 % (w/v); papain-ovalbumin ratio, 1:1000 (w/w); pH of the reaction system, 6.0; temperature, 37°C; and incubation time, 24 hr. The reaction medium contained 10 mM L-cysteine as the papain activator. After incubation the entire reaction mixture was treated with an ultra-filtration membrane (Amicon UM-05) to remove salts, free amino acids, oligopeptides and others having molecular weights lower than 500. Disc electrophoresis on polyacrylamide gel demonstrated that the ovalbumin hydrolysate obtained through these procedures had an average molecular weight of 500 – 4500. This fraction was freeze-dried and used as substrate for the following plastein reaction.

The substrate (300 mg) was dissolved in a small amount of water and adjusted to pH 6.0 with a very small amount of 2 N NaOH. The total volume was adjusted finally to 0.9 ml with additional water. To the solution was added one of the amino acid esters that had been previously prepared according to Boissonas et al. (1956). The concentration of each amino acid ester in the solution was set at 20 mM. Subsequently, the solution was preincubated at 37°C for 15 min. On the other hand, papain (3 mg) was dissolved in 0.1 M L-cysteine (0.1 ml) and the enzyme solution (0.1 ml) combined with the above-mentioned preincubation mixture (0.9 ml). The combined solution was incubated at 37°C for the plastein formation. A time-course check with the method of Yamashita et al. (1970) showed that a 10 % trichloroacetic acid-insoluble fraction increased from 34.5 % to 70.3 % during the incubation for 24 hr. In order to determine the degree of incorporation of each amino acid ester an aliquot (0.1 ml) was pipetted from the incubation mixture and treated with 0.1 N NaOH (0.9 ml) to hydrolyze the ester linkage. The free amino acid thereby produced was determined with an amino acid analyzer. The incorporation was quantified by subtracting this determined value (molar basis) from the initial concentration (20 mM). It should be noted that side-reactions such as ester hydrolysis and polymerization by papain did not occur to any significant extent as the plastein reaction was conducted for only a few hours, and also that the incorporation reaction proceeded generally in a linear fashion within 30 min from the beginning of the incubation. This permitted to obtain the initial velocity of incorporation.

A series of α-amino acid ethyl esters were first determined for their initial velocities of incorporation. Figure 2 attempts plotting the observed initial velocities against the relative hydrophobicities of the amino acid side-chains, giving the result that, except in the cases of the β-branched-chain amino acids, valine and isoleucine (filled triangles), there is a close relationship between the hydrophobicity and the initial velocity, no matter how many different types of neutral α-amino acids are tested including aliphatic (open circles), aromatic (filled circles) and sulfur-containing (open triangle) amino acids.

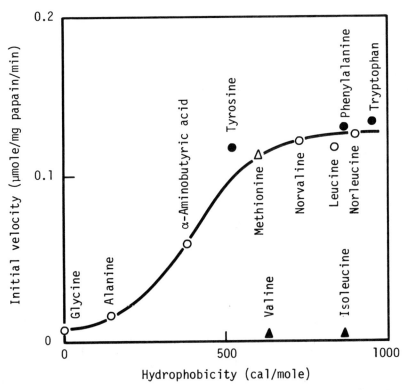

Figure 2. Relationship between the hydrophobicities of amino acid side-chains and the initial velocities of incorporation of amino acid ethyl esters by papain.

Another experiment was carried out to investigate the effect of alcohol chain length on the initial velocity of L-alanine, with the result that this amino acid esterified with a more hydrophobic longer-chain alcohol, i.e., n-butanol, n-hexanol or n-octanol, was more reactive than L-alanine ethyl ester (Table 1). The table includes the data on D-alanine and α-methylalanine, showing that these unusual amino acids are unable to be incorporated even if they have been esterified either with ethanol or with n-hexanol. The superiority of longer-chain alcohols to ethanol was further confirmed by comparing the reactivities of n-hexyl esters of various aliphatic amino acids with those of their ethyl esters.

To evaluate the effects of different alcohol-chain structures Aso et al. (1977) used n-pentanol and its stereoisomers having α-, β- and γ-branches, the structures of which resemble those of the side-chains of norleucine, norvaline, isoleucine and leucine, respectively. Because the α-dimethyl alcohol with the same carbon number was not available, tert-butanol was used instead whose structure was analogous to that of α-methylalanine. As the amino acids to be esterified with these alcohols, glycine and L-norvaline were selected, which, as shown in Table 1, had extremely low and high reactivities, respectively. These amino acids were esterified with the above five alcohols and each of the resulting ten amino acid esters was subjected to the plastein reaction. This experiment gave an expected result in that the initial velocity of glycine n-pentyl ester was distinctly higher than that of glycine ethyl ester (Table 1). Similarly, high velocities were observed also for α-, β- and γ-methylbutyl esters (i.e., sec-pentyl, 2-methyl-1-butyl and isopentyl esters, respectively) of glycine. Almost similar results were obtained with the same kinds of L-norvaline esters. However, an extremely great difference was found between glycine tert-butyl ester and L-norvaline tert-butyl ester; the former was almost completely unreactive whereas the latter showed a very high reactivity comparable with those of other esters.

When we collate the data obtained throughout the study (Aso et al., 1977), we can conclude that the initial velocities of incorporation of α-amino acid esters are specifically different depending on their structures. In particular, the amino acid side-chain structure seems to be of primary importance for any particular amino acid ester to be incorporated effectively (Figure 2). In contrast, the alcohol chain structure can make significant contribution only when the amino acid moiety is either poor in hydrophobicity (as in glycine and alanine) or sterically unfavorable (as in valine and isoleucine) (Table 1). However, an exceptional case was found where even n-hexyl esters of the unusual amino acids, D-alanine and α-methylalanine, were quite unreactive (Table 1). It is also clear that the structure of the alcohol moiety has a less specific effect than that of the amino acid moiety, since L-norvaline which is sufficiently hydrophobic

Table 1

Initial velocities of incorporation of amino acid esters

in the plastein reaction catalyzed by papain.*

(Aso et al., 1977)

Amino acid moiety	Alcohol moiety			
	Ethanol	n-Butanol	n-Hexanol	n-Octanol
L-Alanine	0.016	0.054	0.133	0.135
D-Alanine	0.0	—	0.0	—
α-Methylalanine	0.0	—	0.0	—

	Ethanol	n-Hexanol
Glycine	0.007	0.053
L-Alanine	0.016	0.133
L-α-Aminobutyric acid	0.058	0.132
L-Valine	0.005	0.077
L-Norvaline	0.122	0.151
L-Leucine	0.119	0.140
L-Norleucine	0.125	0.149
L-Isoleucine	0.005	0.048

	A	B	C	D	E
Glycine	0.054	0.057	0.049	0.048	0.001
L-Norvaline	0.144	0.122	0.132	0.138	0.135

A: n-pentanol. B: isopentanol (γ-methylbutanol). C: 2-methyl-1-butanol (β-methylbutanol). D: sec-pentanol (α-methylbutanol) E: tert-butanol. *Data given in μmole/mg papain/min.

and has no β-branch can be effectively incorporated even when esterified with any of the branched-chain alcohols including 2-methyl-1-butanol (analogous to isoleucine) and tert-butanol (analogous to α-methylalanine). In short, the amino acid side-chain and the alcohol chain of any particular L-α-amino acid ester may be ranked as primary and secondary, respectively, with regard to the effect on its initial velocity of incorporation during the plastein reaction.

Meanwhile, Aso et al. (1975) have carried out a model experiment to obtain basic information concerning the incorporation of L-amino acid esters. They used as substrate the authentic compound, ethyl hippurate (i.e., N-benzoylglycine ethyl ester), instead of ovalbumin hydrolysate. Ethyl hippurate (50 mM) was first incubated with papain (17 μM) at pH 6.0 and 37°C. After 15 min an amino acid ester (5 mM) was added and the incubation continued under the same conditions. Analysis of the reaction product indicated that the following reaction occurred:

$$Bz\text{-}Gly\text{-}Papain + AA\text{-}OR \rightarrow Bz\text{-}Gly\text{-}AA\text{-}OR + Papain,$$

where AA-OR refers to the amino acid ester. This thus acted as a nucleophile or aminolysis reagent to react with the acyl-enzyme intermediate, Bz-Gly-Papain, synthesizing a peptide bond to form Bz-Gly-AA-OR. Various L-amino acid esters produced different velocities depending on the amino acid side-chain structure; a more hydrophobic side-chain was more effective except in the case of the β-branched-chain amino acid as in L-valine (Table 2). This observation is similar to that of Alecio et al. (1974). Aso et al. (1975) also found that even the β-branched-chain amino acid could be effectively incorporated when esterified with the hydrophobic alcohol, n-butanol (Table 2). Interestingly enough, it is clear that the reactivity of the amino acid esters does not depend on the maximum velocity (V_{max}) but on the apparent Michaelis-Menten constant of the nucleophilic reaction step (K_N).

The data above indicate that specific affinity of papain for the amino acid ester exists. Perhaps a better understanding of the reaction can be obtained by considering some of the properties of this enzyme. Considerable data are available on the structure of papain, in particular its active site. His-159 is thought to be involved in catalysis as a general acid-base in which Cys-25 becomes acylated in an intermediate step (Glazer and Smith, 1971). Schechter and Berger (1967) and Schechter and Berger (1968) have postulated from data of studies on the specificity of papain for synthetic substrate that binding of substrate occurs by interaction with one or more of the seven subsites designated S_1, S_2, S_3 and S_4 toward the N-terminal from the cutting point of a substrate peptide and S_1', S_2' and S_3' toward the C-terminal from the cutting point. Since any amino acid ester acts as a nucleophile, this must interact with papain by fitting the amino acid side-chain to the S_1' subsite and the alcohol chain to the S_2' subsite.

Table 2

Kinetic parameters for papain-catalyzed aminolysis of

ethyl hippurate by amino acid esters as nucleophiles*

(Aso et al., 1975)

Amino acid ester	v_0 ** (mM/min)	K_N (mM)	V_{max} (mM/min)	$V_{max}/[E]_0$*** (1/sec)
L-Alanine				
ethyl ester	0.17	27.0	0.98	0.96
butyl ester	0.32	9.0	0.91	0.89
L-Norvaline				
ethyl ester	0.59	2.5	0.91	0.89
butyl ester	0.67	2.0	0.93	0.91
L-Valine				
ethyl ester	0.13	33.3	0.95	0.93
butyl ester	0.25	13.9	0.88	0.86
L-Phenylalanine				
ethyl ester	0.63	2.0	0.85	0.83
butyl ester	0.69	1.9	0.80	0.78

* pH 6 (25°C). ** Initial velocity ($[S]_0 = 5$ mM). *** $[E]_0 = 17$ μM.

The observed differences in the incorporation velocities of the
amino acid esters (Table 2) may thus be ascribable to the differences in the chain-subsite affinity.

It is interesting to note that apparently there is a general
similarity between the data in Table 1 and those in Table 2.
Based on this comparison the following speculation may be valid.
In the plastein reaction also each amino acid ester acts primarily
as a nucleophile to be eventually incorporated into the C-terminal
of a peptide. In fact, Yamashita et al. (1972), analyzing a
methionine plastein for its end groups, have disclosed that the
incorporated methionine molecules are located mostly at the C-
terminals of the plastein molecules, as discussed later in more
detail.

INCORPORATION OF ESSENTIAL AMINO ACIDS
BY MEANS OF THE PLASTEIN REACTION

Much attention has been paid to plant proteins as human food, in spite of their relatively low nutritional quality due to insufficient essential amino acids. To improve the nutritive value of plant proteins up to that of common animal proteins it is necessary to supplement them with proper amounts of essential amino acids. The method now in use for this purpose is the addition of free amino acids. Though some sophisticated techniques including encapsulation are actually used for this type of supplementation, there is no great difference — in that the supplemented amino acids still remain in a chemically free state in protein products. Free amino acids per se have a greater or lesser extent of flavor, sometimes causing unpalatability of the protein products. Furthermore, it may be inevitable that parts of the supplemented amino acids in a free state are readily degraded and lost during processing, storage and cooking. These problems may be solved when amino acid molecules are covalently attached to protein molecules. A variety of chemical methods could be available for this way of amino acid incorporation. However, such methods are considered improper when used for food processing, not only because the process is highly expensive, but also because no safety can be warranted since a number of chemicals are used throughout the many unit-processes.

Yamashita et al. (1971) found that the plastein reaction with papain permitted very efficient incorporation of methionine into soy protein under a mild condition, leading to the formation of a plastein product with a highly improved level of methionine. For example, a 10:1 mixture of a peptic hydrolysate of soy protein isolate and L-methionine ethyl ester (HCl salt) was incubated in the presence of papain at 37°C for 24 hr. Dialysis of the entire reaction product against water gave a refined plastein as a non-diffusible fraction. The methionine content of this plastein was found to be 7.22 g%, nearly seven times the original content of methionine in the soy protein isolate. Yamashita et al. (1972) also investigated the location of the incorporated methionine molecules in this kind of plastein. When the plastein was treated with carboxypeptidase A, methionine was liberated much faster than any other amino acid. A second portion of the same plastein was methylated and then treated with lithium borohydride to reduce the COOH to CH_2OH. Hydrolysis of such a chemically treated plastein with 6 N HCl gave aminols in satisfactory yields. Subsequently, the aminols were converted to their dinitrophenyl derivatives, which were separated by thin-layer chromatography and quantified. These experiments, together with some others, showed that 84.9 % (molar basis) of the C-terminals of the plastein molecules were occupied with methionine, whereas only 14.4 % of the N-terminals contained methionine.

This result may provide evidence that the L-methionine ethyl ester added in the plastein reaction system acts primarily as a nucleophile to be eventually incorporated into the C-terminal of each peptide in a manner similar to that described with the hippuryl-papain model system.

A feeding test with rats was made using the methionine plastein (Yamashita et al., 1971). Prior to feeding, this plastein, because of having been overenriched with methionine, was diluted with soy protein to a methionine level of 2.74 %. This sample gave a PER value of 3.38 ± 0.08, compared with a PER value of 2.40 ± 0.05 for casein used as a control. It can be added that according to taste-panel evaluation the methionine plastein was bland in taste and almost completely free from any sulfide flavor. Arai et al. (1974) have prepared a similar plastein from soy protein isolate on an enlarged scale and refined it by precipitation with 70 % ethanol. Table 3 shows the amino acid composition of this refined plastein in comparison with that of the soy protein isolate used as the starting material.

A similar technique applying the plastein reaction by papain has been reported to be useful for enhancing a lysine level of wheat gluten (Yamashita et al., 1976a) and lysine, threonine and tryptophan levels of zein (Aso et al., 1974). A recent study of Yamashita et al. (1976b) has dealt with the preparation, by means of the plastein reaction, of a peptide-type dietetic food for phenylketonuria; this food contains a minor amount of phenylalanine and an adequate amount of incorporated tyrosine.

Attention is now being given to unconventional proteins as potential human food for the future, especially to those of photosynthetic origin. Arai et al. (1976) have tried to improve the quality of proteins from Spirulina maxima (blue-green alga), from Rhodopseudomonas capsulatus (non-sulfur purple bacterium) and from Trifolium repens L. (a type of white clover). What may be important is how to decolor these raw organisms since they are characterized by very high contents of photosynthetic pigments. Each raw sample (10 g on a dry-matter basis) was suspended in 99 % ethanol (250 ml) and the suspension stirred for 3 hr in the dark at room temperature. After filtration the residue was similarly treated with another 250 ml of 99 % ethanol. The extraction residue was suspended in 0.1 N NaOH (1 liter) and the suspension subjected to a mechanically grinding treatment at 5°C for 30 min. Centrifugation gave a clear supernatant, which was then dialyzed in running water at 5°C until the non-diffusible fraction reached a pH value of about 7. This fraction, still somewhat pigmented, was treated with pepsin [3·4·4·1] under the following conditions: protein concentration in medium, 1 % (w/v); enzyme-protein ratio, 1:100 (w/w); pH of the system, 1.5; temperature, 37°C; and incubation time, 24 hr. After incubation the entire product was submitted to gel filtration with a Sephadex G-15 column (3 × 50 cm), the elution being made with 10 % ethanol (400 ml). This column

Table 3

Amino acid compositions of a soy protein isolate
and a methionine plastein
(Arai et al., 1974)

Amino acid	Soy protein isolate	Methionine plastein
	g%	g%
Lysine	5.28	4.78
Histidine	2.04	2.20
Arginine	5.94	5.61
Aspartic acid*	8.70	7.76
Threonine	2.63	2.11
Serine	3.53	2.75
Glutamic acid**	15.00	10.20
Proline	4.32	2.18
Glycine	4.38	2.55
Alanine	3.98	2.65
Valine	3.36	4.29
Isoleucine	3.00	5.72
Leucine	5.17	7.26
Tyrosine	2.83	3.52
Phenylalanine	4.20	5.94
Tryptophan	1.34	1.30
S amino acid***	2.94	9.96
Half-cystine	1.76	1.98
Methionine	1.18	7.98

* Aspartic acid plus asparagine.

** Glutamic acid plus glutamine.

*** Sulfur-containing amino acids.

treatment facilitated the separation between the peptide fraction
eluted before and the pigment fraction remaining adsorbed, giving
a peptic hydrolysate almost completely free from any color. This
hydrolysate was freeze-dried and used as substrate for the plastein reaction. To the substrate was formulated ethyl esters of
the three essential amino acids, L-methionine, L-lysine and L-
tryptophan, which were found insufficient for any of the unconventional proteins used; the proportions of formulation of the ethyl
esters (HCl salt) were determined by taking into consideration
both the nutritional requirements of methionine, lysine and tryptophan and the data on how efficiently their ethyl esters are
incorporated (Table 1). The plastein reaction was carried out
under the following conditions: substrate (peptic hydrolysate)
concentration in medium, 30 % (w/v); enzyme (papain)-substrate
ratio, 1:100 (w/w); pH of the system, 6.0; temperature, 37°C; and
incubation time, 24 hr. After incubation the entire product was
diluted with a 100-fold volume of 10 % ethanol and then treated
with an ultrafiltration membrane (Amicon UM-05). A fraction with
a molecular weight of higher than 500 was obtained by this treatment. Freeze-drying of this fraction gave a final refined product
without any color and flavor. Table 4 summarizes material balances throughout the respective processes. Table 5 shows the amino
acid compositions of the plasteins in comparison with those of
their original proteins.

Table 4

Material balances in the plastein production

from photosynthetic protein sources

(Arai et al., 1976; Yamashita et al., 1976a)

	Alga*	Bacterium**	Leaf***
	g	g	g
Starting material, dried	10	10	—
Decolored protein hydrolysate	4.74	3.90	2.00
L-Methionine ethyl ester·HCl	0.54	0.35	0.25
L-Lysine ethyl ester· 2 HCl	1.18	0.65	0.33
L-Tryptophan ethyl ester·HCl	0.10	0.04	0.04
Plastein, dried	4.96	4.08	2.03

* S. maxima.   ** R. capsulatus.   *** T. repens L.

Table 5

Amino acid compositions of algal, bacterial and leaf proteins
and of the respective plasteins
(Arai et al., 1976; Yamashita et al., 1976a)

Amino acid	S. maxima Protein	S. maxima Plastein	R.capsulatus Protein	R.capsulatus Plastein	T. repens L. Protein	T. repens L. Plastein
	g%		g%		g%	
Lysine	4.59	7.75	5.37	7.39	6.06	8.23
Histidine	1.77	1.91	2.35	2.44	1.94	2.01
Arginine	6.50	6.70	6.27	6.05	3.66	3.84
Aspartic acid*	8.60	11.87	8.57	10.21	11.10	10.45
Threonine	4.56	5.42	5.07	4.36	5.60	5.93
Serine	4.20	4.43	3.16	4.63	4.17	4.00
Glutamic acid**	12.60	14.68	10.03	9.77	16.00	15.54
Proline	3.90	3.62	4.26	3.45	3.75	3.57
Glycine	4.75	4.76	4.53	5.98	5.01	4.79
Alanine	6.80	5.80	8.74	8.32	6.23	6.05
Valine	4.69	6.00	6.59	6.56	7.45	7.00
Isoleucine	6.03	6.32	4.96	5.30	4.98	4.55
Leucine	8.02	8.98	8.45	8.47	8.86	8.24
Ar amino acid***	8.92	8.96	8.09	8.16	9.61	9.00
Tyrosine	3.95	3.98	3.21	3.53	4.11	3.88
Phenylalanine	4.97	4.98	4.88	4.63	5.50	5.12
S amino acid****	1.77	8.75	3.73	9.06	1.82	8.13
Half-cystine	0.40	0.53	0.76	0.77	0.97	0.99
Methionine	1.37	8.22	2.97	8.29	0.85	7.14
Tryptophan	1.40	2.72	2.05	2.56	1.51	2.73

* Aspartic acid plus asparagine. ** Glutamic acid plus glutamine. *** Aromatic amino acids. **** Sulfur-containing acids.

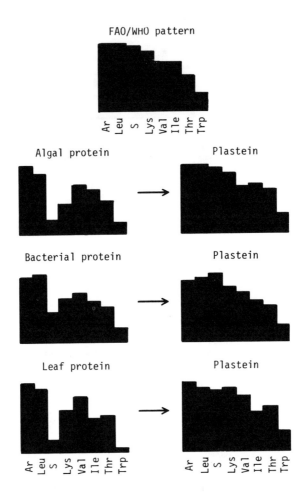

Figure 3. Essential amino acid patterns of algal, bacterial and leaf proteins and of the plasteins produced from them, with the FAO/WHO pattern (1973) on the top. Ar = phenylalanine plus tyrosine. S = methionine plus half-cystine.

It may be interesting to pick out the eight essential amino acids and compare their patterns of the plasteins with the FAO/WHO suggested pattern for male adults (cf. Report of a Joint FAO/WHO Ad Hoc Expert Committee, 1973). In Figure 3 there are the essential amino acid patterns of the proteins and the plasteins, with the FAO/WHO pattern shown uppermost. This comparison makes clear the differences between the proteins and the FAO/WHO suggestion, especially in regard to methionine, lysine and tryptophan levels, and also reveals that the essential amino acid patterns of the plasteins have become almost similar to the FAO/WHO pattern.

The plastein reaction is thus applicable to the nutritional improvement of conventional and unconventional proteins through the incorporation of controlled amounts of essential amino acids, with an even further possibility of maximizing the nutritive value of food proteins. However, what may be of pressing importance in the practical application of the plastein reaction is to find out how to effect the process in a more efficient and economic manner. As pointed out in Figure 1, the plastein reaction always requires the foregoing protein hydrolysis step and therefore the entire process must be composed of the two different steps. Provided that a proper set of reaction conditions is determined, it might be feasible to unify the two steps and permit the amino acid incorporation into protein by only one step.

INCORPORATION OF AMINO ACIDS BY A NOVEL ONE-STEP PROCESS

Our current work is disclosing that amino acid ethyl ester added to ovalbumin (not to its hydrolysate) is generally incorporated with the aid of papain when an unconventional incubation condition is adopted, especially in respect to substrate (protein) concentration and pH. Although more remains to be elucidated than the information we have obtained up to the present, it is likely that the one-step process for the most efficient incorporation of any particular amino acid ethyl ester will require the highest possible substrate concentration and, at the same time, a weakly alkaline pH which is apparently far from the optimum for the hydrolytic activity of papain.

Various kinds of amino acid ethyl esters were evaluated for how efficiently they were incorporated at the initial stage of the one-step process. Each amino acid ethyl ester (0.1 mmole), ovalbumin (200 mg) and papain (2 mg) were dissolved in 1 ml of 1 M phosphate containing 2 mM L-cysteine, and the solution was incubated at 37°C. An initial velocity of incorporation was determined for each of the amino acid ethyl esters according to Aso et al. (1977). This experiment gave the result shown in Figure 4, where, just as in Figure 2, the hydrophobicities of the amino acid side-chains are plotted along the abscissa and the determined initial velocities of incorporation along the ordinate. From this result it is clear that there is a close relationship between the

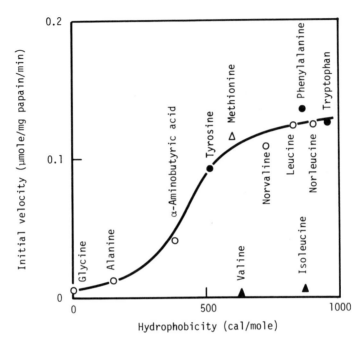

Figure 4. Relationship between the hydrophobicities of amino acid side-chains and the initial velocities of incorporation of amino acid ethyl esters by papain.

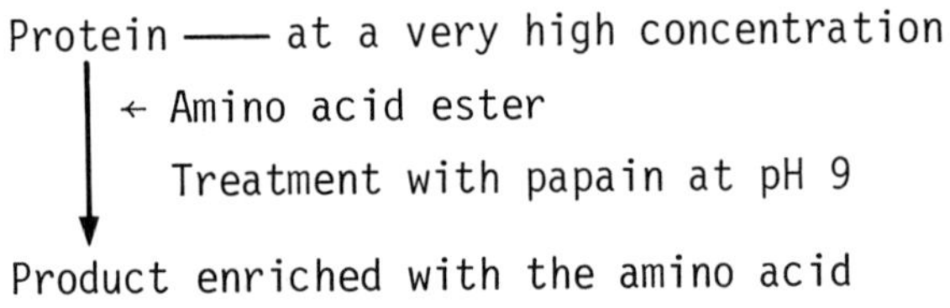

Protein ——— at a very high concentration
        | ← Amino acid ester
        | Treatment with papain at pH 9
        ▼
Product enriched with the amino acid

Figure 5. Simplified scheme of amino acid incorporation by means of the novel one-step process with papain.

hydrophobicity and the velocity, except in the cases of the β-branched-chain amino acids as in valine and isoleucine. It may be interesting to compare this profile with that shown in Figure 2; both profiles seem almost identical. However, compared to the conventional plastein reaction (Figure 1), the one-step process (Figure 5) can be characterized by its easy implementation, although it is essential that further work be done before this procedure will be economically feasible in the field of protein processing.

REFERENCES

Alecio, M. R., Dann, M. L. and Lowe, G. (1974). The specificity of the S$_1'$ subsite of papain. Biochem. J., 141, 495 - 501.

Arai, S., Aso, K., Yamashita, M. and Fujimaki, M. (1974). Note on an enlarged-scale method for preparing a methionine-enriched plastein from soybean protein. Cereal Chem., 51, 143 - 145.

Arai, S., Yamashita, M., Aso, K. and Fujimaki, M. (1975). A parameter related to the plastein formation. J. Food Sci., 40, 342 - 344.

Arai, S., Yamashita, M. and Fujimaki, M. (1976). Enzymatic modification for improving nutritional quality and acceptability of proteins extracted from photosynthetic microorganisms Spirulina maxima and Rhodopseudomonas capsulatus. J. Nutr. Sci. Vitaminol. (Japan), 22, 447 - 456.

Aso, K., Yamashita, M., Arai, S. and Fujimaki, M. (1974). Tryptophan-, threonine- and lysine-enriched plasteins from zein. Agric. Biol. Chem. (Tokyo), 38, 679 - 680.

Aso, K., Yamashita, M., Arai, S. and Fujimaki, M. (1975). Abstracts of Papers, Annual Meeting of the Agricultural Chemical Society of Japan, Sapporo, Japan, 1975, p. 153.

Aso, K., Yamashita, M., Arai, S., Suzuki, J. and Fujimaki, M. (1977). Specificity for incorporation of α-amino acid esters during the plastein reaction by papain. J. Agric. Food Chem. 25, 1138-1141.

Boissonas, A. R., Guttman, St., Jaquenoud, P.-A. and Waller, J.-P. (1956). Synthese d'analogues structuraux de l'oxytocine. Helv. Chim. Acta, 39, 1421 - 1427.

Determann, H. (1966). Peptidsynthesen mit Hilfe von Proteolytischen Enzymen (Plasteinreaktion). In "Peptides", L. Zervas (Editor). Pergamon Press, pp. 89 - 103.

Eriksen, S. and Fagerson, I. S. (1976). The plastein reaction and its application: a review. J. Food Sci., 41, 490 - 493.

Glazer, A. N. (1966). Transesterification reactions catalyzed by papain. J. Biol. Chem., 241, 3811 - 3817.

Glazer, A. N. and Smith, E. L. (1971). Papain and other sulfhydryl proteolytic enzymes. In "The Enzymes", Vol. 3, P.D. Boyer (Editor). Academic Press, New York and London, pp. 501-546.

Hofsten, B. v. and Lalasidis, G. (1976). Protease-catalyzed for-
    mation of plastein products and some of their properties.
    J. Agric. Food Chem., 24, 460 – 465.

Horowitz, J. and Haurowitz, F. (1959). Mechanism of plastein
    reaction. Biochim. Biophys. Acta, 33, 231 – 237.

Mycek, M. J. and Fruton, J. S. (1957). Specificity of papain-
    catalyzed transamidation reactions. J. Biol. Chem., 226,
    165 – 171.

Schechter, I. and Berger, A. (1967). On the size of the active
    site in proteases. I. Papain. Biochem. Biophys. Res. Commun.,
    27, 157 – 162.

Schechter, I. and Berger, A. (1968). On the size of the active
    site in proteases. III. Mapping the active site of papain;
    specific peptide inhibitors of papain. Biochem. Biophys. Res.
    Commun., 32, 898 – 902.

Sluyterman, J. A. AE. and Wijdenes, J. (1972). Sigmoidal progress
    curves in the polymerization of leucine methyl ester cata-
    lyzed by papain. Biochim. Biophys. Acta, 289, 194 – 202.

Tauber, H. (1951). Synthesis of protein-like substances by chymo-
    trypsin. J. Amer. Chem. Soc., 73, 1288 – 1290.

Virtanen, A. I. (1951). Über die enzymatische Polypeptidsynthese.
    Makromol. Chem., 6, 94 – 103.

Yamashita, M., Arai, S., Matsuyama, J., Gonda, M., Kato, H. and
    Fujimaki, M. (1970). Enzymatic modification of proteins in
    foodstuffs. III. Phenomenal survey on α-chymotryptic plastein
    synthesis from peptic hydrolysate of soy protein.
    Agric. Biol. Chem. (Tokyo), 34, 1484 – 1491.

Yamashita, M., Arai, S., Tsai, S.-J. and Fujimaki, M. (1971).
    Plastein reaction as a method for enhancing the sulfur-
    containing amino acid level of soybean protein. J. Agric.
    Food Chem., 19, 1151 – 1154.

Yamashita, M., Arai, S., Aso, K. and Fujimaki, M. (1972).
    Location and state of methionine residues in a papain-
    synthesized plastein from a mixture of soybean protein
    hydrolysate and L-methionine ethyl ester. Agric. Biol. Chem.
    (Tokyo), 36, 1353 – 1360.

Yamashita, M., Arai, S. and Fujimaki, M. (1976a). Plastein re-
    action for food protein improvement. J. Agric. Food Chem.,
    24, 1100 – 1104.

Yamashita, M., Arai, S. and Fujimaki, M. (1976b). A low-phenyl-
    alanine, high-tyrosine plastein as an acceptable dietetic
    food. Method of preparation by use of enzymatic protein
    hydrolysis and resynthesis. J. Food Chem., 41, 1029 – 1032.

33

POTENTIAL FOR THE USE OF GERMINATED WHEAT AND SOYBEANS TO ENHANCE

HUMAN NUTRITION

P. L. Finney

USDA-ARS, Western Wheat Quality Laboratory
Wilson Hall, Rm. 7
Washington State University
Pullman, WA 99164

INTRODUCTION

Wheat and soybeans are the major agricultural exports of the United States. The U.S. sells more of each crop than any other nation. Soybeans are the main staple in China, but the U.S. sells more soybeans than China grows. For hundreds of millions of other people, wheat is the main staple. And yet, most Americans eat whole grains of neither wheat nor soybeans.

In the United States, many nutrients of wheat and soybeans are lost in processing or are fed to animals. A highly significant share of the wheat nutrients are lost from the main foodstream when the germ and bran (with aleurone) portions are separated. Whole soybeans are carefully processed for food by only a handful of Americans.

Ancient Sciences Forgotten or Mistaken

When "maximum nutrients for minimum costs" have dictated, wheat and soybeans have nearly always been eaten whole. For use as food, whole grains were usually treated by selected processes of germination, fermentation, or heat, or both to increase amounts or availability of nutrients. Food processes today are too often selected on the basis of speed, storability and ease of preparation instead of the nutritional value of foods produced. I believe time-proven traditional processes are ignored (as with soybean germination or fermentation) or very crudely approximated (as with wheat flour yeast fermentation).

Time honored processing methods tend to make foods more desirable and more nutritious than many of the newer processes. For
example, when wheat is prepared as a staple food it is steeped,
then mashed and boiled, or leavened with yeast into bread. Soybeans are usually steeped in water overnight (or much longer) then
mashed or fractionated by treatment with salts, acids, heat or
other processes of fermentation or some combination of those
treatments. Soybean fractions are then eaten directly or used as
a base for production of hundreds of highly nutritious and taste-
variable foods [see for example references on tofu (germinated
curd) and miso (fermented soybean paste)].[1]

A critical review of the methods by which wheat and soybeans
are processed in the U.S. is especially pertinent in light of recent advances in the science of human nutrition. Some of those
advances are reflected in the Dietary Goals of the Senate Select
Committee on Nutrition.[2] In those Goals, leading nutritionists
recommend that dietary levels be increased for whole fruits, grains,
and vegetables, and be decreased for animal fat and protein, and
for sugar and salt.

Degenerative Diseases in the U.S.

There is evidence that too much sugar,[3] too much fat, too
much salt, and too little dietary fiber may be associated with
heart disease, obesity, cancer, stroke, or other degenerative
diseases.[4-9] Some of those diseases are for all practical purposes found only in highly industrial nations.[10] Indeed, the U.S.
and England may be plagued with them even more than most other industrial nations.[10]

Some medical researchers link low dietary fiber with cancer
of the colon and rectum,[11] diverticular disease of the colon,[12]
and generally with metabolic and vascular disease.[13,14] For over
20 years, others have attributed the anti-toxic effects of food
and feed to the plant fiber in the diet.[15]

How can Americans begin to rebalance their diets so that the
Senate dietary goals are achieved? Which foods should be eaten
more, which less? If the U.S. eating patterns are "as critical as
any problem now before us,"[2] what short- and long-term modifications
in food processing are most appropriate? By increasing fresh fruits
and vegetables 100%, by eating more whole grains, and by eating more
carbohydrates but less "refined" carbohydrate foods, Americans could
take steps toward achieving the Senate dietary goals and also increase their dietary fiber intake.

Traditional dishes from all over the world could incorporate
those changes. Many Chinese, Japanese, Indian and other national

foods satisfy the dietary goals of the U.S. Senate Committee. However, there are other viable methods of improving U.S. diets utilizing existing American food processing abilities. For example,
over 50 million pounds of white bread are produced each day in the
U.S. Although that bread represents a small fraction of the total
nutrients most Americans now consume, breads (if properly formulated) could easily provide more nutrients and greater bulk, while
helping to reduce food cost.

Purpose of Paper

It is the major purpose of this paper to present information
which shows that carefully controlled germination and fermentation
of wheat and soybeans can: (1) Increase or maximize many otherwise
unavailable nutrients; (2) Decrease or eliminate most known undesirable "antinutritional" factors associated with those seeds;
and (3) Generally provide a range of flavor and structure components so that delicious and interesting foods (including a wide
variety of yeast leavened breads) may be produced from them at a
low cost.

Particularly pertinent is the information which comes from
over 2,000 years of Chinese and 1,000 years of Japanese soybean
processing experience. Also of importance is the information from
the scientific literature of the West, from U.S. commercial bread
production, and from experimental wheat and soybean germination,
fermentation, and breadmaking studies.

WHEAT AND WHEAT PROCESSING

For centuries, millions of people have eaten whole wheat as a
staple. Consequently, they have eaten relatively high concentra-
toins of wheat bran (about 2-5% total diet). Thus as a food, wheat
(including its bran and germ portion) is already time-proven. It
is available and inexpensive. It is high in dietary fiber, and has
a relatively high water carrying capacity to the colon so that it
often decreases transit time through the digestive tract. In
fact, wheat bran has been recommended as a common home remedy for
constipation and associated diseases for years.

Wheat bran and germ portions are excellent sources of vitamins
and minerals, and other important nutrients. Because the wheat
bran includes most of the aleurone layer, it contains about 85% of
the niacin, 70-75% of the pyridoxine, 50% of the pantothenic acid,
42% of the riboflavin, 33% of the thiamine, and about 18-20% of
the protein of the whole wheat (although the bran constitutes only
about 14-15% of the kernel).

Differences among Wheat Brans

Fibrous materials now added in U.S. foods are from sources as diverse as methyl-cellulose (extracted wood pulp), brewers spents, soybean hulls, and white and red wheat bran. Those sources vary in food processability and organoleptic properties as much as they vary in nutritional properties.

Wheat brans also differ markedly. People who eat wheat as a staple generally prefer white wheat, and often express a distaste for the "bitter-brany" red wheats. Some of those flavor differences may be related to nutritional factors. Sandstead et al. (1977) found red and white brans had different effects on mineral balance.[16] Munoz et al. found they have different effects on serum lipids and cholesterol and found that reds increased fecal weight while whites did not.[17] Comparisons of phytic acid level and phytase activity among brans were not found in this literature search.

USDA Researchers (1977) milled and sifted all classes of wheats into three fractions: endosperm (75%), bran (20%), and shorts (5%). Fractions were reconstituted in all combinations and processed into whole wheat breads. Some brans were heat treated at different temperatures for different times so that a range of brans between dehydrated and slightly burnt was produced (120°F, 8 hrs; to 240°F, 2 hrs). Breads made with red bran were distinctly bitter, and those made with white brans had a nut-like aroma. Researchers also studied effects of bran particle size. Finer brans were found to be more detrimental to bread processability.[18]

Kirwin et al. found that the effectiveness of bran as a dietary fiber source was related to particle size. Coarse brans absorbed and carried nearly three times as much water to the colon as the finer brans (throughs). When the coarse bran was remilled, its water-binding capacity to the colon was reduced from 6.15 g/g to 3.54 g/g while the reground fine bran was reduced from 2.63 to 2.16 g/g.[19]

The reminder is that wheats in general and brans in particular differ significantly in their nutritional value even before the wheats are germinated or fermented. For the formulation of breads or other foods with white or red wheat, however, the method of processing affects the palatability, food functionality and nutritive value of the product.

Importance of Phytic Acid to Human Nutrition

One main nutritional disadvantage of wheat bran is its phytic acid content. Phytic acid interferes with digestion or absorption

of various minerals, including zinc, calcium, and iron. Mihailovic
et al. (1965) found the esters of myoinositol phosphate, from mono
to penta, in wheat seedlings.[20] Those esters are produced *in vitro*
when sodium phytate and phytase are combined in solution, as
Tomlinson and Ballou demonstrated during the early 1960s.[21]

Wheat Germination and Phytic Acid

In plants wherever phytic acid is present, phytase appears;
however, germination is sometimes required to activate the enzyme.
In cereal grains a considerable proportion of the total phosphorous
is present as phytate. In wheat, phytin P constitutes 70–75% of the
total P of the grain. In fact a principle function of phytase in
grains is to provide inorganic phosphate from phytate during initial
stages of germination. Shrivastava (1964) found phytase activity
increased 290% with gibberellic acid (GA) and 220% without GA during
96 hours of germination of barley (after steeping 72 hours, $15^{\circ}C\pm$
1°).[24] Matheson and Strother (1969) found that in wheat phytase
activity increased by 320% after 3 days of germination ($25^{\circ}C$).
They also found that fourteen days germination reduced the phytate
to zero.[23] Bianchetti and Sartirana noted that with wheat phytase
activity in germ and scutellum was maximum after about 30 hours
germination (2 hours steeping, $20^{\circ}C$, then $28^{\circ}C$ in dark with 0.5%
glucose.)[24]

Most published reports indicate that in wheat and barley
phytate is reduced and phytase increased during germination; the
net result is an additive or multiplicative increase in nutritionally available Ca, Fe, Zn, and/or P, depending on subsequent food
formulation and processing.

Feeding Studies in Man and Rat

Reinhold *et al.* (1974) showed that yeast fermentation in the
traditional whole wheat bread (naan) of Iran increased zinc solubility two to three fold (pH adjusted between 4.5 to 7.5).[25] Rat
jujunum and ileum absorbed more labeled zinc from leavened than
from unleavened whole meal bread. The solubility of the labeled
zinc in suspensions of leavened and unleavened breads increased
exponentially as pH was decreased from 7.0 to 4.5.[26] Reinhold and
others (1973) studied the effects of purified phytate and of
phytate-rich bread upon zinc, calcium, and phosphorous metabolism
in man. Their results showed that high-phytate intake may be the
cause of zinc- and calcium-related metabolic disturbances that are
common among Iranian villagers.[27]

Reinhold *et al.* stress the applicability of their work to
other populations who eat much unleavened whole wheat meal.

Producers and consumers alike in the United States who are responding to the numerous references in medical, academic, and popular
publications which urge increased consumption of wheat bran and
other dietary fibrous materials should re-evaluate those studies.
It would be unfortunate if the amount of phytate in whole wheat
breads which are produced with little or no fermentation parallels
the amount found in unleavened bread.

Lysine and Wheat Germination

Lysine plays an important role in animal and human nutrition.
Much less certain is the degree of availability of lysine in whole
wheat meal or its fractions. Still less well documented are the
effects of many methods of food preparation. In general, processing profoundly affects the availability of lysine and of other
nutrients. Indeed, differences in methods of food preparation
might be responsible, at least in some degree, for differences of
opinion concerning the need for lysine supplementation. Some well
documented studies suggest that very high concentrations of whole
wheat would maintain optimum human health at nearly all ages.[27]

Dalbi and Tsai (1976) reported that the lysine content of wheat
increased about 50% during 6 days' germination.[28] Those authors also
found that germination increased tryptophan (believed by many to be
the third or fourth limiting amino acid in unprocessed whole wheat).
Mason (1977) found that wheat varieties differed in rate of lysine
increases during germination. During 7 days' germination (24°C)
lysine increased 30% in a Fortuna composite and 50% in Nugaines
(single seed lot).[29]

Wheat Germination and Vitamins

Whole wheat is a valuable source of many vitamins, including
the ones (Table 1) that Michele and Lorenz (1976) studied. Those
authors compared whole wheat and its three major commercial milling
fractions: white flour (endosperm), shorts (most of the germ with
some endosperm and some bran), and bran (mostly the outer fiber
layers of the wheat, including the aleurone layer).[30]

Many of these vitamins listed in Table 1 can increase during
germination: levels of increase depend on germination conditions.
Table 2 summarizes for some of those vitamins the average increases
that were reported by a number of independent workers.[31-38]

Other Changes During Wheat Germination

After 30 minutes of imbibition, adenosine triphosphate (ATP)
increased five-fold.[39] Under usual germination conditions, deoxy-

TABLE 1

Vitamin Contents of Whole Wheat, White Flour, Shorts, and Bran Fractions (g/g, Dry)

Vitamins	Whole Wheat 100%	White Flour 75%	Shorts 5%	Bran 20%
Thiamine	9.9	0.7	10.1	13.2
Riboflavin	3.1	1.5	1.8	5.5
Niacin	48.3	9.5	23.5	171.4
Biotin	0.056	0.013	0.055	0.162
Folacin	0.56	0.09	0.59	1.59
Pantothenic Acid	9.1	2.5	7.0	31.7
Vitamin B_6	4.7	0.48	5.3	13.0

From: Michele & Lorenz. Cereal Chem. 53:853 (1976)

TABLE 2

The Average Increase in Vitamins During Wheat Germination (the average of a number of independent workers), Expressed as % Increase on Dry Weight

Vitamins	% Increase
Riboflavin	300
Niacin	10-25
Pantothenic Acid	40-50
Pyridoxine	200
Ascorbic Acid	500

ribonucleic acid (DNA) began to increase after about 15 hours.[40] Usual commercial malting conditions increase DNA polymerase and DNase about eight-fold.[41,42]

Other important nutritional and food-functional changes that take place during wheat germination include rapid increases in

cellulases, amylases, and proteases, and associated intermediate
compounds. Those enzymes are particularly important to food processing. The cellulases are able (during both germination and subsequent fermentation) to hydrolyze cell walls (primarily cellulose)
and thereby liberate many vital nutrients. If the cell walls of
the aleurone layer of wheat are well hydrolyzed one would expect
the availability of nutrients to increase. Control of amylases
give the processor the ability to produce breads or other fermented
foods by the use of native wheat starch as a source of sugar. In
bread production, the proteases alter certain important physio-
chemical dough properties. If germination is too long or improperly
accomplished, the value of those or other enzymes becomes highly
problematic. Again we are reminded that how wheat is "processed"
is crucial to its food value.

Fermentation and Phytic Acid

During the production of yeast-leavened bread, significant
quantities of phytate are destroyed. The amount destroyed depends
on pH of dough, the nature and quantity of some metal salts present
(particularly Ca salts), and on other apparently less important
factors.[43] Pringle and Moran showed (1942) that as fermentation
time increased from 3 to 8 hours (1% yeast), phytate destruction
increased from 59 to 76%. The pH of the dough is probably the
single most important factor in that destruction. The authors demonstrated that after 5 hours of fermentation, addition of acetic
acid to the doughs lowered the pH to 5.44 and 5.41. Phytate destruction was for all purposes complete.[43]

The effectiveness of fermentation activity and lowering of pH
on the destruction of phytate is not surprising when ordinary solubility principles are considered. Time is obviously required, independent of fermentation activity, to solubilize the phytate. It
is still less surprising in light of Peers work (1952) which showed
that phytase activity of both wheat meal and isolated enzyme was
maximum at 5.15.[44]

Thus, particularly when mineral availability is considered,
the usual U.S. commercial continuous breadmaking processes appear
inadvisable for the production of whole wheat breads, since they
involve relatively little fermentation. Minimum fermentation processes probably are not suitable for phytate-phytase interactions.

Germinated Wheat versus Bread Processability

USDA researchers (1976) found that high percentages of whole
germinated wheat (mashed, fresh, or variously dried and ground)

could replace regular bakers (endosperm) flour or whole wheat flour
in straight-dough and sponge-and-dough (prefermentation) baking procedures. Most of their experimental bread was baked with 7.6% fresh
yeast, no added sugar, 70-minute straight dough fermentation or
45:35 minute sponge-and-dough fermentation, along with a variety of
other baking ingredients. As wheat germination (Peak variety) time
increased from 23 to 55 hours (25°C, 42% hydration), the amount of
ground, germinated wheat substitutable in the formula decreased from
60% to 13%. After another wheat variety (Nugaines) had been germinated 48 hours, 15% could be substituted in the formula. The germinated meal was required to provide amylase because of the lack of
sugar. The amount of germinated wheat meal that could be used in
the formula was inversely related to the alpha-amylase produced with
increasing germination time.[45]
     Mason (1977) studied varieties of a number of wheat composites.
After 5 days germination, the amount of germinated wheat meal required for optimum no-sugar bread baking varied from 0.60% (Twin
wheat variety) to 1.30% (Wared wheat variety), in essentially identical bread baking procedures to USDA researchers. Mason also found
that germinated, dried Nugaines meal replaced only 0.9% formula
flour after 5 days' germination.[29] The amount of germinated wheat
that could be added to bread was limited by its amylase content.

Germination Time Versus Bread Functionality

     After alpha-amylase, the next most limiting factor that governs
the amount of germinated wheat that can be used in the sugar-free
bread formulations appears to be the relative degree to which protein (and associated compounds) is degraded. As germination proceeds, endosperm protein (the protein that affects the quality of
bread) is hydrolyzed and transported to the developing wheat plant.
The first 20 to 35 hours of germination cause some significant
changes, as expressed by the 10 g mixograph, in the mixing and
other rheological properties of the flour dough. Up until about 35
hours, however, there is no apparent loss of mixing strength (as
measured in the mixograph by curve height and width at peak). Beyond 35 hours of germination, those important properties of the
flour begin to diminish rapidly.

SOYBEAN AND SOYBEAN PROCESSING

Soy Flours for Food

     Progress has been made in improving the nutritional, food
functional, and flavor properties of soy flours processed in the
usual U.S. fashion (i.e., steamed, dehulled, flaked, solvent extracted, dehydrated, and/or toasted). Major commercial processing

conditions have been selected to optimize and balance cost, nutrition, flavor, and food processability, but today's improved soy flours can be used to replace only 5-7% of the wheat flour in breadmaking formulae (for example) unless special dough conditioners are also used. Even with conditioners, flavor and flatulence problems remain. Soy flours are included in millions of pounds of U.S. commercially processed foods, but are sought directly by few Americans.

Germinated Soybeans in China

Soybeans can be processed for foods that are less expensive and I believe generally, better than soy flour products. For centuries, Far Eastern peoples have germinated soybeans and mung beans and often fermented their mashes, with success. Today nearly 100% of the bean is carefully processed into high quality, low cost foods that form the main staple for hundreds of millions of people. Usually the bean is germinated a few days and eaten whole (with minimal heating); or it is germinated about 10-14 hours (hydrated to about 60%), cooked, mashed and washed, or salt or acid precipitated. Some of those processing steps are used in a variety of combinations to yield a host of delicious, nutritious, and very inexpensive foods. The salient point is that success is based: (1) on carefully controlled and rather precise germination and/or fermentation processing; (2) on selective fractionation; and (3) on precise heat treatment. Care is taken to assure that sanitary conditions are such that treatment with fungicides is unnecessary.

Those facts and considerations and my recent review of some pertinent Western literature suggested that germinated and fermented soybeans probably could be incorporated into breads and other mass-produced U.S. foods. A review of some of that literature follows and prefaces a discussion of completed, or on-going, studies of germinated soybeans conducted at two USDA research laboratories.

Soybeans as a Source of Vitamin C

Soybean sprouts are often compared nutritionally with mung bean sprouts, which, according to Miller and Hair (1928) are "a fair source of vitamin A in both the raw and the cooked state; a very good source of vitamin B, both raw and cooked; and an excellent source of vitamin C in the raw state and a good source in the cooked" (authors compared sprouts to many common vegetables).[46]

The comparison between the beans is reasonable, particularly with respect to their vitamin C contents, when germinated. Delf (1922) studied South African foodstuffs and found that germinated soybeans were an excellent antiscorbutic source, and implied that their vitamin C content was high (relatively small quantities kept rats scurvy free).[47]   Lee and Read (1936) found that vitamin C increased markedly when soybeans were germinated.[48] Riboflavin is reported to be 0.31 mg/100 g in ungerminated soybeans.[48a] Hsu (1978) found roboflavin increased from 0.26 to 0.49 mg/100 g in cotyledons after five days soybean germination.[48b]

Few studies predate those in which Everson *et al.* (1944) evaluated germinated soybeans for protein nutritional quality. They found the protein of freshly germinated soybeans (60 hours, 26°C) "superior to that of the unheated mature beans, although the percentage of nitrogen absorbed was not increased."[49] Protein efficiency of germinated and ungerminated beans increased with autoclaving. Mattingly and Bird (1945) corroborated Everson's work with rats, but found that germination did not improve soybeans as feed for chickens.[50]

Trypsin Inhibitors in Soybeans

Desikachar and De (1950) reported that the activity of trypsin inhibitor in soybeans did not change with germination.[51] Liener (1977) found that trypsin inhibitor remained unchanged under the 3-day germination conditions studied by USDA researchers.[52]

Lipoxygenase and Trypsin Inhibition

Trypsin inhibitors are generally characterized as proteins;[53] but researchers disagree on the extent to which those inhibitors are responsible for total growth-depressing effects. Kakade *et al.* (1973) associated 40% of the growth-depressing effect with trypsin inhibitors.[54] Studies by Matsushita (1975) may have accounted for some of the remaining growth-depressing effects of soybeans. He showed that the secondary degradation products of linoleic acid (the major fatty acid of soybeans) hydroperoxides reacted with trypsin. In 30-40 minutes, 60% of the trypsin activity was inhibited.[55] Matsushita's work implies that not all trypsin inhibitors are proteins after all, and that some inhibitory activity may be generated after soybean processing has begun.

Lipoxygenase and Soybean Flavor Problems

Work during the last 10-15 years shows that in soybeans the interaction of lipoxygenase with linoleic acid produces off-odors and -flavors, and generates toxic or physiologically active compounds that can damage proteins, enzymes, and amino acids.[56] Those objectionable flavors are reduced, or their development prevented, by a number of treatments including soaking and heating steps. Kon *et al.* (1970) ground soybeans at pH 3.85, cooked and then neutralized the slurry to inactivate lipoxygenase.[57] Nelson *et al.* (1971) found

that a 10-minute blanching step (100°C) was sufficient if beans were
hydrated to 50% (about 4 hours), whereas a 20-minute blanching was
required for unsoaked beans.[58] Certainly the degree to which the
individual soybean components are hydrated is important in reducing
the cooking time. Nelson and co-workers did not explain whether
the germination-related biochemical changes that took place during
the early steeping hours help to reduce cooking time and off-flavors.
Holman[58a] found lipoxidase (lipoxigenase) activity of soybeans
decreased more than 50% between day two and day five of germination.

Soybean Germination and Phytates

As discussed above, germination of seeds generally promotes a
nutritionally favorable phytate:phytase ratio. Soybeans are no exception. Chen and Pan (1977) found that in soybeans phytates
decreased 22% during 5 days of soybean germination.[59]

Experimental Use of U.S. Soy Flour in Bread

Historically some cereal chemists and other researchers have
studied wheat:soybean interactions. At first, they studied them
because even in the 1940s, "it had long been recognized that soybean proteins effectively supplement wheat proteins in animal nutrition and greatly increase their nutritive value by the addition
of lysine and other amino acids in which wheat proteins are relatively low."[60] However, as the work progressed, it became more
generally recognized that the process of breadmaking could be used
to evaluate the techniques used to process soybeans (by assaying
changes in native soybean constitutents in conjunction with frac-
tionation-reconstitution studies) and also to provide a bread for
organoleptic and nutritive studies.[61-64] Thus today much is known
about the interactions between soy flour and specific wheat flour
components that take place during breadmaking.[65]

Germinated Soybeans in Bread

Pomeranz et al. (1977) investigated a commercially available
Mexican flour made from defatted, germinated soybeans.[66] Germinated
soy flour (replacing 10% wheat flour) slightly outperformed a popular, U.S.-produced, defatted, ungerminated soy flour (Ardex 550).
The authors suggested that the production, with the Mexican flour,
of bread with highly satisfactory loaf volume, crumb grain, and texture was particularly interesting in light of earlier observations
that high protein solubility is generally detrimental in breadmaking.
The bread with 10% germinated soy flour was organoleptically acceptable. In fact, "untrained taste panels consistently approved and
preferred the germinated soy flour breads."[66]

In independent germination studies, time, temperature, percent hydration, and hydration procedures were tested with two soybean varieties (Amsoy 71 and Williams).[64] Earliest successful germination was accomplished when beans were soaked in excess distilled water for about 6-7 hours (24°C), drained and rinsed thoroughly, put into a large-mouth jar, which was inverted, then placed in a cabinet with controlled temperature (23°C) and humidity. Beans were allowed to germinate 3 days, rinsed periodically, then mashed for immediate use in bread baking or were freeze dried. Rinsing during germination increased hydration from about 50% to 60%.[67]

In baking tests mashes were used to replace 9.3% wheat flour (14% m.b.). Bread was baked with high-yeast (7.6%), straight- and sponge-type fermentation systems (no formula sugar). In the sponge system (prefermentation prior to dough development), soybean mashes were incorporated either at the beginning of the prefermentation or at the mix step. All three procedures were studied with and without shortening in the formula.[67]

In all tests, the prefermentation step (sponge system) improved the functional and flavor properties of bread. Bread was further improved when the fresh soybean mash was incorporated at the mix step. Whether the improvement was due to the low pH in the sponge, or another factor, was not determined. The pH of the sponge was 5.5 when the fresh (enzyme active) soybean mash was added, and yielded breads that were equal to the 100% white flour standard structurally. At the 9.3% replacement level, breads had no detectable "beany" flavors or odors. Three percent shortening was required for those results.[67]

Improved Soybean Germination

More recent studies by the same researchers accomplished more vigorous and more wholesome soybean germination than reported in the above study. Improvments resulted from steeping beans in a highly aerated, moving water bath (20.5°C) for 12 hours prior to wrapping samples in wetted cloth for the remaining germination period. The 12-hour steeping period raised moisture level of beans from 10 to 60%. Usually rewashing of cloth wrappers or movement of germinating soybeans reduced germination rate, vigor, and wholesomeness. Another degree of improvement in germination vigor and percentage was accomplished by reducing steeping time to 6 hours (23.5°C) and adding excess water to cloth-wrapped samples during subsequent germination. The 6-hour steeping period raised moisture level of beans from 10% to 58.6%.[68]

A wide range in germination properties (Table 3) is attributed to differences in steeping (12 or 6 hours), or rinsing.[68] The variation in germination percentage, vigor, and wholesomeness is likely due to a kind of "water sensitivity", or lack of adequate oxygen. Excess steeping (i.e. more than 10-12 hours), even with vigorous aeration and water movement, is particularly detrimental. Rinsing or wetting beans after steeping is also harmful if the initial moisture of the beans is already near maximum. The Chinese are reputed to rinse beans periodically when germinating long enough for sprout production, which implies to me that their steeping period must limit water intake. Certainly more studies are needed to establish optimal conditions for individual varieties or composites. For the purpose of this paper it will suffice to remind the reader that relatively subtle differences in germination conditions may markedly affect soybean germination percent, vigor, and wholesomeness. I urge researchers, food producers and consumers to keep those facts in mind when evaluating the role germinated soybeans should play in human nutrition. Except for comparative purposes, poorly germinated soybeans should not warrant our investigations.

TABLE 3

Germination percent, final steep hydration percent, final germination hydration percent, average radical length, and general appearance (wholesomeness) of Amsoy 71 soybeans using two procedures of germination

Properties	Steeped 12 Hours Germinated 3 Days Rinsed Periodically (23.5°C)	Steeped 6 Hours Germinated 3 Days No Rinsing (23.5°C)
Final Steep Hydration %	61.4	58.5
Final Germination Hydration %	61.4	59.1
Germination %	25	90
Average Radical Length	1 cm	3 cm
General Appearance	Wet, Sour Smell, Yellow, Yellow-Brown, & Brown (Bruised Look)	Dry, Sweet Smell, No Stickiness, Yellow & Yellow-Tan

SUMMARY

Germination increases many of the nutrients or food functional properties in the wheat kernel, including vitamins, lysine, tryptophan, phytase (mineral availability), protease, amylase, cellulase, and others. Overall benefits are probably maximum after 24 to 48 hours of germination. Lysine does not increase much during 48 hr, but other advantages are realized and bread (wheat protein) functionality is only beginning to deteriorate. Prolonged germination would likely yield still greater nutritional benefits if sprouts were to be eaten stir-fried or steamed and eaten whole or cooked and extruded for inclusion in other foods.

Germination also enhances the nutritive value of soybeans. Levels of vitamins and of protein efficiency increase. Phytase increases while phytate decreases during germination. Objectionable flavors of soybeans are eliminated or do not evolve under optimum processing conditions. Germination may reduce lipoxygenase-linoleic acid degredation. Secondary products of that degredation are definitely related to soybean flavor problems and may be partially responsible for trypsin inhibition.

Yeast fermentation also definitely reduces phytate in wheat flour. The reduction of pH during germination may help to retard the production of off-flavor when soybeans are included in bread formulae.

For incorporation of whole germinated soybeans into bread, fresh mash apparently should be added to a sponge at the mix stage. Prompt introduction of fresh soybean mash into the buffered but lowered pH sponge system may help to avoid lipoxygenase-linoleic acid degradation and to promote phytase activity.

The elevated cellulase activity of germinated seeds should enhance the availability of highly nutritious fractions (such as aleurone layer of wheat), particularly if germination is followed by mashing and fermentation to allow for still greater nutrient disassociation and interaction. For those reasons wheat brans and other fiber sources from seeds probably should be given extra fermentation in a sponge if high-fiber breads are to be most nutritious.

Wheats and their bran fractions differ markedly in their nutritional potential. White brans are generally preferred by those who eat wheat as a staple. Studies designed to elucidate reasons for this preference are incomplete; however, lack of the typical "bitter-brany" flavors and greater digestability may be part of the reason for white wheat preferences.

Many questions, of course, remain. How can we improve wheat and soybean (and other seed) germination conditions to tailor them

for bread and other U.S. foods? After germination, what fractionation procedures (salt, acid, or alcohol extractions) can be used to
still further enhance the functional, nutritional and flavor properties of wheats and soybeans? At what time in the processing is heat
required and which fractions should receive heat treatment? Answers
to those and other questions should benefit human nutrition.

REFERENCES

1. Shurtleff, W., and Aoyagi, A. The Book of Tofu: Food for
    Mankind, Vol. I. Autumn Press, Kanagawa-Ken, Japan (1975).

2. "Dietary Goals for the United States," Select Committee on
    Nutirtion and Human Needs, United States Senate, February (1977).

3. Sugar in the Diet of Man. ed. F. J. Stare, Boston, Mass.
    From World Review of Nutrition and Dietetics 22:237 (1975).

4. Trowell, H. Ischemic Heart Disease and Dietary Fiber. Am.
    J. Clin. Nutri. 25:926 (1972).

5. Burkitt, D. P. Good Fiber--Benefits from a Surgeon's Perspec-
    tive. Cereal Foods World 22:6 (1977).

6. Eastwood, M. A. Physical Characteristics of Fiber Influencing
    the Bowel. Cereal Foods World 22:10 (1977).

7. Anderson, J. W. High Polysaccharide Diet Studies in Patients
    with Diabetes and Vascular Disease. Cereal Foods World 22:12
    (1977).

8. Kimura, K. K. High Fiber Diet--Who Needs It? Cereal Foods
    World 22:16 (1977).

9. AACC Food Fiber Committee. Food Fiber Committee--Update.
    Cereal Foods World 22:18 (1977).

10. Burkitt, D. P. Some Diseases Characteristic of Modern Western
    Civilization. British Medical Journal 3:274 (1973).

11. Reilly, R. W., and Kirsner, J. B. Fiber Deficiency and Colonic
    Disorders. Am. J. Clin. Nutr. 28:293 (1975).

12. Painter, N. S. et al. Unprocessed Bran in Treatment of Diverti-
    cular Disease of the Colon. British Med. J. 15:137 (1972).

13. Trowell, H. C. Dietary Fiber: Metabolic and Vascular Diseases.
    Norgine Ltd., 26-28 Bedford Row. London WCiR 4HJ (1975).

14. Trowell, H. C. Definition of Dietary Fiber and Hypothesis that It Is a Protective Factor in Certain Diseases. Am. J. Clin. Nutr. 29:417 (1976).

15. Ershoff, B. H. Antitoxic Effects of Plant Fiber. Am. J. Clin. Nutr. 27:1395 (1974).

16. Sandstead, H. H. *et al.* Effects of Selected Fiber Sources on Mineral Balance. Presented at the Annual Meeting American Chemical Society, Chicago, Ill. (Aug. 28, 1977).

17. Monoz, J. M. *et al.* Effects of Dietary Fiber on Serum Lipids. Manuscript in preparation for publication. USDA-ARS, Human Nutrition Laboratory, Grand Forks, North Dakota.

18. Unpublished data, USDA-ARS, Western Wheat Quality Laboratory, Pullman, Wash. (Dec.-Jan., 1976-77).

19. Kirwin, W. O. *et al.* Action of Different Bran Preparation on Colonic Function. Brit. Med. J. 4:187 (1974).

20. Mihailovic, M. L. J. *et al.* Chemical Investigation of Wheat: Dynamics of Various Forms of Phosphorus in Wheat during Its Antogensis. The Extent and Mechanism of Phytic Acid Decomposition in Germinating Wheat Grain. Plant Soil. 23:117 (1965).

21. Tomlinson, R. V., and Ballou, C. E. Myoinositol Polyphosphate Intermediates in the Dephosphorylation of Phytic Acid by Phytase. Biochem. 1:166 (1962).

22. Shrivastava, B. I. The Effect of GA on Ribonuclease and Phytase Activity of Germinating Barley Seeds. Canadian J. of Botany 42:1303 (1964).

23. Matheson, N. K., and Strother, S. The Utilization of Phytate by Germinating Wheat. Phytochemistry 8:1349 (1969).

24. Bianchetti, R., and Sartirana, M. L. The Mechanism of the Repression by Inorganic Phosphate of Phytase Synthesis in the Germinating Wheat Embryo. Biochimica et Biophysica Acta 145:485 (1967).

25. Reinhold, J. G. *et al.* Availability of Zinc in Leavened and Unleavened Whole Meal Wheaten Breads as Measured by Solubility and Uptake by Rat Intestine *in vitro*. J. Nutr. 104:976 (1974).

26. Reinhold, J. G. *et al.* Effects of Purified Phytate and Phytase rich Bread upon Metabolism of Zinc, Calcium, Phosphorus, and Nitrogen in Man. Lancet 1:283 (1973).

27. Vaghefi, S. B. *et al.* Lysine Supplementation of Wheat Proteins. A Review. Am. J. Clin. Nutr. 27:1231 (1974).

28. Dalby, A., and Tsai, Y. Lysine and Tryptophan Increases during Germination of Cereal Grains. Cereal Chem. 53:222 (1976).

29. Mason, W. Information from M.S. Thesis (in preparation) Department of Agronomy and Genetics, Washington State University, Pullman, Wash. Work completed in collaboration with ARS-USDA, Western Wheat Quality Laboratory.

30. Michele, P., and Lorenz, K. The Vitamins of Triticale, Wheat and Rye. Cereal Chem. 53:853 (1976).

31. Rudra, M. N. Studies in Vitamin C. Part V. The Vitamin C Content of Some Germinated Cereals and Pulses. J. Indian Chem. Soc. 15:191 (1950).

32. Davis, C. F. *et al.* A Study of the Vitamin C Complex Factors in Malted and Unmalted Barley and Wheat of the 1941 Crop. Cereal Chem. 20:109 (1943).

33. Burkholder, P. R., and McVeigh, I. The Increase of B Vitamin in Germinated Seeds. Proceedings of the National Academy of Science 28:440 (1942).

34. Burkholder, P. R. Vitamins in Dehydrated Seeds and Sprouts. Science 97:562 (1943).

35. Organ, J. G. *et al.* Some Constituents of Malt Extract. Quart. J. of Pharm. 16:275 (1943).

36. Klatzkin, C. *et al.* Riboflavin in Malt Extract. Quart. J. of Pharm. 19:376 (1946).

37. Lemar, L. E., and Swanson, B. G. Nutritive Value of Sprouted Wheat Flour. J. of Food Science 41:719 (1976).

38. Cook, A. H. Barley and Malt Biology, Bichemistry, Technology. Academy Press, New York (1962).

39. Obendorf, R. L., and Marcus, A. Rapid Increase in Adenosine 5'-Triphosphate during early Wheat Embryo Germination. Plant Physiol. 53:779 (1974).

40. Mory, Y. *et al.* Onset of Deoxyribonucleic Acid Synthesis in Germinating Wheat Embryos. Plant Physiol. 49:20 (1972).

41. Mory, Y. *et al.* Deoxyribonucleic Acid Polymerase from Wheat Embryos. Plant Physiol. 53:377 (1973).

42. Mory, Y. *et al.* De Novo Bioshythesis of Deoxyribonucleic Acid Polymerase during Wheat Embryo Germination. Plant Physiol. 55:437 (1975).

43. Pringle, W. J. S., and Moran, T. Phytic Acid and Its Destruction in Baking. J. Soc. Chem. Ind. 61:108 (1942).

44. Peers, R. G. The Phytase of Wheat. Biochem. J. 53:102 (1952).

45. Unpublished Studies, USDA-ARS, Pullman, Washington, Nov. 1975 to March 1976.

46. Miller, C. D., and Hair, D. The Vitamin Content of Mung Bean Sprouts. J. Home Economics 20:263 (1928).

47. Delf, E. M. Studies in Experimental Scurvy. Lancet. 1:576 (1922).

48. Lee, W. Y., and Read, B. E. The Effect of Light on the Production and Distribution of Ascorbic Acid in Germinated Soybeans. J. Chinese Chem. Soc. 4:208 (1936).

48a. Composition of Foods. Agriculture Handbook No. 8. USDA, 1963.

48b. Hsu, From Ph.D. dissertation in preparation. Cooperative work between Department of Food Science, Home Economics Research Laboratory, and the Western Wheat Quality Laboratory, USDA-ARS, Washington State University, Pullman, Washington.

49. Everson, G. L. *et al.* The Effect of Germination, The State of Maturity, and The Variety upon the Nutritive Value of Soybean Protein. J. of Nutrition 27:255 (1944).

50. Mattingly, J. P., and Bird, H. R. Effect of Heating, under Various Conditions, and of Sprouting on the Nutritive Value of Soybean Oil Meals and Soybeans. Poultry Sci. 24:344 (1945).

51. Disikachar, H. S. R., and De, S. S. The Tryptic Inhibitor and the Availability of Cystine and Methionine in Raw and Germinated Soya Beans. Biochimica et Biophysica Acta 5:285 (1950).

52. Liener, I. E. Personal Communication. Inhibitor activity
     assayed on some of the germinated soybean and fractions studied
     by Finney *et al.* (1977).

53. Rackis, J. J., and Anderson, R. L. Isolation of Four Trypsin
     Inhibitors by DEAE-cellulose Chromatography. Biochem. Biophys.
     Res. Commun. 15:230 (1964).

54. Kakade, M. L. *et al.* Contribution of Trypsin Inhibitors to the
     Deleterious Effects of Unheated Soybeans Fed to Rats. J. of
     Nutr. 103:1772 (1973).

55. Matsushita, S. Specific Interactions of Linoleic Acid Hydro-
     peroxides and Their Secondary Products with Enzyme Proteins.
     J. Agr. Good Chem. 23:150 (1975).

56. Wolf, W. J. Lipoxygenase and Flavor of Soybean Protein Products.
     J. Agr. Food Chem. 23:136 (1975).

57. Kon, S. *et al.* PH Adjustment Control of Oxidative Off-Flavors
     during Grinding of Raw Legume Seeds. J. Food Sci. 35:343
     (1970).

58. Nelson, A. I. *et al.* Food Products from Whole Soybeans. Soy-
     bean Dig. 31:32 (1971).

58a. Holman, R. T. Lipoxidase Activity and Fat Composition of
     Germinating Soy Beans. Arch. Biochem. Biophys. 17:459 (1948).

59. Chen, L. H., and Pan, S. H. Decrease of Phytates during Germin-
     ation of Pea Seeds (*Pisum sativa*). Nutritional Reports Inter-
     national 16:125 (1977).

60. Finney, K. F. Loaf Volume Potentialities, Buffering Capacity,
     and Other Baking Properties of Soy Flour in Blends with Spring
     Wheat Flour. Cereal Chem. 23:96 (1946).

61. Bohn, R. T., and Favor, H. H. Functional Properties of Soya
     Flour as a Bread Ingredient. Cereal Chem. 22:296 (1945).

62. Bayfield, E. C., and Swanson, E. C. Effect of Yeast, Bromate,
     and Fermentation on Bread Containing Soy Flour. Cereal Chem.
     23:104 (1946).

63. Finney, K. F. *et al.* Baking Properties and Palatability
     Studied of Soy Flour in Blends with Winter Wheat Flour.
     Cereal Chem. 27:312 (1950).

64. Finney, K. F., Rubenthaler, G. L., and Pomeranz, Y. Chemical Composition and Physical Treatment Are among the Soy-Product Variables Affecting Bread Baking. Cereal Sci. Today 8:166 (1963).

65. Hyder, M. A. *et al.* Interactions of Soy Flour Fractions with Wheat Flour Components in Breadmaking. Cereal Chem. 51:666 (1974).

66. Pomeranz, Y. *et al.* Flour from Germinated Soybeans in High-Protein Bread. J. of Food Sci. 42:824 (1977).

67. USDA-ARS, Western Wheat Quality Laboratory, unpublished data, Jan.-Feb., 1977.

68. USDA-ARS, Western Wheat Quality Laboratory, unpublished data, Mar.-Jan., 1978.

34

IMPROVING PROTEIN QUALITY OF BREAD - NUTRITIONAL BENEFITS AND REALITIES

Antoinette A. Betschart

Western Regional Research Center, United States
Department of Agriculture, Berkeley, California 94710

ABSTRACT

The bases for improving bread protein quality are critically examined. Protein consumption is shown to be directly related to total calorie intake in many countries, with a correlation coefficient (r) of $\geq$ 0.90. Concentration of protein in bread, % kilocalories, is similar to that of mixed diets in many parts of the world. Quality of bread protein, when evaluated by male weanling rats, may be improved by supplementation with lysine and threonine, as well as with many protein sources. Human adults, on bread diets, may be maintained in nitrogen equilibrium or slightly positive nitrogen balance. Increases, however, in nitrogen retention have been reported when lysine was added to bread. Laboratory studies with infants and young children, often hospitalized and recovering from severe malnutrition, show that lysine supplementation of wheat flour and gluten diets enhanced nitrogen retention and weight gain. No effect was observed when whole wheat diets were supplemented with lysine. Several field studies with children indicate that the addition of lysine to either supplemental breads provided at school, or to all wheat products consumed, resulted in no observed beneficial effects. Other field studies report an increase in either weight or height with addition of lysine to breads. A laboratory study with human adults suggests that a wheat flour: soy flour mixture has a higher biological value than wheat flour alone. The role, in human nutrition, of breads with improved protein quality remains somewhat obscure.

INTRODUCTION

Bread has been an integral part of the human diet for at
least six thousand years. Early recordings of the addition of
various cereal and legume flours are described by Hulse (1974).
In response to emergencies, the Romans, as well as more recent
civilizations, added various legumes including beans and peas
to wheat flour in order to provide a less costly bread for the
poor and/or to extend the wheat supply. In fourteenth century
England, bread was reported to contain beans, peas, oats, and
acorns in combination with wheat, barley and rye. Sour dough
recipes in the seventeenth century included wheat, barley, rye
and peas. A value judgement regarding the nutritional value
of wheat bread mixtures is discussed by Hulse (1974) whereby
Stubbs in 1585 "considered that men who loved on brown bread
containing rye, peas, beans and oats were healthier, stronger,
and 'longer living'".

Although long term trends indicate that consumption of
cereal products is decreasing in the U.S., cereal grains,
including wheat, are being consumed in increasing quantities
in many other areas of the world. The disappearance of wheat
in the U.S. which includes food and feed uses, has decreased
slightly during the last two decades from 168 to 156 lbs per
capita (ERS, 1976). U.S. per capita consumption of wheat flour,
during the period 1909 - 1970, decreased from 217 to 111 pounds.
This trend is also reflected in changes in consumption of food
energy, protein, fat and carbohydrate. In the period 1910-1973,
per capita consumption of carbohydrates decreased $\simeq$ 25%, food
energy and protein remained relatively constant, and fat
increased $\simeq$ 25% (Gortner, 1977). These trends in dietary
patterns have prompted a U.S. Senate Select Committee on
Nutrition and Human Needs to recommend dietary goals including
the following: (McGovern, 1977).

Goal 1: Increase carbohydrate consumption to account for
         approximately 55 to 60% of the energy intake,
Goal 2: Reduce overall fat consumption from approximately
         40 to 30 percent of energy intake.

In contrast to changes in the U.S. consumption of cereals,
many countries in Latin America, Asia, Oceana and Africa have
experienced increases in consumption. Data for 1975-1976
indicate that per capita consumption of wheat was as follows:
500 lbs., Turkey; 400-499 lbs., Morocco, Syria and Tunisia;
300-399 lbs., Afghanistan, Algeria, Chile, Cyprus, Egypt, Jordan,
and Uruguay; 200-299 lbs., Trinidad and Tobago; and 100-199 lbs.,
Bolivia, Fiji, Guyana, Mauritiua, Paraguay, Peru, Singapore,
and Sri Lanka (FAS, USDA, 1976). Thus, wheat is a major constituent of the diet of many countries with diverse cultural
food patterns.

PROTEIN ALLOWANCES

A premise for altering the protein quantity and/or quality of a food such as bread is that either the food, or the diet, is inadequate in protein. Although this was frequently suggested in the past for entire populations, more recently it is seen by some as a problem of specific target or age groups. Since the protein adequacy of a diet is based upon certain criteria, a brief examination of such criteria is essential.

Protein allowances have been the center of much controversy, especially since the suggested levels of protein intake were modified downward by both the Food and Agriculture Organization (1973) and The National Academy of Sciences, National Research Council (Recommended Dietary Allowances, RDA, 1974). Suggested levels of protein intake are influenced by various factors including variations in growth and maintenance requirements as a result of age, pregnancy, and lactation; stress resulting from infectious diseases; quality and digestibility of dietary protein; protein-energy relationships, efficiency of utilization, and many others. FAO has made an effort to quantitate the effect of protein quality upon safe levels of protein intake. Safe level of intake is defined as "the amount of protein considered necessary to meet the physiological needs and maintain the health of nearly all persons in a specific group" (FAO, 1973). As a result, this level is greater than that of the average requirement for protein. Protein quality is defined in reference to milk or egg, with the amino acid score serving as the criteria. As shown in Figure 1, the suggested safe levels of protein, calculated from FAO (1973) data as g/Kg body weight/day, increase as the score decreases. A mixed diet with a score of 70 would require 43% more protein than would a diet consisting mainly of egg or milk. Differences in suggested intake levels as a function of age are also clearly illustrated in Figure 1. On the basis of g protein/Kg body weight/day, it is apparent that the 1-3 year old needs more than twice as much protein as does the adult, with the 6-11 month old infant requiring ≃ 3 times that of the adult. The importance of obtaining accurate information on population distribution by age, and protein quality of a mixed diet (both difficult, and sometimes impossible to obtain) in estimating the protein needs of a population, is apparent (Cf. also Abernathy and Ritchey, 1978).

It is noteworthy that the RDA for protein for most age groups is similar to the FAO (1973) suggested safe level of intake for proteins with a score of 70. It should be stressed that the criteria and means of calculating RDA are somewhat different from those of the FAO data. Criteria for RDA are "levels of intake of essential nutrients . . . to be adequate

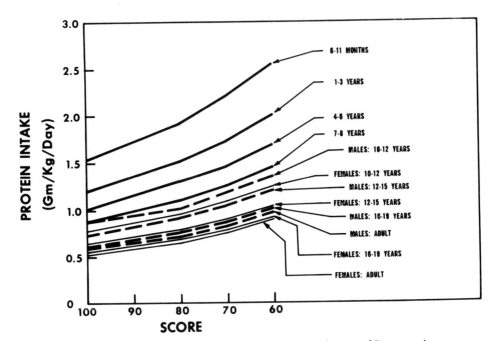

FIGURE 1.   Influence of protein quality (amino acid score) upon
            safe levels of intake calculated from FAO (1973) data.

to meet the known nutritional needs of practically all healthy
persons"(NAS/NRC, 1974).   Protein allowances are calculated to
allow for individual variability and 75% efficiency of utilization.   For example, a figure of 0.47 g protein/Kg body weight/day
is increased by 30% to 0.6 g protein to allow for individual
variability, and to 0.8 g to allow for 75% efficiency of
utilization.

In addition to variation in protein intake as a function of
age, amino acid requirements are also influenced by age.   Suggested patterns of requirements calculated from FAO (1973) data as
mg/g nitrogen (Table 1) serves to illustrate the point that
essential amino acids required/g of protein decrease markedly
with age.

TABLE 1

RECOMMENDED AMINO ACID PATTERNS AND AMINO ACID COMPOSITION OF SELECT FOODS

Amino Acid	FAO[a] (1973)	Wheat Flour[b]				Suggested Patterns of Requirements[a]			Milk		Egg
		Wheat	80-90%	70-80%	60-70% Extraction Rates	Infant	Child (10-12)	Adult	Human	Cows	
					mg amino acid/ g nitrogen						
Histidine		143	121	130	121	88			163	169	138
Isoleucine	250	204	232	228	217	219	231	113	288	294	338
Leucine	440	417	379	440	400	500	350	156	581	594	538
Lysine	340	179	159	130	113	325	469	138	413	488	438
Methionine + Cystine	220	253	224	250	229	181	213	150	263	206	356
Phenylalanine + Tyrosine	380	469	462	449	423	394	213	156	450	638	581
Threonine	250	183	192	168	153	275	275	81	269	275	294
Tryptophan	60	-	68	67[m]	58[m]	53	29	41	106	88	106
Valine	310	276	270	258	240	294	256	113	344	400	413

a FAO. 1973. Energy and Protein Requirements.
b FAO. 1970. Amino Acid Content of Foods and Biological Data on Proteins.
m Microbiological method.

EVALUATION OF PROTEIN QUALITY

Chemical, in vitro and/or in vivo methods are commonly used to evaluate protein quality. Chemical methods are limited by their inability to detect anti-nutritional factors or to reflect digestibility. The difficulties and shortcomings of the many methods used to determine protein quality have been treated extensively in the literature. The reader is referred to various texts, reviews and symposia on the topic (Porter and Rolls, 1973; McLaughlan and Campbell, 1974; Hegsted, 1974; Friedman, 1975; Hackler, 1977; Hegarty, 1975; Young, et al., 1977; Bodwell, 1977; Steinke, 1977). The limitations of methods used to evaluate protein quality should be considered as data resulting from such methods are evaluated.

ENERGY PROTEIN RELATIONSHIPS

Against a background of debate regarding recommended protein allowances and limitations of methods used to evaluate protein quality, is superimposed another degree of complexity, i.e., the polarization of views regarding the relative importance of energy and/or protein deficits as causative agents of malnutrition. That energy needs have priority and must be met has been a long accepted principle. The direct influence of energy intake upon efficiency of utilization of protein has been reviewed (Miller, 1973). The supplementation of a diet with protein in the face of a caloric deficit would be expected to gain little support, even from the most avid protein technologists. In reality, the diets of the malnourished are most often limiting, in varying degrees, in both calories and protein. In addition, foods and food mixtures used to improve diets provide both additional calories and protein when they are not merely substituted for other foods. Initially, the nature and magnitude of deficits in a diet should be defined. It should then be possible to identify the most appropriate food(s) and/or mechanisms of redistribution to most effectively alleviate such deficits. The issue then focuses upon questions of "What proportion of calories, protein and other essential nutrients should be provided? To whom should they be provided? In what form should they be provided? Who will bear the cost?"

The former Protein Advisory Group (PAG) of the United Nations is concerned that the FAO (1973) recommendations for protein are too low, since they were developed for "healthy" individuals in a somewhat less than healthy world. Scrimshaw (1977) noted that the FAO protein requirements for adults (in terms of egg or milk protein) are less than the amount required to maintain healthy Caucasian adults. The concern relates to the many parts of the world where infectious diseases and other such stresses are often encountered.

Others, less enamored with the emphasis upon protein requirements, suggest that disproportionate attention placed upon protein deficits may obscure problems of caloric deficits (Harper et al., 1973). Calloway (1976) summarized several concepts in support of the latter position.

The hypotheses that protein is present in most diets in relatively constant proportions has been tested by various methods. The ratio of protein to calories in the diet was examined by Perisse and coworkers (1969) using food balance sheets for some 85 countries. Total protein consumption seemed to be independent of income and, generally, accounted for ≈ 11% of the total caloric intake. Consumption of animal protein was, however, closely associated with income. If data from dietary surveys conducted by the Interdepartmental Committee on Nutrition For National Defense (ICNND) and others (Beaton and Swiss, 1974; Beaton, 1975; PASB, 1976) are used, the majority of the diets contain levels of protein which represent 10-14% of total caloric intake (Figure 2). Whether this relatively constant ratio of protein to calories is a result of a selection process or merely unavoidable when consuming a wide variety of mixed diets, is unclear.

When the RDA (1974) and FAO human nutritional requirements are examined, and protein as % of calories are calculated for specific age groups (Table 2), it is apparent that these values are less than values observed with dietary surveys for mixed diets (Figure 2). The protein requirements, as % calories, range from 6.3 to 7.5% of the calorie requirements for all FAO recommendations, except for that of the < 1 year old, for which the value is 9.8%. This suggests that the diet of the infant should be more concentrated in protein than diets for the general population. The comparable values, protein as % calories, are somewhat higher for the RDA. However, even for these recommended allowances, all but one of the values are < 10% (Table 2).

For comparison, protein as % of calories, was calculated for whole and milled wheat flours and for breads baked from both types of flours (Figure 2). These data were obtained from food composition tables prepared for the U.S. (USDA, 1975), Africa (US HEW and FAO, 1969) and Sri Lanka. Descriptions and compositions of these wheat products are included in Table 3. For both flours and breads, the whole wheat products contained from 13 to 17%, calories contributed by protein. The comparable values for the milled products were generally 11 to 13%. Thus, it appears that wheat flours or breads contain protein, as % of total calories, in quantities similar to those found in most mixed diets (Figure 2). Neither digestibility nor protein quality have entered into the criteria of protein as % of caloric intake.

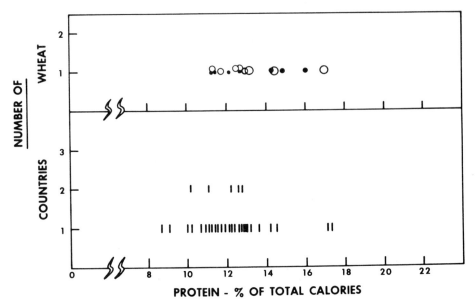

FIGURE 2.   Distribution of mixed diets and wheat and wheat products by protein concentration calculated as protein % of kilocalories.   Data on countries taken from dietary surveys conducted by ICNND and others (PASB, 1976; Beaton & Swiss, 1974). Data for wheat and wheat products taken from USDA (1975), US HEW & FAO, (1969) and FAO, (1973).   / = individual countries; ● and . = whole wheat and milled wheat, respectively; O and o = breads made from whole wheat and milled wheat, respectively.

The proportion of protein in most diets was examined by Calloway (1976) who found that in earlier work, dietary protein intake varied with total energy intake in self-selected diets of young, pregnant women (Calloway, 1974).   On the basis of dietary surveys in Latin America and the Caribbean, simple linear regression equations and correlation coefficients (r) were calculated for available calories and protein (I) and consumption of calories and protein (II) (Figure 3).   For total protein intake, the correlation coefficients were identical for both available and consumption data (0.90).   For animal protein, however, the linear function accounted for significantly less of the trend with consumption than with availability data.

TABLE 2. PROTEIN CONCENTRATION - % of Kilocalories

RECOMMENDED DIETARY ALLOWANCES (1974)			SAFE LEVEL OF PROTEIN INTAKE SCORE 70 (FAO, 1973)		
AGE (years)	% Kcal	% Kcal	AGE (years)	% Kcal	% Kcal
0 - 0.5	7.5				
0.5 - 1	7.4		<1	9.8	
1 - 3	7.1		1 - 3	6.8	
4 - 6	6.7		4 - 6	6.3	
7 - 10	6.0		7 - 9	6.4	
	Male	Female		Male	Female
11 - 14	6.3	7.3	10 -12	6.6	7.0
15 - 18	7.2	9.1	13 - 15	7.3	7.2
19 - 22	7.2	8.8	16 - 19	7.0	7.4
23 - 50	8.3	9.2	Adult	7.1	7.5
51 +	9.3	10.2			

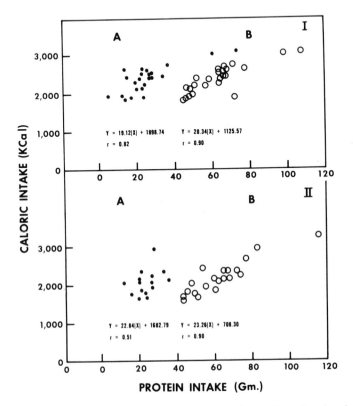

FIGURE 3. Relationship between protein and caloric intake.
Data from dietary surveys conducted in Latin American and
the Caribbean I = Based upon available calories and protein,
II = based upon consumption of calories and protein. A (●)
= animal protein, B (o) = total protein.

TABLE 3

WHEAT FLOURS & BREADS	CALORIES (Kcal)	PROTEIN (g)	PROTEIN % Kcal	FAT (g)	CARBOHYDRATE (g)
FLOURS					
USDA, 1975. U.S.					
Whole Wheat (hard wheat), 72% Extraction	333	13.3	16.0	2.0	71.0
	364	10.5	11.5	1.0	76.1
US HEW & FAO, 1968. AFRICA					
Whole Wheat	319	11.9	14.9	1.7	70.0
80-90% Extraction	348	10.5	12.1	2.0	74.6
75-80% Extraction	370	11.2	12.1	1.3	75.8
72% Extraction	367	10.4	11.3	1.0	76.8
MEDICAL RESEARCH INSTITUTE					
SRI LANKA					
95% Extraction	347	12.4	14.3	1.7	70.6
70% Extraction	385	12.2	12.7	1.0	81.9
BREADS					
USDA, 1975. U.S.					
Whole Wheat	254	10.8	17.0	3.3	49.5
White	274	8.9	13.0	3.7	50.3
US HEW & FAO, 1968. AFRICA					
Whole Wheat	254	8.4	13.2	1.7	55.3
White	275	8.1	11.8	2.1	54.5
Ballady					
90% Extraction	261	8.2	12.6	1.5	55.2
72% Extraction	272	7.8	11.5	1.3	55.9
MEDICAL RESEARCH INSTITUTE					
SRI LANKA					
Whole Wheat, 85% Extraction	273	9.8	14.4	1.6	54.6
White, 70% Extraction	249	7.9	12.7	0.7	52.9

To examine similar trends in an individual country, dietary survey data on cultural, socioeconomic and geographic sectors of Bolivia and Morocco were evaluated. On the bases of these data, summarized by Fellers et al. (1977) for Bolivia and by Betschart et al. (1977) for Morocco, linear equations and correlation coefficients were calculated (Figure 4). Although the slopes relating calories and total protein intake differed from that obtained with data from many countries (Figure 3), the correlation coefficients were $\geq$ 0.92. As with the data on several countries, relatively poor correlation coefficients were obtained when animal protein was related to calorie intake. These data support the general hypothesis that calorie and protein consumption are related by a linear function. From country to country, the slope of this function may vary considerably. Such a linear function does not exist between calorie and animal protein intake.

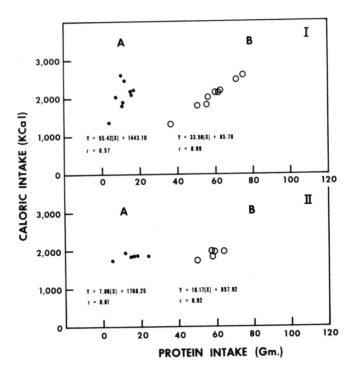

FIGURE 4. Relationship between protein and caloric intake for select countries. I = Morocco, II = Bolivia. A (.) = animal protein, B (o) = total protein.

PROTEIN QUALITY OF BREAD

An examination of the protein quality of white flour and breads, hereafter referred to as flour and bread unless otherwise specified, seems appropriate prior to reviewing various method of altering protein quality. Emphasis will be placed upon breads made mainly from the endosperm since it is such breads which are most often the subject of studies in altering protein quality.

The nutritional quality of wheat protein has been extensively reviewed by Bolourchi et al. (1974), Carpenter (1975), Widdowsen (1975) and Moran (1959). When considering protein quality, it was calculated that white breads with 11.5-13.0% protein contain concentrations of protein (% of calories) similar to that of the mixed diets of many countries (Figure 2). Wheat flour was also calculated to contain sufficiently more protein, as a function of calories, for all age groups for FAO (1973) except, perhaps, those <1 year of age, and for RDA for all but the adults >51 years old (Table 2 and Figure 2). Although many areas of the world produce wheat flour containing 8-9% protein, the protein concentration would still be adequate to meet nearly all of the FAO and RDA recommendations. It should be stressed that these calculations do not consider digestibility which is especially important for the very young and the aging.

On the basis of amino acid composition, the quality of wheat flour (70-80% extraction, FAO, 1970) may be compared with the FAO (1973) Provisional Amino Acid Pattern, and suggested levels of consumption for various age groups (FAO, 1970) (Table 1). Disregarding a factor for digestibility, these data indicate that 70-80% extraction flour would be deficient in the following amino acids, for the criteria, or age group indicated:

AMINO ACID	FAO PROVISIONAL PATTERN	INFANT	CHILD 10-12
Isoleucine	X		
Leucine		X	
Lysine	X	X	X
Threonine	X	X	X
Valine	X	X	

Wheat flour provides sufficient quantities of essential amino acids to meet the suggested level for adults except for lysine where the suggested level is only 8 mg/g nitrogen more than that found in wheat flour. For practical purposes wheat flour protein appears to be adequate for the adult.

Amino acid data indicate that wheat flour would be an adequate source of protein for the adult, but somewhat less than adequate for the infant and child. Evaluations of protein based upon amino acid composition alone tend to be higher than may actually be the case, since a factor for digestibility is not included.

Rat Studies. The quality of wheat protein has often been evaluated by rats and much less frequently evaluated by human studies. Osborne and Mendel (1914) in their study of wheat proteins including gluten as the sole source of protein, used rats to determine protein quality. Their results could be interpreted to indicate that wheat and other plant proteins had lower biological values than did animal proteins.

The limitations of data obtained with weanling rats, and the pitfalls of directly applying these data to human situations, are critically reviewed by Bolourchi et al. (1974). Protein Efficiencey Ratios (PER), and other biological data obtained with rats, provide useful information on relative protein values within the specific conditions of the experiment and for the species being studied.

Studies with growing rats generally indicate that Net Protein Utilization (NPU) of wheat is 40-50% that of good animal protein sources (Carpenter, 1975). Even when different levels of protein were fed and slope ratios of incremental growth were compared, the Relative Nutritive Value (RNV) of wheat flour was only 24% when compared with lactalbumin. In contrast, the RNV of various portions of the wheat kernel were significantly higher, i.e., whole wheat, 39; bran, 51; middlings, 57; and germ, 79 (Miladi et al., 1972). The relative concentration of albumins and globulins within the germ and the glutelins in the endosperm, influence these marked differences in protein quality. When PER is used as the criteria, values for white bread tend to fall between 0.70 and 0.95 (Betschart, et al., 1976; Ranhotra et al., 1971; Stillings et al., 1971; and Tsen and Reddy, 1977).

Weight gain (g gained/g protein consumed, or uncorrected PER) was used by Chick (1946) in studies with weanling rats to evaluate the protein quality of wheat flours milled to varying degrees of extraction. The respective weight gain observed for the 100%, 85% and 70% extraction flours were 1.77, 1.67, and 1.48 g. The variation in response of the rat as a function of age was demonstrated by Hutchinson et al. (1956). When whole wheat and white flours were compared, the male weanling rats did best on the whole wheat flour. Older (5-6 weeks after weanling) male rats showed a less pronounced difference between the flours, and older female rats grew equally well with either type of flour. The scientific literature on wheat protein quality may have been profoundly different, had rats at less rapid growth periods than that of the weanling, been chosen to evaluate protein quality.

As with most heated proteins, some alterations in protein value occur during the baking of breads and cakes. Studies indicate that the decrease in protein quality is usually approximately 15% (Carpenter, 1975) and this decrease in quality is directly related to temperature. Thus, these alterations are localized mainly in the crust (Morgan, 1931; Hutchinson et al., 1960).

Human Studies. The importance of sufficiently long adjustment periods to allow for accurate reflection of nitrogen retention in humans was emphasized by Bolourchi (1974).

Investigations with humans indicate that the protein digestibility of wheat flour and bread is ≃ 90% with either infants or school children (Bressani et al., 1960; Daniel et al., 1968; Graham et al., 1969). Increases in fecal nitrogen, observed with high extraction flours, have been argued to be mainly due to bacteria and cell walls, as a result of the more fibrous diet (McCance, and Widdowson, 1947). Hegsted, (1954) emphasizes that the apparent digestibility coefficient is lower for high extraction wheat products. Thus, breads made from 75% extraction flour seem quite digestible, whereas those of higher extraction rates are associated with increases in fecal nitrogen and undigested fat (McCance and Walsham, 1948).

Human studies which evaluate wheat protein in the form of unsupplemented flour or bread are limited. Hegsted et al. (1954) proposed that wheat protein could maintain nitrogen equilibrium for adults. Theoretical evidence, presented by the same authors in 1962, suggested that essential amino acids for those >7 years of age could be provided by wheat if most of the calories were also provided by wheat.

Experimental data have been reported in which wheat protein has been evaluated by adults (Bolourchi et al., 1968; Bricker et al., 1945; and Edwards, et al., 1971). Twelve normal men, aged 19-27, were maintained in a slightly positive nitrogen balance during the last 40 days of a 50 day experimental period in which wheat flour and other wheat products provided 90-95% of the protein. The subjects were in negative balance during the first 10 days, even though there had been a 20 day adjustment

period. The experimental diet provided 1.0 g crude protein/Kg
body weight. Although fecal nitrogen remained constant, the
wet fecal weight nearly doubled when the subjects changed from
the control period to the experimental diet. Although fecal
weight did decrease slowly, it never reached the weight observed
with the control diet. In a study with nine adult women, Bricker
et al. (1945) found that the biological value of milk and wheat
flour were 74 and 41, respectively. Feeding the protein sources
at various levels of the diet, they found that 2.76 and 4.76 mg
protein/basal calorie of milk and wheat flour, respectively
were required to attain nitrogen equilibrium. More recently,
Edwards et al. (1971) reported that young men could be maintained in positive nitrogen balance for three months with bread,
when sufficient calories were provided. Thus, under the appropriate conditions of calorie and protein consumption, wheat can
meet the protein needs of human adults.

Studies with children do not provide such consistent evidence. Begum et al. (1970) conducted a two year study with two
groups of 13 children ranging in age from 2 to 5 years. Wheat
provided ≈ 90% of the protein (26 g/day) for one group, and rice
was the major protein source for the other. Although there were
no differences in nitrogen retention or weight gain between the
two groups, those consuming wheat grew less rapidly than did
those eating rice (2.6 and 4.04 cm, respectively).

The study of Widdowson and McCance (1954) in which they
studied large numbers of children 4 to 15 years of age for one
year, has received much attention. The purpose was to observe
effects of adding breads made with flours of various extraction
rates, some fortified, to the diets of children living in two
German orphanages. The flours including whole wheat and those
milled to 85 and 70% extraction, contained 12.0, 11.8, and 10.9%
protein, respectively. Up to 75% of the calories were provided
by the bread which could be eaten ad libitum. All breads,
irrespective of flour used, were equally effective in promoting
growth. Addition of 500 ml milk/day to the diet resulted in no
improvement in growth, suggesting that lysine was not limited
in the diet.

Limitations of the data of Widdowson and McCance (1954) need
to be considered. The study was conducted with "undernourished"
children who were below average in both height and weight. The
preface of the report (Widdowson and McCance, 1954) stated, in
part, "It remains an open question, however, whether the flours
were equally nutritious, or whether differences existed between
them which were obscured by the exceptionally rapid growth rate
of undernourished children when receiving a diet adequate in

calories." Another concern is that quantities of breads consumed by the various groups may not have been constant, i.e., taste preference may have favored greater consumption of the lower extraction breads. Also, in addition to the protein from wheat, the children also consumed varying quantities of animal protein in the forms of milk, butter, meat, fish, sausages and cheese. Finally, the British had difficulties interpreting data since the wheat, a blend of 57 1/2% Manitoba, 12 1/2% Hard Winter (American), and 30% English, bore little resemblance to those milled in Britain. Sinclair (1968) reported that the 70% extraction flour from the above blend more nearly resembled an 80% rather than a 70% extraction of flour commonly used. Thus, conclusions based on extraction rates were somewhat less significant to the British, when applied to their wheat supply.

AMINO ACID SUPPLEMENTATION OF BREAD

The vast body of data in support of supplementing wheat protein with lysine and, perhaps threonine, has been based mainly on studies with male weanling rats. Fewer studies, and less conclusive data, are available for humans. Amino acid supple- mentation, as a means of improving protein quality of wheat in the human diet, should be viewed with some reservations. This is especially the case in view of limited available data for humans, cost, varying rates of absorption of free amino acids as opposed to proteins, susceptability of free lysine to damage during baking, relative merits of increasing nitrogen retention in adults, possible problems resulting from amino acid imbalance and/or toxicity, and the relative impact of this type of dietary intervention upon the complex problem of calorie-protein defi- cits. Major advantages of this approach are simplicity of the process and, generally, minor effects upon acceptability of the fortified product.

Amino acid fortification of cereals has been reviewed by Jansen (1974), and of wheat flour and bread by Bolourchi et al., (1974) and Carpenter (1975).

Limitations of applying data on amino acid supplementation based upon weanling rats to the human infant have been emphasized by several authors (Bolourchi et al., 1974, Carpenter, 1975). Following a brief summary of the voluminous data available on rats, major emphasis will be placed upon human studies.

Rat Studies. Male weanling rats were used in studies discussed, unless indicated otherwise. What appears to be uncorrected PER values for rats consuming whole wheat breads (1.0 and 1.6) may be increased to from 1.6 to 2.0 through the addition of 0.25

to 0.36% L-lysine monohydrochloride (L-lysine). The further
addition of 0.2-0.5% DL-threonine in various studies, significantly improved PER above that obtained with lysine alone, e.g.,
PER of 2.0-3.0. The RNV of wheat gluten, which contains less
lysine than does the protein of wheat flour, may be increased
from 15 to 48 with addition of lysine (lactalbumin value, 100).
The RNV of wheat flour, 24, was increased to 38 after supplementation with 0.2% L-lysine. The NPU of wheat flour 36.0, was
improved to 52.8 by the addition of 0.4% L-lysine (Stillings
et al., 1971). PER of wheat flour, 0.65-0.68, was increased to
≈ 1.5 with addition of 0.4% L-lysine and further increased to
2.3-2.7 by adding 0.3-0.5% threonine. Still another improvement in PER was observed when DL-valine was added in combination
with the lysine and threonone (Jansen, 1974).

The protein quality of wheat breads may also be improved by
adding L-lysine and DL-threonine. For example, breads with a
PER of ≈ 0.5 may have PER values of ≈ 1.7-2.1 as a result of
adding 0.5% L-lysine and 0.3% DL-threonine. Ericson (1960)
noted significant increases in weight gain when rats being fed
breads received supplements of 0.4% L-lysine which were further
increased by adding 0.2% DL-threonine. Hutchinson et.al., (1956)
studied the effect of lysine supplementation of whole wheat and
white flour. Increased rates of growth were observed when whole
wheat or white flours were supplemented with 0.62% and 0.72%
L-lysine, respectively.

Human Studies. Most studies on amino acid supplementation of
wheat have been conducted with young children in which growth
indices and nitrogen retention are used as criteria. Those
studies with human adults are based mainly upon nitrogen balance
data. Nitrogen balance studies are not without limitations, some
of which have been summarized by Jansen (1974). This index of
protein quality is a reflection of many factors including total
calories (Garza et al., 1976), protein and nitrogen in the diet;
previous health and nutritional status of the individual; and
previous nature and quantity of protein in the diet (Bolourchi
et al., 1974).

Most cereals seem to be adequate sources of protein for the
adult. This is consistent with the lower essential amino acid
requirement of the adult as compared with the infant and child
(Table 1).

Improvements in nutritional value of gluten for adults have
been reported by the addition of lysine (Hoffman and McNeil,
1949; Scrimshaw et al., 1973). The biological value of this
fraction of wheat protein was increased by lysine supplementation

(Hoffman and McNeil, 1949). Scrimshaw et al. (1973) observed that NPU of gluten in adult men was increased by approximately 8% when lysine was added to the diet.

Since Rice et al. (1970) concluded that nitrogen balance was significantly increased when lysine, as opposed to glycine, was added to wheat bread diets of adults, this study has been most often thoroughly reviewed by others. Twenty-two male adults received 86-87% of their dietary protein from bread, at levels of both 0.75 and 1.1 g/Kg body weight. The breads were supplemented with 0.15, 0.25 and 0.4% (w/w) L-lysine, as a % of wheat flour. These treatments were compared with isonitrogenous diets containing glycine. Although the authors concluded that there was a statistically significant positive response to lysine supplementation, there were no differences between three levels of lysine supplementation. Concern regarding experimental design and interpretation of data have been reported (Bolourchi et al., 1974; and Carpenter, 1975). The nitrogen balance seemed to increase in an almost linear fashion as a function of time and did not appear to be effected by a change in the amino acid supplement. Thus, nitrogen retention during the glycine treatment (first 9 days) was less than that observed with the lysine supplementation (last 12 days) (Bolourchi et al., 1974). Subjects were somewhat different for the two amino acid treatments, and characteristic differences in nitrogen retention patterns for individuals have been reported by others (Kies, et al., 1978). A preliminary control with adjustment periods of 21 days when protein intake is altered, 10 days when protein sources are changed, has been recommended by Bolourchi et al., 1974). The purpose is to obtain nitrogen balance data which are more indicative of long term rather than short term responses. Had the study of Bolourchi et al. (1968) been conducted for only 9 or 12 days, the conclusion would have been that wheat protein could not maintain human adults in nitrogen equilibrium. The importance of experimental design in human and other biological studies is apparent.

Both laboratory and field studies have been conducted with children to evaluate effects of amino acid supplementation of wheat. The data suggest that positive results may be obtained with lysine supplementation when children are fed under controlled laboratory conditions (Bressani et al., 1960; 1963; Graham et al., 1969; 1971). Field studies have shown less consistent results (King et al., 1963; Krut et al., 1961; Hedayat et al., 1970; and El Lozy & Kerr, 1976).

Lysine supplementation of whole wheat in diets providing
2 g protein and 100 Kcal/Kg body weight had no obvious beneficial
effects upon nitrogen retention of 2-5 year old children (Reddy,
1971. Graham et al. (1969) found that lysine addition to air
classified white flour (≃ 21% protein), at levels of 0.12, 0.20
and 0.40%, improved weight gain and nitrogen retention of 6
infants, 10-24 months of age. Diets, which were fed 15-36 days,
contained 1.5-2.0 g protein and 90-125 Kcal /Kg body weight.
Some of the subjects reportedly suffered from infectious diseases
during the study. In a subsequent study these authors (Graham
et al., 1971) examined the interactions between protein concentration in the diet and lysine levels (0.12, 0.20, and 0.4%)
required to maintain normal linear growth and nitrogen retention.
At 8% protein, % of calories, all three levels of lysine were
adequate, whereas at 6.4 and 7.3% protein (% calories), 0.2%
and/or as high as 0.4% were recommended. These data apply to an
air classified fraction of wheat flour, higher in protein and,
presumably, different in other aspects of composition than the
original flour.

In studies with 6 hospitalized children, recently recovered
from protein malnutrition, nitrogen retention was improved with
lysine supplementation of a wheat flour (85%) and gluten (5%)
diet (Bressani et al., 1960). Approximately 2 g protein and
80-100 Kcal/Kg body weight were supplied by the diet. Data was
gathered from the subjects, aged 1 year to 5 years 6 months, as
a result of 6-9 day balance studies. The nutritional status of
the subjects and the duration of the studies may somewhat limit
the interpretation of results.

Daniel et al. (1968), concluded that threonine was the
second limiting amino acid for 7 children, 10-12 years old, on a
whole wheat diet (300 g/day). Experimental periods were 10 days
each with 1.5 g L-lysine, and 0.86 g DL-threonine in combination
with L-lysine, as levels of supplementation. Thus, under various
conditions, and within the constraints of experimental procedures,
improvements in nitrogen retention and weight gain have been
observed in children as a result of amino acid supplementation
of wheat flour.

Data obtained from field studies are somewhat less respon-
sive to amino acid supplementation (El Lozy and Kerr, 1976;
Hedayat et al., 1970; King et al., 1963; Krut et al., 1961).
In a study with 45 children, 2-8 years of age, effects of supplementing a diet of wheat bread (6.4% protein), supplying 89% of
the dietary protein, with the equivalent of 0.27-0.30% L-lysine
were evaluated (Krut et al., 1961). Weight gain of the group
receiving lysine was reported to be greater than that of the

group receiving glycine. It may be significant that the lysine was administered separately as a drink and, thus, was not subjected to baking temperatures. This is one of the few field studies indicating a positive response to the addition of lysine

Statistically significant improvements in height of Indian schoolchildren were reported when a diet in which wheat supplied 85% of the protein, was supplemented with 0.25% L-lysine as a % of flour (Pereira et al., 1969). No significant differences were observed in this 6 month study in nitrogen retention, weight gain, serum albumin or total serum protein levels, as a result of lysine supplementation. It should be noted that the children also received concentrated calories in the form of > 40 g peanut oil per day.

Approximately 350 malnourished Haitian schoolchildren, 4-18 years of age, were provided with either two wheat buns made from enriched flour, or these same buns supplemented with 0.632% L-lysine (King et al., 1963). The buns, which provided ≈ 390 Kcal and 13 g protein/day, were supplied on 150 of the 261 days in the 9 months study. Initially, the lysine supplement appeared to be correlated with an increase in both height and weight. However, only increases in weight were associated with feeding of buns at the end of the study. Little, if any, advantage was attributed to the lysine. The relatively small quantities of lysine provided by the buns in proportion to the total diet, and lack of information on the diet and on nutritional status of the subjects, make interpretation of data difficult.

Iranian children, 6-12 years old, were provided with unfortified or fortified bread (0.3% L-lysine) (Heyadat et al., 1970). The breads, which provided ≈ 50% of the caloric and protein needs, caused an increase in the weight of those receiving them compared with the control group who did not receive the bread. There were, however, no beneficial effects due to lysine supplementation on the basis of anthropometric and biochemical criteria. The results of the Haitian and Iranian studies have been explained to be a consequence of lower essential amino acid requirements of the older child, compared with those <5 years (Jansen, 1974).

Most recently, El Lozy and Kerr (1976) conducted an extensive study in Southern Tunisia in an attempt to clarify the issue regarding the impact of lysine supplementation of wheat protein in field studies. The ≈ 3,000 children <5 years of age were examined every 6 months from 1970-1975. Treatments included 1) unfortified wheat products, 2) wheat products fortified with vitamins A,D, thiamine, riboflavin and niacin, and iron, and

3) the latter treatment with 0.3% L-lysine. The authors,
conclude, in part, "It is clear that this study failed to
demonstrate any improvement following fortification". Several
"possible" explanations for this outcome were provided, in
part, as follows:

    a. "No nutritional intervention can, in isolation,
        have any effect....

    b. Low caloric intake may be responsible for the
        lack of response....

    c. Protein quality is a less important factor than
        has been believed in the past....

    d. Failure to demonstrate an effect was due to a
        specific, uncorrected, dietary deficiency...".

Most field studies suffer from lack of control between treatment
groups, e.g., different villages, and lack of detailed information and control of the total diet. These field studies serve
to illustrate some of the many complexities of nutrition intervention programs.

PROTEIN FORTIFICATION OF BREAD

As a result of the implication that wheat is deficient in
lysine and many other factors, a wide variety of protein
sources, rich in lysine, have been studied as fortificants of
bread. Protein fortification of breads has as its objective
the improvement of both quality and quantity of protein. Use
is being made of such protein sources as: animal protein,
animal byproducts (animal blood, cheese whey); fish, wheat germ
and protein concentrates from wheat milling byproducts (shorts,
millrun); rice bran, defatted corn germ, and potato; legumes
including fababean, field pea and soy; oilseeds such as cottonseed, peanut, sunflower, and safflower; yeast and coconut
(Betschart, 1978; Betschart et al., 1978; Chastian et al.,
1975; Fellers et al., 1976; Fleming and Sosulski, 1977; Hulse,
1974; Jansen, et al., 1974; Knorr, 1977; Luh et al. 1975;
Mizrahi et al., 1967; Ranhotra et al., 1971; Saunders et al.,
1976; Womack et al., 1954, and Yanez et al., 1973). Studies
with plant protein sources will be emphasized since they are most
often given consideration by economically developing countries.
Barrett (1975) reviewed the general concept of bread as a vehicle
in international nutrition programs. Although the nutritional
evaluation of protein fortification of bread has been conducted
mainly with rats, those few studies with human subjects will be
discussed in greater detail.

Protein fortification, as compared with amino acid supplementation, is more likely to have adverse effects upon the

quality and acceptability of bread. The functional considerations of protein enriched bread have been reviewed (Pomeranz,
1970). Hulse (1974) presents an extensive review of the effects
of protein fortification upon bread baking quality as well as
protein quality.

Rat Studies. Coconut flour (20.9% crude protein), when added to
flour at levels of 15 and 20%, produced PER values of 1.21 at
both levels, as compared to 0.99 for the control (Chastian et al.,
1975). Lysine values of the flour and mixtures were 348,413, and
431 mg/100g bread for the control and breads containing 15 and
20% coconut flour, respectively. Chilean workers (Yanez et al.,
1973) incorporated the yeast Candida utilis into breads at levels
of 1-10%. The PER for the 10% level was 1.74 as opposed to 0.84
for the control bread.

Protein concentrates prepared by various methods from wheat
shorts and millrun have been studied. Ranhotra et al., (1971)
added a wheat protein concentrate (15.4% protein, N x 5.7) prepared by dry milling to breads. Lysine values of .0.265, 0.303,
0.365, and 0.372% lysine were reported for the control and breads
including 15, 30 and 45% of the protein concentrate, respectively.
The respective PER value reported for these four treatments were
0.95, 1.10, 1.19, and 1.22. Betschart et al. (1976) added wheat
protein concentrates prepared by alkaline extraction of wheat
millrun (51-63% protein, N x 5.7) to breads at levels of 10, 15,
and 20%. Lysine values were 112, 177, 187 and 206 mg/g nitrogen
for the control and breads with 10, 15, and 20% wheat protein
concentrate, respectively, whereas corrected PER were 0.76, 1,71,
1.57, and 1.44 for the respective replacement levels. In these
two studies, PER was not correlated linearly with lysine content.

Fleming and Sosulski (1977) found that the PER of bread
containing vital gluten (1.09) was increased to 1.27, 1.69, 1.67,
and 1.81 when 12 parts of sunflower concentrate, and 15 parts
of soy flour, fababean concentrate, and field pea concentrate,
respectively, were added to 100 parts of flour.

Hulse (1974) reviewed reports on work with cottonseed
(Womack et al., 1954) and soy flour (Westerman et al., 1954).
Significantly higher weight gain/g nitrogen was observed when
rats were fed breads containing 10 parts cottonseed flour/100
parts wheat flour, when compared with the control. The addition
of soy flour and wheat germ to breads containing enriched flour
promoted similar rates of growth in rats for two generations.

Fellers et al. (1976) reported an increased PER from 0.91 for the control to 1.21 and 1.44 when 6 and 12% defatted soy flour were added to breads. Mizrahi et al. (1967) evaluated the addition of soy protein isolates to breads at from 2-10%. PER increased with increasing concentrations of the protein isolate, with the PER of the 6% bread being ≈ 50% greater than that of the control. There was a linear relationship between the PER increases and lysine content of the breads. Thus, it does not seem to be difficult to increase PER values of wheat bread with the addition of any one of several plant protein sources.

Human Studies. Available studies are very limited and include brief reports from Russia and the Phillippines (Efremov et al., 1970; Formacion et al., 1974). Workers in the Phillippines (Formacion et al., 1974) examined the effect of supplementing "nutribuns" with coconut flour. The six adult women on low protein diets could consume these products with up to 11% coconut flour without adverse effects upon protein utilization or acceptability.

Bricker et al. (1945) evaluated the biological value of milk, wheat flour, soy flour, and a mixture of soy (13%) + wheat flour for adult women. Biological values of 74, 41, 65, and 55 were obtained for the milk, wheat flour, soy flour, and soy-wheat mixture, respectively. The quantity of nitrogen from each of the protein sources required to attain equilibrium differed with 2.76, 4.76, 2.88, and 3.38 mg/basal calorie being required from milk, wheat flour, soy flour and the soy-wheat flour mixture, respectively. By both criteria, the soy flour appears to be a valuable supplementary protein source.

More recently Graham et al. (1970), with a limited number number of infant subjects, 4-12 months old, evaluated a mixture (18.8% protein) of unbleached flour-wheat protein concentrate (1:1 w/w) in which the protein concentrate was prepared by milling wheat shorts. Corrected PER of the mixture was 1.31, whereas NPU was 47. Casein was the protein source supplied 9 days before and after the mixture which was fed for 15-30 day periods. The nitrogen retention observed with the mixture was an average of 60% that of casein, as compared with a value of 63% for wheat flour obtained in an earlier study by the same authors (Graham et al., 1969). Lysine supplementation of the flour-wheat protein concentrate mixture increased the nitrogen retention values ≈ 50%. Weight gain of the infants on the mixture was 74% that of casein, as compared with 67% for wheat flour. The authors suggest that such a response, in light of the theoretically available lysine, higher PER and NPU, is the

result of an inferior digestibility of the wheat flour-wheat
protein concentrate mixture. Caution should be excercised when
referring to the data in the earlier study (Graham et al., 1969)
as being indicative of wheat flour. Since the flour had been
air classified into a high protein fraction ($\approx$ 21% protein),
this fraction would not be expected to reflect the response of
subjects to the original flour. Another concern is that the
absorptive processes of the subjects, hospitalized and recovering from severe malnutrition, may have been partially impaired.
These factors should be considered when interpreting the results
of the latter study (Graham et al., 1970).

Removing less of the bran during the milling of wheat, i.e.,
producing a higher extraction flour, is another possible method
of enhancing the protein quality of bread. The study of
Widdowson and McCance (1954) in which there were no significant
differences in German children fed breads made from flours of
various extraction rates, provides some insight into this
approach. However, the limited digestibility of protein in the
bran portion of the wheat kernel (Saunders and Kohler, 1972;
Hegsted, 1954) suggests that the additional protein recovered
with higher extraction may be less available than that of the
endosperm.

FUTURE DIRECTIONS

The addition of protein and amino acids to bread has been
studied by two, sometimes closely related, groups, i.e., food
technologists and nutritionists. Most of the studies relate
mainly to technological considerations. Since the purported
function is to improve protein nutritional value, somewhat
similar effort should be devoted to this end. In addition,
future studies evaluating the protein quality of bread would be
improved if specific descriptions of the wheat and wheat products were included, e.g., composition and degree of milling.

Programs designed to improve nutritional status should
respond to the needs of the target population(s). Therefore,
critical analyses of diets and limiting nutrients should precede
any decision on methods used to combat nutritional problems.
If a specific protein deficit is identified in a target group,
several nutrition-related alternatives including the following
exist: 1) to increase the total consumption of food, 2) to
increase the consumption of protein rich food(s), and/or
3) to fortify commonly consumed foods with protein or amino
acids. The food vehicle chosen in #3 may be selected because it
is widely consumed by the target group, rather than because of
its deficiency in the specific fortificant. If a protein source

is required it should, ideally, be an indigenous crop, familiar and acceptable to the population. If the protein fortification of foods is to be pursued, there appears to be a need for a systematic approach in which protein quality and quantity, technical problems, and acceptability are consdiered concurrently in arriving at various levels of incorporation.

The ultimate impact of any nutrition intervention program is likely to be affected by a) the existence and integration of other concurrent programs designed to improve the health and well being of individuals, b) governmental philosophy and commitment to support c) the support of other decision makers who will be directly effected, d) the availability, effective marketing, and acceptability of foods involved in these programs, and e) the cost of such a program, including the retail cost of the food vehicle(s).

The addition of indigenous cereals and legumes to breads may be pursued for reasons other than nutritional benefits. Such reasons might include extension of the wheat supply, savings of foreign exchange by decreasing the importation of foods including wheat, and/or stimulation of the agricultural sector as well as food processing, marketing and distribution functions.

Although much effort has been devoted to improving the protein quality of bread through plant breeding, amino acid supplementation and protein fortification, the role of breads with improved protein quality in human nutrition, as part of a mixed diet, remains somewhat obscure.

REFERENCES

Abernathy, R. P. and Ritchey, S. J. 1978. Position paper on RDA for protein for children,This volume.

Barrett, F. 1975. The role of bread in international nutrition. Cereal Foods World 20:323.

Beaton, G. H. 1975. Protein:energy ratios--guidelines in the assessment of protein nutritional quality. In "Protein Nutritional Quality of Foods and Feeds. Part 2. Quality Factors--Plant Breeding, Composition, Processing, and Antinutrients", M. Friedman, Ed., Dekker, New York, pp. 619-634.

Beaton, G. H., and L. D. Swiss. 1974. Evaluation of the nutritional quality of food supplies: prediction of "desirable" or "safe" protein:calorie ratios. Amer. J. Clin. Nutrs. 27: 485.

Begum, A., Radhakrishnan, A. N., and S. M. Pereira. 1970. Effect of amino acid composition of cereal bread diets on growth of preschool children. Amer. J. Clin. Nutr. 23: 1175.

Betschart, A. A., Enochian, R. V., and R. M. Saunders. 1977.
Potential for fortification of wheat foods in Morocco.
Western Regional Research Center/U.S. Agency for International
Development PASA Agreement #931-11-560-231-73-3168048, USDA
ARS, Berkeley, Calif.

Betschart, A. A., Saunders, R. M., and F. N. Hepburn. 1976.
Supplementation of one pound loaves with wet alkaline process
wheat protein concentrate: baking and nutritional quality.
J. Food Sci. 41: 820.

Betschart, A. A. 1978. Preparation of protein isolates from
safflower seeds. U.S. Patent No. 4,072,669. February 7.

Betschart, A. A., Hanamoto, M. M., and R. M. Suanders. 1978.
Protein concentrates from rice bran as ingredients in wheat
breads. Presented at the 17th Rice Technical Working Group
Meeting, College Station, TX, February 14-16.

Bodwell, C. E. 1977. Application of animal data to human
protein nutrition: A review. Cereal Chem. 54: 958.

Bolourchi, S., Makdani, D. D., and O. Mickelsen. 1974. Lysine
supplementation of wheat proteins. A review. Amer. J. Clin.
Nutr. 27: 1231.

Bolourchi, S., Friedmann, M., and O. Mickelsen. 1968. Wheat
flour as a source of protein for adult human subjects.
Amer. J. Clin. Nutr. 21: 827.

Bressani, R., Wilson, D., Behar, M., Chung, M., and N. S.
Scrimshaw. 1963. Supplementation of cereal proteins with
amino acids. IV. Lysine supplementation of wheat flour fed to
young children at different levels of protein intake in the
presence and absence of the other amino acids. J. Nutr. 79:
333.

Bressani, R., Wilson, D., Behar, M., and N. S. Scrimshaw. 1960.
Supplementation of cereals with amino acids. III. Effect of
amino acid supplementation of wheat flour as measured by
nitrogen retention of young children. J. Nutr. 70: 176.

Bricker, M., Mitchell, H. H., and G. M. Kinsman. 1945. The
protein requirements of adult human subjects in terms of the
protein contained in individual foods and food combinations.
J. Nutr. 30: 269.

Calloway, D. H. 1976. Protein and energy-nutritional need and
demand. In: Opportunities to Improve Protein Quality and
Quantity for Human Food. P. 26. Division of Agriculture
Science, Special Publication No. 3058.

Calloway, D. H. 1974. Nitrogen balance during pregnancy. In;
"Nutrition and Fetal Development". Ed. M. Winick. Vol. 2:
29. John Wiley and Sons, Inc. New York.

Carpenter, K. J. 1975. The nutritive value of wheat protein.
In: "Bread Social, Nutritional and Agricultural Aspects of
Wheat on Bread". Ed., A. Spicer. p. 93. Applied Science
Publishers, London.

Chick, H., 1946. Nutritive value of proteins contained in wheat flour of different degrees of extraction. Proc. Nutr. Soc. 4: 6.

Chastian, M. G., Sheen, S.J.S., Cooper, T. J., and D. R. Strength. 1975. Coconut bread as a means of improving protein nutrition. J. Food Sci. 40: 1014.

Daniel, V. A., Doraiswamy, T. R., Rao, S. V., Swaminathan, M., and Parpia, H.A.B. 1968. The effect of supplementing a poor wheat diet with L-lysine and DL-threonine on the digestibility coefficient, biological value and net utilization of protein and nitrogen retention in children. J. Nutr. Dietet. 5: 134.

Edwards, C. H., Booker, L. K., Rumph, C. H., Wright, W. G., and S. N. Ganapathy. 1971. Utilization of wheat by adult man: nitrogen metabolism, plasma amino acids, and lipids. Amer. J. Clin. Nutr. 24: 181.

Efremov, W., Maslenikova, E. M., Nemenovia, Y. M., Gvozdava, L. G. Kraiko, E. A., Krums, L. S., Penar, O. I., and A. S., Vaineman. 1970. Biological value of wheat bread containing various enriching additions. Giglenai Sanitarya 35: (6): 80.

El Lozy, M., and G. G. Kerr. 1976. Results of lysine fortification of wheat products in southern Tunisia. In: Improving the Nutrient Quality of Cereals. II. p. 113. Ed., H. W. Wilcke. U.S. Agency for International Development.

Ericson, L. E. 1960. Studies on the possibility of improving the nutritive value of Swedish white bread. II. The effect of supplementation with lysine, threonine, methionine and tryptophan. Acta Physiol. Scand. 48: 295.

ERS. Economic Research Service. 1976. Food consumption prices and expenditures. Agriculture Economic Report No. 138. Washington, D.C.

FAO. Food and Agriculture Organization. 1973. Energy and protein requirements. FAO Nutrition Meeting Report Series No. 52. FAO. Rome.

FAO. Food and Agriculture Organization. 1970. Amino acid content and biological data on proteins. FAO. Rome.

FAS. Foreign Agriculture Service. 1976. Washington, D.C.

Fellers, D. A., Betschart, A. A., and Enochian, R. V. 1977. Potential for protein fortification of wheat foods in Bolivia. Western Regional Research Center/U.S. Agency for International Development, PASA #931-11-560-231-73-3168048, ARS, USDA, Albany, Calif.

Fellers, D. A., Mecham, D. K., Bean, M. M., and Hanamoto, M. M. 1976. Soy-fortified wheat flour blends. I. Composition and properties. Cereal Foods World 21: 75.

Formacion, C. S., Wentworth, J., and R. P. Abernathy. 1974. Wheat and coconut flour protein utilization by six young college women. Phillippine J. Nutr. 27(1): 42. Nutr. Abstr. Rev. 45(11) #8175, 1975.

Fleming, S. E., and F. W. Sosulski. 1977. Nutritive value of bread fortified with concentrated plant proteins and lysine. Cereal Chem. 54: 1238.

Friedman, M., Ed. 1975. "Protein Nutritional Quality of Foods and Feeds. Part 1. Assay methods--Biological, Biochemical, and Chemical." Dekker, New York. 624 pages.

Garza, C., Scrimshaw, N. S., and V. R. Young. 1976. Human protein requirements: the effect of variations in energy intake within the maintenance range. Amer. J. Clin. Nutr. 29: 280.

Gortner, W. A. 1977. U.S. Dietary Trends and Implications. Cereal Foods World. 22(4): 165.

Graham, G. G., Cordano, A., Morales, E., Acevedo, G., and R. P. Placko. 1970. Dietary protein quality in infants and children. V. A wheat flour-wheat concentrate mixture. Pl. Fds. Hum. Nutr. 2: 23.

Graham, G. G., Morales, E., Cordano, A., and R. P. Placko. 1971. Lysine enrichment of wheat flour: prolonged feeding of infants. Amer. J. Clin. Nutr. 24: 200.

Graham, G. G., Placko, R. P., Acevedo, G., Morales, E., and A. Cordano. 1969. Lysine enrichment of wheat flour: evaluation in infants. Amer. J. Clin. Nutr. 22: 1459.

Hackler, L. R. 1977. Methods of measuring protein quality: A review of bioassay procedures. Cereal Chem. 54: 984.

Harper, A. E., Payne, P. R., and J. C. Waterlow. 1973. Human protein needs. Lancet. p. 1518.

Hedayat, A., Sarkissian, N., Lankarini, S., and G. Donosco. 1968. The enrichment of whole wheat flour and Iranian bread with lysine and vitamins. Acta Biochimica Iranica 5: 16.

Hegarty, P.V.J. 1975. Some biological considerations in the nutritional evaluation of foods. Food Tech. 29(4): 52.

Hegsted, D. M. 1962. The potential of wheat for meeting man's nutrient needs. In: Role of Wheat in World's Food Supply. Conference, USDA, ARS, Albany, Calif.

Hegsted, D. M., Trulson, M. F., and F. Stare. 1954. Role of wheat products in human nutrition. Physiol. 34: 221.

Hulse, J. H. 1974. The protein enrichment of bread and baked products. In: New Protein Foods, IA. p. 155. Ed. A. M. Altschul. Academic Press, New York.

Hutchinson, J. B., Moran, T., and J. Pace. 1960. The quality of the protein in germ and milk breads as shown by the growth of weanling rats: the significance of the lysine content. J. Sci. Food Agr. 11: 576.

Hutchinson, J. B., Moran, T., and J. Pace. 1956. Nutritive value of the protein of white and wholemeal bread in relation to the growth of rats. Proc. Royal Soc. B., 145: 270.

Jansen, G. R. 1974. The amino acid fortification of cereals. In: New Protein Foods IA. Ed. A. M. Altschul. p. 39. Academic Press, New York.

Kies, C., Fox, H. M., Mattern, P. J., Johnson, V. A. and Schmidt, J. W. 1978. Comparative protein quality as measured by human and small animal bioassays of three lines of winter wheat. This volume.

King, K. W., Sebrell, W. H., Severinghaus, E. L., and W. O. Storvick. 1963. Lysine fortification of wheat bread fed to Haitian school children. Amer. J. Clin. Nutr. 12: 36.

Knorr, D. W. 1977. Potato protein as partial replacement of wheat flour in bread. J. Food Sci. 42: 1425.

Krut, L. H., Hansen, J.D.L., Trusweld, A. S., Schendel, H. E., and J. F. Brock. 1961. Controlled field trials of a bread diet supplemented with lysine for children in an institution. S. African J. Lab. Clin. Med. 7: 1.

Luh, B. F., Maneepun, S. and Rucker, R. B. 1975. Biological quality and functional properties of lima bean protein for bread enrichment. In "Protein Nutritional Quality of Foods and Feeds", Part 2. Ed. M. Friedman, Marcel Dekker, pp. 135-160.

McCance, R. A., and C. M. Walsham. 1948. The digestibility and absorption of the calories, protein, purines, fat and calcium in wholemeal wheat bread. Brit. J. Nutr. 2: 26.

McCance, R. A. and E. M. Widdowson. 1947. The digestibility of English and Canadian wheats with special reference to the digestibility of wheat protein by man. J. Hygiene, Cambridge, 45: 39.

McGovern, G. 1977. Dietary goals for the United States. Report of the U.S. Senate Select Committee on Nutrition and Human Needs. Nutrition Today, 12(5): 20.

McLaughlan, J. M., and J. A. Campbell. 1974. Methodology for evaluation of plant protein for human use. In: "Triticale Protein". p. 27. Ed. J. H. Hulse and E. M Laing. International Development Research Centre, Ottawa, Canada.

Medical Research Institute. Sri Lanka. Food Tables. Farm Women's Extension, Department of Agriculture, Peradeniya, Sri Lanks.

Miladi, S., Hegsted, D. M., Saunders, R. M., and G. O. Kohler. 1972. The relative nutritive value, amino acid content and digestibility of the proteins of wheat mill fractions. Cereal Chem. 49: 119.

Miller, D. S. 1973. Protein energy interrelationships. In: "Proteins in Human Nutrition". p. 93. Ed. J.W.G. Porter, and B. A. Rolls. Academic Press, New York.

Mizrahi, S., Zimmermann, G., Berk, Z., and U. Cogan. 1967. The use of isolated soybean proteins in bread. Cereal Chem. 44: 193.

Moran, T. 1959. Nutritional significance of recent work on wheat, flour and bread. Nutr. Abst. Rev. 29: 1.

Morgan, A. F. 1931. The effect of heat upon the bilogical value of cereal proteins and casein. J. Biol. Chem. 90: 771.

NAS. National Academy of Sciences, National Research Council. 1974. Recommended dietary allowances. 8th edition. Washington, D.C.

Osborne, T. B., and L. B. Mendel. 1914. Amino acids in nutrition and growth. J. Biol. Chem. 17: 325.

PASB. Pan American Sanitary Bureau. 1976. Situacion nutricional alimentaria en los paises de American Latina y el Caribe. Boletin de la Officina Sanitaria Pan America. LXXX (6): 498.

Pereira, S. M., Begum, A., Jesudian, G., and R. Sundararaj. 1969. Lysine supplemented wheat and growth of preschool children. Amer. J. Clin Nutr. 22: 606.

Perisse, J., Sizaret, F., and P. Francois. 1969. FAO Nutr. Newsletter 7(3): 1.

Pomeranz, Y. 1970. Protein-enriched bread. Critical Reviews in Food Technology 1: 453.

Porter, J.W.G., and B. A. Rolls. (ED). 1973. "Protein in Human Nutrition." Academic Press, New York.

Ranhotra, G. S., Hepburn, F. N., and W. B. Bradley. 1971. Supplemental effects of wheat protein concentrate on the protein quality of white wheat flour. Cereal Chem. 48: 699.

Reddy, V. 1971. Lysine supplementation of wheat and nitrogen retention in children. Amer. J. Clin. Nutr. 24: 1246.

Saunders, R. M., Betschart, A. A., Edwards, R. H., and G. O. Kohler. 1976. Nutritive assessment and potential food applications of protein concentrates prepared by alkaline extraction of wheat millfeeds. Proc. 9th National Conference on Wheat Utilization Research, ARS NC-40, USDA.

Saunders, R. M., and G. O. Kohler. 1972. In vitro determination of protein digestibility in wheat millfeeds for monogastric animals. Cereal Chem. 49: 98.

Scrimshaw, N. S. 1977. Through a glass darkly: Discerning the practical implications of protein-energy interrelationships. Nutr. Rev. 35: 321.

Scrimshaw, N. S., Taylor, Y., and V. R. Young. 1973. Lysine supplementation of wheat gluten at adequate and restricted energy intakes in young men. Amer. J. Clin. Nutr. 26: 965.

Sinclair, H. M. 1968. Nutritional aspects of high-extraction flour. Proc. Nutr. Soc. 17(1): 1958.

Steinke, F. H. 1977. Protein efficiency ratio: Pitfalls and causes of variability - A review. Cereal Chem. 54: 949.

Stillings, B. R., Sidwell, V. D., and O. A. Hammerle. 1971. Nutritive quality of wheat flour and bread supplemented with either fish protein concentrate or lysine. Cereal Chem. 48: 292.

Tsen, C. C., and P.R.K. Reddy. 1977. Effect of toasting on the nutritive value of bread. J. Food Sci. 42: 1370.

USDA. United States Department of Agriculture. 1975. Nutritive value of American foods. Agriculture Handbook No. 456. Agricultural Research Service, Washington, D.C.

US HEW and FAO. United States Department of Health, Education and Welfare, and Food and Agriculture Organization. 1969. "Food Composition Table for Use in Africa". Bethesda, Maryland.

Widdowson, E. M. 1975. Extraction rates – nutritional implications. In: Bread: Social, Nutritional and Agricultural Aspects of Wheaten Bread. p. 235. Ed. A. Spicer. Applied Science Publishers, London.

Widdowson, E. M., and R. A. McCance. 1954. Studies on the nutritive value of bread and on the effect of variations in the extraction rate of flour on the growth of undernourished children. Med Res. Council Spec. Rep. Ser. No. 287, HMSO, London.

Womack, M., Marshall, M. W., and J. C. Summers. 1954. Cottonseed food supplement. Nutritive value of bread and cookies containing cottonseed flour. J. Agr. Food. Chem. 2: 138.

Yanez, E., Wulf, H., Ballester, D., Fernandez, N., Battas, V., and F. Monckeberg. 1973. Nutritive value and baking properties of bread supplemented with Candida utilis. J. Sci. Food Agric. 24: 519.

Young, V. R., Rand, W. M., and N. S. Scrimshaw. 1977. Measuring protein quality in humans. A review and proposed method. Cereal Chem. 54: 929.

35

FORTIFICATION OF SOFT DRINKS WITH PROTEIN FROM COTTAGE CHEESE WHEY

V. H. Holsinger

Eastern Regional Research Center, Agricultural Research
Service, U.S. Department of Agriculture, 600 East
Mermaid Lane, Philadelphia, Pennsylvania 19118

ABSTRACT

Cottage cheese whey protein concentrates, prepared by precon-
centration by ultrafiltration followed by gel permeation to remove
low molecular weight materials, have the solubility, stability and
flavor that make them suitable for fortification of soft drinks
and related products. These concentrates are characterized by
high levels of "available" lysine and by amino acid compositions
indicating good nutritional value. Carbonated beverages prepared
with conventional beverage ingredients and containing up to 1% by
weight of the total beverage of added whey protein maintained
clarity, color, and flavor during 203 days storage at room temperature. Spray dried whey protein concentrates were incorporated
without adverse effects into commercial "ade" type powders. Clarity
of 1% protein solutions at pH 2-3.5 was not impaired by heating for
6h at 80°, but some structural change occurred since an average of
37% of the protein present precipitated on shifting pH to 4.7.
Increased stability against heat denaturation under acidic conditions was conferred by some soft drink ingredients. Added sucrose
reduced protein denaturation by 1/2 but sodium saccharin had no
effect. The type of acid used also altered protein denaturation
rate. While properly isolated whey protein concentrates have
functional properties necessary for soft drink fortification,
feasibility of use will depend upon cost.

INTRODUCTION

The soft drink industry in the United States can serve as a
model of successful merchandizing as Americans of all ages and

walks of life consume its products. Most of these are purchased
along with the family's weekly food requirements; in 1975, 2.45%
of the average food dollar spent at the supermarket went for soft
drinks (Anon., 1976). Although soft drinks contribute only about
4.3% of the caloric requirement of the population and therefore
should be of little national concern, many nutritionists consider
them to be a type of dietary pollutant because of their strong
appeal to the young. As more nutritious beverages such as milk
and fruit juice are replaced in the diets of children and teenagers,
nourishing materials such as calcium and protein are replaced by
carbohydrate calories.

Consequently, the soft drink companies have been under great
pressure from consumer advocates and nutritionists to improve not
only the nutritional quality of their product (Nader, 1972) but
also the quality of their advertising (Morris, 1973). Steps which
can be taken to alleviate these criticisms would be either to
fortify the familiar beverages with valuable nutrients without
detectable change in flavor or appearance or to develop new types
of beverages for the snack trade.

The U.S. Department of Agriculture has concerned itself for
many years with the development of foods high in protein. The
unique functional properties of proteins isolated from cheese whey
make them suitable for the fortification of carbonated beverages.

Traditionally, whey, the byproduct of cheese manufacture, has
been fed to pigs or dumped into streams and municipal sewage
systems. Because the disposal of whey is a growing problem in the
United States due to the large increase in cheese production in
recent years (USDA, 1977), increasing concern over pollution has
led to stricter environmental controls. Consequently, research
efforts have been expanded toward developing new uses for whey,
particularly acid whey, which is more difficult to process because
of its high lactic acid content (Table 1). Since acid whey is now
being wasted and is a serious pollutant in some areas, a soft
drink fortification program could yield benefits to both snack
drink consumers and cheese manufacturers.

USE OF WHEY IN BEVERAGES

The manufacture of both alcoholic and nonalcoholic beverages
from whey has been attempted for many years, particularly in
Europe (Holsinger et al., 1974). As early as the seventeenth
century, medicinal properties were ascribed to whey; this led to
the growth of "whey houses" designed for the treatment of a variety
of human ailments, especially those related to digestion.

Some commercial success has been achieved with the development
of drinks containing whey components. Perhaps the most successful

TABLE 1

Composition of whey solids[a]

	Cheddar whey (sweet)	Cottage cheese whey (acid)
% Total protein	11.5	11.4
% Lactose	74.4	66.8
% Ash	7.4	10.2
% Lactic Acid	< 1.0	9.6
% Fat	2.7	< 1.0
pH	6.5	4.7

[a]Holsinger (1976).

is Rivella, a sparkling, crystal clear herbal infusion in deproteinized whey that appeared on the market in Switzerland in 1952
(Susli, 1956). This product is currently sold in most of Western
Europe, being promoted as a therapeutic tonic. Rivella resembles
ginger ale in flavor and appearance; it has been pasteurized and
must be refrigerated after opening.

Alcoholic beverages produced from whey include beer-like
drinks that have been marketed with some success in Russia and a
champagne-like product in Poland (Holsinger et al., 1974). In the
United States, Yang et al. (1975) developed a process for making
wine from whey which is undergoing commercialization trials in
California. By adding dextrose to the whey, they use a non-lactose
fermenting organism to produce the alcohol.

A conventional type nonalcoholic orange flavored carbonated
beverage fortified with 1.5% whey protein was test marketed in
Brazil in 1971 (Anon., 1973). Since the whey protein concentrate
used contained milkfat, lactose, and whey salts, these were also
present in the drink. This product, although resembling the
carbonated soft drinks that dominate the American beverage market,
did not advance beyond the test market stage.

RESEARCH TOWARD SOFT DRINK FORTIFICATION

Protein fortification offers a means of increasing the nutritive value of soft drinks. The possible magnitude of a fortification program using protein isolated from cheese whey may be
estimated from a consideration of the volume of soft drinks consumed
in the United States. In 1976, 459 8-oz. bottles of soft drinks
were consumed per capita, representing an estimated nine billion

dollars in sales (Anon., 1977). In addition, beverage powders
were consumed after reconstitution at a rate of 7.7 gallons/capita,
representing an estimated one billion dollars in sales (Anon.,
1977).

Acid cheese whey represents about 18% of the total whey
production (USDA, 1977). The estimated amount of recoverable
protein in this wasted byproduct is 64 million pounds. A price
quotation of $1.50 per pound has been made for a whey protein
isolate containing 75% protein (Stauffer Chemical Co., 1977). If
a market existed for protein recovered from all the whey produced
annually, this could represent a sizeable potential income for
protein processors.

Considering the volume of soft drinks manufactured in the
United States, the potential amount of acid whey protein available
and its projected price, one can calculate that 13% of the total
soft drink production in the United States could be fortified with
1% cheese whey protein at an added materials cost of about one
cent per 8-oz. bottle. Fortification at this level would increase
the nutritional value of soft drinks. Therefore, research was
carried out to determine if proteins isolated from cottage cheese
whey, regardless of cost, had functional characteristics that made
them suitable for soft drink manufacture (Holsinger et al., 1973a).
Fortification with only whey proteins represents a different
approach than that taken by previous researchers. The development
of new methods to isolate the whey proteins from the lactose and
salts made this approach possible.

A large-scale process was developed to permit the isolation
of undenatured proteins from cottage cheese whey (Holsinger et
al., 1975). The whey proteins were preconcentrated by ultrafiltration at pH 4.7; low molecular weight materials were then removed
from the preconcentrate by gel permeation on Sephadex G-25. The
high protein eluate obtained was condensed under vacuum and spray
dried. In order to produce a highly soluble protein, centrifugal
clarifiers were used to remove residual milkfat and insoluble
material formed during the purification steps. The isolates produced contained 75-90% protein after dehydration. Whey proteins
are exceptionally rich in the essential amino acid lysine; isolates
prepared by this procedure had over 90% of the total lysine in a
nutritionally available form as measured by chemical means (Holsinger
et al., 1973b). This was one indication that the quality of the
dried products was excellent.

Carbonated soft drinks were formulated and fortified with a
whey protein concentrate containing 81.4% protein, 10.2% lactose,
and 1.5% ash (Table 2). Solid carbon dioxide was used to achieve
carbonation.

TABLE 2

Composition of protein-fortified carbonated soft drinks, percent by weight[a]

	Flavor			
Ingredient	Strawberry	Orange	Lemon	Lime
Sucrose	12.0	14.0	13.0	13.0
Flavoring	0.37	0.37	0.37	0.37
Citric acid	0.37	0.185	0.74	0.74
Protein	1.0	1.0	1.0	1.0
Water	86.26	84.44	84.89	84.89
Carbon Dioxide Volumes	2	1	1	1
pH before carbonation	2.50	2.66	2.35	2.46

[a]Holsinger et al. (1973a).

Beverages fortified with 1% whey protein maintained clarity and color over one year of storage in colorless glass bottles on shelves and in glass-fronted cabinets in the laboratory. However, compared with a freshly made control, the lime-flavored drink had faded slightly in color after 203 days of storage, but the flavor remained unchanged; after one year, a slight stale whey flavor was tasted in the fortified product.

Carefully prepared spray dried whey protein concentrates are also well suited for the fortification of the sweetened powders that are dissolved in water to form the popular "ade" type drinks. Seven flavors of these products were fortified with 0.5% and 1.0% whey protein, and the reconstituted beverages along with unfortified controls were then submitted to trained dairy products judges. One flavor was tested per panel. Using the 9-point hedonic scale of Peryam and Pilgrim (1957), the judges were asked to rate acceptance; on this scale, the higher the number, the more acceptable the flavor (Table 3).

Analysis of variance (Larmond, 1970) showed that at the 5% confidence level, only the scores of the cherry and lemon-lime· flavored drinks fortified with 1% whey protein deviated significantly from their controls. However, no dislikes were registered, even though some products neared the indifferent response, a score of 5.0, at the highest protein concentration. Even though fortification with 1% whey protein was not readily detectable in some

TABLE 3

Organoleptic evaluation of protein fortified noncarbonated
soft drinks[a]

| | Average hedonic ranking | | |
Flavor	Control	0.5% Protein	1.0% Protein
Cherry	7.0	6.5	5.5[b]
Grape	7.2	6.8	6.3
Tart Lemon	5.7	5.2	5.5
Lemon-Lime	7.2	6.5	6.2[b]
Orange	6.2	5.9	6.0
Raspberry	6.3	6.7	6.4
Strawberry	6.5	5.9	6.0

[a]Holsinger et al. (1973a).

[b]Significantly different, P < .05.

instances even by experienced judges, it might be difficult to
produce soft drinks with protein levels approaching the 3.3-3.9%
protein found in fluid milk (Posati and Orr, 1976).

An unpublished report suggests that the type of acid used in
the soft drink formulation could have an effect on the detection
of off-flavors brought about by fortification with whey protein
(Berger, 1977). Citric acid was used in the formulation of the
beverages studied by Holsinger et al. (1973a). Malic acid, which
is known in the food trade for its ability to mask and smooth out
off-flavors (Gardner, 1966), has reportedly effected considerable
flavor improvement when used in whey drink formulations. As malic
acid is an ingredient in many present-day "ade" powders, fortification with whey proteins above the 1% level may be possible.

WHEY PROTEIN BEHAVIOR IN THE SOFT DRINK SYSTEM

Little information is available about the solubility and
stability of the mixed whey proteins at the low pH values characterizing most carbonated beverages. Guy et al. (1967) examined
the denaturation of cottage cheese whey proteins by heat but did
not investigate the behavior of protein solutions of pH below 3.4.

While empirical studies showed that soft drink fortification
with whey protein isolates was possible, more fundamental data
were needed to make commercialization feasible. Holsinger et al.

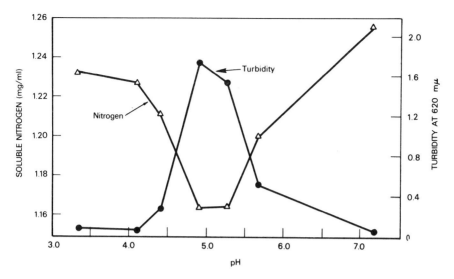

Figure 1.   Change in solubility and turbidity of a high protein
isolate from acid cheese whey with pH (Holsinger et al., 1973a).

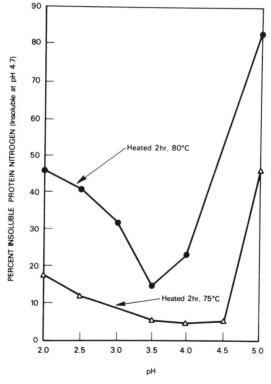

Figure 2.   Effect of acid pH on the heat denaturation of a 1% whey
protein solution (Holsinger et al., 1973a).

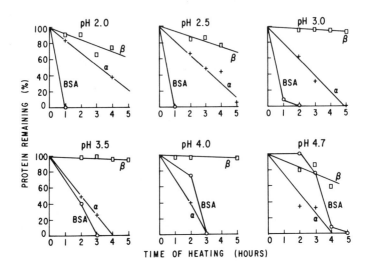

Figure 3.   Effect of pH on concentration of whey proteins remaining after heating at 80°.   BSA = bovine serum albumin, β = β-lacto-globulin, α = α-lactalbumin.

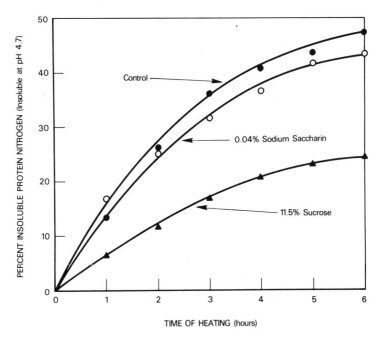

Figure 4.   Effect of added sucrose and sodium saccharin on protein stability at 80° and pH 3.3 when acidified with citric acid (Holsinger et al., 1973a).

(1973a) studied the solubility and stability of whey proteins under acid conditions to provide some of the additional information required.

The solubility and turbidity of a whey protein concentrate dissolved in water varied over the pH range from 3.5 to 7.5 (Figure 1). Decrease in solubility was accompanied by a sharp increase in turbidity around pH 4.7, the region of the proteins' isoelectric points. Quite unexpected was the clearing of the protein solution in the more acid pH ranges typical of carbonated soft drinks. These results explain beverage clarity when whey proteins were added to the soft drink formulations.

Heating at elevated temperatures indicated that beverage clarity could be maintained over long periods of time (Figure 2). The whey proteins were most resistant to thermal denaturation at pH 3.5. As the pH of most commercial carbonated drinks is near this value, solubility changes on storage should be of little concern.

Prolonged heating at different pH's produced changes in the relative concentrations of the individual whey proteins in the mixed system (Figure 3). Heated samples containing equivalent amounts of protein were examined electrophoretically and quantified by densitometry. An unheated sample served as the control. The curves show that, as the pH became more acid, bovine serum albumin (BSA) became increasingly less heat stable, while the heat stability of α-lactalbumin increased. At pH 3.5, BSA and α-lactalbumin showed approximately equivalent heat stabilities. β-lactoglobulin, comprising about 70% of the whey proteins, seemed little affected by heat in the pH range 3-4.

After one year of storage at room temperature, chemical changes had occurred in the fortified carbonated drinks. When bottles of a lime-flavored carbonated drink were opened for tasting, no sediment was visible. However, 9% of the protein precipitated when the pH of the drink was raised from 2.5 to 4.7. During the storage period 84% of the sucrose present in the beverage had inverted. In spite of the presence of the reducing sugar formed, only 3% of the total lysine in the protein had been destroyed and 95% of the lysine remaining was nutritionally available as measured by chemical means.

Many of the soft drink ingredients themselves stabilize the added protein against heat damage. Sucrose, a popular sweetener in soft drinks, retarded the heat denaturation of whey proteins (Figure 4). After heating for 6h at 80°, the sucrose containing solution had only half the amount of denatured protein found in the unsweetened control. Sodium saccharin, however, conferred

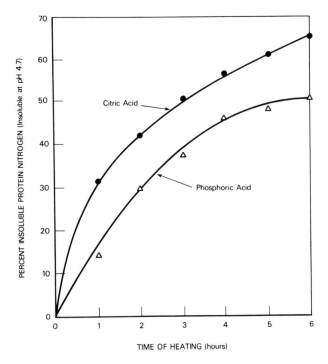

Figure 5. Effect of type of acid on protein stability at 80° and pH 2.68 (Holsinger et al., 1973a).

little protection against heat denaturation. At the present time, there is no information available about the behavior of whey protein concentrates in the presence of the high fructose corn sweeteners that are finding increased use in many soft drink formulations.

   The type of acid used in the soft drinks also influences protein stability. The rate of denaturation of the whey proteins in phosphoric acid solutions of pH 2.68 was less than that noted in solutions brought to the same pH by addition of citric acid (Figure 5).

   The whey proteins showed good heat stability when heated at 80° in two popular commercial soft drinks (Figure 6). The proteins were less stable in the cola beverage, which had a pH lower than the point of greatest heat stability. The pH of the citrus beverage was very close to the point where the proteins are most stable to heat denaturation. The electrophoretic behavior of the individual whey proteins in the two beverages (Figure 7) was similar to that observed in the samples previously described (Figure 3). This suggests that the presence of flavorings and colorings

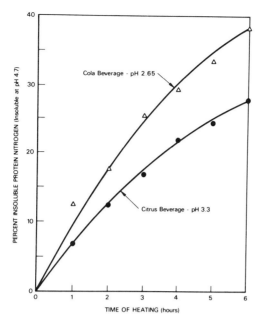

Figure 6. Protein stability in commercial soft drinks heated at 80° (Holsinger et al., 1973a).

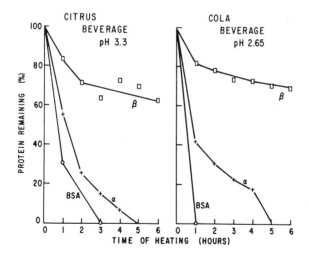

Figure 7. Concentration of whey proteins remaining in two commercial soft drinks after heating at 80°. BSA = bovine serum albumin, β = β-lactoglobulin, α = α-lactalbumin.

affected the protein stability only slightly, if at all, in these particular products.

From these results, Holsinger et al. (1973a) concluded that most soft drinks of pH below 4 could be successfully fortified with undenatured cheese whey proteins. Precipitation problems might be encountered with the protein fortification of those drinks containing natural fruit juices high in tannins; some caramel colorings also act as protein precipitants. However, with only slight formula modifications, a stable system should be attainable.

The success of a fortification program of this magnitude is strongly dependent upon cost. Several commercial concerns are currently producing high quality whey protein isolates of varying protein content. Consumer interest in improved nutrition could provide the necessary impetus leading to the commercial production of protein fortified soft drinks.

REFERENCES

Anonymous. (1973). Tomorrow's pop bottles may be loaded - with protein. Ind. Week, 177(4), 42.

Anonymous. (1976). Summary of 1975 sales of food store products. Supermarketing, 31(9), 38.

Anonymous. (1977). The beverage market index. Beverage World, 96(1240), 46-59.

Berger, S. E. (1977). Personal communication.

Gardner, W. H. (1966). Food Acidulants. Allied Chemical Corporation, New York, p.38-45, 97-117.

Guy, E. J., Vettel, H. E. and Pallansch, M. J. (1967). Denaturation of cottage cheese whey proteins by heat. J. Dairy Sci., 50, 828-832.

Holsinger, V. H. (1976). New dairy products for use in candy manufacture. Manufacturing Confectioner, 56(1), 25-28.

Holsinger, V. H., DeVilbiss, E. D., McDonough, F. E., Posati, L. P., Vettel, H. E., Becker, D. E., Turkot, V. S. and Pallansch, M. J. (1975). Production and utilization of high protein concentrates from acid cheese whey. Abstracts of papers of the 169th national meeting of the American Chemical Society, Philadelphia, Pa., April 6-11, #41, ACFD.

Holsinger, V. H., Posati, L. P. and DeVilbiss, E. D. (1974). Whey beverages: a review. J. Dairy Sci., 57, 849-859.

Holsinger, V. H., Posati, L. P., DeVilbiss, E. D. and Pallansch, M. J. (1973a). Fortifying soft drinks with cheese whey protein. Food Technol., 27(2), 59-65.

Holsinger, V. H., Posati, L. P., DeVilbiss, E. D. and Pallansch, M. J. (1973b). Variation of total and available lysine in dehydrated products from cheese wheys by different processes. J. Dairy Sci., 56, 1498-1504.

Larmond, E. (1970). Methods for sensory evaluation of food. Publication 1284, Canada Department of Agriculture, Ottawa, Ontario, Canada, p. 19.

Morris, B. (1973). Ads that tell you nothing rapped by consumer group. The Evening Star and Washington Daily News, Washington, D.C., February 28, p. A-24.

Nader, R. (1972). Coke replacing water? The Sunday Star and Washington Daily News, Washington, D.C., July 30, p. B-2.

Peryam, D. R. and Pilgrim, F. J. (1957). Hedonic scale method for measuring food preferences. Food Technol., 11, Insert 9.

Posati, L. P. and Orr, M. L. (1976). Composition of foods: Dairy and egg products; raw .. processed .. prepared. Agricultural Handbook No. 8-1. USDA, Washington, D.C., November, Item No. 01-077-01-088.

Stauffer Chemical Company. (1977). Personal communication.

Susli, Hans. (1956). Neue art der Molkenverwertung: Ein Lacto-minerales Tafelgetrank. XIV Internat. Dairy Congr., Rome, Vol. 1, Part II, 477-485.

USDA, Crop Reporting Board, SRS. (1977). Dairy Products Annual Summary 1976. DA 2-1(77), Washington, D.C., p. 3-5.

Yang, A. Y., Bodyfelt, F. W., Berggen, K. E. and Larson, P. K. (1975). Utilization of cheese whey for wine production. Progress report, U.S. EPA grant R-803301.

Reference to brand or firm name does not constitute endorsement by the U.S. Department of Agriculture over others of a similar nature not mentioned.

36

SOY PROTEIN UTILIZATION IN FOOD SYSTEMS

G. N. Bookwalter

Northern Regional Research Center, Agricultural
Research Service, U.S. Department of Agriculture,
1815 N. University Street, Peoria, Illinois 61604

ABSTRACT

Soy protein products are utilized in food systems as
whole beans, flours and grits, concentrates and isolates,
and textured products. Soy proteins play a significant role
in food systems as a source of supplementary and complementary
protein and contribute functional properties such as solubility,
water absorption, viscosity, emulsification, texture, and
antioxidation. Whole soybeans are processed into snack
foods, beverages, and fermented foods. Soy protein is an
ideal supplement for cereal protein because it corrects
lysine and other amino acid deficiencies. Blends of soy
flour or grits with cereals such as corn, wheat, or sorghum
are widely used in world feeding programs. The blends are
also valuable in domestic food systems such as breakfast
cereals and baked foods. Concentrates and isolates are
utilized in processed meats and baby foods. Isolates are
employed as whipping agents and coffee whiteners. Thermoplastic
extrusion of defatted flours or protein concentrates produces
an expanded type of textured protein. Isolated soy protein
is converted to meat analogs by a spun fiber process.
Textured soy protein products are used to extend or replace
meat products in food systems.

INTRODUCTION

Soybean products have been consumed for centuries in
the Orient. A variety of soybean foods including tofu,
shoyu (soy sauce), miso, and tempeh have been developed
(Hesseltine and Wang, 1972). Processes used include cooking,
grinding, extraction, fermentation, and even sprouting. In
contrast to these well-established food patterns in the
Orient, it was not until the 20th Century that the Western
World recognized soybeans for their human food value. In
the last few decades, the soybean has become a major element
of world commerce. By 1973, soybeans were the No. 1 cash
crop in the United States.

Soybeans are now our major source of edible oil.
Introduction of the solvent extraction process, replaced the
expeller to yield the maximum amount of oil and also produced
a higher quality oil and defatted meal (Weiss, 1970). Most
of the extracted oil is consumed in the form of salad and
cooking oils, shortening, and margarine. Of the approximately
18-19 million metric tons of defatted soybean meal produced
annually in the United States, the majority is utilized in
animal feeds. Only about 3% of the defatted meal is used
directly in human food.

In 1973 (Lockmiller), soy proteins in food systems were
increasing at the rate of about 5-7% per year. Currently
the annual growth rate is estimated to be about 10% (Anton,
1975). New product types with a wide range of functionality,
high nutritive value, and low costs relative to animal
proteins contribute to this growth. Slower market growth
rates are found in some high quality soy products that
require specialized processing which puts the product in the
same cost range as animal protein. Although use of soy
proteins is still relatively small, many of the major food
companies are now incorporating them into some of their
products. This paper will consider various soy protein
products and characteristics relative to their application
in food systems.

PRODUCTION OF COMMERCIAL FORMS OF SOYBEAN PROTEINS

Soybean proteins available to the food industry are
conveniently classified into three major groups based on
protein content. Flour and grits are further classified
into products based on fat content (Wolf, 1970). Typical

analyses for these products are shown in Table 1. The products range from flours and grits to textured isolates.

Full-fat products. Several methods can be used to produce full-fat soy flour. In one, soybeans are treated with live steam in a conveyer, followed by cooling, drying, and milling to flour (Horan, 1967). In another (Bookwalter et al., 1971a), milled grits are dry heat-treated at 105° for 6-8 min to inactivate lipoxygenase. Then the grits are adjusted to about 20% moisture and extrusion-cooked at about 135°, 1.25 min retention time, followed by cooling, drying, and milling to flour. Cooking of soybean products is necessary to inactivate lipid enzymes and antinutritional factors. Foods in which the whole soybean is used, including the seed coat, have been described by Nelson et al., 1971. Whole soybean food prototypes such as canned chicken and soybeans have been prepared. Whole soybeans can also be roasted for use as a snack food (Lockmiller, 1973).

TABLE 1

Commercial forms of soybean proteins and their analyses*
(Wolf, 1970)

Form	Protein %	Fat %	Moisture %
Flours and grits			
Full-fat	41.0	20.5	6.0
High-fat	46.0	14.5	6.0
Low-fat	52.5	4.0	6.0
Defatted**	53.0	0.6	6.0
Lecithinated	51.0	6.5	7.0
Concentrates**	66.2	0.3	6.7
Isolates**	92.8	<0.1	4.7

*"As is" basis.
**Base materials for textured protein products.

Defatted flours and grits. Defatted soy flour and
grits are processed from cleaned, whole soybeans which have
been dehulled, flaked and then defatted by hexane. Precise
control of the heat treatment given the defatted soy flakes
during the desolventizing process and during subsequent
steps is critical in that both the nutritive value and
functionality are directly dependent upon the degree to
which the product is heat treated (Kellor, 1974). An untoasted,
defatted soy flour retains high protein solubility and is
useful for preparation of concentrates, isolates, and as a
base material for thermoplastic extruded textured protein.
A fully toasted soy flour is low in protein solubility, but
the antinutritional factors are minimized. Defatted soy
flour of various combinations of heat treatment, with various
levels of added fat and lecithin, are produced for special
uses (Table 1). Defatted soy flour proteins are also hydrolyzed
by acid, enzymatic, or fermentation treatment to break them
down into amino acids, peptides, and polypeptides. The
products, hydrolyzed vegetable proteins, are useful as
flavoring agents (Lockmiller, 1973).

TABLE 2

Typical composition (%) of soy flours, concentrates, and isolates*
(Horan, 1974)

Component	Defatted flour	Concentrates	Isolates
Protein	56.0	72.0	96.0
Fat	1.0	1.0	0.1
Ash	6.0	5.0	3.5
Oligosaccharides (soluble)**	14.0	2.5	0
Polysaccharides (insoluble)†	19.5	15.0	0.3
Fiber (cellulose)	3.5	4.5	0.1

*Moisture-free basis.
**Sucrose, stachyose, raffinose, verbascose.
†Acidic polysaccharides, arabinogalactan, starch.

Protein concentrates. Soybean protein concentrates are refined forms of defatted soy flour (Table 2). The undenatured, 50% protein, defatted flakes are upgraded to the higher protein product by leaching out soluble carbohydrates, the oligosaccharides (sucrose, stachyose, raffinose, verbascose), part of the ash, and some of the minor components. This is done by washing the defatted flakes with either 60-80% aqueous alcohol or dilute (pH 4.5) acid. Another method involves moist heat to insolubilize the proteins, followed by a water wash (Horan, 1974). Several new modifications of these methods are described by Wolf (1976). Protein concentrates are useful in food systems to contribute functionality and also as a base material for thermoplastic extruded textured protein.

Protein isolates. The most refined forms of soybean proteins are the isolates, which contain 90% or more protein (Table 2). They are prepared by removing the water-insoluble polysaccharides, as well as the water soluble oligosaccharides and other low-molecular-weight components that are separated in making protein concentrates. Defatted flakes are treated with a mild alkaline solution to dissolve the proteins, and the insoluble carbohydrate residue is separated. The proteins are then acid coagulated into a curd at the isoelectric point (pH 4.5). By this treatment the proteins are separated from the soluble carbohydrates. The precipitated proteins are then washed and dried to give the isoelectric protein which is insoluble in water (Horan, 1974). Usually the protein is neutralized before drying to yield the proteinate form which is water dispersible. Isolates are now available which have processing modifications to make them suitable for different food applications (Wolf, 1976). Isolated soy protein is utilized as a base material for the production of textured vegetable protein by the spinning process.

Textured soy proteins. Defatted soy flours, concentrates, and isolates can be transformed from a flaky or powdery material to one which has "chewiness" and a fibrous texture. Two principal processes are utilized, thermoplastic extrusion and fiber spinning. In the thermoplastic extrusion process, either defatted soy flour, concentrates, isolates, or combinations of these are blended with steam and water, flavors, colors, or chemical additives to control density or structure (Atkinson, 1970; Reinhart and Sair, 1975; Puski and Konwinski, 1976). While mixing, mechanical heat is developed, and steam heat is applied which causes a high pressure near the die outlet. Then as this mixture is extruded rapidly into atmospheric pressure, the moisture expands to form tiny air pockets throughout the mass. It is the thin wall structure between these air pockets which creates the texture of the product. Isolated soy protein is converted to textured protein by a spinning process. Isolated soy protein is solubilized in an alkaline medium and passed through a spinnaret to form fibers by coagulation in an acid bath and then stretched by means of a series of rolls revolving at increasing speeds. Bundles of fibers are held together with edible binders and treated with other ingredients such as colors, flavors, seasonings, and supplementary nutrients to give fabricated slices, cubes, bits, or granules with an oriented fibrous structure to simulate animal tissues (Horan, 1974).

More recently, meat-like textures have been produced with pressure-molded mixtures of thermoplastically extruded concentrate, stabilized fat, binder, and flavor (Howard, 1976). Chewy meat-like textures also result from precipitating soy protein isolates into meat-like pieces, followed by heating in an oil bath, cooling, and stabilizing in a water bath (Kumar, 1976). Levinson (1976) produced a fibrous chewy texture by placing compacted defatted soy grits in a mild acidic solution containing propylene glycol which was heated to 120°, followed by filtration and drying.

CHARACTERISTICS RELATIVE TO FOOD USES OF SOYBEAN PROTEINS

Flavor and color. The bitter flavor of raw legumes, including soybeans, is readily eliminated by mild cooking (Moser et al., 1967). The residual "beany" flavor of soybean proteins is more difficult to remove and has been a limiting factor to their use in food systems. The objective of soy protein manufacture is the production of a bland material, but this has not always been the case (Kalbrener et al., 1971). New processing methods are being developed to minimize "beany" flavor characteristics. A combination of toasting and hexane:ethanol azeotrope extraction can be used to produce soy flours and concentrates with flavor scores which are similar to wheat flour (Honig et al., 1976). Azeotrope extraction effectively removes residual lipids (Sessa et al., 1976) which have been associated with undesirable flavors in soy products. Substantial progress has been made toward soy proteins with improved flavors. For example, soy protein isolates are being substituted for milk proteins in coffee whiteners, a food system which requires a bland flavor and light color.

In addition to flavor, the dark color of soy flours had previously limited their application in some food systems. For instance, the use of soy flours of the mid-1940's in bakery goods resulted in poor colored finished products (Hoover, 1975). Considerable improvements in product color have been brought about through process developments such as carefully controlled desolventizing and toasting, chemical treatments, and further purified products such as concentrates and isolates.

Biological and physiological factors. The diverse biological and physiological characteristics of soy protein products have been reviewed by Rackis (1974). The flatulence element has prompted considerable research interest. The gas-producing factor resides mainly in the low- molecular- weight carbohydrate fractions, soy whey solids, and aqueous alcohol extractives. These fractions contain 60-80% water- soluble, alcohol-soluble oligosaccharides, primarily as sucrose, raffinose, and stachyose. Thus, the removal of oligosaccharides in the production of concentrates and isolates also removes the flatus factor. The production of intestinal gas appears to be related to the intake levels of soybean products which contain the oligosaccharides. Flatulence was not indicated in a feeding study of a cereal blend containing 38% full-fat soy flour (Graham, 1973). During 11 years of feeding cereal blends fortified with as much as 27.5% defatted, toasted soy flour, no cases of flatulence have been reported. Little or no flatus activity is present in the hulls, fat, protein, or the water-insoluble high- molecular-weight polysaccharides.

Nutritional aspects. Raw soybean meal contains antinutritional factors such as trypsin inhibitor and other heat-labile components (Rackis, 1974). The adverse effects of these factors have been demonstrated in rat feeding studies. Although their effects on humans are unknown, soybean protein products are heat-treated to optimize their nutritional value. The relationship between heat treatment, nutritive value, and activity of antigrowth factors is shown in Table 3. With increased heat, protein efficiency ratios increase as the antigrowth factors decrease. The decrease in protein dispersibility indicates heat denaturation of the protein. In food systems which require a further cooking step after formulation, it may not be necessary to use a fully cooked soy protein.

TABLE 3

Relationships between heat treatment, nutritive value, and activity
of selected antigrowth factors in soybean flour
(Kellor, 1974)

Heat treatment			Antigrowth factor activity*	
Degree	PDI**	PER†	SBTI	Hemagglutinin
Untoasted	85+	1.31	500	52
Lightly toasted	60-75	1.59	150	51
Fully toasted	20-40	2.19	15	14

*SBTI = soybean trypsin inhibitor.
**PDI = protein dispersibility index.
†PER = protein efficiency ratio (corrected to 2.50 casein
control).

TABLE 4

Essential amino acid content of soybean proteins
(Wolf, 1970)

Amino acid	Grams amino acid per 16 grams nitrogen		
	Defatted flour	Concentrate	Isolate
Lysine	6.9	6.6	5.7
Methionine	1.6	1.3	1.3
Cystine	1.6	1.6	1.0
Tryptophan	1.3	1.4	1.0
Threonine	4.3	4.3	3.8
Isoleucine	5.1	4.9	5.0
Leucine	7.7	8.0	7.9
Phenylalanine	5.0	5.3	5.9
Valine	5.4	5.0	5.2

The essential amino acid compositions of defatted flour, concentrate, and isolate are shown in Table 4. Processing has little effect on the essential amino acid distribution. Although the essential amino acids are well balanced, methionine is the first limiting amino acid of soybean proteins (Coppock, 1974). Fortification with 0.48% DL-methionine to full-fat soy flour results in significantly higher protein efficiency ratios (Bookwalter et al., 1975). Soybean proteins being high in lysine, the first limiting amino acid in cereals (Kato and Muramatsu, 1971), are useful as supplementing blends. Soy flours are a major factor in producing nutritious food mixtures with cereals such as corn, wheat, sorghum, and oats (Bookwalter, 1977; Crowley, 1975; Horan, 1973). Table 5 lists cereal-based blended food mixes which are supplemented with various defatted, toasted, or full-fat soy products in the form of flours, flakes, and grits. These commodities are donated to nutritionally deprived people overseas under Public Law 480. In addition to increasing the protein content, the protein quality also improves by combining cereal with soybean proteins. By addition of 15% soy flour to degermed corn meal, protein efficiency ratios (PER) increase from about 0.4 to 2.0 (Bookwalter et al., 1971b). Addition of the same level of soy protein to sorghum meal results in a PER increase from about 0.3 to 1.8 (Bookwalter et al., 1977). PER does not respond to the addition of DL-methionine in these and other tests (Bookwalter et al., 1975), which indicates that adequate sulfur amino acids are supplied by the cereal components. In 12% soy-fortified bread, the PER value is 1.95 compared to 1.00 in regular white bread (Marnett et al., 1973). Human feeding studies by Graham et al. (1972, 1973) indicate satisfactory biological values for cereal-soy blends. Other food systems, such as breakfast cereals, pasta products, specialty breads, and snack items utilize the complementary effects of soy protein (Wolf and Cowan, 1975).

Textured flours, concentrates, and isolates have been used extensively in the human diet with meat products. Wilding (1974) reported on hydrated textured soy protein at levels of 0, 12, 21, and 30% in chicken patties, meat loaf, meat balls, and other meat preparations. PER values at levels of 12-30% were higher than casein. With human subjects, Kies and Fox (1971) compared textured vegetable protein (TVP) and TVP containing 1% DL-methionine with ground beef at 4.0 or 8.0 g of nitrogen per person daily. At the 4.0 g

TABLE 5

Cereal-based blended food mixes* supplemented with soybean
protein products

Commodity	Soybean protein %	Type
Soy-fortified corn meal	15	DT**-flour
Corn-soy blend	22	DT-flour-E†
Corn-soy-milk (CSM)	17.5	DT-flour-E
Instant CSM	23.7	DT-flour-E
Instant CSM, sweetened	27.5	DT-flour-E
Soy-fortified bread flour	12	LT‡-flour
Soy-fortified bulgar	15	DT-grit
Soy-fortified sorghum	15	DT-grit
Soy-fortified rolled oats	15	DT-flake
Wheat-soy blend	20	DT-flour

*Public Law 480, Title II commodities.
**DT = defatted, toasted.
†E = equivalent (full-fat) soy flour optional.
‡LT = defatted, lightly toasted.

nitrogen intake level, beef was superior to TVP on
the basis of nitrogen balance. Methionine fortification was
partially effective in improving the nitrogen balance,
demonstrating that it is the first limiting amino acid in
TVP. However, at 8.0 g of nitrogen intake, no significant
differences were observed between nitrogen balances of
subjects who consumed one of the three sources of nitrogen.
It was concluded from these studies that below a critical
level of intake, soy proteins had a lower protein value than
beef; but at more liberal levels, soy proteins could meet
the protein requirements of adult men. Greater quantity of
soy protein compensated for lower quality.

Soy proteins are also being utilized in special dietary
foods. In infant formulas, they provide nutrients for
infants who are allergic to cow's milk (Decock, 1974). Soy
proteins are also utilized to fabricate foods for segments

of the population who require a low cholesterol diet such as simulated meats derived from spun fibers or in dietary wafers which provide balanced nutrition along with controlled caloric intake (Kolb, 1974).

Functionality. The soy flours, concentrates, and isolates are further modified into a large number of other products for specific functional and nutritional uses (Smith and Circle, 1972; Wolf and Cowan, 1975). The functional properties of the specialized soy protein forms enhance their usefulness and generally limit their application to specific food systems. Table 6 lists the wide range of functional properties which may be achieved with various forms of soy protein and their contribution to food systems. Functional properties such as emulsification, fat absorption, water absorption, solubility, texture, dough formation, and film formation are utilized in food systems such as bakery goods, meats, infant formulas, pasta products, and specialty items.

TABLE 6

Functional properties of soybean proteins in food systems

Functional property	Protein* form used	Contribution to food system
Emulsification	F, C, I	Formation and stabilization
Fat absorption	F, C, I	Promotion or prevention
Water absorption	F, C	Controlled uptake and retention
Solubility	I	Homogenous, nonsettling
Texture	F, C, I	Viscosity, gelation, formation of chips, chunks, shreds, and fibrils
Dough formation	F, C, I	Cohesion, elasticity
Film formation	C, I	Packaging (e.g. frankfurters)
Color control	F	Bleaching or browning
Aeration	I	Whippability, foam stabilizer
Antioxidation	F, C, I	Rancidity protection

*F, C, and I represent flours, concentrates, and isolates, respectively.

In bakery items, soy flours improve the water absorption of bread doughs, cake batters, and other products. Moisture retention after baking is also improved and this results in longer shelf life. Inclusion of soy proteins increases the rate of browning and crust color is improved (Levinson and Lemancik, 1974). Lipoxygenase-active full-fat soy flour is also available which will produce a whiter crumb color through bleaching when added to bread doughs (Cotton, 1974). Defatted soy flour added to bread doughs has been found to decrease the mixing requirements and fermentation time (Hoover, 1975). Soy proteins improve the cohesion and elasticity of bread doughs and pie crusts. This results in improved pliability and reduced stickiness which facilitates high-speed machine handling (Levinson and Lemancik, 1974). However, decreased loaf volume, coarse grain and texture, and darker crumb color results from the addition of high levels of defatted soy flour to bread formulas. High-quality bread containing as much as 12% soy flour is facilitated by the addition of dough conditioners such as sodium stearoyl-2-lactylate (Marnett et al., 1973) or fatty esters of polyalkoxylated polyol glycosides (Bookwalter and Mehltretter, 1976). In doughnut mixes, soy flour (defatted, full-fat, or lecithinated) is added to decrease fat absorption during frying. Soy flours, concentrates, and isolates contribute emulsification in cake batters. Cake formulations containing soy flour are more tolerant to process and ingredient variations (Cotton, 1974). It is interesting to note (Table 6) that soy proteins function to prevent fat absorption in doughnut frying while promoting fat absorption in other food systems. The reasons for this are not clear, but illustrates the necessity for testing each specific application for functionality.

In meat systems, flour and grits, concentrates, and isolates are utilized for a variety of functional properties. Soy flour and grits have been utilized for many years as meat extenders. It was recognized early that soy flour has the advantage of holding both the meat juices and fat. Soy flour is used in sausage and nonspecific loaves while soy grits are utilized in coarse ground meat products (Rakosky, 1974). Concentrates and isolates are incorporated into processed meat products such as frankfurters, luncheon loaves, patties, meat loaves, and meat balls, and meat-in-sauce items (Meyer, 1971). Concentrates are used both for meat extension and functionality. In the formation and stabilization of emulsions, the absorption of fat and water provide a juicy texture and reduce shrinkage during cooking. Soluble isolates are used in processed meat products for their emulsifying capacity, emulsion stabilizing effect, and increased viscosity and gel formation on heating. Soy proteins provide a natural film which is formed during the processing of frankfurters. Isolates are suitable for canned meats because they are not adversely affected by high processing temperatures. During heat processing there is an additional stabilizing effect which results from gelling. Fat globules are entrapped to prevent their coalescence (Schweiger, 1974).

Methods of providing texture include chewy gel formation (Anson and Pader, 1959), curd formation (Watanabe et al., 1974) and yuba film formation (Wu and Bates, 1975). However, the development of textured proteins through thermoplastic extrusion and fiber spinning provided a new dimension of functionality for soybean proteins. These products are finding application in food systems based on meat (Horan, 1974). Extruded soy flours and concentrates can be produced in chips, chunks, flakes, and a variety of other shapes. The extruded textured soy protein has a "crunchy" or "chewy" texture along with fat and water absorbing properties and may be used in a wide variety of product applications, either flavored or unflavored. The flavored dry form may be added to salads or dips. The unflavored form is often hydrated when used in meat applications such as patties, loaves, meat balls, tacos, chili, meat spreads, and many others. The extruded textured protein functions as an extender and retains the desirable juices and flavors that would be lost during cooking. In meat-like products, textured proteins improve the consistency and appearance by reducing the floating fat and increasing the meat-like texture (Wilding, 1974). The fiber spinning process requires an isolated soy protein with high solubility. Soy proteins textured by this process are fabricated into analogues. These products are engineered to resemble conventional meat, poultry, and fish products in flavor, color, texture, and appearance. Spun-fiber type textured proteins are also used as extenders in combination with traditional products. Of the textured products, the spun-fiber type more closely simulate the structural and textural characteristics of animal protein (Rosenfield and Hartman, 1974).

Soy proteins provide functionality in a wide variety of other food systems. In soups and gravies, flours, concentrates, and isolates furnish viscosity or thickening. Caramels and toffee-type confections containing soy flour are less sticky on a high-speed wrapping machine. In fudge, soy flour will slow the rate of rehydration and thereby aid in preventing sugar crystallization (Levinson and Lemancik, 1974). Pasta products containing soy flour are firmer after being subjected to long cooking periods (Paulson, 1961). Soy protein isolates may be modified with pepsin to improve water solubility and aeration properties. The modified isolates are useful as coffee whiteners (Claus, 1974) or can be aerated to produce whipped toppings. Modified isolates utilize the ability to produce stable foams in nougats, frappes, mazettas, and marshmallows. They are also used in the foam mat drying of fruits (Levinson and Lemancik, 1974). The solubility of soy protein isolates is utilized to provide simulated milks (Circle, 1974) and infant formulations (Decock, 1974; Johnson, 1975). Dehulled soybeans or an extracted lipid-protein concentrate can be processed into dry, water-dispersible beverages (Mustakas et al., 1971; 1974).

Soybean proteins also provide antioxidant activity in food systems. Soybean flour has been shown to be a basic source of such antioxidant compounds as isoflavone glycosides and their derivatives, phospholipids, tocopherols, amino acids, peptides, as well as compounds of uncertain origin and/or composition. Residual antioxidant activity has been reported in food systems containing soy protein concentrates, isolates, textured proteins, and protein hydrolyzates (Hayes et al., 1977).

TABLE 7

Estimated production of edible soy protein products and future projections in millions of pounds

| | 1974 | | 1980* | 1985** |
	I*	II**		
Soy flour and grits	300	900	600	2000
Textured soy proteins	160	100	1080	450
Soy protein concentrate	175	70	350	600
Soy protein isolate	75	60	400	450
Soy milk-type products	---	nil	---	200
Total	710	1130	2340	3700

*Anton, J. (1975).
**Johnson, D. (1976).

FUTURE PROSPECTS

U.S. Department of Agriculture projections cited by Milner (1975) estimated that the demand for U.S. soybeans will increase 73% by 1985 over the 1970-1972 average annual production of about 35 million metric tons. Soybean production may increase to 85 million metric tons per year by the year 2000. As shown in Table 7, Anton (1975) and Johnson (1976) predict that 1974 production of 0.71 and 1.13 billion pounds of edible soy protein products, respectively, could more than double by 1980 and 1985.

Although the potential for increased utilization of soy proteins in food systems is enormous, further research and development are necessary. The concept of proper usage demands increased product application studies coupled with technical service support efforts. Further flavor studies are needed to increase the compatability of soy proteins in a wider range of food systems. Additional research is also required on detection methods for soy in foods, antinutritional factors, color, flatulence, solubility, and sulfur amino acid content.

REFERENCES

Anson, M. L. and Pader, M. (1959). Method of preparing a meat-like product. U.S. Patent 2,879,163.

Anton, J. J. (1975). Good market climate nurtures soy industry growth. Food Prod. Dev., 9(8), 96-99.

Atkinson, W. T. (1970). Meat-like protein food product. U.S. Patent 3,488,770.

Bookwalter, G. N., Mustakas, G. C., Kwolek, W. F., McGhee, J. E., and Albrecht, W. J. (1971a). Full-fat soy flour extrusion-cooked: properties and food uses. J. Food Sci., 36(1), 5-9.

Bookwalter, G. N., Kwolek, W. F., Black, L. T., and Griffin, E. L. (1971b). Corn meal/soy flour blends: characteristics and food applications. J. Food Sci., 36(7), 1026-1032.

Bookwalter, G. N., Warner, K., Anderson, R. A., Mustakas, G. C., and Griffin, E. L. (1975). Fortification of dry soybean based foods with DL-methionine. J. Food Sci., 40(2), 266-270.

Bookwalter, G. N. and Mehltretter, C. L. (1976). Dough conditioners for 12% soy-fortified bread mixes. J. Food Sci., 41(1), 67-69.

Bookwalter, G. N., Warner, K., and Anderson, R. A. (1977). Fortification of dry-milled sorghum grits with oilseed proteins. J. Food Sci., 42(4), 969-973.

Bookwalter, G. N.   Corn-based foods used in food aid programs; stability characteristics--a review. J. Food Sci., 42, 1421-1424 (1977).

Circle, S. J. (1974). Soy proteins in dairy-type foods, beverages, confections, dietary, and other foods. J. Am. Oil Chem. Soc., 51(1), 198A-199A.

Claus, W. S. (1974). Soy products in other applications. J. Am. Oil Chem. Soc., 51(1), 197A-198A.

Coppock, J. (1974). Soy proteins in foods--retrospect and prospect. J. Am. Oil Chem. Soc., 51(1), 59A-62A.

Cotton, R. H. (1974). Soy proteins in bakery goods. J. Am. Oil. Chem. Soc., 51(1), 116A-119A.

Crowley, P. R. (1975). Practical feeding programs using soy protein as base. J. Am. Oil Chem. Soc., 52(4), 277A-279A.

Decock, A. (1974). Soy protein isolates in hypoallergenic infant formulations and humanized milks. J. Am. Oil Chem. Soc., 51(1), 199A-200A.

Graham, G. G., Baertl, J. M., Placko, R. P., and Cordano, A. (1972). Dietary protein quality in infants and children VIII. Wheat- or oat-soy mixtures. Am. J. Clin. Nutr., 25(8), 875-880.

Graham, G. G., Baertl, J. M., Placko, R. P., and Morales, E. (1973). Dietary protein quality in infants and children. IX. Instant sweetened corn-soy-milk blend. Am. J. Clin. Nutr., 26(5), 491-496.

Hayes, R. E., Bookwalter, G. N., and Bagley, E. B. Antioxidant acitvity of soybean flour and derivatives. J. Food Sci., 42, 1527-1532 (1977).

Hesseltine, C. W. and Wang, H. L. (1972). Fermented soybean food products. In, "Soybeans: Chemistry and Technology, Vol. I, Proteins," A. K. Smith and S. J. Circle (Editors). Avi Publishing Co., Westport, Conn., pp. 389-419.

Honig, D. H., Warner, K., and Rackis, J. J. (1976). Toasting and hexane:ethanol extraction of defatted soy flakes. Flavor of flours, concentrates, and isolates. J. Food Sci., 41(3), 642-646.

Hoover, W. J. (1975). Use of soy proteins in bakery products. J. Am. Oil Chem. Soc., 52(4), 267A-269A.

Horan, F. E. (1967). Defatted and full-fat soy flour by conventional processes. In "Proceedings of International Conference on Soybean Protein Foods," Peoria, Illinois, October 1966. U.S. Dep. Agric. ARS-71-35, pp. 129-141.

Horan, F. E. (1973). Wheat-soy blends--high quality protein products. Cereal Sci. Today, 18(1), 11-14.

Horan, F. E. (1974). Soy protein products and their production. J. Am. Oil Chem. Soc., 51(1), 67A-73A.

Howard, N. B. (1976). Protein food product. U.S. Patent 3,935,319.

Johnson, D. W. (1975). Use of soy products in dairy product
    replacement. J. Am. Oil Chem. Soc., 52(4), 270A-271A.
Johnson, D. W. (1976). Marketing and economic production--
    summing up. In "World Soybean Research," L. D. Hill
    (Editor). Proceedings of the World Soybean Conference,
    The Interstate Printers and Publishers, Inc., Danville,
    Illinois, pp. 1014-1017.
Kalbrener, J. E., Eldridge, A. C., Moser, H. A., and Wolf,
    W. J. (1971). Sensory evaluation of commercial soy
    flours, concentrates, and isolates. Cereal Chem.,
    48(6), 595-600.
Kato, J. and Muramatsu, N. (1971). Amino acid supplementation
    of grain. J. Am. Oil Chem. Soc., 48(8), 415-419.
Kellor, R. L. (1974). Defatted soy flour and grits. J. Am.
    Oil Chem. Soc., 51(1), 77A-80A.
Kies, C. and Fox, H. M. (1971). Comparison of protein
    nutritional value of TVP, methionine enriched TVP and
    beef at two levels of intake for human adults. J. Food
    Sci., 36(6), 841-845.
Kolb, E. (1974). Use of soy protein isolate in slimming
    food. J. Am. Oil Chem. Soc., 51(1), 200A-202A.
Kumar, S. (1976). Textured protein product and process.
    U.S. Patent 3,962,335.
Levinson, A. A. and Lemancik, J. F. (1974). Soy protein
    products in other foods. J. Am. Oil Chem. Soc., 51(1),
    135A-137A.
Levinson, A. A. (1976). Vegetable protein product and
    process. U.S. Patent 3,966,977.
Lockmiller, N. R. (1973). Increased utilization of protein
    in foods. Cereal Sci. Today, 18(3), 77-81.
Marnett, L. F., Tenney, R. J., and Barry, V. D. (1973).
    Methods of producing soy-fortified bread. Cereal Sci.
    Today, 18(2), 38-50.
Meyer, E. W. (1971). Oilseed protein concentrates and
    isolates. J. Am. Oil Chem. Soc., 48(9), 484-488.
Milner, M. (1975). How can science expand world protein
    resources? In Conference Papers "Soya Protein Conference
    and Exhibition 1975." London, United Kingdom, October,
    American Soybean Association, Hudson, Iowa.
Moser, H. A., Evans, C. D., Campbell, R. E., Smith, A. K.,
    Cowan, J. C. (1967). Sensory evaluation of soy flour.
    Cereal Sci. Today, 12(7), 296-314.
Mustakas, G. C., Albrecht, W. J., Bookwalter, G. N., Sohns,
    V. E., and Griffin, E. L. (1971). New process for low-
    cost, high protein beverage base. Food Technol.,
    25(5), 80-86.
Mustakas, G. C. (1974). A new soy lipid-protein concentrate
    for beverages. Cereal Sci. Today, 19(2), 62-73.

Nelson, A. I., Wei, L. S., and Steinberg, M. P. (1971). Food products from whole soybeans. Soybean Dig., 31(3), 32-34.

Paulson, T. M. (1961). A study of macaroni products containing soy flour. Food Technol., 15(3), 118-121.

Puski, G. and Konwinski, A. H. (1976). Process of making a soy-based meat substitute. U.S. Patent 3,950,564.

Rackis, J. J. (1974). Biological and physiological factors in soybeans. J. Am. Oil Chem. Soc., 51(1), 161A-174A.

Reinhart, R. R. and Sair, L. (1975). Simulated meat products. U.S. Patent 3,925,566.

Rakosky, J. (1974). Soy grits, flour, concentrates, and isolates in meat products. J. Am. Oil Chem. Soc., 51(1), 123A-127A.

Rosenfield, D., and Hartman, W. E. (1974). Spun-fiber textured products. J. Am. Oil Chem. Soc., 51(1), 91A-94A.

Schweiger, R. G. (1974). Soy protein concentrates and isolates in comminuted meat systems. J. Am. Oil Chem. Soc., 51(1), 192A-194A.

Sessa, D. J., Warner, K., and Rackis, J. J. (1976). Oxidized phosphatidylcholines from defatted soybean flakes taste bitter. J. Agric. Food Chem., 24(1), 16-21.

Smith, A. K. and Circle, S. J. (Editors) (1972). Soybeans: Chemistry and technology. Vol. I. Proteins. Avi Publishing Co., Westport, Conn.

Watanabe, T., Ebine, H., and Okada, M. (1974). New protein food technologies in Japan in new protein foods. A. Altschul (Editor). Academic Press, New York, p. 414.

Weiss, T. J. (Editor) (1970). Food oils and their uses. pp 48-49. Avi Publishing Co., Westport, Conn.

Wilding, M. D. (1974). Textured proteins in meats and meat-like products. J. Am. Oil Chem. Soc., 51(1), 128A-130A.

Wolf, W. J. (1970). Soybean proteins: their functional, chemical, and physical properties. J. Agric. Food Chem., 18(6), 969-976.

Wolf, W. J. (1976). Chemistry and Technology of Soybeans, Chapter 6. In "Advances in cereal science and technology, Vol. I," Y. Pomeranz (Editor). American Association of Cereal Chemists, St. Paul, Minn., pp. 325-377.

Wolf, W. J. and Cowan, J. C. (Editors) (1975). Soybeans as a food source. Revised edition. CRC Press, Cleveland, Ohio.

Wu, L. C. and Bates, R. P. (1975). Protein-lipid films as meat substitutes. J. Food Sci., 40(1), 160-163.

37

COTTONSEED PROTEIN DERIVATIVES AS NUTRITIONAL AND FUNCTIONAL SUPPLEMENTS IN FOOD FORMULATIONS

John P. Cherry, Leah C. Berardi, Zigrida M. Zarins,
James I. Wadsworth, and Carolyn H. Vinnett

Southern Regional Research Center, Science and Education
Administration, U. S. Department of Agriculture,
P. O. Box 19687, New Orleans, Loiusiana 70179

ABSTRACT

Cottonseeds contain protein with desirable food functional and nutritional properties. Storage globulins make up most of the protein stored in cottonseed and can be separated into five fractions by gel filtration chromatography. Each fraction is distinguishable from the other by its amino acid and polyacrylamide gel electrophoretic properties. Proteins of cottonseed contribute greatly to the functional properties of emulsions, co-isolates, and texturized derivatives. For example, increasing the amount of high protein cottonseed flour in water suspensions from 2% to 10% improved the capacity (54-97 ml of oil) and viscosity (5,000-100,000 cps) of emulsions. The 10% suspension formed emulsions with increasing oil capacity (84-100 ml) and viscosity (28,000-100,000 cps) as the pH was adjusted from 4.5 to 9.5. Consistencies of the products ranged from that of salad dressing (low percent suspensions, or acid pH) to that of mayonnaise (high percent, or basic pH). These data were utilized to derive a multiple regression model to predict optimum use of cottonseed proteins in emulsions of varying consistencies. A coprecipitated isolate containing greater than 94% protein was prepared from a blend of cottonseed and peanut flours. Amino acid content of the co-isolate reflected that of the protein in the two flours of the composite. The co-isolate has lower gossypol level and improved color and functional properties than a cottonseed protein isolate.

Storage protein isolate of cottonseed suspended in aqueous
solution and heated with constant stirring forms a texturized
product; the quality of the product depends on heat, pH, salt,
and the quantity of nonstorage proteins. Protein and amino
acid content of meat products were improved by the addition of
the texturized protein of cottonseed.

INTRODUCTION

Fundamental investigations have brought about recognition of
cottonseeds as potential sources of edible vegetable proteins.
Extraction of cottonseed proteins with water, salt, and/or alkaline
solutions was initially completed by Osborn and Voorhees (1894),
and Jones and Csonka (1925). Fontaine and coworkers (1945, 1946)
recognized that cottonseed proteins were potentially important
commercially, and examined the relationship between varying pH
conditions and solubilization of these storage constituents.
Arthur and Karon (1948) showed that the efficiency of isolating
cottonseed protein in dispersions is dependent upon concentration
of sodium hydroxide in the extractant.

Cottonseed proteins became widely known as potential sources
of nutrients for human consumption during the 1960's, when they
were incorporated into a low cost vegetable protein product
called Incaparina (Scrimshaw et al., 1962). Bressani (1965)
noted the potential value of cottonseed as a source of edible
food because it contained protein of nutritional quality and was
grown in practically all areas of the world where deficits of
these components existed. However, two disadvantages were also
noted that would affect the use of cottonseed as a food. These
problems were the presence of gossypol, which was shown to be
toxic when ingested by nonruminant animals, and the green-to-gold
colors of cottonseed products (Berardi and Goldblatt, 1969).
Edible-grade cottonseed flours were being produced for use in
blends with cereal products to feed the malnourished in several
countries (Bressani et al., 1966; Bressani, 1965).

While these efforts were under way to characterize and
utilize cottonseed protein as an edible food ingredient, engineers
and geneticists were developing practical methods for removing
gossypol from cottonseeds, at the same time maintaining their
nutritional value. Two scientific breakthroughs resulted from
these efforts: (a) the development of the liquid cyclone process,
which has become the first economical and workable process
capable of removing pigment glands from cottonseed to consistently
produce high protein, low gossypol, edible flour, or concentrate
(Gardner et al., 1976; Ridlehuber and Gardner, 1974; Vix et al.,
1971; Gastrock, 1968; Vix, 1968; Vix et al., 1949); and (b)
breeding of cotton cultivars with glandless cottonseed, and fiber
quality similar to that of commercial glanded cottons (Hess,

1977, 1976; Vix, 1968). Glandless kernels can be processed to edible, nut-like products by toasting, roasting, or frying; they can be used in spreads, candies, cookies, and other bakery items, and in direct consumption snack foods (Lawhon et al., 1970).

Since cottonseed was a potential source of edible food, Berardi et al. (1969) evaluated available data on protein fractionation from cottonseed and developed a two-step extraction procedure that isolated water-soluble proteins (nonstorage) of low molecular weight, precipitable at pH 4, and high molecular weight, alkali-soluble globulins (storage), precipitable at pH 7. This work resulted in the development of the commercially feasible, selective precipitation and selective extraction procedures for preparing nonstorage and storage protein isolates from cottonseed (Martinez et al., 1970a). Studies showed that these isolates differed in solubility properties, number of molecular species, average molecular weights, amino acid composition, and select functional characteristics (Martinez et al., 1970a,b). Moreover, these cottonseed products can make a significant nutritional contribution to the diet (Cater et al., 1977; Castro et al., 1976; Martinez and Hopkins, 1975; Harden and Yang, 1975).

Processing method and pH were shown to affect yields of protein concentrates and functionality in various food products (Lawhon and Cater, 1971). A low-fat concentrate was produced by aqueous extraction of the protein from full-fat cottonseed flour at the isoelectric pH (Lawhon et al., 1972a). Tests showed that this cottonseed concentrate had excellent functional properties in protein-fortified bread and in meat loaf to reduce juice and fat cook-out during baking, as well as to supplement the meat. Organoleptic testing of these products produced scores equal to or better than the all-meat patties.

Proteolytic enzyme-chemical methods improved solubilization of protein from cottonseed flours (Childs, 1975; Arzu et al., 1972). Enzymatic solubilization worked effectively with a lower ratio of liquid to meal than that of conventional treatments, resulting in low amounts of whey (cf. Childs, 1975 and Berardi et al., 1969). A major deterrent to use of wet-extraction procedures to form protein concentrates and isolates has been the byproduct whey, which posed processing and/or pollution problems. Lawhon et al. (1976) showed that ultrafiltration membrane processing of whey-type liquids, followed with concentration either by reverse osmosis membrane processing or by vacuum evaporation, was an economically feasible way to recover valuable constituents and simultaneously remove a serious water pollution threat. Whey extracts from cottonseed flour were shown to contain a whippable substance with commercial potential as an egg white extender or substitute (DeVilbess et al., 1974; Lawhon et al., 1974, 1972b).

This finding greatly enhanced the economic attractiveness of protein isolation processes.

This chapter examines key research presently under way with cottonseed products, to improve understanding of their food properties and maintain interest in using this material as vegetable protein ingredients in foods.

STORAGE PROTEINS

The major portion of protein in cottonseed is that stored in protein bodies and extracted as alkaline- or salt-soluble globulins (Martinez et al., 1970a). Therefore, these proteins contribute considerably to most of the functional and nutritional properties of cottonseed flour. Characterizing some of their chemical properties can assist in understanding certain of the basic food properties of cottonseed.

Sephadex gel filtration chromatography of alkaline or salt soluble extracts (after removal of the water soluble nonstorage proteins) on a G-200 column separates the storage proteins into five major fractions (peaks I to V; Figure 1). Proteins in these fractions range in molecular weight from greater than 600,000 (Peak I) to less than 1,000 (Peak V). A small fraction, Peak IIIA, is not separable from Peak III by the method of gel filtration used in this study.

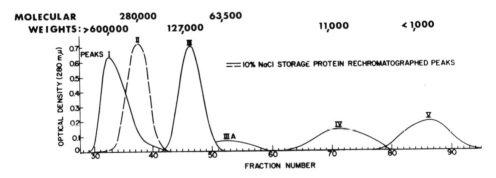

Figure 1. Sephadex G-200 gel filtration of 10% salt-soluble storage proteins of cottonseed after removal of water-soluble nonstorage proteins. Peaks I to V are of fractions from the original column run, rechromatographed to the purity shown.

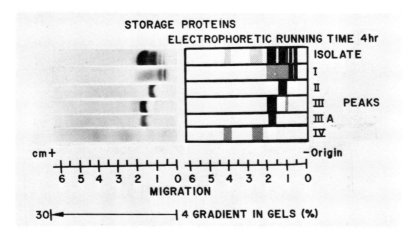

Figure 2. Gradient polyacrylamide (4% to 30%) slab gel
electrophoretic patterns (actual and diagramatic) of the initial
10% salt-soluble storage protein isolate, rechromatographed to
purity of peaks I to IV shown in Figure 1. Electrophoretic methods
were similar to those of Cherry et al. (1975).

Polyacrylamide gel electrophoresis on gradient gels (4% to
30% pore sizes) shows the number of protein components in each
fraction isolated by gel filtration (Figure 2). The proteins of
each of peaks I to V can be compared to individual components in
the initial storage protein isolate. The data show that gel
filtration has fractionated the storage proteins of cottonseed
into distinct components, enabling comparison of their amino acid
composition (Table 1). The data show that quantities of most
amino acids vary considerably among fractions.

Data on amino acids of individual proteins, qualitatively
separated by gel filtration and electrophoretic techniques, can
be used in cooperative studies with geneticists in an attempt to
breed cottonseed with improved protein quality (Cherry et al.,
1978). Cultivars of cottonseed that have high quantities of
certain proteins and desirable amino acid composition can be
selected for in plant breeding programs. In addition, genetic
and agronomic variables, as well as processing techniques, can be
interrelated to functional properties of cottonseed and their
products for their more efficient utilization in food formulations
(Cherry and McWatters, 1975).

Table 1. Amino acid composition of glandless cottonseed flour
          storage proteins and their isolated constituents
          prepared as shown in Figure 1.

| Amino Acids | Amino Acid Analyses[1] (g/100 g protein) | | | | | |
| | | Peaks | | | | |
	Isolate	I	II	III	IV	V
Aspartic acid	9.46	9.58	9.69	9.18	8.75	7.85
Glutamic acid	21.29	18.06	20.45	20.04	19.25	11.91
Alanine	3.73	4.78	5.26	3.57	4.20	4.80
Isoleucine[3]	3.67	3.58	3.75	3.26	2.75	3.02
Phenylalanine[3]	8.35	6.05	5.46	10.54	5.94	3.85
Threonine[3]	3.02	4.00	2.63	3.04	3.38	4.19
Proline	1.08	3.51	1.26	1.48	3.60	0.80
Valine[3]	4.69	4.00	4.86	5.49	3.76	4.12
Leucine[3]	6.34	6.80	6.72	6.36	4.99	5.45
Histidine	3.10	2.63	2.97	3.71	3.29	2.49
Arginine	12.67	12.13	15.99	12.46	9.67	23.06
Serine	5.00	6.21	4.33	5.37	8.31	7.31
Glycine	4.19	5.68	5.38	3.85	5.91	6.66
Methionine[3]	1.45	1.14	1.22	0.21	0.63	1.46
Tyrosine	3.88	4.27	0.66	4.06	4.11	2.56
Lysine[3]	3.13	2.10	2.27	3.12	2.65	8.43
Half Cystine	1.53	2.03	–[2]	0.57	–	–

[1] Method according to Kaiser et al. (1974).

[2] Not determined.

[3] Essential amino acid.

EMULSIFYING PROPERTIES

Cottonseed flour suspended in water can be emulsified to
viscosities that simulate salad dressing and mayonnaise (Figure 3).
Suspensions that are low in protein and/or solubility (isoelectric
pH) do not form emulsions (e.g., 2% suspension, shown in Figure 3).
Varying percentages of flour-in-water suspensions, and their pH
values, greatly influence emulsifying capacity and viscosity of
cottonseed flour (Figure 4). These data can be related to

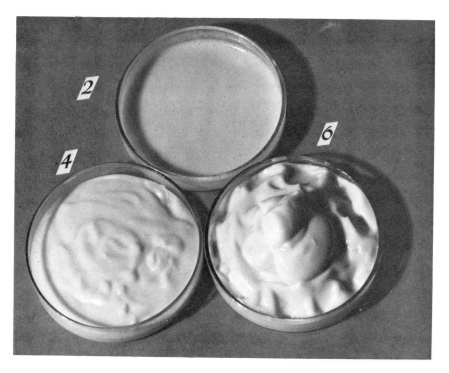

Figure 3. Emulsifying properties of 2%, 4%, and 6% defatted
flour suspensions of glandless cottonseed, prepared according to
the method of McWatters and Cherry (1975).

percentage of protein, carbohydrate, ash, and fiber of the soluble
and insoluble portions obtained from the suspensions by centrifugation at 18,000 x g for 30 min (Figure 4; Table 2).

Emulsion capacity of 10% suspensions, adjusted to pH values
between 1.5 and 11.5, ranged between 85-110 ml oil/25 ml suspension
(Figure 4). The lowest and highest values were noted at isoelectric
pH (4.5) and 11.5, respectively; solubility of proteins in
the suspension was lowest and highest, respectively, at these pH
values. Emulsion capacity increased from 54 ml to 110 ml oil for
suspensions of 2% to 10%, then declined to 74 ml for the 30%
mixture. Relative to pH, emulsion viscosity was highly correlated
with the percentage protein in the soluble fraction; i.e., declining between pH 1.5 and 4.5, and increasing at first gradually, then

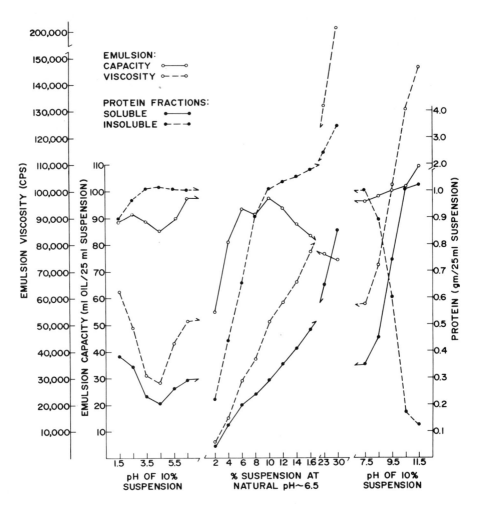

Figure 4. Emulsion viscosity and capacity and protein solubility relative to pH and percentage of glandless cottonseed flour in the suspensions. Emulsifying properties were determined according to the methods of McWatters and Cherry (1975) and McWatters et al. (1976). Protein is macro-Kjeldahl determined nitrogen x 6.25.

Table 2. Components[1] of soluble and insoluble fractions of various cottonseed flour suspensions at different pH values.

pH	% Suspension	Fractions (g/25 ml Suspension)					
		Carbohydrate		Ash		Fiber	
		Soluble	Insoluble	Soluble	Insoluble	Soluble	Insoluble
1.5	10	.27	.24	.14	.31	.003	.062
2.5	10	.31	.19	.13	.33	.005	.063
3.5	10	.34	.20	.18	.34	.002	.060
4.5	10	.32	.20	.18	.33	.002	.064
5.5	10	.37	.26	.16	.28	.002	.063
6.5	2	.09	.08	.02	.02	.002	.015
6.5	4	.17	.16	.03	.04	.004	.029
6.5	6	.26	.23	.06	.05	.009	.040
6.5	8	.32	.33	.06	.08	.010	.053
6.5	10	.41	.47	.07	.11	.009	.072
6.5	12	.46	.56	.08	.13	.018	.082
6.5	14	.54	.63	.09	.16	.020	.102
6.5	16	.62	.71	.11	.18	.015	.116
6.5	23	.83	1.24	.13	.29	.018	.170
6.5	30	1.00	1.46	.15	.40	.022	.214
7.5	10	.41	.31	.08	.27	.002	.075
8.5	10	.42	.33	.08	.25	.002	.073
9.5	10	.40	.38	.09	.20	.008	.057
10.5	10	.47	.41	.11	.14	.004	.036
11.5	10	.47	.38	.14	.14	.006	.032

[1]Analyses completed by official AOCS methods (1976).

rapidly, to pH 11.5. Emulsion viscosity increased from 5000 cps
to greater than 200,000 cps (estimated by multiple regression
analysis) for 2% to 30% suspensions.

Percentage of protein, carbohydrate, ash, and fiber (g/25 ml
suspension) in soluble and insoluble fractions increased continuously for 2% to 30% suspensions (Figure 4; Table 2). These fractions
compared extractability of seed storage components from water-
flour suspensions at their natural pH of approximately 6.5. Thus,
less protein and fiber were noted in water-soluble fractions (nonstorage proteins; Martinez et al., 1970a) than in the insoluble or
storage protein portions. Water-soluble and insoluble fractions
from 2% to 10% suspensions had similar quantities of carbohydrate
and ash. Values of these components were higher in insoluble than
in soluble fractions of 12% to 30% suspensions.

Quantities of proteins in soluble and insoluble fractions, relative to pH, resembled typical solubility curves for cottonseed
protein; these values, over the pH profile, were the inverse of
each other (Figure 4). For example, protein quantity declined in
soluble fractions from suspensions at pH values between 1.5 (acid
dissociated polypeptides) and 4.5 (isoelectric point), then
gradually increased as water-soluble components were extracted at
neutral pH, and amounts of storage globulins increased as the pH
rose to 11.5. The soluble fraction contained greater quantities
of carbohydrate than the insoluble portion, throughout the pH
range. Values for ash and fiber were higher in the insoluble
than in the soluble fraction for these same pH values.

Empirical multiple linear regression models were developed to
describe emulsion capacity and viscosity as a function of pH and
suspension concentration (Tables 3 and 4). These statistical
analyses and emulsifying procedures were modeled after those of
McWatters et al. (1976), McWatters and Cherry (1975), and
Cherry et al. (1975). The multiple R^2 values for these models,
0.823 and 0.996, were very high, indicating that approximately 82%
and 99% of the variability in emulsion capacity and viscosity,
respectively, were accounted for by the seven variables used in
the empirical multiple regression equations.

Further studies were conducted to determine multiple linear
regression equations of emulsion capacity and viscosity based on
pH and composition of soluble and insoluble fractions in the
cottonseed flour suspensions (Tables 5 and 6). Multiple R^2
values of 0.902 and 0.994 were obtained for the capacity and
viscosity equations, respectively. The relative importance of
each respective partial regression coefficient was determined by
comparison of β values (Steel and Torrie, 1960). These comparisons
indicated that the most important variables in the two models for
emulsion capacity and viscosity were pH, pH squared, soluble and

Table 3. Empirical multiple linear regression model[1] describing emulsion capacity as a function of pH and suspension concentration.

Variable Y	Component	Regression Coefficient
	Intercept	112.390
X_1	pH	− 20.917
X_2	Suspension concentration	− 0.091
X_3	pH squared	2.158
X_4	Suspension concentration squared	− 0.201
X_5	pH times concentration	1.905
X_6	pH squared X concentration	− 0.209
X_7	pH squared X concentration squared	0.002

[1]Multiple R^2 = 0.823.

Table 4. Empirical multiple linear regression model[1], describing emulsion viscosity as a function of pH and suspension concentration.

Variable Y	Component	Regression Coefficient
	Intercept	46044.000
X_1	pH	− 7233.300
X_2	Suspension concentration	2780.500
X_3	pH squared	68.250
X_4	Suspension squared	225.810
X_5	pH times concentration	− 0.020
X_6	pH squared X concentration	306.840
X_7	pH squared X concentration squared	− 2.169

[1]Multiple R^2 = 0.996

Table 5.   Multiple linear regression analysis[1] of emulsion
            capacity on composition of glandless cottonseed flour.

Variable Y	Component	Beta Value
X_1	pH	−2.414
X_2	pH squared	2.821
X_3	Soluble protein	0.839
X_4	Soluble carbohydrate	3.215
X_5	Soluble ash	−0.188
X_6	Soluble fiber	−0.259
X_7	Insoluble protein	1.025
X_8	Insoluble carbohydrate	−1.687
X_9	Insoluble ash	−0.486
X_{10}	Insoluble fiber	−0.740
X_{11}	Soluble carbohydrate X soluble protein	−2.038

[1]Multiple R^2 = 0.902

Table 6.   Multiple linear regression analysis[1] of emulsion

Variable	Component	Beta Value
X_1	pH	−0.171
X_2	pH squared	0.349
X_3	Soluble protein	0.331
X_4	Soluble carbohydrate	−0.648
X_5	Soluble ash	−0.062
X_6	Soluble fiber	0.069
X_7	Insoluble protein	0.115
X_8	Insoluble carbohydrate	−0.016
X_9	Insoluble ash	0.140
X_{10}	Insoluble fiber	0.567
X_{11}	Soluble carbohydrate X soluble protein	0.675

[1]Multiple R^2 = 0.994

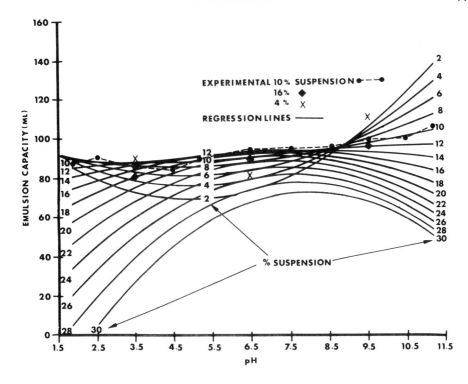

Figure 5. Experimentally observed and mathematically simulated
regression lines of emulsion capacity of different percentages of
cottonseed flour in suspensions at various pH values. Experimental
4%, 10%, and 16% suspensions were run at pH 3.5, 6.5, and 9.5 to
test the reliability of the multiple linear regression analysis.

insoluble protein and carbohydrate, and the product of soluble
carbohydrate x soluble protein. Because the other variables
represented small quantities of soluble and insoluble fractions,
they had little influence on the emulsion properties; only insoluble fiber had a representative β value (Table 6).

The limited experimental data (Figure 4; Table 2) were
used in multiple regression equations to predict emulsion capacity
and viscosity of 2% to 30% suspensions adjusted to pH values of
1.5 to 11.5 (Figures 5 and 6). Observed and predicted data were
similar for the 10% suspension at different pH values and the 2%
to 30% suspensions at pH 6.5. Observed and predicted emulsion
capacities and viscosities of 4%, 10%, and 16% suspensions at
pH 3.5, 6.5, and 9.5, serving as checks, were comparable.
Some variability was noted in emulsion viscosity for all three
suspensions at pH 3.5. Table 7 shows the percentages of proteins,
carbohydrates, ash, and fiber of soluble and insoluble fractions
from these additional tests.

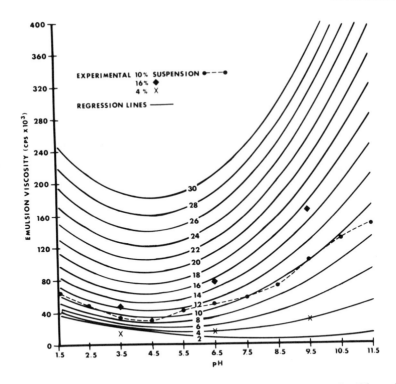

Figure 6. Experimentally observed and mathematically simulated regression lines of emulsion viscosity of different percentages of cottonseed flour in suspensions at various pH values. See Figure 5 for further explanation of data.

Statistical studies including multiple regression analysis may be useful in the prediction of the effect of pH, suspension percentage, and composition of soluble and insoluble fractions on emulsion capacity and viscosity. The regression equations presented in this study are not considered optimal, and predicted values outside the range of the experimental data should be used only with caution. These values can give an estimate of the degree of predictability if such a study were conducted with other samples. In addition, developing methods to measure emulsion properties (or any other functional property) that are highly correlated with pH and suspension percentage dimensions would seem a logical way for producing valued measures; other effects of this type with peanuts include those of McWatters et al. (1976), McWatters and Cherry (1975), and Cherry et al. (1975). Samples which do not follow the predicted curves such as those of pH 3.5 need to be further evaluated in future experiments. Poor correlations at pH 3.5 may be related to the low solubility properties of proteins when they are near their isoelectric point.

Table 7. Components[1] of soluble and insoluble fractions of cottonseed flour suspensions.

| | | Fractions (g/25 ml Suspension) | | | | | | | |
| | | Protein | | Carbohydrate | | Ash | | Fiber | |
pH	% Suspension	Soluble	Insoluble	Soluble	Insoluble	Soluble	Insoluble	Soluble	Insoluble
3.5	4	.09	.43	.17	.15	.05	.08	.000	.025
3.5	10	.23	1.08	.34	.20	.18	.34	.002	.060
3.5	16	.38	1.56	.50	.67	.16	.26	.009	.090
6.5	4	.13	.44	.17	.16	.03	.04	.004	.029
6.5	10	.29	1.06	.41	.47	.07	.11	.009	.072
6.5	16	.48	1.77	.62	.71	.11	.18	.015	.116
9.5	4	.55	.03	.27	.06	.05	.02	.002	.011
9.5	10	.74	.60	.40	.38	.09	.20	.008	.057
9.5	16	1.03	1.04	.70	.57	.15	.21	.004	.121

[1]Analyses completed by Official AOCS methods (1976).

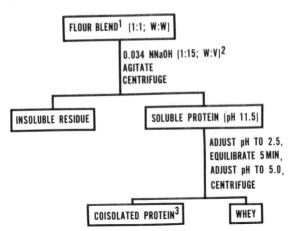

Figure 7. Method for preparation of cottonseed and peanut protein isolates and co-isolates.

CO-ISOLATES

Hsu et al. (1977) summarized the importance of utilizing vegetable protein sources as composites with the following statement: "No single protein possesses chemical, nutritional, and functional properties that would permit its use in all cases of food fortification and extension to give products with both improved amino acid profile and desirable organoleptic character- istics. Blending of protein concentrates or isolates might optimize these properties and enhance the use of unconventional proteins."

Figure 7 presents a method for preparing co-isolates from flour blends (1:1; w:w) made with any combination of vegetable proteins. In general, the method involves extraction of proteins from a flour blend with dilute aqueous sodium hydroxide, acidifi- cation of the extract to pH 2.5, and adjustment of the resulting mixture to pH 5.0 to precipitate protein curds. The protein curds were removed, resuspended in water, washed free of contami- nants, neutralized, and lyophilized or spray dried as co-isolate.

With the formation of co-isolate with liquid cyclone processed (LCP) cottonseed flour and peanut flour as an example, poly- acrylamide disc gel electrophoresis suggests that the proteins in

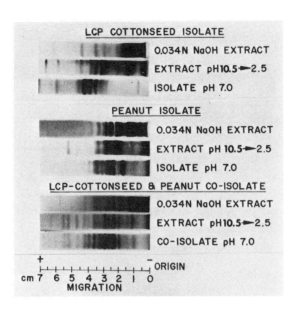

Figure 8. Polyacrylamide disc gel electrophoretic patterns of protein changes during preparation of isolates and co-isolates in Figure 7. Method of gel electrophoresis similar to that of Cherry et al. (1975). Analyses are for experimental test runs in Figures 5 and 6.

the extract dissociate into subunits at pH 2.5, then reassociate into their original and/or new protein forms as the pH is adjusted to 7.0 (Figure 8). Dissociation and reassociation can also be noted for isolates of peanut and LCP cottonseed flours processed by this method. Verification of these changes will have to await future characterization of each protein band in the gel patterns of preparations at the various steps of the method. The presence of some new protein forms, as well as original proteins in the co-isolate, suggests new derivatives were made that may differ in solubility, functional, and nutritional properties from those of the isolates.

Approximately 90% of the total nitrogen in individual and blended flours was extracted with 0.034 N NaOH (Table 8). The co-isolate accounted for 72% of the total nitrogen in the initial alkaline extract. This percentage was similar to that of the peanut isolate and approximately 4% higher than the value for the LCP cottonseed isolate. The percentage of protein going to the whey and residue fractions during formation of the co-isolate was intermediate between the values of the two isolates.

Table 8. Recovery of total nitrogen (%) in fractions during
          isolate and co-isolate formation[1].

| Fractions | Isolates | | Co-isolate |
	LCP Cottonseed	Peanut	LCP Cottonseed-Peanut
0.034 N NaOH Extract[2]	89.8	89.7	89.7
Isolates[3], Coisolate[3]	67.8	71.6	72.0
Wheys[3]	16.7	5.5	10.7
Residues[3]	4.6	12.1	6.2

[1]Fractions obtained by the methods outlined in Figure 7; nitrogen
determined by Official AOCS methods (1976).

[2]Percent total nitrogen in flours and blend.

[3]Percent total nitrogen in 0.034 N NaOH Extract.

     The co-isolate and isolates contained more than 95% protein,
small amounts of lipid, ash, and carbohydrates, and less than
0.1% crude fiber (Table 9). The gossypol pigments were concentrated
in the LCP cottonseed isolate (0.03% free and 0.17% total gossypol).
Coprecipitation of the LCP cottonseed proteins with peanut proteins provided a co-isolate with low gossypol content (0.01%
free, 0.05% total).

     Only small amounts of sugars originally present in the
flours were present in the co-isolate and isolates (Table 10).
Centrifugation of the protein-precipitated mixtures at pH 5.0
allowed the soluble carbohydrates in the wheys to be recovered,
thereby eliminating most of the sugars that produce flatulence
from the final protein products.

     Amino acid values (g/100 g protein) of the co-isolate were
either greater than or intermediate to those of the LCP cottonseed
and peanut flours (Table 11). Half of the essential amino acids
in the co-isolate had values greater than those of the starting
flours. The higher levels of certain amino acids in the
co-isolate, compared to the flours, adds further support to the
gel electrophoretic data, indicating that proteins dissociate at
pH 2.5 and reassociate at pH 5.0 into new forms. Since the
nonstorage proteins are richer in essential amino acids than
storage globulins (Martinez and Hopkins, 1975), the former may
have contributed to this improvement. Table 11 also shows that,
in most cases, amino acid values of the co-isolate are intermediate
to those of the two isolates. In other cases, values of the
co-isolate resemble either those of the peanut or the LCP cottonseed isolate.

Table 9. Components[1] (%) of flours, isolates, and co-isolates.

	Flours		Isolates		Co-isolate
	LCP		LCP		LCP Cotton-
Components	Cottonseed	Peanut	Cottonseed	Peanut	seed-Peanut
Protein[2]	68.1	67.2	96.2	96.8	95.5
Lipid	0.3	0.6	0.3	0.3	0.6
Carbohydrate	24.0	27.7	0.7	0.7	1.1
Crude Fiber	2.2	3.4	<0.1	<0.1	<0.1
Ash	7.6	4.5	2.7	2.1	2.7
Free Gossypol	0.02	0	0.03	0	0.01
Total Gossypol	0.14	0	0.17	0	0.05

[1] Analyses completed by Official AOCS methods (1976).
[2] $N \times 6.25$.

Table 10. Sugar content[1] (%) of flours, isolates, and co-isolate.

	Flours		Isolates		Co-isolate
	LCP		LCP		LCP Cotton-
Sugar	Cottonseed	Peanut	Cottonseed	Peanut	seed-Peanut
Raffinose	11.17	0.14	0.44	0.01	0.54
Sucrose	1.73	9.26	0.26	0.69	0.45
Stachyose	trace[2]	0.36	–	trace	0.23
Fructose	–[3]	0.11	–	–	–
Glucose	trace	0.08	–	–	–

[1] Gas liquid chromatographic analysis by Official method of AOCS (1976).
[2] <0.01%
[3] Not detected at level of analysis.

Table 11. Amino acid composition[1] (gm/100 gm protein) of flours, isolates and co-isolate.

| Amino Acid | Flours | | Isolates | | Co-isolate |
	LCP Cottonseed	Peanut	LCP Cottonseed	Peanut	LCP Cotton-seed-Peanut
Alanine	3.49	3.60	3.57	3.69	3.70
Valine[2]	3.35	3.28	3.99	3.29	3.15
Glycine	3.60	4.93	3.91	4.07	3.87
Isoleucine[2]	2.42	2.56	3.19	2.87	3.28
Leucine[2]	4.98	5.94	6.13	6.38	5.93
Proline	3.23	3.95	4.91	4.21	3.87
Threonine[2]	2.96	2.28	3.32	2.77	2.84
Serine	4.17	5.35	4.72	5.28	4.89
Methionine[2]	1.15	1.00	1.41	0.83	1.23
Phenylalanine[2]	4.64	4.56	6.24	5.25	5.55
Aspartic acid	8.21	11.18	8.96	12.48	10.59
Glutamic acid	17.39	17.17	20.77	21.71	22.94
Tyrosine	2.59	3.75	3.17	4.09	3.65
Lysine[2]	4.14	3.19	3.80	2.91	3.24
Histidine	2.01	1.93	3.52	1.94	2.86
Arginine	10.85	10.22	11.05	12.85	11.54
Half cystine	1.34	1.16	1.15	1.28	1.14

[1] Method according to Kaiser et al. (1974).

[2] Essential amino acid.

Some functional properties are compared for LCP cottonseed and peanut flours, isolates, and co-isolate in Table 12. More specifically, water absorption and emulsion capacity were greater for the co-isolate than for the isolates and flours. Total color difference, oil absorption, and foaming properties were similar to either one of the isolates or the flours. The co-isolate had better solubility properties than the LCP cottonseed isolate. The poor solubility of the LCP cottonseed isolate typifies that prepared by the "classical method," where the initial alkaline

Table 12. Some functional properties of LCP cottonseed and peanut derivatives.

Test	Flours		Isolates		Co-isolate
	LCP Cottonseed	Peanut	LCP Cottonseed	Peanut	LCP Cotton-seed-Peanut
Color:					
Total Color Difference[1]	14.0	6.9	25.1	15.3	23.2
Water absorption[2]	2.0	1.6	1.7	2.8	3.4
Oil absorption[2]	1.4	1.4	1.2	3.2	3.1
Emulsion capacity[2]	50.5	28.2	64.4	60.1	65.8
Foaming properties (%):					
Volume increase	450	86	500	8	416
Foam stability (60 min)	9	54	162	24	56
Protein solubility (% total):					
pH 2.5	33.8	56.6	83.0	95.0	92.5
4.0	13.6	3.8	12.5	27.5	14.0
7.0	23.7	88.9	8.5	33.0	14.0
9.0	76.3	92.1	15.0	95.0	39.0

[1] Method of Hunter (1976).

[2] ml/gm product.

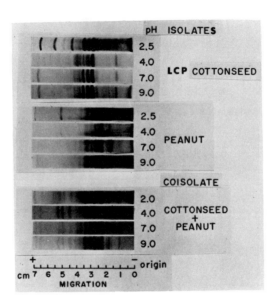

Figure 9. Polyacrylamide disc gel electrophoretic patterns of soluble proteins in isolates and co-isolates at different pH values as shown in Table 11. Method of Cherry et al. (1975).

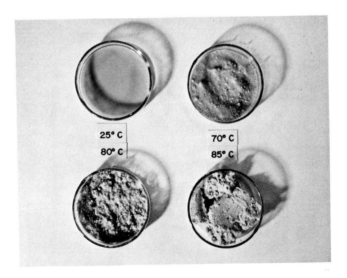

Figure 10. Observable changes in storage protein suspension constantly stirred on being heated from 25°C to 85°C to induce texturization. Textured product shown in plate labeled 85°C.

Table 13. Texturizing or gelling properties of storage and
classical (nonstorage and storage) protein isolates
from cottonseed.

pH	Storage ± Salt[2]	Classical (Storage & Nonstorage)	
		− Salt	+ Salt
3.0	gelled	gelled	gelled
4.0	gelled	gelled	texturized
5.0–9.0	texturized	thick paste	texturized
10.0	gelled	gelled	gelled

[1]20% and 16% aqueous suspensions of storage and classical
isolates, respectively, stirred constantly and heated slowly
from 25°C to 85°C in 20 min.

[2]0.3% salt added to suspensions.

Table 14. Composition[1] (%) of cottonseed protein products.

Component	Storage Protein	Textured Storage Protein	Uncooked Meat	% Textured Storage Protein in Cooked Meat Loaf		
				0	10	30
Moisture	4.97	1.78	62.05	61.83	61.47	52.56
Protein[2]	99.25	98.62	18.38	23.19	26.81	30.13
Lipid	0.41	0.34	18.50	13.90	11.90	6.70
Ash	0.73	2.16	0.81	1.78	1.34	1.19
Fiber	0.67	0.38	0.09	0.28	0.14	0.12

[1]Analyses by Official Methods of AOCS (1976).

[2]N x 6.25.

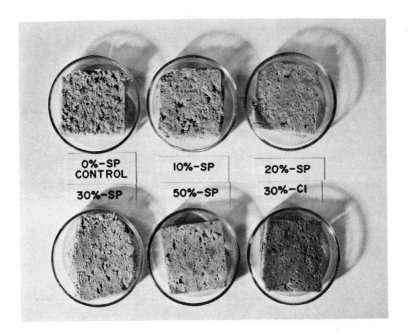

Figure 11. Meat loaf products containing varying amounts of textured cottonseed protein. SP = storage protein; CI = classical isolate or mixture of storage and nonstroage protein (Berardi et al., 1969).

Table 15. Amino acid content[1] (g/100 g sample) of cottonseed
protein products.

Amino Acids	Storage Protein	Textured Storage Protein	Uncooked Meat	% Textured Storage Protein in Cooked Meat Loaf		
				0	10	30
Alanine	3.55	4.10	1.16	1.38	1.37	1.56
Valine[2]	4.25	3.78	0.82	1.14	1.17	1.63
Glycine	3.79	4.13	1.31	1.53	1.48	1.58
Isoleucine[2]	2.84	2.34	0.71	0.99	0.95	1.21
Leucine[2]	5.97	6.24	1.28	1.66	1.73	2.32
Proline	3.48	4.00	0.96	1.25	1.20	1.51
Threonine[2]	2.87	3.22	0.73	0.88	0.98	1.23
Serine	4.92	5.72	0.69	0.82	1.08	1.80
Methionine[2]	0.95	1.08	0.37	0.48	0.52	0.46
Hydroxyproline	-[3]	-	0.39	0.36	0.28	0.11
Phenylalanine[2]	6.67	6.80	0.66	0.90	1.30	2.13
Aspartic Acid	9.20	10.21	1.57	1.95	2.40	3.33
Glutamic Acid	19.80	20.95	2.48	3.40	4.24	6.32
Tyrosine	2.91	2.80	0.51	0.65	0.73	1.16
Lysine[2]	2.99	2.82	1.41	1.66	1.57	1.53
Histidine	2.77	3.62	0.50	0.62	1.04	0.77
Arginine	12.41	11.62	1.32	1.68	2.01	4.04
Half Cystine	0.90	0.95	0.23	0.29	0.33	0.44

[1] Method according to Kaiser et al. (1974).

[2] Essential amino acid.

[3] Not detected.

extract contains both storage and nonstorage proteins (Berardi et al. 1969).

Polyacrylamide disc gel electrophoretic patterns show the qualitative composition of soluble proteins in the co-isolate and isolates when they are adjusted to pH 2.5, 4.0, 7.0, and 9.0 (Figure 9). The patterns show dissociated polypeptides in the pH 2.5 extract and similar patterns for the pH 4.0, 7.0, and 9.0 preparations. Additional protein components in the co-isolate patterns, compared to those of the LCP cottonseed isolate, probably account for the higher solubility values noted in the latter over those of the former (cf. Figure 9 and Table 12).

TEXTURED PROTEINS

Increasing the temperature (25°C to 85°C) of a constantly stirred suspension of cottonseed storage protein isolate and water results in a textured product (Figure 10). The textured protein product has the appearance and mouth feel of extruded products and meat. Formation of the textured product is pH-related, occurring only when the suspension of storage protein isolate is between pH 5.0 and 9.0 (Table 13). At other pH values, this suspension forms heat-stable, gelatin-like substances. Additionally, the textured product cannot be made if the isolate contains nonstorage protein (classical method of Berardi et al., 1969). However, addition of as little as 0.3% salt overcomes this problem (Table 13).

The textured cottonseed products produce acceptable meat loaves when used instead of the protein ingredient in a commercial meat extender (Figure 11). Proximate and amino acid composition of the storage and textured cottonseed protein, meat, and vegetable protein-meat blends (0%, 10%, and 30%) are presented in Tables 14 and 15. Compared to meat alone, addition of textured cottonseed protein improves the composition of the final product.

We have attempted in this work to present data reinforcing what has been known a long time, i.e., cottonseed has excellent potential as a source of edible vegetable protein. Moreover, an understanding of the chemical and functional properties of cottonseed can assist in the production of new products such as emulsions, co-isolates, and nonextruded meat extenders from this vegetable protein source.

REFERENCES

American Oil Chemists' Society (1976). Official and tentative methods (3rd ed., additions and revisions). The Society, Chicago, Ill.

Arthur, J. C. and Karon, M. K. (1948). Preparation and properties of cottonseed protein dispersions. J. Am. Oil Chem. Soc., 25, 99-102.

Arzu, A., Mayorga, H., Gonzalez, J. and Rolz, C. (1972). Enzymatic hydrolysis of cottonseed protein. J. Agric. Food Chem., 20, 805-809.

Berardi, L. C. and Goldblatt, L. A. (1969). Gossypol. In, Toxic Constituents of Plant Foodstuffs, I. E. Liener (Editor). Academic Press, New York, N. Y.

Berardi, L. C., Martinez, W. H. and Fernandez, C. J. (1969). Cottonseed protein isolates: two step extraction procedure. Food Technol., 23 (10), 75-82.

Bressani, R. (1965). The use of cottonseed protein in human foods. Food Technol., 19 (11), 51-58.

Bressani, R., Elias, L. G. and Braham, E. (1966). Cottonseed protein in human foods. In, 'World Protein Resources,' R. F. Gould (Editor). Advances in Chemistry Series 57, 75-100. Am. Chem. Soc., Washington, D. C.

Castro, C. E., Yang, S. P. and Harden, M. L. (1976). Supplemental value of liquid cyclone processed cottonseed flour on the proteins of soybean products and cereals. Cereal Chem., 53, 291-298.

Cater, C. M., Mattil, K. F., Meinke, W. W., Taranto, M. V. and Lawhon, J. T. (1977). Cottonseed protein food products. J. Am. Oil Chem. Soc., 54, 90A-93A.

Cherry, J. P. and McWatters, K. H. (1975). Solubility properties of proteins relative to environmental effects and moist heat treatment of full-fat peanuts. J. Food Sci., 40, 1257-1259.

Cherry, J. P., McWatters, K. H. and M. R. Holmes. (1975). Effect of moist heat on solubility and structural components of peanut proteins. J. Food Sci., 40, 1199-1204.

Cherry, J. P., Simmons, J. G. and Kohel, R. J. (1978). Potential for improving cottonseed quality by genetic and agronomic practices. In, 'Improvement of Protein Nutritive Quality of Foods and Feeds,' M. Friedman (Editor). Plenum Publishing Co., New York, N. Y.

Childs, E. A. (1975). An enzymatic-chemical method for extraction of cottonseed protein. J. Food Sci., 40, 78-80.

DeVilbiss, E. D., Holsinger, V. H., Posati, L. P. and Pallansch, M. J. (1974). Properties of whey protein concentrate foams. Food Technol., 28 (3), 40-48.

Fontaine, T. D., Detwiler, S. B. and Irving, G. W. (1945). Improvement in the color of peanut and cottonseed proteins. Ind. Eng. Chem., 37, 1232-1236.

Fontaine, T. D., Irving, G. W. and Markley, K. S. (1946). Peptization of peanut and cottonseed proteins. Effect of dialysis and various acids. Ind. Eng. Chem., 38, 658-662.

Gardner, H. K., Hron, R. J. and Vix, H. L. E. (1976). Removal of pigment glands (gossypol) from cottonseed. Cereal Chem., 53, 549-560.

Gastrock, E. A. (1968). The application of liquid cyclone to production of high quality cottonseed concentrate. Oil Mill Gazet., 73 (9), 18-20.

Harden, M. L. and Yang, S. P. (1975). Protein quality and supplementary value of cottonseed flour. J. Food Sci., 40, 75-77.

Hess, D. C. (1977). Genetic improvement of gossypol-free cotton varieties. Cereal Foods World, 22, 98-105.

Hess, D. C. (1976). Prospects for glandless cottonseed. Oil Mill Gazet., 81 (11), 20-26.

Hsu, H. W., Satterlee, L. D. and Kendrick, J. G. (1977). Computer blending predetermines properties of protein foods. Food Prod. Dev., 11 (7), 52-58.

Hunter, R. S. (1976). The measurement of appearance. John Wiley and Sons, New York, N. Y.

Jones, D. B. and Csonka, F. A. (1925). Proteins of the cotton-seed. J. Biol. Chem., 64, 673-683.

Kaiser, F. E., Gehrke, C. W., Zumwalt, R. W. and Kuo, K. C. (1974). Amino acid analysis. Hydrolysis, ion-exchange cleanup, derivatization, and quantitation by gas-liquid chromatography. J. Chromatogr., 94, 113-133.

Lawhon, J. T., Cater, C. M. and Mattil, K. F. (1970). Preparation of a high-protein low-cost nut-like food product from glandless cottonseed kernels. Food Technol., 24 (6), 77-94.

Lawhon, J. T., Rooney, L. W., Cater, C. M. and Mattil, K. F. (1972a). Evaluation of a protein concentrate produced from glandless cottonseed flour by a wet-extraction process. J. Food Sci., 37, 778-782.

Lawhon, J. T., Cater, C. M. and Mattil, K. F. (1972b). A whippable extract from glandless cottonseed flour. J. Food Sci., 37, 317-321.

Lawhon, J. T., Hensley, D. W., Cater, C. M. and Mattil, K. F. (1976). An economic analysis of cottonseed whey processing. J. Food Sci., 41, 365-369.

Lawhon, J. T., Lin, S. H. C., Rooney, L. W., Cater, C. M. and Mattil, K. F. (1974). Utilization of cottonseed whey protein concentrates produced by ultrafiltration. J. Food Sci., 39, 183-187.

Lawhon, J. T. and Cater, C. M. (1971). Effect of processing method and pH of precipitation on the yields and functional properties of protein isolates from glandless cottonseed. J. Food Sci., 36, 372-377.

Lawhon, J. T., Cater, C. M. and Mattil, K. F. (1970). Preparation of a high-protein low-cost nut-like food product from glandless cottonseed kernels. Food Technol., 24(6), 77-94.

Martinez, W. H., Berardi, L. C. and Goldblatt, L. A. (1970a). Potential of cottonseed: products, composition, and use. 3rd Internat. Congr. Food Sci. Technol., 3, 248-260.

Martinez, W. H., Berardi, L. C. and Goldblatt, L. A. (1970b). Cottonseed protein products - composition and functionality. J. Agric. Food Chem., 18, 961-968.

Martinez, W. H. and Hopkins, D. T. (1975). Cottonseed protein products: Variation in protein quality with product and process. In, '14th Nutritional Quality of Foods and Feed. Part II. Quality Factors: Plant Breeding, Composition, Processing, and Anti-Nutrients,' M. Friedman (Editor). Marcel Dekker, New York, N. Y.

McWatters, K. H. and Cherry, J. P. (1975). Functional properties of peanut paste as affected by moist heat treatment of full-fat peanuts. J. Food Sci., 40, 1205-1209.

McWatters, K. H., Cherry, J. P. and Holmes, M. R. (1976). Influence of suspension medium and pH on functional and protein properties of defatted peanut meal. J. Agric. Food Chem., 24, 517-523.

Osborne, T. B. and Voorhees, C. G. (1894). The proteins of cottonseed. J. Amer. Chem. Soc., 14, 778-785.

Ridlehuber, J. M. and Gardner, H. K. (1974). Production of food-grade cottonseed protein by the liquid cyclone process. J. Am. Oil Chem. Soc., 51, 153-157.

Scrimshaw, N. S., Bressani, R., Wilson, D. and Behar, M. (1962). All-vegetable protein mixtures for human feedings. X. Effect of torula yeast on the protein quality of INCAP vegetable mixture 9. Am. J. Clin. Nutr., 11, 537-550.

Steel, R. G. D. and Torrie, J. H. (1960). Multiple and partial regression and correlation. In, 'Principles and Procedures of Statistics.' McGraw-Hill Book Co., Inc., New York, N. Y.

Vix, H. O. E. (1968). High protein flour products from glandless and glanded cottonseed. Oil Mill Gazet., 72 (6), 53-56.

Vix, H. L. E., Eaves, P. H., Gardner, H. K. and Lambou, M. G. (1971). Degossypolized cottonseed flour - the liquid cyclone process. J. Am. Oil Chem. Soc., 48, 611-615.

Vix, H. L. E., Spadaro, J. J., Murphey, C. H., Persell, R. M., Pollard, E. F. and Gastrock, E. A. (1949). Pilot-plant fractionation of cottonseed. II. Differential settling. J. Am. Oil Chem. Soc., 26, 526-530.

38

YEAST PROTEINS: RECOVERY, NUTRITIONAL AND FUNCTIONAL PROPERTIES

J.E. Kinsella and K.J. Shetty

Dept. of Food Science, Cornell University

Ithaca, New York   14853

ABSTRACT

The future need for supplementary sources of food grade functional proteins is emphasized and the potential role of yeasts as a source of protein is discussed. The problems of proteolysis and nucleic acid contamination can be circumvented by succinylation or derivatization of the yeast protein during extraction. Succinylated yeast proteins demonstrate improved functional properties though their nutritional value needs to be investigated.

INTRODUCTION

People in many of the developing regions of the world suffer from protein-calorie malnutrition and as the world population continues to expand at an increasing rate toward 7 billion by the 21st century the need for more protein will become accentuated. It has been estimated that by that time the world demand for protein will range from 130-150 million metric tons per annum. Though the "average" world protein supply exceeds statistical requirements by approximately 70 percent (Anonymous 1974, Burrows et al. 1972) marked inequities in distribution and in the capacity to redistribute this protein prevails. Many approaches for increasing protein supply and nutritive value have been proposed and research is in progress on several novel sources.

Excluding energy, the two major factors determining the adequacy of the world's food supply are population and availability of arable land. At the present level of food production and with a

world population of 3.6 billion, approximately 0.4 hectare of land
per person is in use. Malnutrition is common; 50 percent of the
world's population may be undernourished (White et al. 1970).   If
the world population continues to grow at the present rate, it is
anticipated that three times the area of cultivated land (i.e. 5
billion hectares) will be needed by 2025. This far exceeds available arable land. Though crop productivity can be expanded some
and waste reduced, the overall need for food cannot be totally met
using conventional approaches. Sustaining present food production
by conventional agriculture will require the expenditure of the
most important nonrenewable resource in crop food production, viz.
energy. Because of the very limited area of new arable land available, expanded food production will depend increasingly on increasing energy inputs. But because energy is a very finite resource the
most efficient methods must be employed and alternative, supplementary sources of protein must be fully developed as expeditiously as
possible.

As real demand for protein expands with a burgeoning population and as the emphasis changes from animal agriculture to more
direct consumption of plant and microbial proteins the necessity
for new processes and new products will increase, thereby accentuating the critical physicochemical properties required in proteins.
Such properties, generally referred to as functional properties are
important in determining the potential uses of new proteins for the
development of new food products.

Functional Properties

Functional properties is a collective term for those physico-
chemical properties of proteins which govern their composite performance in foods during manufacturing, processing, storage, and
consumption. They reflect the properties of the protein that are
influenced by its composition, conformation, and interactions with
other food components and they are also affected by the immediate
environment (Kinsella 1976).

Typical functional properties include emulsification, which is
important in sausage-type processed meats and coffee whiteners;
hydration and water binding, which are critical in doughs and meat
products; viscosity, important for beverages, e.g. liquid instant
breakfast; gelation, required in marshmallows and cold meat products; foaming/whipping, vital in whipped toppings; cohesion, which
is important in manufacture of textured products; and color control,
which is important in several products, particularly breads. Thus,
the range of properties is very broad, i.e. in a beverage, solubility and viscosity are desired; in breads, compatibility with gluten
and dough formation is desired, and in meat, several functionalities,
e.g. emulsification, water holding capacity, and gelation, are
required.

These criteria are frequently overlooked in studies concerned with new protein sources where quantity of protein and its biological value are considered. The successful supplementation of existing foods, the replacement or simulation of traditional proteinaceous foods and the fabrication of new foods will depend on the availability of new proteins with the critical functional characteristics which enable them to be successfully used. Food proteins should have good nutritional value, satisfactory intrinsic properties (i.e. color, odor, flavor, texture) and possess additional functional properties (solubility, surface activity, thermal stability, adsorption properties, etc.) for successful performance in a variety of specific applications in the food industry.

Because of the limitations on land, energy, the burgeoning population, and the increasing cost of production, food crops may become limited in time. Therefore the development of supplementary sources of food protein, e.g. microbial proteins or single cell protein (SCP) is prudent.

PROTEIN FROM MICROBES

The advantages of SCP, a source which can complement the conventional methods of food production, have been well documented (Cooney et al. 1975, Lipinski 1974, McLaren 1975, Tannenbaum 1971, Tannenbaum et al. 1973, 1977). Production can be continuous and is relatively independent of climate, land, etc. A multitude of different microbes can be grown on a wide range of substrates, many of which are by-products (waste effluents from food processing plants, sulfite liquor, etc.). Microbes have a short generation time (1-2 hrs) which ensures a rapid biomass increase. Genetic flexibility via induced mutations, recombination and selection can be exploited to obtain desirable strains in terms of growth, essential amino acid composition, etc. Microbes are rich in protein (7-12% nitrogen) compared to other natural sources. These, and other reasons warrant the continued research on microbial sources of protein (Bellamy 1974, Cooney et al. 1975, Hockenhull 1971, Humphrey 1974, Kihlberg 1972, Lipinski, 1974, McLaren 1975, Rose and Morrison 1971, Mateles and Tannenbaum 1968, Tannenbaum and Wang 1975.

Much of the research and development has concentrated on production of biomass, frequently referred to as SCP. However for potential food use biomass from microbial fermentations should be regarded as a protein rich raw material, analogous to a harvested crop, requiring further processing before becoming valuable as a high protein food ingredient. Many economic, processing, nutritional, safety, regulatory, and functional criteria must be fulfilled before microbial protein is generally available and acceptable. A popular rationalization for SCP is that it may be a significant source of food protein for developing countries with poor agricultural bases and chronic food shortages, however, in reality the successful use of unconventional proteins in foods may be much more closely related to their compatibility with highly sophisticated food systems (McLaren 1975).

The general status, technical aspects and economics of biomass production has been extensively discussed and reviewed (Bellamy 1974, Cooney 1975, Hockenhull 1971, Humphrey 1974, Kihlberg 1972, Lipinski 1974, Litchfield 1977, Rose and Morrison 1971, Seeley et al. 1974, Shacklady 1970, Tannenbaum 1971, 1973, 1977). A wide range of microbes (bacteria, yeasts, fungi) have been grown as appropriate for the wide range of substrates that have been exploited (Cooney 1975, Kihlberg 1972, Litchfield 1977, Rose and Morrison 1971, Shacklady 1970, Tannenbaum 1973, 1977). Microbes have been successfully grown on hydrocarbons, cellulose, carbohydrates, waste by-products (whey, sulfite liquor), ethanol and methanol (Cooney 1975, Litchfield 1977, Tannenbaum 1973, 1977). For eventual food use the acceptable substrates may be limited to well-defined materials devoid of actual or potential toxins. Cells are usually harvested by centrifugation though flocculation, foam separation and filtration may be used in certain cases (Kihlberg 1972). The cell mass is dried and this biomass, called SCP actually corresponds to a raw material requiring further processing and refining. Yeast has been a traditional food item though as a potential protein source it has received much attention recently (Litchfield 1977).

Composition. Microbes and yeasts are good sources of protein (7.5-8.5% nitrogen dry weight) and also contain 2-6, 5-9, and 6-12 percent fat, ash and nucleic acid respectively (Kihlberg 1972, Tannenbaum 1973).

The most popular yeasts are of the genera Saccharomyces and Candida because of their long tradition of use in foods.

The amino acid composition of microbial proteins are generally well balanced except they are deficient in sulfur containing amino acids especially methionine, when compared to egg protein (Kihlberg 1972). The concentration of most amino acids is higher than in the original intact dried cells. Nelson et al. (1960) studied the methionine content of 271 strains of yeast and found values of 0.4 - 1.7 g/16g of nitrogen. The total essential amino acid content of yeast (S. fragilis) protein was 44, compared to 52 (grams of amino essential acids per 100g of protein) for egg protein (Vananuvat and Kinsella 1975)a). The lower biological value is attributed to the limiting amounts of methionine and tryptophan in these yeast proteins.

Nutritional. The general digestibility of yeast is good but several problems, i.e. potential (acute and chronic) toxicity, gastrointestinal upsets, nausea, vomiting, diarrhea rashes, caused by ingredients (endotoxins, metabolites) emphasize the general need

for refining yeast protein for human diets. Young et al. (1976) listed some of the concerns requiring study before microbial protein
should be used in human foods. These included physiological aspects
i.e. nutritional value as a major and/or supplementary protein source;
physiological effects of cell wall materials and their constituents;
examination of safety, allergenicity, intolerance and effects of
nucleic acids and purines; palatability and acceptability.

The nutritional value (and safety) of SCP biomass has been
studied to a relatively limited extent and conflicting reports
exist (Scrimshaw 1975, Tannenbaum 1973, Young et al. 1976). There
have been numerous reports of gastro-intestinal problems following
ingestion of intact cells and cell homogenates rather than refined
protein. Conflicting reports exist on this problem and these may
to some extent be attributed to the various strains fed, contam-
inants of various kinds and different processing of the biomass before consumption. Feeding trials have shown that C. utilis cells
are not as good as animal protein partly because of cell wall
materials and low methionine. Isolation of the protein improves
digestibility 50 percent over the homogenized cells (Kihlberg 1972,
Worgan 1974). Supplementation with methionine enhanced protein
value. The protein utilization values of only a limited number of
microbial species have been reported (NPU ranged from 0.38 to 0.6)
(Worgan 1974). Human tolerance tests are essential to determine if
SCP will cause allergic reactions or digestive disturbances when
ingested by man (Young and Scrimshaw 1975).

Cell wall material in unfractionated SCP is undesirable because
it reduces the bioavailability of proteins; may contain antigenic,
allergenic agents and factors causing nausea, gastro-intestinal disturbances (flatulence diarrhea); the cell wall materials may also
cause darkening, i.e. off coloring, of the SCP (Scrimshaw 1975,
Tannenbaum 1973, 1975, Young et al. 1976, Young and Scrimshaw 1976).
The presence of cell wall material also impairs the desirable functional properties of the proteins in various food applications.
For the above reasons and for many potential applications of the
protein(s) it is very desirable to separate cell wall material from
the protein(s) for food applications, and much research is needed
to develop a practical method for isolation of yeast proteins in an
intact, undenatured state from the yeast cell wall material.
    Cell Rupture. The most effective utilization of yeast protein
is not possible until the rigid, indigestible cell wall is removed.
The cell wall of the yeast amounts to approximately 15% of the dry
weight of the cell and is made up of 30 to 40% mannans, 30 to 60%
glucans, 5 to 10% proteins and about 1% chitin. The composition of
the cell wall is influenced by growth conditions and species of
yeast (Phaff 1977).

The principal methods used for rupturing yeast cells are mechanical disruption and enzymatic digestion of the cell walls. The

latter approach is attractive because of its low energy requirement
and enhanced efficiency compared to mechanical cell breakage. Enzymatic digestion of the cell wall components is a feasible approach
(Carenburg 1970, Mogren and Lindblom 1974). This may be achieved
by endogenous β glucanases produced within the yeast or by exogenous
enzymes obtained from microbes (Phaff 1977). Yeasts contain auto-
lytic enzymes which can slowly digest the cell wall once they are
activated. Non-polar organic solvents (chloroform, ethyl acetate)
or inorganic salts (sodium chloride) activate these endogenous enzymes and accelerate autolysis. Autolysis may also be stimulated
by heat shock and resuspension of the cells at 45°C (Johnson 1977).
Studies in our laboratory have demonstrated that low molecular
weight thiol compounds are effective for activating endogenous enzymes which degrade yeast cell walls (Shetty and Kinsella 1978).

    Yeast cells exposed to monothioglycerol, 2-mercaptoethanol or
dithiothreitol and incubated at 37° showed a progressive release of
glucose, indicating the gradual autolysis of the cell wall. Mono-
thioglycerol (50 mM) was most effective in causing the release of
glucose. These treatments also markedly facilitated the extractability of proteins from the yeast cell. The increased extractability of protein following treatment of the cells with thiol
reagents was associated with breakage of the cell wall. However,
there was concomitant degradation of the yeast protein as incuba-
tions were continued, indicating that the thiol reagents also reac-
tivated the endogenous proteases in the yeast cells. Thus the
quantity of protein with a molecular weight, above 100,000, progressively decreased from 80% to 20% after 10 hours incubation.
This hydrolysis of proteins epitomizes one of the major problems
confronting the food chemist concerned with the recovery of proteins from yeast cells, i.e. treatments which facilitate cell rupture activate endogenous proteases which in turn hydrolyze the proteins resulting in significantly reduced yields of protein.

    Effective disintegration of yeast cell walls has been achieved
using mechanical methods (Cunningham 1977, Dunhill and Lilly 1975,
Vananuvat and Kinsella 1975b). They demonstrated the effectiveness
of various methods, i.e. grinding, homogenization, freeze thawing,
pressure-cell, sonic oscillation and milling on release of protein
from yeast. The Manton-Gaulin homogenizer is widely used for disintegration on commercial scale (Newell et al. 1975, Robbins 1975).
For commercial processing, efficient and complete cell breakage is
highly desirable for ensuring maximum extractability and recovery
of protein. Mechanical methods require large energy expenditures
to achieve efficient rupture of the cell wall. Thermal denaturation of the protein during cell breakage is frequent.

    Treatment of yeast cells with alkali pH 11 weakens the cell

wall and facilitates the rupture by mechanical methods. This is a common procedure used for the recovery of yeast proteins, however alkali treatment of food grade proteins is undesirable because it may cause hydrolysis of the protein, depolymerization, racemization of component amino acids, β elimination reactions, and subsequent cross linking and denaturation (Cheftel et al. 1977, Friedman 1977a).

Another significant problem associated with consumption of microbial cells is the high content of nucleic acid (NA) which ranges from 8 to 25 gms nucleic acid per 100 gms protein in various cells. Most of the nucleic acid is present as RNA (Sinskey and Tannenbaum 1975). Before single cell protein can be used as a major source of protein for human consumption, the content of nucleic acid must be reduced, so that the daily intake of nucleic acid from yeast would not exceed 2 g on dry weight basis. Higher quantities cause uricemia and continued ingestion of SCP may result in gout (Miller 1968, Waslien et al. 1970).

TABLE 1

Summary of methods available for reduction of RNA in yeast

Method	Advantages	Disadvantages
Control of growth rate by substrate limitation	Simplest method, no added chemicals	Limited reduction, economics
Base-catalyzed hydrolysis	Simple and rapid	Loss of protein, salt addition deleterious effects of high pH on amino acids
Chemical extraction	Simple, rapid, remove polymerized RNA	Chemical residues, loss of weight and protein
Cell disruption	Only if protein isolate desired	Economics, others specific to process used
Exogenous RNase	Rapid, simple, choice of enzyme	Cost and availability of enzyme, loss of dry matter; proteolysis
Endogenous RNase heat shock, anions	Simple, cells direct from fermentor	Proteolysis, poor yield, slow, only certain organisms

from Tannenbaum 1977

Nucleic acid content of yeast cells can be reduced by decreasing the growth rate, but this is not practical since rapid growth is obligatory in most processes for economic cell production. Thus, reduction of the nucleic acids present in cells or protein preparations is necessary if SCP is to be used in reasonable quantities as source of food protein. Tannenbaum (1977) discussed the possible advantages and disadvantages of the various methods used for removal of nucleic acids from SCP (Table 1). The two principle approaches have employed ribonclease (endogenous and exogenous) or chemical (usually alkali) treatments.

The heat-shock process for reducing NA of Candida utilis was developed by Ohta et al. (1971). This consists of an initial heat-shock, at 68°C for 1 to 6 sec, of the yeast cells followed by incubation for 2 hrs around 52°C at pH 5-6. Hydrolysis of RNA by endogenous RNase and leaking of accumulated hydrolysis products into the suspending medium occurs. The nucleic acid content is reduced from an initial value of 8 percent to less than 2 percent. The addition of carboxylic anions during the heat-shock process facilitate the reduction of the nucleic acids (Sinskey and Tannenbaum 1975). Sodium chloride improves the degradation of NA by endogenous RNase (Lindblom 1977).

Lindblom and Mogren (1977) reported the use of sodium chloride to enhance the ribonuclease activity in homogenized yeast cells. The salt (4%) added after homogenization caused a remarkable reduction in RNA at incubation temperature between 48 and 62°C ar pH between 5 to 9. At the lower pHs, precipitation of the protein occurred during the incubation, hence the pH should be in the neighborhood of 9. Acidic precipitation should be slow so that large flocs of protein are formed. This facilitates separation of the protein with a NA content of 1-3 per cent.

Castro et al. (1971) showed that exogenous pancreatic RNase could be used for the reduction of nucleic acid in yeast. Newell et al. (1975) patented a process of making isolated yeast protein low in nucleic acid by adding exogenous nuclease from malt sprouts to proteins separated from ruptured yeast cells. Robbins et al. (1975) patented a process of making yeast protein isolate having below 3 percent nucleic acid using endogenous RNase to solubilize the nucleic acid of the yeast. This process consists of extracting the proteins and nuclease from the disrupted cells at alkaline pH. The extracted soluble proteins plus NA were separated by centrifugation. Then the pH of the supernatant was decreased to 5-6 and this preparation was incubated at 52°C for 2 hrs to allow the endogenous nuclease to digest the nucleic acids. The protein precipitated from this incubated supernatant contained less than 1 percent nucleic acid.

A limited amount of information is available concerning the

preparation of SCP concentrate with reduced nucleic acid content
using chemical extraction methods. Hedenskog and Ebbinghous (1972)
prepared protein concentrates from yeast by acid precipitation of
the alkali-extracted protein after cell wall removal. Alkaline
extraction combined with high ionic strength (NaCl), heat treatments and acid precipitation can be used to significantly reduce
NA contamination of yeast protein (Hedenskog and Ebbinghous 1972,
Lindblom 1977).

     There are serious drawbacks associated with all of these
methods. The heat-shock process and use of RNase is disadvantageous
because of the extensive proteolysis, which proceeds concurrently
and significantly reduces the yield of protein. In addition, these
processes are time consuming and exogenous enzyme is very expensive.
The chemical methods, while effective result in degradation and denaturation of the protein and possible chemical alteration, with
reduction of nutritive value. The alterations of the yeast protein
is a serious drawback because it destroys many of the critical functional properties of the protein (Kinsella et al. 1976).

     Thus, better method(s) for the reduction of nucleic acids while
preventing or minimizing proteolysis and avoiding denaturation of
the proteins are needed.

                        Protein Extraction

     Ideally microbial cells should be consumable directly as food
or food ingredients. However, because of their nucleic acid content; the presence of undesirable physiologically active components;
the deleterious effects of cell wall material on protein bioavailability and the lack of requisite and discrete functional properties of intact cells rupture of cells and extraction of the protein is a necessary step. Importantly, for many food uses (particularly as a functional protein ingredient) an undenatured protein is
required. Therefore, there exists an immediate need to develop a
practical procedure for the isolation of intact, undenatured protein with a low nucleic acid content, or if this is not feasible to
isolate proteins with useful functional properties.

     The few studies to date indicate that dried cells have limited
functional properties (Labuza 1972, Labuza and Jones 1973). Thus,
to improve nutritional value and exploit functional properties,
extraction and concentration of the protein is necessary. Numerous
techniques have been developed for the extraction of yeast proteins
(Dunhill and Lilly 1975, Hedenskog and Mogren 1973, Mateles and
Tannenbaum 1968, Tannenbaum and Wang 1975, Vananuvat and Kinsella
1975), but few produce a protein with the properties that meet the
necessary nutritional and functional criteria. For the extraction

TABLE 2

Methods used for release of cell components

Methods	Disadvantages
Autolysis	Slow process. Poor yield (50-60%)
Plasmolysis	Less efficient
Hydrolysis (acid)	High salt concentration in the finished product (>25%)
Lytic enzymes and thiol reagents	Cost. Activation of proteolytic enzymes. Significant weight loss.
Chemicals	Effective only at high concentrations. Requires longer period. Denaturation and degradation of proteins.
Mechanical	Cost

of protein from microbial cells extensive chemical treatment of physical rupture is necessary to render the cell contents available to the extractant. Lysis of cell wall with endogenous or exogenous β-1,3 glucanases has been employed (Carenburg and Heden 1970, Hockenhull 1971, Johnson 1977, Mogren and Lindblom 1974, Phaff 1977). This approach results in poor yields of protein because of extensive proteolysis.

For maximizing protein yield and minimizing contaminant nucleic acids, alkali extraction at elevated temperatures is the most practical procedure (Cunningham 1977, Lindblom 1977, Vananuvat and Kinsella 1975b). Hedenskog and Mogren (1973) reported that by heating (80°C for 8 sec. an alkaline extract (pH 9 - 11.5) of mechanically disintegrated yeast cells, a protein concentrate (70-75%) with good nutritive value (PER 2.1) and low nucleic acid (<2%) could be obtained. Lomdblom (1974) showed that extraction disintegrated yeast at pH 6 and pH 11 and precipitation with acid pH 4, or heat 80°C at pH 8, in presence of 5 percent NaCl, yielded proteins with low NA but possessing poor solubility below pH 8.

The most common method for obtaining protein isolate with low nucleic acid consists of extracting the protein from mechanically disrupted cells with concentrated alkali followed by precipitating the extracted protein either by decreasing the pH to 4.5 (Lindblom 1974) or by heating at 80°C (Vananuvat & Kinsella 1975b) (Table 3).

The high concentration of alkali inactivates the proteolytic enzymes of the yeast, thereby controlling the weight loss due to proteolysis and causes reduction of the ribonucleic acid, but these

TABLE 3

Methods used for protein isolation with reduced nucleic acid

Methods	Description	Disadvantages	References
DRASTIC CONDITION	Alkaline extraction (0.2M NaOH) followed by heat precipitation of protein [80°]	Loss of weight and nitrogen. Degradation and denaturation of proteins. Formation of new substances because of the side reaction, i.e. lysinoalanine, sulphones, etc. Deleterious effects of high pH.	Hedenskog and Ebbinghaus (1972) Cunningham et al. (1977) Hedenskog and Mogren (1973) Vananuvat and Kinsella (1975 Lindblom (1974)
MILD CONDITION	Extraction of protein from mechanically disrupted cells at slightly alkaline pH and incubating the extract for RNA reduction by making use of endogenous RNase and exogenous RNase	Loss of protein because of proteolysis during incubation process (more than 50%), cost.	Newell et al. (1975) Robbins et al. (1975) Lindblom (1977)

drastic conditions cause degradation and denaturation of the isolated protein.

Denaturation of proteins during extraction is a serious problem because it significantly destroys functional properties and therefore limits the food applications of the extracted protein (Kinsella 1977, Vananuvat and Kinsella 1978). Exposure of protein to alkaline treatments, in addition to denaturation, may also cause other undesirable effects, i.e. racemization of amino acids, β-elimination and cross-linking of certain amino acids and formation of potentially antinutritive compounds (Cheftel 1977, Feeney 1977b, Friedman 1977a). While these changes are reputedly minimal under mild processing conditions, the possibility of their occurrence under the more drastic conditions (time, temperature, pH) prevailing during large scale processing is a matter of concern.

The drawbacks associated with the conventional methods of protein extraction from yeast revealed the need for novel methods for the extraction of functional protein low in nucleic acid in high

yield from yeast cells. We have developed such a method employing
succinylation (Kinsella and Shetty 1978) to render the yeast protein
resistant to proteolysis during extraction and nucleic acid reduction. The chemistry of succinylation is reviewed later. In this
process, yeast cells are ruptured in aqueous buffer, pH 8.5, and
extracted (Shetty and Kinsella 1978). However the inclusion of
succinic anhydride, and maintenance of the pH at 8.5, during extraction resulted in a significant increase in protein extractability, i.e. from the usual 55–60% to 90% of the protein of the
yeast cell. This was significant because the pH of extract represented very mild conditions compared to conventional procedures.
Maximum extraction was obtained when 100 per cent of all free amino
groups were succinylated.

During conventional extraction of yeast protein, and incubation
at 55°C (pH 6) to reduce nucleic acid, there is a progressive precipitation of protein as hydrolysis of RNA proceeds. This coagulated protein is very difficult to resolubilize and has limited
functional properties. Furthermore, during the incubation extensive
proteolysis by endogenous proteases reduces the total yield of protein. Both of these events limit the practical use of this approach
for reducing RNA. However succinylation of 80% of amino groups
eliminated this precipitation of the protein. In addition the degradation of proteins by endogenous proteases during incubation was
eliminated resulting in increased yields of intact soluble protein,
i.e. negligible proteolysis occurred compared to the 70% that occurs
during normal extraction and incubation (Lindblom 1977) (Fig. 1).
However succinylation also inactivated the ribonuclease thereby im-
pairing the hydrolysis of nucleic acid during extraction. Nevertheless, by precipitating the succinylated protein at pH 4.5 a protein
isolate (>90% protein) with less than 1.8% nucleic acid was obtained
(Fig. 2).

This procedure is a significant and practical discovery in developing a process for the isolation of a soluble protein, low in
nucleic acid, in high yields from yeast cells (Fig. 3). The procedure is rapid, it eliminates the incubation (4–5 hr) step, avoids
proteolysis, and is amenable to current extraction procedures. The
method is effective when dicarboxylic residues are introduced but
is less successful with acetylation. The functional properties of
these succinylated proteins are described below.

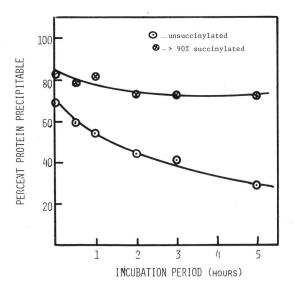

Figure 1. The relative recoveries of protein from yeast cells following incubation after extraction with and without succinylation.

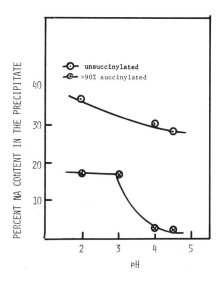

Figure 2. The nucleic acid content of proteins precipitated at different pHs following extraction in the presence and absence of succinic anhydride.

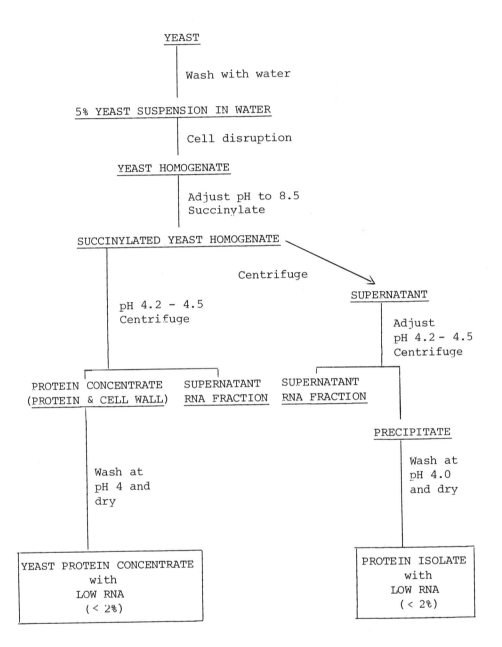

Figure 3.   Schematic outline of the succinylation procedure for
             the isolation of yeast protein concentrate (72% protein)
             or yeast protein isolate 92% protein with low (<2%)
             nucleic acid.

FUNCTIONAL PROPERTIES OF YEAST PROTEINS

Yeast proteins, in addition to being nutritionally good and safe, must possess functional properties to be adopted by the food industry and to gain general consumer acceptance. Information on functional properties of SCP is needed to evaluate and predict how these new proteins behave in specific food systems and if they can be used to complement, replace or simulate conventional proteins in different foods. The successful adoption of SCP will depend upon their acceptance by the food manufacturing industry. To achieve adoption (in addition to availability, cost, nutritive value, safety) the physicochemical properties and processing characteristics of the protein(s) must be fully described. These properties must be known to determine (and predict) how these proteins will behave in a variety of food applications, if they can be used to replace more expensive proteins, and their capacity for the fabrication of new proteinaceous foods.

There is a limited amount of information published concerning the functional properties of yeast proteins intended for food applications, though proprietary knowledge exists (Akin 1976, Newell et al. 1975). Tannenbaum (1971) alluded to the importance of functional properties and the need for study of physical properties of SCP. The information on various functional properties has been reviewed (Vananuvat and Kinsella 1978).

Flavor, color, texture are important primary properties of proteins. In novel proteins the absence of flavors or odors is desired to render the new protein compatible with the food to which they are added. Off-flavors frequently limit the use of new protein preparations including SCP (Lipinsky and Litchfield 1974). Frequently these arise from the lipid materials which are associated with the isolated proteins.

Solubility is a critical functional characteristic because many functional properties depend on the capacity of proteins to go into solution initially, e.g. gelation, emulsification, foam formation. Data on solubility of a protein under a variety of environmental conditions (pH, ionic strength, temperature) are useful diagnostically in providing information on prior treatment of a protein (i.e. if denaturation has occurred) and as indices of the potential applications of the protein. Determination of solubility is the first test in evaluation of the potential functional properties of proteins and retention of solubility is a useful criterion when selecting methods for isolating and refining protein preparations (Kinsella 1976).

Several researchers have reported on the solubility of extracted microbial proteins (Lindblom 1974 & 1977, Robbins et al. 1975, Vananuvat and Kinsella 1975c). In many instances yeast proteins

demonstrate very inferior solubility properties below pH 7.5
because of denaturation.

The foaming and emulsifying capacity of yeast proteins have
been studied (Lindblom 1974, Vananuvat and Kinsella 1975c).
Rha (1975) has summarized the limited information on the
fiber forming ability of proteins from C. utilis.

The available data indicate that yeast proteins extracted by
the current, conventional methods lack the requisite functional
properties for many applications. Therefore, in conjunction with
the need for research on extraction methods to isolate functional
proteins there is a concurrent and justifiable need for the development of methods (physical, chemical, enzymatic) for imparting
specific functional properties to yeast proteins.
    Protein Modification: Several approaches have been used to
improve the functional properties of proteins by physical, enzymatic or chemical agents (Kinsella 1977). Modification may be viewed
as an approach to improve functionality and expand the applications
of novel proteins, and also as a means of facilitating the selection
of the most practical methods of extraction and preparation of protein.

The recent development of physical methods for texturizing
novel proteins significantly expanded their potential use in foods
and simulated foods (Kinsella 1978). Rha (1975) has reviewed the
information concerning the spinning of protein fibers from S.C.P.
Tannenbaum (1974) patented a process for texturizing single cell
protein pastes by extrusion. The textured, chewy extrudate which
had a permanent structure could be flavored or fried, or added to
products as a filler.

During isolation from single cells by conventional methods,
proteins frequently become insolubilized and nonfunctional. These
proteins can be rendered more soluble by limited hydrolysis with
acid, alkali or proteolytic enzymes. Protein hydrolyzates are
most commonly prepared by partial acid hydrolysis and yeast hydrolyzates are popular as food flavorings and ingredients (Johnson 1977).
Acid hydrolyzates have flavors resembling cooked meats and are widely
used by canners to impart brothy, meaty flavors to soups, gravies,
sauces, canned meats. Recently the use of protein hydrolyzates in
the formulation of proteinaceous, acidic soft drinks has received
intensive study (Johnson 1977).

Alkali treatment has been used for improving the functional
properties of the insoluble protein prepared by heat precipitation
of an alkaline extract of broken yeast cells (Hedenskog and Mogren
(1972). Heating this protein (60°C for 20 min) at pH 11.8
followed by acid precipitation (pH 4.5) yielded a protein with
increased aqueous solubility and significantly increased the

protein nitrogen content of these preparations which was composed of polypeptides with a wide range of molecular weights. It also increased foaming capacity of the protein 20-fold and the foam was also stable. The emulsion capacity of the modified protein was good whereas the original insoluble protein was incapable of forming an emulsion. However, alkaline treatment resulted in a loss (60%) of cysteine. Heating in the presence of alkali adversely affects the nutritive value of protein by causing racemization of amino acids, destruction of amino acids, threonine, serine, cystine and formation of reactive dehydroalanine (Table 4). These adversely affect the nutritive value of proteins (Cheftel 1977, De Groot et al. 1977, Friedman, 1977b)

TABLE 4

Effect of severe alkali treatment of proteins

---

1. Racemization of amino acids, e.g. methionine, lysine

2. Destruction of amino acids, e.g. lysine, cysteine, serine, threonine

3. Splitting of peptide bonds

4. Formation of new amino acids, e.g. dehydroalanine, lysinoalanine via β-elimination and condensation reactions

---

Enzyme hydrolysis is occasionally used to modify the functional properties of proteins, and yeast autolyzates are used commercially as food flavorants (Johnson 1977, Reed and Peppler 1973). Partial proteolysis of novel proteins improves their solubility and foaming properties (Hermansson et al. 1974). The problem associated with enzyme hydrolysis are excessive hydrolysis, especially under batch conditions; the generation of bitter peptides and the cost of enzymes. Fujimaki and co-workers (1977) have summarized their extensive work on enzyme hydrolysis and the plastein reaction as a means of improving the functional properties of novel proteins. Plastein synthesis effectively debittered pepsin hydrolyzates of yeasts (Saccaromyces, Candida); aided the release of lipid materials responsible for the development of off-flavors and reduced pigments and heme materials present in the original SCP. Transesterification of proteins from various sources via the plastein reaction can be used to incorporate superior nutritional and functional polypeptides. Several food proteins, casein, ovalbumin, zein, gluten, soybean, fish, yeasts and various oilseed proteins can be successfully exploited in this reaction. Thus, proteins from widely different sources can be interesterified, though yields from this reaction depend on protein source and the particular combination of enzymes used (Fujimaki et al. 1977).

Chemical Modification. Intentional chemical alteration of
proteins by derivatization of functional groups on the side chains
offers numerous opportunities for the development of new functional
ingredients and improved processing procedures.

The conformation of a protein is governed by its amino acid composition and their sequence as influenced by the immediate environment. The secondary, tertiary and quaternary structures of proteins
are mostly due to noncovalent interactions between the side chains
of contiguous and apposed amino acid residues. Covalent disulfide
bonds may be important in the maintenance of tertiary and quaternary
structure. The non-covalent forces are hydrogen-bonding, electrostatic interactions, Van der Waals interactions and hydrophobic
associations. The relative importance of these in relation to protein structure and function has been discussed by Ryan (1977). Because of the side chains of component amino acids and their involvement in noncovalent interactions markedly influence structure and
function of proteins, the chemical modification of specific functional groups should facilitate alteration of functional properties.
This also may provide useful information concerning the role of
specific amino acid groups in conformation and functionality of
a protein.

Modification of proteins is widely practiced in fundamental
research on proteins (Cohen 1968, Friedman 1977b, Hirs and Timasheff
1972, Knowles 1974, Means and Feeney 1971, Glazer 1976, Stark 1970,
Vallee and Riordan 1969) and a broad range of reagents (mostly
unsuitable for use with food proteins) have been developed (Hirs
and Timasheff 1972).

Knowles (1974) summarized the chemistry of residue modification.
With regard to side chain reactivity, amino acid side chains may be
divided into three classes - electron rich, electron deficient and
neutral. Chemical modification predominantly involves nucleophilic
or reductive reactions of electron rich side chains. There are
several types of electron rich nucleophilic groups: the nitrogen
of the ε-amino, imidazole and guanidino groups of lysine, histidine
and arginine, respectively; the oxygen nucleophiles of the hydroxyl,
phenolic and carboxyl groups of serine, threonine, tyrosine, glutamic
and aspartic acids, respectively; the sulphur nucleophile of
cysteine and the thioether group of methionine. Reagents susceptible to nucleophilic attack may react with any of these groups.
However, the reactivity of nucleophilic groups are greatly influenced by pH, via the pKa values of these electron rich groups. In
addition, the reactivity of these groups depends upon their accessibility, the size of the modifying agent and reaction conditions,
i. e. temperature and solvent used. Most side chain groups are modified when they are non-protonated, i.e. nucleophilic. The pH (pK)
determines reactivity. Thus, α-amino and thiol groups are reactive
above pH 7.5, the ε-amino group of lysine above pH 8.5, where they

are mostly non-protonated (Feeney 1977a, Friedman 1977b), and the
phenolic group of tyrosine above pH 10. These pKa values may vary
in different proteins depending upon their microenvironment (Knowles
1974). Reagents used to modify proteins should have a reasonable
half-life in aqueous solution at the pH values of the reaction to
enable the protein to react with the active derivative (Knowles
1974, Means and Feeney 1971).

Common methods of derivatization are acylation of amino,
hydroxyl and phenolic residues; alkylation of amino, indole, phenolic, sulfhydryl and thioether groups; esterification of carboxyl;
oxidation of indole, thiol and thoether groups and reduction of
disulfide groups (Feeney 1977a).

Protein acylation reactions presumably follow the carbonyl
addition pathway (Means and Feeney 1971) as shown below:

$$
\underset{X}{\overset{O}{\underset{|}{\overset{||}{R-C}}}} \longleftarrow :NH_2 \;\rightleftharpoons\; \left[\underset{X}{\overset{O^-}{\underset{|}{\overset{|}{R-C-NH_2^+}}}} \right] \pm H^+ \rightleftharpoons \left[\underset{X}{\overset{O^-}{\underset{|}{\overset{|}{R-C-NH}}}} \right] \rightleftharpoons \underset{NH}{\overset{O}{\overset{||}{R-C}}} + X^-
$$

The rates of reaction depend upon the rate of nucleophilic attack
and upon the percentage of tetrahedral intermediates which undergo
fission at the carbonyl-X bond. Except at very high pH (> 11) acylation rates for homologous nucleophiles are inversely related to pK
values. Where steric effects or pH render nucleophilic amino acid
residues resistant to reaction, hydrolysis of the active derivative
becomes the favored reaction because of the presence of large
amounts of water in the reaction media.

The number of nucleophilic residues acylated is influenced by
the level of acylating reagent used; the amino acid composition of
the protein, ease of reactivity (i.e. accessability) of amino acids
with acylating agent (protein size and conformation, extent of
protein denaturation) and the reaction conditions, i.e. temperature,
agitation, purity of reagents, and particularly pH. The phenolic
groups of tyrosine are readily acylated compared with the other
amino acid residues. The tyrosine phenolic groups, however, have
a higher pK and are ususally more protected from reaction (buried
in the interior of the protein) than the free amino groups. Acylation of histidine and cysteine residues is seldom observed because
the reaction products hydrolyze in aqueous solution. Serine and
threonine hydroxyl groups are weak nucleophiles and are not easily
acylated in aqueous solution. Under most conditions prevailing
in foods, the ε-amino group of lysine residues are most reactive
(Means and Feeney 1971, Friedman 1977b). The reaction rate of lysine
in aqueous solution increases in proportion to the concentration of
unprotonated amino groups(ε-NH$_2$, pKa 10.5).

Chemical modification may be used for several purposes in food proteins to block reactive groups involved in deteriorative reactions; to improve nutritional properties, to enhance digestibility; to impart thermal stability; to modify physicochemical properties; to facilitate study of structure-function relationships and to facilitate separationk processing and refining of proteins (Bjarnason and Carpenter 1970, Feeney 1977a, Kinsella and Shetty 1978).

Numerous undesirable reactions that result in organoleptic, nutritional and functional deterioration may occur in food proteins during processing and storage. These include the non-enzymatic or Maillard reactions, transamidation; condensation reactions with dehydroalanine forming cross-links, and carbonyl amine interactions, all of which may involve the free ε-amino group of lysine (Feeney 1977b, Friedman 1977b). To minimize these reactions a significant volume of work has been done on the protective modification of the ε-NH$_2$ of lysine. Bjarnason and Carpenter (1970) reported that formylation, acetylation and propionylation considerably reduced the extent of the Maillard reaction in food proteins. The formyl and acetylated derivatives were available nutritionally whereas propionylated lysine was not utilized. Feeney (1977a, 1977b) reviewed modification of ε-NH$_2$ groups by reductive methylation to protect the ε-NH$_2$ group from Maillard reactions. In vitro studies revealed that peptides containing dimethylated residues significantly inhibited hydrolysis by chymotrypsin (Feeney 1977a, Galembeck et al. 1977).

Modification to directly enhance the nutritive value of protein has received little attention. The possibility of introducing essential amino acids into vegetable proteins deficient in specific amino acids warrants study. Recently Whitaker (1978) reported the successful introduction of methionine residues into proteins thereby improving nutritional value.

The acylation (and alkylation) of various chemical groups into proteins provides a method whereby a broad spectrum of functional compounds may be incorporated into proteins. Studies of chemically derivatized food proteins have only recently been undertaken as a result of the critical need for proteins with improved and controlled functional properties (Kinsella 1977). Generally derivatization enhances the thermal stability of food proteins and reduces thermal coagulation and precipitation (Barman et al. 1977, Gandi et al. 1968, Groniger 1973).

For the modification of vegetable or yeast proteins acetic and succinic anhydrides have been the most common derivatives used and under the conditions employed the ε-NH$_2$ is the principal site of acylation. Acetylation does not significantly enhance functional properties of proteins, but it does improve thermal stability. By virtue of its susceptibility to in vivo enzyme hydrolysis it affords a useful reagent for protection of ε-NH$_2$ groups of lysine in food proteins during heating or storage (Feeney 1977a).

Succinylation of amino acid residues, e.g. α- and ε-amino groups, has three major effects on the physical character of proteins: it increases net negative charge (Habeeb 1967), changes conformation (Gounaris and Perlmann 1967, Habeeb et al. 1958, Shetty and Rao 1978); and increases the propensity of proteins to dissociate into subunits (Table 5).

Electrostatic repulsion(s) resulting from the introduction of succinate anions alter the conformation of the protein and penetration by water molecules is physically easier because of the expanded loosened state of the polypeptides. The structural instability of succinylated proteins results from their high net negative charge and the replacement of short range attractive forces in the native molecule with short range repulsive ones with subsequent unfolding of polypeptide chains. This is accentuated if two negatively charged carboxyl groups are juxtaposed in the succinylated molecule where an ammonium and carboxyl group had been formerly apposed in the unmodified form. This probably accounts for the looser texture, higher bulk density, lighter color, and enhanced solubility and pronounced thermal stability of succinylated food proteins (Kinsella and Shetty 1978).

TABLE 5

Molecular properties of protein affected by succinylation

Increased negative charges

Dissociation into subunits

Conformational changes

Increased viscosity, i.e. swelling

Changes in difference spectra

Chemical modification of yeast protein has received limited attention though as described above it has potential as a method for facilitating recovery of yeast protein.

No off-odors or flavors are imparted by succinylation (Franzen and Kinsella 1976). The proteins hydrate rapidly on the tongue, taste clean, but slightly acidic. It is not known if derivatization facilitates the removal of off-flavors from modified proteins. Currently, the changes in the flavor binding capacity of proteins and the effects of modification on binding characteristics are being studied. It is conceivable that derivatization may facilitate the removal of adsorbed off-flavors from vegetable proteins.

The pH solubility profile of succinylated proteins revealed the typical increased solubility between pH 4 to 6. The succinylated samples became increasingly insoluble below the isoelectric point as the degree of succinylation was increased (Vananuvat and Kinsella 1978). Significantly succinylated yeast proteins were very stable to heat precipitation above pH 5, i.e. they remained soluble at temperatures up to 100°C. As the degree of succinylation was increased the rate of precipitation of the derivatized protein increased in the neighborhood of the isoelectric point and much larger protein flocs were obtained, facilitating their recovery.

The emulsifying capacity of the yeast proteins was significantly and progressively improved with the extent of succinylation as measured by the turbidimetric technique (Pearce and Kinsella 1978). The modified yeast proteins had excellent emulsifying activities compared to several other common proteins (Table 6). McElwain et al. (1975) observed that succinylation of yeast protein increased emulsion viscosity but decreased emulsion stability.

Succinylation during extraction significantly improved the foaming capacity of yeast protein. The succinylated protein was almost equivalent to ovalbumin whereas the unmodified yeast was

TABLE 6

Emulsifying activity index values for various proteins[*]

Protein	Emulsifying Activity Index $(m^2 \cdot g^{-1})$	
	pH 6.5	pH 8.0
Yeast protein (88%) succinylated	322	341
Yeast protein (62%) succinylated	262	332
Sodium dodecylsulfate (0.1%)	251	212
Bovine serum albumin	–	197
Sodium caseinate	149	166
β-lactoglobulin	–	153
Whey protein powder A	119	142
Yeast protein (24%) succinylated	110	204
Whey protein powder B	102	101
Soy protein isolate A	41	92
Hemoglobin	–	75
Soy protein isolate B	26	66
Yeast protein (unmodified)	8	59
Lysozyme	–	50
Egg albumin	–	49

[*]Protein concentration 0.5% in phosphate buffer pH 6.5; I = 0.1. Determined by turbidometric procedure (Pearce and Kinsella 1978).

very inferior and failed to retain gas efficiently during expansion.
The rate of drainage of water from the foam was appreciable for all
proteins being least for ovalbumin which lost 50 percent of water
after 10 minutes and greatest for the unmodified yeast protein which
had collapsed after 10 minutes.

Maximum foam strengths of succinylated yeast protein and ovalbumin occurred slightly above the isoelectric points of these two
proteins. The ovalbumin foam was significantly (100 fold) stronger
than the succinylated yeast protein at similar concentrations of
protein.

The major proteins from yeast have molecular sizes greater than
100,000 daltons. Upon succinylation extensive dissociation of these
high molecular proteins occurred and sedimentation velocity studies
revealed that the succinylated yeast proteins sedimented as a single
band with a sedimentation coefficient of 1S corresponding to molecular weight of 10,000 daltons.

The succinylated yeast proteins were susceptible to hydrolysis
by both α-chymotrypsin and trypsin though the α-chymotrypsin was
more effective than trypsin which tended to be inhibited in time.

These studies demonstrated that chemical derivatization provides a practical approach for facilitating the recovery of highly
functional proteins from yeast cells.

NUTRITIONAL ASPECTS OF MODIFIED PROTEINS

For chemically derivatized proteins to be successfully accepted
as food ingredients they must be digestible, nontoxic, and ideally
the modified amino acid residues should be available nutritionally.
Nutritional studies using modified food proteins are limited and
have been mostly done with modified casein and fish protein. Succinylated and acetylated derivatives have been investigated since
succinic and acetic acids are normal metabolites in the tricarboxylic
acid cycle and thus are least likely to be toxic.

The nutritional effects of proteins with acylated lysine residues were tested by Bjarnason and Carpenter (1969, 1970) who fed
lysine-deficient rats ε-N-acetyl-L-lysine and ε-N-propionyl-L-lysine
as well as acetylated and proprionylated proteins. The ε-N-acetyl
lysine promoted the growth of lysine-deficient rats but demonstrated
only half the activity of lysine. The ε-N-propionyl-L-lysine provided
no detectable growth activity for the rat. Acylated proteins gave
lower responses than equivalent supplements of unmodified protein;
however the differences were not statistically significant with
acetylated bovine albumin. The smallest growth response was obtained with exhaustively propionylated lactalbumin. Creamer et al.

(1971) reported that casein, acetylated casein and succinylated
casein gave PER values of 2.5, 1.6 and 0.3, respectively.

The nutritional impact and safety of chemical modified proteins
should be adequately tested for each derivative. However, it must
be recognized and appreciated by all interested parties, i.e. food
processor, nutritionists, and regulatory agents, that it is unlikely
that a modified protein would be consumed as a significant, much
less a sole source of dietary protein for any particular population
group. Research should be continued even though modification may
reduce the availability of some amino acid residues. Highly functional proteins may well facilitate the incorporation of nutritionally superior, but functionally inferior, proteins into a
variety of foods appealing to a broad range of consumers. Research
to develop functional derivatives that specifically react with non-
limiting amino acids should be encouraged.

ACKNOWLEDGMENT - Some of this work was supported by Grant # Eng
                 75-7273 from the National Science Foundation.

REFERENCES

Akin, C. 1976. Water soluble whippable protein product and process
     for making same. U.S. Patent 3,833,552.
Anon. 1974. "A Hungry World", General Report, Univ. California,
     Berkley, California Task Force.
Barman, B. G., Hansen, J. and Mossey, A. 1977. Modification of the
     physical properties of soy protein isolate by acetylation.
     J. Agr. Food Chem. 25: 638.
Bellamy, W. D. 1974. Single cell protein from cellulosic wastes.
     Biotechnol. Bioeng. 16: 869.
Bjornason, J. and Carpenter, K. J. 1969. Mechanism of heat damage
     in proteins. I. Models with acylated lysine units. Br. J. Nut.
     23: 859.
Bjornason, J. and Carpenter, K. J. 1970. Mechanism of heat damage
     in proteins. Chemical changes in pure proteins. Br. J. Nutr.
     24: 313.
Burrows, V., Green, A. H., Korol, M. A., Melnychyn, P., Pearson, G.
     and Sibbald,I. 1972. Food protein from grains and oilseeds.
     Can. Wheat Board, Ottawa, Canada.
Carenberg, C. O. and Heden, C. G. 1970. Experiments with lysis of
     living cells of Eremothecium   ashbyii and of Methanomonas by
     microbial enzymes. Biotechnol. & Bioeng. 12: 167.
Castro, A. C., Sinskey, A. J. and Tannenbaum, S. R. 1971. Reduc-
     tion of nucleic acid content in Candida yeast cells by bovine
     pancreatic ribonuclease A treatment. Appl. Microbiol. 22: 422.
Cheftel, J. C. 1977. Chemical and nutritional modifications of
     food proteins due to processing and storage. In Food Proteins.
     Whitaker and Tannenbaum, Eds. Avi Publ. Co., Westport, Conn.

p. 404.

Cohen, L. A. 1968. Group-specific reagents in protein chemistry. Ann. Rev. Biochemistry 37: 695.

Cooney, C. L., Levine, D. W. and Snedecor, B. 1975. Production of single cell protein from methanol. Food Technol. 29: 32.

Creamer, L., Roeper, J. and Lohry, E. 1971. Preparation and evaluation of some acid soluble casein derivatives. N.Z.J. Dairy Science and Technol. 6: 107.

Cunningham, S. D., Cater, C. M. and Mattil, K. F. 1977. Rupture and protein extraction of petroleum grown yeast. J. Food Sci. 40: 732.

DeGroot, A. P., Slump, P., Van Beek, L. and Feron, V. J. 1977. Severe alkali treatment of protein in evaluation of proteins for humans. Bodwell C., Ed. Avi Publ. Co., Westport, Conn. p. 270.

Dunhill, P. and Lilly, M. D. 1975. Protein extraction and recovery from microbial cells. In Single Cell Protein II. Tannenbaum and Wang, Eds. M.I.T. Press, Cambridge, Mass. p. 179.

Feeney, R. E. 1977a. Chemical modification of food proteins in food proteins. Feeney and Whitaker, Eds. Am. Chem. Soc., Washington, D. C. p. 3

Feeney, R. E. 1977b. Chemical changes in food proteins in evaluation of proteins for humans. Bodwell, Ed. Avi Publishing Co., Westport, Conn. p. 233.

Franzen, K. L. and Kinsella, J. E. 1976. Functional properties of succinylated and acetylated soy protein. J. Agric. Food Chem. 24: 788.

Friedman, M. 1977a. Protein crosslinking -- stereochemistry and nomenclature. In Protein Crosslinking: Nutritional and Medical Consequences. Friedman, Ed. Plenum, New York, p. 1-26.

Friedman, M. 1977b. Effects of lysine modification on chemical, physical, nutritive and functional properties of proteins. In Food Proteins, Whitaker and Tannenbaum, Eds. Avi Publ. Co., Westport, Conn. p. 446.

Fujimaki, M., Arai, S., Yamashita, M. 1977. Enzymatic protein degradation and resynthesis for protein improvement. In Food Proteins. Feeney and Whitaker, Eds. Am. Chem. Soc., Washington, D. C. p. 156.

Galembeck, F., Ryan, D. S., Whitaker, J. R. and Feeney, R. E. 1977. Reaction of proteins with formaldehyde in the presence and absence of sodium borohydride. J. Agr. Food Chem. 25: 238.

Gandhi, S. K., Schultz, J. R., Boughey, F. W. and Forsythe, R. H. 1968. Chemical modification of egg white with 3,3-dimethylglutaric anhydride. J. Food Sci. 33: 163.

Glazer, A. N. 1976. The chemical modification of proteins by group-specific and site-specific reagents. In The Proteins, Vol. 2, Neurath, Mill & Boeder, Eds. Academic Press., N. Y.

Gounaris, A. and Perlmann, G. E. 1967. Succinylation of

pepsinogen. J. Biol. Chem. 242: 2739.

Groninger, H. S. 1973. Preparation and properties of succinylated fish myofibrillar protein. J. Agr. Food Chem. 21: 978.

Habeeb, A.F.S.A. 1967. Quantification of conformational changes on chemical modification of proteins: Use of succinylated proteins as a model. Arch. Biochem. Biophys. 121: 652.

Habeeb, A.F.S.A., Cassidy, H., Singer, S. 1958. Molecular structural effects produced in proteins by reaction with succinic anhydride. Biochim. Biophys. Acta 29: 587.

Hedenskog, G. and Ebbinghaus, L. 1972. Reduction of the nucleic acid content of single-cell protein concentrates. Biotechnol. Bioeng. 14: 447.

Hedenskog, G. and Mogren, H. 1973. Some methods for processing of single-cell protein. Biotechnol. Bioeng. 15: 129.

Hermansson, A. M., Olsson I. and Holmberg, B. 1974. Functional properties of proteins for foods: Modification of rapeseed protein concentrates. Lebensmitt Wiss. Technol. 7: 176.

Hirs, C. M., Timmasheff, S. 1972. Methods in Enzymology, Vol. 25. Academic Press, N. Y.

Hockenhull, D. J. 1971. Yeast production. Progr. Indust. Microb. 10: 129.

Humphrey, A. E. 1974. Production of food and feed by fermentation. Proc. Roy. Aust. Chem. Inst. 41: 285.

Johnson, J. C. 1977. Yeasts for food and other purposes. Noyes Data Corp., Park Ridge, N. J.

Kihlberg, R. 1972. The microbe as a source of food. Ann. Rev. Microbiol. 26: 427.

Kinsella, J. E. 1976. Functional properties of proteins in foods: A survey. CRC Critical Revs. in Food Sci. and Nutr. 7: 219.

Kinsella, J. E. 1977. Functional properties in novel proteins: Some methods for improvement. Chemistry & Industry. March. p. 177.

Kinsella, J. E. 1978. Protein texturization and fabrication. In Handbook Food and Nutrition. CRC Press, Cleveland, Ohio (in press)

Kinsella, J. E. and Shetty, K. J. 1978. Chemical modification for the improvement in fucntional properties of vegetable and yeast proteins. Proc. ACS Symp. Pour-El A., Ed. ACS Publications. Am. Chem. Sco., Washington, D. C. (in press).

Kinsella, J. E., Vananuvat, P. and Pearce, K. 1976. Chemical modification to improve functional properties of novel proteins. Joint Conference on Single-Cell Protein of US-USSR Groups. Unpubd. Proc., MIT, Cambridge, Mass.

Knowles, J. R. 1974. Chemical modification and the reactivity of amino acids in proteins. In MTP Intl. Rev. of Science and Biochemistry. Series one. Chemistry of macromolecules. Gutenfreund, Ed., Vol. I. Uni Park, Baltimore, Md. p. 149.

Labuza, T. P. and Jones, K. A. 1973. Functionality in bread-making of yeast protein dried at two temperatures. J. Food Sci. 38: 177.

Labuza, T. P., Jones, K. A., Sinskey, A. J., Gomez, R., Wilson, S. and Miller, B. 1972. Effect of drying conditions on cell viability and functional properties of single cell protein. J. Food Sci. 37: 103.

Lindblom, M. A. 1974. Alkali treatment of a yeast protein concentrate. Lebensmittel.-Wiss μ-Technol. 7: 295.

Lindblom, M. 1974. The influence of alkali and heat treatment on yeast protein. Biotechnol. Bioeng. 16: 1495.

Lindblom, M. 1977. Properties of intracellular ribonuclease utilized for RNA reduction in disintegrated cells of Saccharomyces cerevisiae. Biotechnol. Bioeng. 19: 199.

Lindblom, M. and Mogren, H. L. 1977. Process for preparing a protein concentrate from a microbial cell mass and the protein content thus obtained. Br. Patent 1,474,313.

Lipinsky, E. S. and Litchfield, J. H. 1974. Single-cell protein in perspective. Food Technol. 28: 16.

Litchfield, J. H. 1977. Single cell proteins. Food Tech. 31: 175.

Mateles, R. T. and Tannenbaum, S. R. (Eds.) 1968. Single Cell Protein. MIT Press, Cambridge, Mass.

McElwain, M. D., Richardson, T. and Amundson, C. H. 1975. Some functional properties of succinylated single-cell protein concentrate. J. Milk Food Technol. 28: 521.

McLaren, D. D. 1975. Single cell protein: New processes open wider food uses. Food Prod. Devt. 9: 26.

Means, G. E. and Feeney, R. E. 1971. Chemical modification of proteins. Holden-Day, Inc., San Francisco.

Miller, S. A. 1968. Nutritional factors in single-cell protein. In Single-Cell Protein. Mateles and Tannenbaum, Eds. MIT Press, Cambridge, Mass. p. 77

Mogren and Lindblom, M. 1974. Mechanical disintegration of microorganisms in an industrial homogenizer. Biotechnol. & Bioeng. 16: 261.

Nelson, G.E.N., Anderson, R. F., Rhodes, R. A., Shekleton, M. C. and Hall, H. H. 1960. Lysine, methionine and tryptophan content of microorganisms. II. Yeasts. Appl. Microbiology 8: 179.

Newell, J. A., Robbins, A. E. and Seeley, R. D. 1975. Manufacture of yeast protein isolate having a reduced nucleic acid content by an alkali process. U.S. Patent #3,867,555.

Ohta, S., Maul, S., Sinskey, A. J. and Tannenbaum, S. R. 1971. Characterization of heat shock process for reduction of the nucleic acid content of Candida utilis. Appl. Microbiol. 22: 415.

Pearce, K. P. and Kinsella, J. E. 1978. Emulsifying properties of proteins: A turbidimetric technique. J. Agr. Food Chem. 26: (in press)

Phaff, H. J. 1977. Enzymatic yeast cell wall degradation in food proteins. Feeney and Whitaker, Eds. Am. Chem. Soc., Washington, D. C. p. 244.

Reed, G. and Peppler, J. H. 1973. Yeast Technology. Avi Publishing Co., Westport, Conn.

Rha, C. 1975. Utilization of single-cell protein for human food. In Single-Cell Protein II. Tannenbaum and Wang, Eds. MIT Press, Cambridge, Mass. p. 587.

Robbins, E. A., Sucher, R. W., Schuldt, Jr., E. H., Sidoti, D. R., Seeley, R. D., and Newell, J. A. 1975. Yeast protein isolate with reduced nucleic acid content and process of making same. U.S. Patent #3,887,431.

Rose, A., Morrison, J. S. 1971. The Yeasts, Vol. 1-3. Academic Press, New York.

Ryan, D. S. 1977. Determinants of the functional properties of proteins and protein derivatives in foods. In Food Proteins. Feeney and Whitaker, Eds. J. Am. Chem. Soc., Washington, D. C. p. 67,

Scrimshaw, N. S. 1975. Single-cell protein for human consumption - An overview. In Single-Cell Protein II, Tannenbaum and Wang, Eds. MIT Press, Cambridge, Mass. p. 24.

Seeley, R. D., Robbins, E. A., Sucher, R. W., Newell, J., Sidoti, D., Clayton, R. A. IV Intl. Congr. Food Science & Tech., Inst. Food Tech., Chicago, Ill. p. 73. 1974.

Shacklady, C. 1970. Single cell proteins from hydrocarbons. Outlook on Agric. 6: 102.

Shetty, K. J. and Kinsella, J. E. 1978. Effect of thiol reagents on rupture of yeast cells. Biotech. Bioeng. 20: (in press).

Shetty, K. J. and Rao, M.S.N. 1974. Studies on groundnut proteins. III. Physicochemical properties of arachin prepared by different methods. Anal. Biochemie 62: 108.

Shetty, K. J. and Rao, M.S.N. 1978. Effect of succinylation on oligomeric nature of arachin. Int. J. Peptide Protein Res. (in press).

Sinskey, A. J. and Tannenbaum, S. R. 1975. Removal of nucleic acids in SCP. In Single Cell Protein II. Tannenbaum and Wang, Eds. MIT Press, Cambridge Mass. p. 158.

Stark, G. R. 1970. Recent developments in chemical modification and sequential degradation of proteins. Adv. Protein Chem. 24: 261.

Tannenbaum, S. 1968. Factors in processing single-cell protein. In Single-cell Protein. Mateles and Tannenbaum, Eds. MIT Press, Cambridge, Mass. p. 343.

Tannenbaum, S. 1971. Single-cell protein: Food of the future. Food Tech. 25: 962.

Tannenbaum, S. 1977. Single cell proteins. In Food Proteins. Whitaker and Tannenbaum, Eds. Avi Publishing Co., Westport, Conn. p. 315.

Tannenbaum, S. 1974. Texturizing process for single cell protein. U.S. Patent 3,845,222.

Tannenbaum, S. R., Sinskey, A. J., and Maul, S. B. 1973. Process of reducing the nucleic acid content in yeast. U.S. Patent #3,720,585.

Tannenbaum, S. and Wang, D. I. 1975. Single Cell Protein II.
    MIT Press, Cambridge, Mass.
Vallee, B. L. and Riordan, J. F. 1969. Chemical approaches to
    the properties of active sites of enzymes. Ann. Rev. of
    Biochem. 38: 733.
Vananuvat, P. and Kinsella, J. E. 1975a. Amino acid composition
    of yeast S. fragilis. J. Agr. Food Chem. 23: 595.
Vananuvat, P. and Kinsella, J. E. 1975b. Extraction of protein,
    low in nucleic acid, from Saccharomyces fragilis grown con-
    tinuously on crude lactose. J. Agric. Food Chem. 23: 216.
Vananuvat, P. and Kinsella, J. E. 1975c. Some functional proper-
    ties of protein isolates from yeast, Saccharomyces fragilis.
    J. Agr. Food Chem. 23: 613.
Vananuvat, P. and Kinsella, J. E. 1978. Succinylation of yeast
    protein. I. Preparation and composition. Biotech. Bioeng.
    (in press).
Waslien, C. I., Callaway, D., Margen, S. and Costa, F. 1970. Uric
    acid levels in men fed algae and yeasts as protein sources.
    Food Tech. 35: 294.
Whitaker, J. R. 1978. Chemical modification of casein through
    covalent attachment of hydrophilic and hydrophobic amino
    acids. Amer. Chem. Soc. Ann. Mtg., Anaheim, Calif. (abstract)
White, P. and Selvey, N. 1970. Proceed. Western Hemisphere Nutri-
    tion Congress IV. Publ. Science Group Inc., Acton, Mass.
Worgan, J. T. 1974. Single cell protein. Plant Foods for Mars 1:
    99.
Young, V. R. and Scrimshaw, N. S. 1975. Clinical studies on the
    nutritive value of single-cell proteins. In Single-Cell
    Proteins II, Tannenbaum and Wang, Eds. MIT Press, Cambridge,
    Mass. p. 566.
Young, V. and Scrimshaw, N. S. 1976. Nutritional value and safety
    of single-cell protein in man. Unpubl. Proceedings of Joint
    US-USSR Conference on Single-Cell Protein.
Young, V. R. and Scrimshaw, N. S. and Milner, M. S. 1976. Food
    from plants. Chem & Industry (July) p. 588.

39

DESIGN AND ASSEMBLY OF AN INEXPENSIVE, AUTOMATED MICROBORE AMINO ACID ANALYZER: SEPARATION AND QUANTITATION OF AMINO ACIDS IN PHYSIOLOGICAL FLUIDS[1]

G. R. Beecher

Protein Nutrition Laboratory, Nutrition Institute
Federal Research, Science and Education Administration
U. S. Department of Agriculture, Beltsville, MD 20705

ABSTRACT

An amino acid analyzer capable of separating and quantitating 0.5 to 20 n moles of each ninhydrin-positive compound in physiological fluids has been designed and assembled from commercially available components. The buffer sequence, column temperature change and sample application are controlled by an automatic programmer constructed from a series of timers. The liquid delivery portion of the instrument consists of a series of polystyrene and stainless steel chambers pressurized with argon and connected through valves and manifolds to conventional positive displacement pumps. The column is highly polished stainless steel tubing (0.21-cm ID) packed with 9-μ cation exchange resin. Micro colorimeters, equipped with appropriate interference filters and small-volume (2-8 μl) flow cells, are used as detectors. The sample loader is a dual 20-port automatic valve containing 25-μl sample loops. Small-bore teflon tubing (32 AWG), interconnected with tubing adapters and connectors, is used for buffer lines and reaction coil (100° C); ninhydrin lines are 1/16-inch stainless steel tubing. Separation of 42 ninhydrin positive compounds, including column equilibration, is accomplished in 5 hours. Procedures for the extraction of amino acids from physiological fluids and tissues as well as the preliminary clean-up of these extracts are also described.

---

[1] Mention of a trademark or proprietary product does not constitute a guarantee or warranty of the product by the U. S. Department of Agriculture, and does not imply its approval to the exclusion of other products that may also be suitable.

INTRODUCTION

A change in the protein nutritive quality of foods and feeds is ultimately manifest in the perturbation of amino acid(s) levels in certain fluids and tissues of mammalian organisms. In order to rapidly assess the impact of altering the protein quality of foods and feeds on the protein nutriture of animals or humans, low cost, short, sensitive amino acid analyses of physiological fluids and tissue extracts are required. Since the description of the first automatic amino acid analyzer (Spackman et al., 1958), reduction in resin particle diameter, as suggested by Hamilton (Hamilton et al., 1960), has resulted in instruments with dramatic increases in sensitivity and significant decreases in analysis time. Coincidental with these technical advances, the cost of sensitive instruments has risen to the extent that many small laboratories or departments cannot withstand or justify such an investment.

Hare (1969) developed a simple, yet sensitive amino acid analyzer characterized by a 1.5 mm inside diameter column and the use of nitrogen pressure to force buffers and ninhydrin through the system. Several modifications of the original instrument shortened analysis time and increased sensitivity to the extent that amino acids in geological samples are routinely analyzed (Hare 1971, 1972, 1973). These instruments as well as others constructed from commercially available components (Liao et al., 1973) were optimized to separate and quantitate only the amino acids commonly found in proteins. The separation and accurate quantitation of amino acids in physiological fluids or tissue extracts, however, requires additional capabilities both in terms of sensitivity and number of column eluents. This report details the assembly of a microbore amino acid analyzer capable of separating and quantitating low levels of ninhydrin positive compounds in samples of physiological origin.

APPARATUS AND PROCEDURES

General. A schematic of the microbore amino acid analyzer is shown in Figure 1. The column reagent is forced, by argon pressure, from the appropriate reagent reservoir (A, B, C, D, E, LiOH) through a filter/ammonia trap, on-off valve and seven-port manifold to the pump. The pump delivers the column reagent, at a constant flow rate, through a flow meter and the sample injector to the ion-exchange column. The column eluent is mixed with the ninhydrin reagent, pumped at a constant flow rate by a system similar to the column reagent system, after which it goes through the reaction bath, equilibration coil, colorimeters and bubble suppressor and finally is deposited in waste. Reagent and ninhydrin reservoirs are stored at 4° C. Gas-actuated on-off valves, controlled by the programmer, select the appropriate reagent in sequence for the elution of amino acids from the ion-exchange resin in the column.

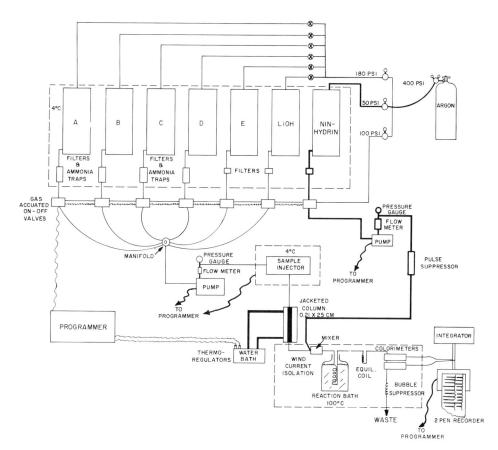

Figure 1.   Schematic of microbore amino acid analyzer.

The sample injector is also maintained at 4° C to minimize the loss
of glutamine from samples prior to application to the column.   All
of the tubing and components involved in post-column chemistry and
color detection are placed in a cabinet to minimize temperature
changes of the solution in the small-bore tubing resulting from
wind currents.   Analog signals from both colorimeters are sent, in
parallel, to a dual, drag.pen recorder[2] and a computing integrator[3].
The details of the component parts are described below.

---

[2]Omniscribe, Houston Instrument Co., Austin, TX.

[3]System AA, Spectra Physics Corp., Santa Clara, CA.

Reagent and Ninhydrin Reservoirs. Column reagent reservoirs, capable of withstanding 400 PSIG[4], were constructed[5] from 10.5-cm diameter polystyrene rod. The body of each reservoir was formed by boring a 34-cm segment of rod to 5.3-cm diameter; ends were machined from 3.2-cm thick segments of rod and fastened to the body with ten 1/4 X 2-inch stainless steel cap screws. Teflon gaskets, cut from 1/32-inch thick sheet teflon[6], provided a liquid seal between the body and each end. The top was bored and threaded 3/4 NPT to allow easy introduction of solutions; the bottom was bored and threaded 1/4 X 28 flat-seat for Cheminert[7] fittings. A liquid channel was bored from the flat-seat to the body of the reservoir. A Kel-F adapter was machined to serve as a plug for the top of each reservoir and also to allow Cheminert fittings to be attached.

The ninhydrin reservoir was constructed from a 1 liter stainless steel sample cylinder[8] (Fig. 2). A liquid level indicator was assembled from polycarbonate tubing[6] and attached to the ninhydrin chamber with appropriate stainless steel connectors[8] (see Figure 2 for details).

Tubing and Connectors. Cheminert teflon tubing systems[7] were used throughout the analyzer except for the ninhydrin system in which stainless steel tubing was used. One-sixteenth inch OD X 0.031-inch ID tubing was used to supply argon to the reagent reservoirs and gas-actuated valves and to connect the reagent reservoirs to the ammonia traps and line filters. Thin-wall 32-AWG teflon tubing[6] in conjunction with microbore adapters[9] was used to carry reagents from the line filters through the valves, manifold, pumps and injector to the column and from the column through the mixer, reaction bath and colorimeters to waste. A seven-port manifold with 1/4 X 28 flat-seat connections and 0.031-inch connecting ports was machined from Kel-F[6]; tees were Cheminert type with

---

[4]Abbreviations used: AWG, american wire gauge; NPT, national pipe thread; PSI, pounds per square inch; PSIG, pounds per square inch gauge.

[5]William R. Reed Co., Rockville, MD.

[6]Read Plastics Inc., Rockville, MD.

[7]Cheminert tubing systems consisting of 1/4 X 28 threaded connectors and flanged teflon tubing are available from several suppliers including Durrum Chemical Corp., Sunnyvale, CA and Laboratory Data Control, Riviera Beach, FL.

[8]Potomac Valve and Fitting, Inc., Rockville, MD.

[9]Durrum Chemical Corp., Sunnyvale, CA.

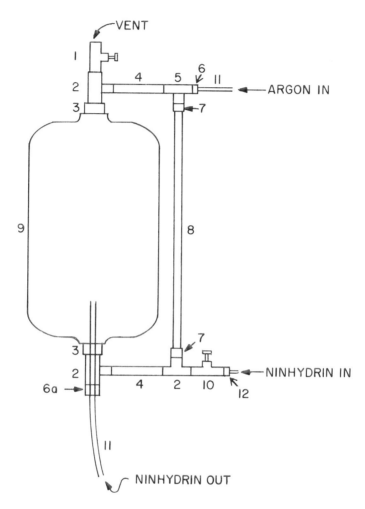

Figure 2.   Schematic of stainless steel ninhydrin reservoir.
All components are stainless steel unless otherwise noted: 1, 1/8
NPT male X 1/8 Swagelok shutoff valve; 2, 1/8 street-tee; 3, 1/4 to
1/8 NPT reducing bushing; 4, 1/8 NPT X 1-1/2-inch hex long nipple;
5, 1/8 NPT tee; 6, 1/16 tube to 1/8 NPT male connector; 6a, 1/16
tube to 1/8 NPT male connector drilled to allow 1/16-inch tube to
pass through; 7, 3/8 tube to 1/8 NPT male connector; 8, 3/8-inch OD
X 1/4-inch ID polycarbonate tube; 9, one liter sample cylinder; 10,
1/8 NPT female shutoff valve; 11, 1/16-inch OD X 0.030-inch ID
stainless steel tubing; 12, 1/8 NPT male to 1/4 X 28 male teflon
adapter.   Insertion of the outlet tubing into the chamber approximately 3-cm provided a settling basin and prevented particulate
material from entering the outlet tubing.

0.031-inch ports. The ninhydrin column-effluent mixer was machined
from teflon to allow the column effluent to be completely encapsulated with ninhydrin.

Stainless steel tubing[10] (1/16-in OD X 0.030-in ID) was used
to supply argon to the ninhydrin reservoir and to carry ninhydrin
from the reservoir through the filter, valve, pump and pulse
suppressor to the ninhydrin column-effluent mixer. Stainless steel
tubing connectors[7,8] were used to connect the tubing to 1/4 X 28
ports and Cheminert fittings. Argon distribution manifolds were
assembled from 1/8 NPT brass street-tees and, where applicable,
brass shut-off valves[8].

Ammonia Traps and Filters. Ammonia traps were placed in line
for buffers A through D (Fig. 1). The traps consisted of 5-cm
segments of 1/4-inch OD stainless steel tubing fitted with a bed
support[11] (2-μ pore stainless steel frit encapsulated in Kel-F) and
stainless steel bottom-drilled end-fittings[10,11]. Resin type DC-3[9]
was added to each trap to retain ammonia dissolved in the buffers.
For those reagents not requiring ammonia traps, in-line filters
were assembled from bottom-drilled end-fittings, bed supports and
metal to plastic tubing adapters[7] (3-cm segment of 1/4-inch OD
stainless steel tubing threaded 1/4 X 28). Stainless steel tubing
(1/16-in) and connectors[7,8] were used to connect the traps and
filters to Cheminert fittings. The ninhydrin-line filter was a
stainless steel inline removable filter[8] with a 7-μ pore filter
element.

Reagent Selection Valves. Cheminert on-off valves (0.031-in[7]
bore) automated with pneumatic actuators[7] and solenoid gas-valves[7]
were used to control the flow of reagents and ninhydrin. Each
valve was supplied with provision for manual control as well as
automatic control from the programmer.

Pumps. Standard Milton Roy minipumps[12], designed to deliver
13 to 130 ml per hr, were used to pump buffer and ninhydrin in the
analyzer. These pumps were capable of accurately pumping at flow
rates of 3 to 4 ml per hr when two criteria were met. First, the
reagents on the inlet side of the pump were maintained under pressure
and, second the pressure applied to the reagents on the inlet side
of the pump was at least 50 PSIG lower than the outlet pressure of
the pump. Thus the reagent reservoirs were pressurized to 180 PSIG
since the ion-exchange column developed a minimum of 250 PSIG

[10]Alltech Associates, Inc., Arlington Heights, IL.

[11]Altex Scientific, Inc., Berkeley, CA.

[12]Laboratory Data Control, Riviera Beach, FL.

backpressure when buffer E at high temperature was pumped. Similarly, the ninhydrin reservoir was pressurized to 50 PSIG since the pulse suppressor in the ninhydrin line produced 100 PSIG back pressure. A flowmeter[13], encased in a polycarbonate shield[5], and a pressure gauge[9] (1000 PSI range) were installed in the outlet line of each pump.[9] The ninhydrin-line pulse suppressor was filled with DC-1A resin[9] which provided 100 PSIG backpressure.

Sample Injector. A modified dual deck 20-port rotary valve complete with drive unit was used as the sample injector[12]. The rotary valve was modified by substituting 29-cm segments of 32-AWG thin-wall teflon tubing complete with microbore adapters for the 1/16-inch OD teflon tubing sample loops supplied with the valve. The volume of each loop (about 25-μl) was accurately determined[14]. The inlet and outlet lines, also 32-AWG tubing, were connected to a sample injection valve[12]. The sample injection valve was automated (see description for the reagent selection valves) and programmed to connect a sample loop of the rotary valve inline for only 5 min during the injection phase of each analysis. During the major portion of the analysis, reagents were pumped through the bypass loop of the sample injection valve. This feature allowed sample loops to be loaded at any time during a run, except during the 5 min injection period, and alleviated operating the rotary valve at continuous high pressure.

Column. The column was a 25-cm segment of 2.1 mm ID X 1/4-inch OD "Li-chroma" finished precision tubing[10] with 1/4 X 28 threads machined on each end. The bed support[11] (2-μ pore stainless frit encapsulated in Kel-F) was held firmly to the bottom of the column by a Cheminert fitting containing a microbore adapter. It was not necessary to place a frit on the top of the column since the continuous flow of buffer from the pressurized reservoirs (when buffer pump was off) prevented the resin from expanding into the small-diameter teflon tubing. The feature of buffer slowly flowing through the column when the pumps were off also minimized "start-up" procedures after a period of non-use. The column was enclosed in a glass jacket[12] which was connected to a circulating water bath[15]. The water bath was modified to use two temperature controllers; details of the electrical connections are described in the programmer section of the apparatus.

---

[13]Gilmont No. 10, Roger Gilmont Instruments, Inc., Great Neck, NY.

[14]Each loop was filled with a solution of p-nitroaniline (A_{380} known). The p-nitroaniline was then washed from each loop with water, diluted to a known volume, the A_{380} of the dilute solution determined and the volume of each loop calculated.

[15]Haake model FJ, Haake, Inc., Saddle Brook, NJ.

Reaction Bath and Colorimeters. Color of the column-effluent ninhydrin mixture was developed in 25-ft of 32-AWG tubing immersed in a water bath maintained at a low boil. The water bath consisted of a 1 liter resin kettle, fitted with a cover and condenser, and a heating mantle controlled by an autotransformer. Immediately after color development, the temperature of the column-effluent ninhydrin mixture was equilibrated to ambient temperature in 10-ft of tubing. Color intensity at 440 and 570 nm was measured in micro-colorimeters having optical pathlengths of 20 and 6 mm, respectively. The design and construction of the micro-colorimeters have been described by Hare (1971, 1977). Maximum outputs from the 440 and 570 nm colorimeters were 10 and 100 mv, respectively, when the photo-resistors were biased at 7 v and the lamps operated at 2.5 v. A 25-ft segment of tubing between the colorimeters and waste prevented bubble formation in the micro-colorimeters.

Automatic Programmer. The wiring schematic of the automatic programmer is shown in Figure 3[16]. As many components as possible were mounted on a standard telephone rack to provide a convenient bench assembly (Hamilton, 1963). Power to the programmer is controlled by switch S1 through fuse F1. Switch S2 allows the programmer to be operated in either automatic mode (position shown in diagram) or manual mode; switch S3 (momentary contact) is used to start the programmer in automatic mode. In the automatic mode, timers 1 to 5 control the length of time that each of buffers A to E, respectively, flow to the pump and subsequently to the column. Timer 6 controls the length of time lithium hydroxide flows and timer 7 controls the duration of the regeneration (Buffer A). Timer 8 is wired parallel to timers 1 to 7 and controls the column temperature change. Timers 9 and 10, also wired in parallel to timers 1 to 7, control the delay before sample injection (establish-ment of baseline) and the duration that the sample loop is maintained in line, respectively. Switches S4 to S11 provide a bypass for each of the timers 1 to 8, respectively; these switches eliminate the need to set a timer to 0 when an elution program requires that a particular buffer not be used. When switch S2 is set for manual operation, all of the timers are bypassed and switches S12 to S18 control the flow of buffers A to E, lithium hydroxide and ninhydrin, respectively. Similarly, switch S19 controls the column tempera-ture change, switch S22 controls the recorder and switches S20 and S23 control the ninhydrin and buffer pumps, respectively.

The timers used to assemble the automatic programmer were either Cramer[17], model 474A-AE (timers 1 to 8, 120 min maximum

---

[16]A large blueprint of the wiring schematic is available from the author.

[17]Conrac Corp., Old Saybrook, CT.

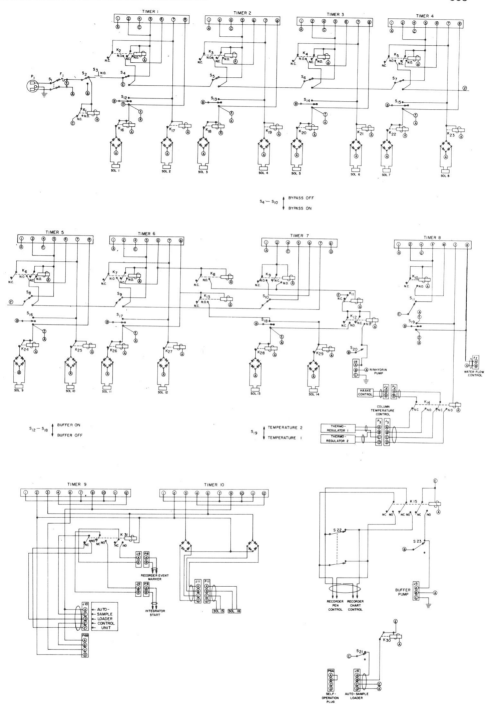

Figure 3. Schematic of automatic programmer for microbore amino acid analyzer.

setting) or Industrial Timer[18], model GP2 (timers 9 and 10, 60 min.
and 5 min., respectively) timers. Relays K2 to K13 (Potter and
Brumfield[19], KRP series) isolate the signal and timers when the
instrument is operated in the manual mode; relays K14, K15 and K31
(Potter and Brumfield[19], KNP series) provide contact closure for
operation of the sample injector, recorder, integrator and the
appropriate thermoregulator of the circulating water bath. Power
to the buffer pump is turned on through relay K15, when the automatic
sequence is initiated and turned off when the timed sequence is
completed. Ninhydrin flow and the ninhydrin pump are also turned
on, through relays K11 and K12, when the automatic sequence is
initiated but turned off through relays K8 and K13, when timer 6
(lithium hydroxide) is started. Relays K16 to K29 (Amperite min-
iature delay relay[19], 15-sec delay) were installed to provide only
a 15-sec pulse of power, rather than continuous power, to the
solenoid gas valves (labelled SOL. 1 etc. in Fig. 3). Full-wave
bridge rectifiers (1 amp.) provided 110 v DC to the solenoid gas
valves. Relays K1 (Potter and Brumfield[19], 0 to 10 sec delay on
release) and K30 (Amperite minature delay relay[19], 5-sec delay)
interrupt the supply of power to the timers at the end of each run
so that each timer resets to the preprogrammed time. Switch S21
provides for continuous recycling through the program (position
shown) or a single cycle through the program. Installation of plug
P6A permits the analyzer to be operated in the automatic mode when
the sample injector is disconnected. The connection of two thermo-
regulators to the control circuit of the circulating water bath is
shown in Figure 3. Timer 8 and switch S19 also control a water
flow valve[20] which allows tap water to flow through the cooling
coil of the circulating water bath during the low temperature phase
of the analysis.

Resin and Reagents. The ion-exchange resin, DC-4A[9] (9.0 $\pm$ 0.5 μ
diameter), was washed and converted to the lithium form as outlined
by the manufacturer. The column was packed with the washed resin
following the procedures described by Hare (1977). Iso-pH, lithium
buffer concentrates[9], diluted and pH adjusted as shown in Table 1,
were used to elute amino acids from the column. A dilute ninhydrin
reagent in dimethyl sulfoxide (Liao et al., 1973) was used to
quantitate amino acids after elution from the column. All reagents
were prepared with freshly deionized distilled water.

---

[18] Industrial Timer, Parsippany, NJ.

[19] Capitol Radio Wholesalers, Inc., Rockville, MD.

[20] Mark Instrument Co., Villanova, PA.

TABLE 1

Microbore Amino Acid Analyzer Operating Parameters

Buffer	pH	Duration
Pico IV A	2.94	60 min
Pico IV B	3.30	30 min
Pico IV C	3.10	20 min
Pico IV D	3.85	20 min
Pico IV E[1]	3.30	100 min
0.3 N LiOH	-	10 min
Pico IV A	2.94	60 min

Temperature	Time
36.7°	0-65 min
64.0°	66-300 min

[1]Diluted to 125% of recommended volume.

Sample Preparation. All samples were extracted with sulfosalicylic acid (Peters and Berridge, 1970; Saifer, 1971). Tissue samples were lyophilized and subsequently homogenized (Potter-Elvehjem all-glass homogenizer) in 10 volumes of 5% (w/v) sulfosalicylic acid. Plasma, prepared from heparinized blood, was treated with 0.25 volumes of 20% (w/v) sulfosalicylic acid. Whole blood and frozen red blood cell packs were diluted with 2 volumes of deionized water, then treated with 0.75 volumes of 20% (w/v) sulfosalicylic acid. All samples were centrifuged for 15 min at 1000 X g max and the supernatants removed for subsequent treatment. In order to eliminate sulfosalicylic acid which indirectly alters the resolution of the acidic amino acids from the analyzer column (Peters and Berridge, 1970), aliquots of supernatants containing sulfosalicylic acid were processed through 0.8 X 10 cm columns[21,22] of AG-2 X 8[23] (200-400 mesh) as described by Stein and Moore (1954). During this treatment, sulfosalicylic acid is bound to the resin (Vanderslice, 1977) while amino acids and other cations are eluted. The eluent was lyophilized and redissolved in amino acid analyzer sample

[21]Disposable polypropylene columns, Kontes, Vineland, NJ.

[22]Glass chromatography columns, Wheaton Scientific, Millville, NJ.

[23]Bio-Rad Laboratories, Richmond, CA.

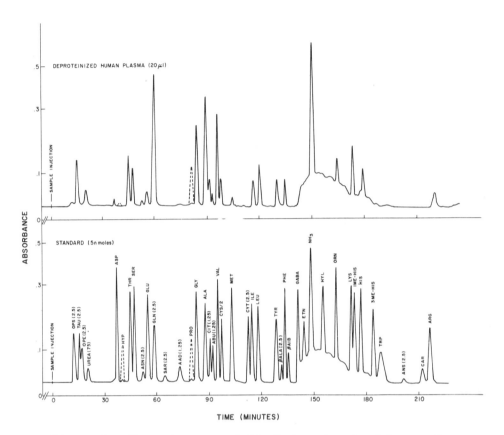

TIME (MINUTES)

Figure 4.   Chromatograms of 20 μl deproteinized human plasma
(top) and amino acid standard (bottom).   Absorbance at 570 nm shown
by solid line; absorbance at 440 nm shown by broken line for imino
acid peaks only.   Concentration of each amino acid in 25 μl standard
was either 5 nmoles or value shown in parentheses following amino
acid or peptide abbreviation.   Amino acid and peptide abbreviations
are as follows: OPS, O-phosphoserine; TAU, taurine; OPE, O-phos-
phoethanolamine; ASP, aspartic acid; HYP, hydroxyproline; THR,
threonine; SER, serine; ASN, asparagine; GLU, glutamic acid; GLN,
glutamine; SAR, sarcosine; AAD, α-amino adipic acid; PRO, proline;
GLY, glycine; ALA, alanine; CIT, citrulline; ABU, α-amino-n-butyric
acid; VAL, valine; CYS/2, half-cystine; MET, methionine; CYT,
cystathionine; ILE, isoleucine; LEU, leucine; TYR, tyrosine; βALA,
β-alanine; PHE, phenylalanine; βAIB, β-amino isobutyric acid; GABA,
γ-amino butyric acid; ETN, ethanolamine; HYL, hydroxylysine; ORN,
ornithine; LYS, lysine; 1ME-HIS, N^{π}-methylhistidine (1-methyl
histidine); HIS, histidine; 3ME-HIS, N^{τ}-methylhistidine (3-methyl
histidine); TRP, tryptophan; ANS, anserine; CAR, carnosine; ARG,
arginine.

buffer (0.15 M Li$^+$ as lithium citrate, pH 2.20); the AG-2 X 8 resin was discarded. It was found necessary to process sulfosalicylic acid extracts of sucrose washed red blood cells through 0.8 X 2.5 cm columns[21,22] of AG-50W-X-8[23] (200-400 mesh, hydrogen form), as described by Asatoor (1969), because sucrose interfered with both lyophilization and resolution on the amino acid analyzer.

RESULTS AND DISCUSSION

Figure 4 shows chromatograms of a standard amino acid mixture and a sample of human plasma. The operating parameters of the analyzer used to obtain these chromatograms are outlined in Table 1; buffer and ninhydrin were each pumped at 4.0 ml per hr. The total time required for each analysis was 300 min, 230 min for elution of the amino acids and 70 min for washing and equilibration of the column. The baseline shift in the region where ammonia elutes is apparently caused by the slow bleeding of ninhydrin positive compounds from the resin. Accurate quantitation ranges from 0.5 to 20 nmoles for each amino acid, except urea. The precision of the system is $\pm$ 3% for those amino acids eluted while the baseline is stable and $\pm$ 5% for amino acids eluted during the baseline shift.

When the level of amino acid detection is reduced to the nanomole range, contamination of the sample presents a serious problem and precautions suggested by Hamilton (1967, 1972) and Hare (1977) must be considered. Use of the present analyzer for the analysis of extracts from samples having modest levels of amino acids has minimized the contamination problem (Hare, 1977). In addition, the processing of all samples through either Dowex 2 or Dowex 50 columns, prior to analysis, removes a considerable amount of non-amino acid contamination. These precautions have permitted 600-900 runs on the analyzer before the backpressure of the column exceeds 600 PSIG, which demands that the resin be cleaned and color factors recalculated.

This amino acid analyzer has been in continuous operation for over two years. It has been a realistic compromise of initial cost ($15,000), operation and maintenance. The microbore column not only provides nanomole sensitivity but buffer and ninhydrin consumption are considerably less than in conventional large column instruments.

REFERENCES

Asatoor, A. M. (1969). The occurrence of E-N-methyllysine in human urine. Clin. Chim. Acta, 26, 147-154.

Hamilton, P. B. (1963). Ion exchange chromatography of amino acids.
    A single column, high resolving, fully automatic procedure.
    Anal. Chem., 35, 2055-2063.
Hamilton, P. B. (1967). Micro and submicro determinations of amino
    acids by ion-exchange chromatography. In, 'Methods in
    Enzymology', C. H. W. Hirs (Editor). Vol. 16, pp 15-27.
    Academic Press, New York.
Hamilton, P. B., Bogue, D. C. and Anderson, R. A. (1960). Ion
    exchange chromatography of amino acids. Analysis of diffusion
    (mass transfer) mechanisms. Anal. Chem., 32, 1782-1792.
Hamilton, P. B., and Nagy, B. (1972). Problems in the search for
    amino acids in lunar fines. Space Life Sci., 3, 432-438.
Hare, P. E. (1969). Geochemistry of proteins, peptides and amino
    acids. In 'Organic Geochemistry', G. Eglintion and M. T. J.
    Murphy (Editors). Springer-Verlag, New York.
Hare, P. E. (1971). Ultrasensitive amino acid analyzer. Carnegie
    Inst. Wash. Year Book, 70, 268-269.
Hare, P. E. (1972). Ion-exchange chromatography in lunar organic
    analysis. Space Life Sci., 3, 354-359.
Hare, P. E. (1973). Fluorescent method for the analysis of amino
    acids and peptides. Carnegie Inst. Wash. Year Book, 72, 701-
    704.
Hare, P. E. (1977). Subnanomole-range amino acid analysis. In,
    'Methods in Enzymology', C. H. W. Hirs and S. N. Timasheff
    (Editors). Vol. 47, pp 3-8. Academic Press, New York.
Liao, T. H., Robinson, G. W. and Salnikow, J. (1973). Use of
    narrow-bore columns in amino acid analysis. Anal. Chem., 45,
    2286-2288.
Peters, J. H. and Berridge, B. J., Jr. (1970). The determination
    of amino acids in plasma and urine by ion-exchange chromatog-
    raphy. Chromatog. Rev., 12, 157-165.
Saifer, A. (1971) Comparative study of various extraction methods
    for the quantitative determination of free amino acids in
    brain tissue. Anal. Biochem. 40, 412-423.
Spackman, D. H., Stein, W. H. and Moore, S. (1958). Automatic
    recording apparatus for use in the chromatography of amino
    acids. Anal. Chem., 30, 1190-1206.
Stein, W. H. and Moore, S. (1954). The free amino acids of human
    blood plasma. J. Biol. Chem., 211, 915-926.
Vanderslice, J. T. (1977). Personal communication.

40

GLOSSARY OF ABBREVIATIONS AND DEFINITIONS OF NUTRITIONAL TERMS

Mendel Friedman

Western Regional Research Center, Science and Education Administration, U.S. Department of Agriculture, Berkeley, California 94710

INTRODUCTION

Publications in food science, and animal and human nutrition use many abbreviations and technical terms that are sometimes not defined. This compilation, which emphasizes protein nutriture, is intended to explain all that may be used in this book and in published papers that I have read. The glossary of nutritional terms is an expanded and revised version of earlier lists by the National Academy of Sciences (NAS, 1963), Kofranyi (1972), and Friedman (1975), so I hope it may be more widely useful. References to the definitions are given as available, although these do not necessarily show their origin. A few botanical identifications are offered for various food plants that may be unfamiliar to some readers. Corrections and suggestions are invited.

AA   Amino acid(s)
AAAC   American Association of Cereal Chemists
AAN   Amino acid nitrogen (Tamminga, 1975)
ABOMASAL SUPPLEMENTS   Postruminal infusion of amino acids and supplemented proteins (Reis and Tunks, 1976)
ADF   Average daily feed intake (Costa et al., 1976; Fenderson and Bergen, 1975)
ADG   Average daily gain (Garling and Wilson, 1976)
AEA   Apparent energy absorbed (Costa et al., 1976)
A/G   Albumin to globulin ratio in plasma as a measure of nutritional status of the aged (Higgons, 1959)
AGFD   Agricultural and Food Chemistry Division of the American Chemical Society
AIB α-Aminoisobutyric acid (Tews and Harper, 1976)

841

AID   United States Agency for International Development

ALAT   Alanine aminotransferase (Aycock and Kerksey, 1976)

AMINO ACID EFFICIENCY % (Gaby and Chawla, 1976)

$$\frac{\underline{\text{moles amino acid required for specific growth rate}}}{\text{moles of analogue required for same growth rate}}$$

AMINO ACID AVAILABILITYY % (Sarwar, et al.,1978; Bragg et al., 1969)

$$= \frac{\text{Total intake of amino acid-(Fecal excretion of amino}}{\text{acid-metabolized amino acid)}}{\text{Total intake of amino acid}} \text{ x 100}$$

AMINO ACID SCORE (FAO, 1973)

$$= \frac{\underline{\text{mg of amino acid in 1 g of test protein}}}{\text{mg of amino acid in reference pattern}}$$

ANA   Apparent nitrogen absorbed (Costa et al., 1976)

ANP   Applied Nutrition Programmes (FAO, 1976)

ANRC   Animal Nutrition Research Council

AOAC   American Association of Official Agricultural Chemists

APDN   % added N digested in acid-pepsin stage (Barry, 1976)

ARC   Agricultural Research Council (United Kingdom)

ARNOULD'S INDEX   Measure of protein quality calculated from
          essential and nonessential amino acid composition
          (Arnould, 1971; Hansen, 1975). See also IEP.

ATSP   Alkali-treated soybean protein isolate (Struthers et al.,
          1978)

ATE   Ratio of specific essential amino acids to the sum of all
          essential amino acids

AVL   Available lysine; determination of chemically and
          presumably nutritionally available lysine by chemical
          modification (Carpenter, 1960; Schwenke et al., 1975)

AVLenz   Available lysine measured by an enzymatic method
          (Finot et al., 1977)

BCAA   Branched chain amino acids (Beisel, 1977)

BCM   Body cell mass (Uauy et al., 1978)

BENGAL GRAM   Chick-pea; sometimes also cow gram;
          garbanzo; Cicer arietinum Linn.

BLACK GRAM   Phaseolus mungo Roxb. (Chavan and Duggal, 1978)

BMR   Basal metabolic rate (Uauy et al., 1978)

BV   Biological value; proportion of absorbed nitrogen that
          is retained (Thomas, 1909; Mitchell, 1923; NAS, 1973;
          Schelling, 1975; Dvorak, 1975; Bodwell, 1975; 1977)

Δ BW   Daily body weight gain (Chawala et al., 1976)

CFTRI   Central Food Technology Research Institute, Mysore, India

CHD   Coronary heart disease (Oldfield, 1977; Yudkin, 1978)

CIAT   International Centre for Tropical Agriculture, Guatemala

CIMMYT   Centro Internacional de Mejoramiento de Maiz y Trigo
          (International Maize and Wheat Improvement Center, Mexico)

CONPAN   Consejo Nacional para la Alimentacion y Nutricion (Chile)

COW GRAM   Catjang; catjang cowpea; Jerusalem pea; marble pea;
          Vigna Catjang (Burm. f.) Walp.; Vigna unguiculata subsp.
          cylindrica (L.) Van Eselt ex Verdc.

CPE   Complete protein evaluation
CPER   See PER
CRUDE PROTEIN VALUE = Protein N x 6.25
CS   Chemical score; content of each of the essential amino
         acids expressed as a percent of a standard (NAS, 1963;
         FAO, 1973)
CSIRO   Commonwealth Scientific and Industrial Research Organiza-
         tion (Australia)
CSM   Corn-soy-milk
CSM   Cottonseed meal
C_T Per capita calorie consumption (Reutlinger and Selowsky, 1977)

DBC   Dye-binding capacity (Brunckhorst et al., 1974; Pomeranz
         and Moore, 1975)
DCP   Digestible crude protein (Ranawana and Kellaway, 1977)
DE   Digestible energy (Barry, 1976)
DFB-LYS   Lysine in food protein available for reaction with
         2,4-dintrofluorobenzene (Carpenter, 1960; Carpenter and Booth,
         1973; Knipfel, 1975; Tanaka et al., 1977; Labuza et al., 1977)
DNA/RNA   Ratio of deoxyribonucleic acid to ribonucleic acid;
         measure of protein utilization (Miller, 1969; von der Decken
         et al., 1975)
DNPOM   Digestible non-protein organic matter (Ferguson, 1975)
DOM   Digestible organic matter (Knipfel, 1977)
DOMD   % organic matter in dry weight (Allison and Borzucki, 1978)
DP   Digestible protein (Fitzhugh, 1976)
DSA   Dairy Science Abstracts
DSM   Dry skim milk

EAA INDEX   Essential amino acid index; geometric mean or ratios
         of essential amino acids in a protein to their amounts in
         whole egg protein (Oser, 1951; Hansen and Eggum, 1973; Hansen,
         1975; Dreyer, 1976; Schwerdfeger and Schuphar, 1976; Clark
         et al., 1978)
EAAN   Essential amino acid nitrogen (Tamminga, 1975)
EAF-LYS Epsilon amino group free or "available" lysine (Martinez
         and Hopkins, 1975)
EGOT   Erythrocyte glutamic-oxalacetic transaminase (Edozien
         et al., 1976)
EGPT   Erythrocyte glutamic-pyruvic transaminase (Edozien et al.,
         1976)
E/N   Essential-to-nonessential amino acid ratio in plasma
         (Swenseid et al., 1963; Bodwell, 1975). See also PAA
ES   Enzyme score (Stahmann and Woldegiorgis, 1975)
E/T   Ratio of essential to total amino acids (FAO, 1973)
E/T_N Ratio of total essential amino acids to total nitrogen
         in foods (Scrimshaw and Young, 1972)
EUN   Endogenous urinary nitrogen (Okumura and Tasaki, 1973)
EVS-LYS   Lysine in food protein available for reaction with
         ethyl vinyl sulfone (Friedman and Wall, 1966; Friedman and
         Finley, 1975a, b; Millard and Friedman, 1976; Friedman, 1977)

FAO/WHO   Food and Agricultural Organization and World Health
             Organization of the United Nations
FCE   Food conversion efficiency (Nitsan and Nir, 1977)
FDA   Food and Drug Administration (USA)
FER   Feed efficiency ratio (Kies et al., 1978)
FFA   Free fatty acid
FFP   Functional fish protein (Lalasidis et al., 1978)
FM   Fish meal (Gjøen and Njaa, 1977)

FORMULAS FOR PROTEIN QUALITY (Dworak, 1975)

True absorption $\quad A = I-(F-F_O)$

Digestibility $\quad D = \dfrac{I-(F-F_O)}{I}$

Nitrogen balance $\quad B = I-(F + U)$

Nitrogen balance index $\quad NBI = \dfrac{B -B_O}{I} \times 100$

Biological value $\quad BV = \dfrac{B -B_O}{A} \times 100$

Net protein utilisation $\quad NPU = \dfrac{R -(R_O-I_O)}{I} \times 100$

I, I_O - N intake of animals fed with- and without proteins,
F, F_O - N in faeces of animals fed with- and without proteins,
U - N in urine,
B_O - N balance of animals fed without proteins,
R, R_O - N of whole animals fed with- and without proteins.

FPC   Fish protein concentrate
FSTA   Food Science and Technology Abstracts

GEC   Galactose elimination capacity (Vilstrup and Keiding 1976)
G/F   Gain to feed ratio (Costa et al., 1976)
GNM   Groundnut meal (Ostrowski, 1978)
FPC   Fish protein concentrate
GPV   Gross protein value (Heiman et al., 1939; NAS, 1963)
GREEN GRAM   Golden gram; mung bean; Phaseolus aureus Roxb.;
             Vigna radiata (L.) R. Wilcz.
GROUNDNUT; Peanut; Arachis hypogaea Linn

HDL   High density lipoproteins (Nicolosi et al., 1976)
HORSE GRAM   Horse grain; Dolichos biflorus Linn

IBP   Isolated beef protein
ICARDA   International Centre for Agricultural Research in Dry
             Areas, Aleppo, Syria
ICNND   Interdepartmental Committee on Nutrition for National
             Defence (Beaton, 1975)

ICRISAT   International Crops Research Institute for the Semi-arid
          Tropics, Hyderabad, India
I/D   Ratio of indispensable to dispensable amino acid
          nitrogen (Stucki and Harper, 1962)
IEP   Index d'equilibre de la proteine (Arnould, 1971; Bock,
          1974); see Arnould's Index
IFIS   International Food Information Service
IITA   International Institute for Tropical Agriculture, Nigeria
INCAP   Institute of Nutrition of Central America and Panama
IRRI   International Rice Research Institute (Philippines)
ISOPEPTIDE BOND   Amide bond between the σ-NH$_2$ group of lysine
          and either the β-COOH group of aspartic acid or the γ-COOH
          group of glutamic acid (Otterburn et al., 1977; Hurrell
          and Carpenter, 1977)
IVD   In-vitro digestibility (Allison and Borzucki, 1978)
IVDMD   In vitro dry matter disappearance (Britton, 1978)
IVPD   In vitro protein disappearance (Schaffert et al., 1974)

JAGGERY   Brown sugar mainly from the jaggery palm or sago palm,
          Caryota urens Linn.

LAL   Lysinoalanine (Friedman, 1977)
LBM   Lean body mass (Waterlow, 1969)
LBP   Lima bean protein
LCP   Liquid cyclone process (Martinez and Hopkins, 1975)
LDL   Low density lipoprotein
LEM   Leukocytic endogenous mediator (Beisel, 1977)
LIMITING AMINO ACID   Essential amino acid in a protein that
          shows the greatest difference in concentration from the
          same amino acid in a reference, high quality protein such
          as casein (Kofranyi, 1972)
LP DIET   Low protein diet (Kabadi et al., 1976)
LPC   Leaf protein concentrate (Bickoff et al., 1975)
LPI   Lysinuric protein intolerance (Simell et al., 1975)
L/T   Lysine to tryptophan ratio of food proteins as a measure
          of protein quality (Albanese, 1959)
LWG   Live-weight gain per day (Armstrong and Annison, 1973)

MA-LYS   Lysine in food protein available for reaction with methyl
          acrylate (Friedman and Wall, 1966; Finley and Friedman;
          1973; Friedman, 1977b)
MAIZE   Corn; Indian corn; Zea Mays Linn
MBM   Meat and bone meal (Ostrowski, 1978)
MCHC   Mean corpuscular hemoglobin concentration (Fisher et al.,
          1978)
MCH-FP   Maternal and child health-family planning
MDN   % added N digested in microbial stage (Barry, 1976)
ME   Metabolizable energy (Eggum et al., 1971)
MEAA   Modified essential amino acid index (Markakis, 1975)
3-MEH   3-Methylhistidine; measure of muscle protein catabolism
          and meat protein content of foods (Long et al., 1977;

Rangeley and Lawrie, 1977)

MEI   Metabolizable energy intake (Canolty and Koong, 1976)
MFAA   Metabolic fecal amino acids (Sarwar, 1978)
MFN   Metabolic fecal nitrogen (Okumura and Tasaki, 1973)
MHA   Methionine hydroxy analog

NAA   Neutral amino acid (Arroyave, 1975)
NAN   Nonammonia nitrogen (Bergen, 1978; Offer et al., 1976)
NAS   National Academy of Science (USA)
NBI   Nitrogen balance index (Harper, 1974; Calloway, 1975;
         Bodwell, 1977; Zezulka and Calloway, 1976; Lautzerheiser
         and Pellet, 1977; Navarrete et al., 1977; Garza et al.,
         1977; 1978)
NDP   Net dietary protein (Beaton, 1975)
ND-pV   Net dietary-protein value (Miller and Naismith, 1958;
         Platt and Miller, 1959; Miller and Payne, 1961; Jacquot
         and Peret, 1972; Beaton, 1975)

         = Protein concentration x Net protein utilization (NPU)
         $= \dfrac{\text{Nitrogen retained (g) X 6.25}}{\text{Total intake}}$

NDPCal % = NPU x P, where P is percentage of energy supplied by
         protein (Miller and Payne, 1962; Jacquot and Peret,
         1972; Beaton, 1975)
         $= \dfrac{\text{NDpV X4}}{\text{Total intake (g) X kcal per g of diet}}$

NE/GE   Nitrogen energy to gross energy efficiency (Fitzhugh, 1976)
NEAA   Non-essential amino acid (Clark et al., 1978)
NEAAN   Non-essential amino acid nitrogen (Tamminga, 1975)
NER   Nitrogen efficiency ratio, defined as ratio between
         weight gained and weight of dietary nitrogen consumed
         (Rosenberg, 1959; Eggum et al., 1971; Eggum, 1973; Bock, 1975)
NFDM   Nonfat dry milk (Sherbon et al., 1978)
NFE   Nitrogen-free extract
NGI   Nitrogen growth index; slope of line relating growth rate
         to nitrogen index (NAS, 1963; Bodwell, 1977)
NIE   Nitrogen incorporation efficiency; a measure of nitrogen
         utilization (Stucki and Harper, 1962)
NIRS   Near infrared reflectance spectroscopy (Williams, 1978)
NITROGEN-CONVERSION FACTORS   Factors used to convert nitrogen
         content of foods to protein content; range from 5.18 to
         6.38 (Merril and Watt, 1955; Heidelbaugh et al., 1975)
N/MJ-ME Nitrogen of metabolizable energy fermentable by rumen
         microorganisms (Miller, 1973)
NPN   Nonprotein nitrogen (Arroyave, 1962; Bergen, 1978)
NPOM   Non-protein organic matter (Ferguson, 1975)
NPR   Net protein ratio (Bender and Doell, 1957; NAS, 1963;
         McLaughlan and Keith, 1975; Schelling, 1975; Hackler,
         1977; Lachance et al., 1977)

NPU   Net protein utilization; per cent of dietary nitrogen consumed (Payne, 1972; Kaba and Pellet, 1975; Bodwell, 1977)

NPV   Net protein value; product of crude protein times NPU as obtained with diets containing 10% protein; CP % x NPU_{10} (Mitchell, 1922; NAS, 1963)

NQF   Nitrogen quality factor (N-Qualitätsfaktor) (Rufeger, 1972; Bock, 1975)

$$= \frac{assimilierbarer\ exogener\ N}{aufgenommener\ N};\ ratio\ of\ assimilable\ to\ utilized\ N$$

NR   Nitrogen retained (Costa et al., 1976)

NR   Nutritional rating (Bodwell, 1977)

NRC/NAS   National Research Council of the National Academy of Science (USA)

NSI   Nitrogen solubility index (Gutcho, 1977)

NSP   Nonstorage protein

OCT   Ornithine-carbamyl transferase

PAA RATIO   Plasma amino acid ratio; expression of relative changes in concentrations of each of free essential amino acids of plasma after consumption of a protein food as a function of specific amino acid requirements of the animal or human (Longenecker and Hause, 1961; McLaughlan, 1964; Young and Scrimshaw, 1972; Bodwell, 1975; McLaughlan and Keith, 1975; Vaughn et al., 1977; McLaughlan, 1978)

PAG/UN   Protein Advisory Group of the United Nations

PAH   p-Aminohippuric acid (Bergman and Heitmann, 1978)

PBI   Protein-bound iodine (Edozien et al., 1976)

PC   Protein concentrate

PCM   Protein-calorie malnutrition (Anderfelt, 1962; Arroyave, 1975; Rao and Naidu, 1977)

Pcal%   Protein-calorie per cent (Kaba and Pellet, 1975)

PDR INDEX   Pepsin digest residue amino acid index (Stahmann and Woldegiorgis, 1975)

PE   Protein energy expressed as a percentage of total energy

$$= \frac{Protein\ consumed\ (g)\ X\ 4.00\ (kcal/g)}{total\ diet\ consumed\ (g)\ X\ 4.25\ (kcal/g)}\ (Ashley\ and$$
Anderson, 1975)

PEC   Pyridylethylcysteine; concentration in hair as a measure of nutritional status of children (Friedman and Orracca-Tetteh, 1978)

PEM   Protein-energy malnutrition (Beaton, 1975; Lodatan and Reeds, 1976)

PER   Protein efficiency ratio (Osborne and Mendel, 1917; McLaughlan and Keith, 1975; Hurt et al., 1975; Jansen and Verburg, 1977)

$$PER\ =\ \frac{weight\ gain\ of\ test\ group\ (g)}{protein\ consumed\ (g)}$$

$$\text{PER MODIFIED} = \frac{\text{wt. gain of test group} + 0.1 \text{ (initial wt of test group)}}{\text{protein consumed}}$$

relative to a standard protein (lactalbumin)
(McLaughlan and Keith, 1975; Womack et al., 1975)

PER CORRECTED $\dfrac{\text{PER Test Protein}}{\text{PER Casein Control}}$

(Steinke, 1977; Satterlee et al., 1977)

PFAA   Plasma free amino acids (Chi and Speers, 1976)
PKU   Phenylketonuria
PLASMA AMINO NITROGEN INDEX (Higgons, 1959)

$$= \frac{\text{Maximal plasma amino N level} - \text{Fasting plasma amino N level}}{\text{Fasting plasma amino N level}}$$

PLP   Pyridoxal phosphate (Aycock and Kirksey, 1976)
PNG   Plant nitrogen in grain (Bhatia and Rabson, 1976)
PO   Polyunsaturated vegetable oils (Garrett et al., 1976)
PPC   Protein polysaccharide complex (Carlisle, 1976)
PPD INDEX   Pepsin pancreatin digest index (Stahmann and Woldegiorgis, 1975)
PPDD INDEX   Pepsin pancreatin digest dialysate (Stahmann and Woldegiorgis, 1975)
PPO   Polyphenol oxidase
PPV   Productive protein value (produktiver Eiweisswert, PEW)

$$= \frac{\text{N-increase of the body}}{\text{N-consumption}} \text{ (Hötzel, 1958; NAS, 1963)}$$

PROTEIN CALORIES PER CENT (Kofranyi, 1972)

$$= \frac{\text{protein calories X 100}}{\text{total metabolizable calories}}$$

PQI   Protein quality index (Arroyave, 1975; Cf. also, Almquist et al., 1935; Lyman et al., 1953)

$$= \frac{\text{Requirement of protein (N X 6.25) for age}}{\substack{\text{Amount of test protein to satisfy requirement of}\\ \text{most limiting amino acid of subjects of the same age}}}$$

PRE   Protein retention efficiency; = NPR x 16 (Bender and Doell, 1957)
PROTEIN DIETARY REQUIREMENT (FAO, 1974)

$$\frac{\text{safe level of protein intake X protein value of egg}}{\text{protein value of dietary protein}}$$

PROTEIN RATING   Product of PER and g protein consumed in "reasonable daily intake" (Campbell, 1959)
PSMF   Protein-sparing modified fast (Bistrian et al., 1977)
PU   Protein Utilization; correlates with utilization determined by nitrogen balance measurements (Closa et al., 1977).

PUFA   Polyunsaturated fatty acid (Carroll, 1978)
PUN   Plasma urea nitrogen (Pelaez et al., 1978)

RBP   Retinol-binding protein (Venkataswamy et al., 1977)
RDA   Recommended daily allowance
% ReCal   Per cent recommended calories (Mata et al., 1977)
% RecPro   Per cent recommended protein (Mata et al., 1977)
RED GRAM   Cajanus cajan (Chavan and Duggal, 1978)
RNR   Relative nitrogen requirement (Young et al., 1977)
RNU   Relative nitrogen utilization (Bodwell, 1977)
RNV   Relative nutritive value

$$\frac{\text{wt gain of test group} + 0.1 \text{ (initial} + \text{final wt of test group)}}{\text{N consumed}}$$

relative to a standard protein (lactalbumin)
(McLaughlan and Keith, 1975)

$$= \frac{\text{sample organism count}}{\text{ANRC reference casein count}} \qquad \text{(Landers, 1975; Ford, 1962)}$$

RNV-AVL   Relative nutritive value available lysine (Landers, 1975)

$$= \frac{\text{test sample available lysine (g/16 g N)}}{\text{ANRC reference casein available lysine (g/16 g N)}}$$

RPG   Relative per cent gain (Schelling, 1975)
RPV   Relative protein value (Bodwell, 1977)
REFERENCE PROTEIN   A protein of high biological value such as
          casein or lactalbumin containing a specified pattern of
          essential amino acids (NAS, 1963)
REPLACEMENT VALUE   The extent to which a dietary protein will
          supply the same nitrogen balance as an equal quantity of
          a standard protein (NAS, 1963)

SAA   Sulfur amino acids
SAAN   Sulfur-containing amino acid nitrogen (Tamminga, 1975)
SACS   S-Allycysteine sulfoxide (Itokawa et al., 1973)
SAM   S-Adenosyl-L-methionine (Case and Benevenga, 1976)
SBH   Soybean hemagglutinin (Liener, 1975)
SBM   Soybean meal (Ostrowski, 1978)
SBOM   Soybean oil meal
SCP   Single cell protein
SCS   Simplified chemical score (Bressani et al., 1972)
SESAME   Sesame indicum Linn.
SGOT   Serum glutamic-oxalacetic transaminase (Edozien et al., 1976)
SGPT   Serum glutamic-pyruvic transaminase (Edozien et al., 1976)
SI   Soybean isolate (Kamat et al., 1978)
SMCS   S-Methylcysteine sulfoxide (Itokawa et al., 1973)
SORGHUM   Broom corn; durra; Sorghum vulgare Pers.; Sorghum
          bicolor (L.) Moench, possibly var. durra (Forssk.)
SOYBEAN   Soya bean; Soja Max Piper; Glycine Max Linn.
SP   Storage protein
SR   Slope ratio method for protein assay (McLaughlan and
          Keith, 1975; McLaghlan, 1978)
SRL   Strained ruminal liquor (Broderick, 1978; Friedman and
          Broderick, 1977)

SUNFLOWER   Helianthus annuus Linn.
TAAA   Total aromatic amino acids (Arroyave, 1975)
TAC   Total available carbohydrate (daSilveira et al., 1978)
TAAV   Total amino acid value; can be calculated for different
        proteins using multiple regression equations with Biological
        Value (BV) as a dependent variable and the quantity of each
        amino acid in g/16g N as independent variables (Hansen and
        Eggum, 1973; Hansen, 1975; Eggum, 1978)
TBK   Total body potassium (Garza et al., 1978; Waterlow, 1969)
TCB   Trypsin carboxypeptidase–B
TD   True digestibility (Slump and van Beek, 1975; Holmes, (1962)

$$= \frac{AA\ intake - (fecal\ AA - metabolic\ AA)}{AA\ intake}$$

TDAA   Modified true digestibility (Slump and Van Beek, 1975)
TDN   Total digestible nutrients (Ostrowski, 1978)
TEAA/TAA Ratio of total essential amino acids to total amino acids
        in plasma; measure of adequacy of protein from different
        diets (MacLean et al., 1976)
TIBC   Serum total iron binding capacity (Kies and Fox, 1978)
TMBV   Thomas Mitchell biological value (Asplund, 1975). See BV.
TNC   Total nonstructural carbohydrate (daSilveira et al., 1978)
TPE   Total protein efficiency, defined as grams of weight per
        gram protein consumed (Benevenga and Cieslak, 1978;
        Woodham, 1978)
TPN   Total parenteral nutrition
TRP/ NAA   Ratio of plasma tryptophan to neutral amino acids
        (Ashley and Anderson, 1975; Munro, 1978)
TSAA   Total sulfur amino acids (Arroyave, 1975)
TSP   Textured soy protein
TVP   Textured vegetable protein (Kies and Fox, 1971)

UHS   Ultra–high sulfur proteins (Campbell, et al., 1975)
U_N Urinary nitrogen (Garza et al., 1977; 1978)
UN   Utilizable nitrogen (Eggum, 1978)
UNICEF United Nations Children's Fund
UP   Utilizable protein (Eggum, 1978)
U_{TN} Total urinary nitrogen (Garza et al., 1978
U_{UN} Urinary urea nitrogen (Garza et al., 1978)
UUN   Unmetabolizable urinary nitrogen

VFA   Volatile fatty acid
VLDL   Very low density lipoproteins (Nicolosi et al., 1976)

WBK   Whole body potassium. See TBK
WNSP   Water–soluble nonstarchy polysaccharide (Ciacco and
        D'Appolonia, 1978)

REFERENCES

Albanese, A.A. (1959). Protein and amino acid requirements of
  children. In "Protein and Amino Acid Nutrition", A.A. Albanese,
  Ed., Academic Press, New York, pp. 419-470.
Allison, J.B. (1955). Biological evaluation of proteins.
  Physiol. Rev., 35, 664-700.
Allison, M. and Borzucki, R. (1978). Cellulase methods for the
  efficient digestion of grasses and brassicas. J. Sci. Fd.
  Agric., 29, 293-297.
Almquist, H.J., Stokstad, E.L.R. and Halbrook, E.R. (1935).
  Supplementary values of animal protein concentrates in chick
  rations. J. Nutr. 10, 193-211.
Anderfelt, L. (1962). Nutrition research and food production.
  In "Mild-Moderate Forms of Protein-Calorie Malnutrition",
  G. Blix, Ed., Bastad, Sweden, pp. 9-31.
Armstrong, D.G. and Annison, E.F. (1973). Amino acid requirements
  and amino acid supply in sheep. Proc. Nutr. Soc., 32, 107-113.
Arnould, R. (1971). La supplementation des proteins par des acides
  amines. Communication du Centre de Recherches Zootechniques de
  l'Universite de Louvain, nr. 14, Lovenjoel, Belgique, pp. 1-43.
Arroyave, G. (1962). Biochemical signs of mild-moderate forms
  of protein-calorie malnutrition. In "Mild-Moderate Forms of
  Protein-Calorie Malnutrition", G. Blix, Ed., Bastad, Sweden,
  pp. 32-46.
Arroyave, G. (1975). Amino acid requirements and age. In
  "Protein-Calorie Malnutrition", R.E. Olson, Ed., Academic
  Press, New York, pp. 1-18.
Ashley, D.V.M. and Anderson, G.H. (1975a). Food intake regulation in the weanling rat: effects of the most limiting
  essential amino acid of gluten, casein, and zein on the
  self-selection of protein and energy. J. Nutr., 105, 1405-1411.
Ashley, D.V.M. and Anderson, G.H. (1975b). Correlation between
  the plasma tryptophan to neutral amino acid ratio and protein
  intake in self-selecting weanling rat. J. Nutr., 105, 1412-1421.
Asplund, J.M. (1975). The determination and significance of
  biological values of proteins for ruminants. In "Protein
  Nutritional Quality of Foods and Feeds", Part 1, M. Friedman,
  Ed., Dekker, New York, pp. 37-49.
Aycock, J.E. and Kirksey (1976). Influence of different levels
  of dietary pyridoxine on certain parameters of developing and
  mature brains in rats. J. Nutr., 106, 680-688 (1976).
Barry, T.N. (1976). Evaluation of formaldehyde-treated lucerne
  hay for protecting protein from ruminal degradation, and for
  increasing nitrogen retention, wool growth, live-weight gain
  and voluntary intake when fed to young sheep. J. Agric. Sci.,
  Camb., 86, 379-392.
Beaton, G. H. (1975). Protein: energy ratios—guidelines in the
  assessment of protein nutritional quality. In "Protein
  Nutritional Quality of Foods and Feeds:", Part 2, Friedman,
  Ed., Dekker, New York, pp. 619-634.

Beisel, W.R. (1977). Resume of the discussion concerning the
    nutritional consequences of infection. Am. J. Clin. Nutr.
    30, 1294-1300.
Benevenga, N.J. and Cieslak, D.G. (1978). Some thoughts on amino
    acid supplementation of proteins in relation to improvement of
    protein nutriture. This volume.
Bender, A.E. and Doell, B.H. (1957). Biological evaluation of
    proteins: a new aspect. Brit. J. Nutr., 11, 140-148.
Bergen, W.G. (1978). Postruminal digestion and absorption of
    nitrogenous components. Fed. Proc., 37, 1223-1227.
Bergman, E.N. and Heitmann, R.N. (1978). Metabolism of amino
    acids by the gut, liver, kidneys, and peripheral tissues.
    Fed. Proc., 37, 1228-1232.
Bhatia, C.R. and Rabson, R. (1976). Bioenergetic considerations
    in cereal breeding for protein improvement. Science, 194,
    1418-1420.
Bickoff, E.M., Booth, A.N., DeFremery, D., Edwards, R.H.,
    Knuckles, B.E., Miller, R.E., Saunders, R.M. and Kohler,
    G.O. (1975). Nutritional evaluation of alfalfa leaf
    protein concentrate. In "Protein Nutritional Quality of
    Foods and Feeds", Part 2, M. Friedman, Ed., Dekker, New York,
    pp. 319-340.
Bistrian, B.R., Winterer, J., Blackburn, G.L. and Scrimshaw,
    N.S. (1977). Failure of yellow fever immunization to produce
    a catabolic response in individuals fully adapted to a
    protein-sparing modified fast. Am. J. Clin. Nutr., 30,
    1518-1522.
Bock, H.D. (1975). Zur Proteinqualitatsbeurteilung von Nahrungs-
    und Futtermitteln. Die Nahrung, 19, 875-884.
Bodwell, C.E. (1975). Biochemical parameters as indices of
    protein nutritional value. In "Protein Nutritional Quality
    of Foods and Feeds" Part 1, M. Friedman, Ed., Dekker, New York,
    pp. 261-310.
Bodwell, C.E.(1977). Application of animal data to human protein
    nutrition: a review. Cereal Chem., 54, 958-983.
Bressani, R., Elias, L.G. and Gomez Brenes, R.A.G. (1972).
    Improvement of protein quality by amino acid and protein
    supplementation. In "Protein and Amino Acid Functions",
    E.A. Bigwood, Ed., Pergamon Press, Oxford, England, pp. 475-540.
Britton, R. (1978). Removal of the growth inhibotor(s) from acid
    and pressure hydrolyzed sawdust. J. Ag. Fd. Chem., 26, 761-763.
Broderick, G.A. (1978). In vitro procedures for estimating rates
    of ruminal degradation and proportions of proteins escaping
    the rumen undegraded. J. Nutr., 108, 181-190.
Brunckhorst, K., Lein, K.A. and Schon, W.J. (1974). Determination
    of lysine content and selection of the character of Hiproly
    after back-crosses in barley. I. Testing and development of
    methods of analysis. Z. Pflanzenzuchtung 73, 269-283 (German).
Buamah, T.F. and Singsen, E.P. (1975). Studies on the protein
    efficiency ratio method for the evaluation of poultry feed
    supplements. Modifications associated with choice of dietary

protein level assay. J. Nutri., 105, 688-700.

Calloway, D.H. (1975). Nitrogen balance of men with marginal intakes of protein and energy. J. Nutri., 105, 914-923.

Campbell, J.A. and Chapman, D.G. (1959). Evaluation of protein in foods-criteria for describing protein value. J. Canad, Diet. Ass., 21, 51-60.

Campbell, M.E., Whiteley, K.J. and Gillespie, J.M. (1975). Influence of nutrition on the crimping rate of wool and the type and proportion of constituent proteins. Aust. J. Biol. Sci., 28, 389-397.

Canolty, M.L. and Koong, L.J. (1976). Utilization of energy for maintenance and for fat and lean gains by mice selected for rapid postweaning growth rate. J. Nutr., 106, 1202-1208.

Carlisle, E.M. (1976). In vivo requirements for silicon in articular cartilage and connective tissue formation in the chick. J. Nutr., 106, 478-484.

Carpenter, K.J. (1960). The estimation of the available lysine in animal protein foods. Biochem. J., 77, 604-610.

Carpenter, K.J. and Booth, V.H. (1973). Damage to lysine in food processing: Its measurement and its significance. Nutr. Abst. and Rev., 43, 424-451.

Carroll, K.K. (1978). The role of dietary protein in hypercholesterolemia and atherosclerosis. Lipids, 13, 360-365.

Case, G.L. and Benevenga, N.J. (1976). Evidence for S-adenosylmethionine independent catabolism of methionine in the rat. J. Nutr., 106, 1721-1736.

Cavins, J.F., and Friedman, M. (1967). New amino acids derived from reactions of ε-amino groups in proteins with α, β-unsaturated compounds. Biochemistry, 6, 3766-3770.

Chavez, J.F. and Pellet, P.L. (1976). Protein quality of some representative Latin American diets by rat bioassay. J. Nutr., 106, 792-801.

Chavan, J.K. and Duggan, S.K. (1978). Synergistic effect of different pulses on the protein quality of rice. J. Sci. Fd. Agric., 29, 230-233.

Chawala, R.K., Hersh, T., Lambe, Jr., D.W., Wadsworth, A.D. and Rudman, D. (1976). Effect of antibiotics on growth of the immature rat. J. Nutr., 106, 1737-1746.

Chi, M.S. and Speers, G.M. (1976). Effects of dietary protein and lysine levels on plasma amino acids, nitrogen retention and egg production in laying hens. J. Nutr., 106, 1192-1201.

Ciacco, C.F. and D'Appolonia, B.L. (1978). Baking studies with cassava and yam flour. I. Biochemical composition of cassava and yam flour. Cereal Chem., 55, 402-411.

Clark, H.E., Brewer, M.F. and Bailey, L.B. (1978). Effect of nitrogen retention by adults of different proportions of indispensable amino acids in isonitrogenous cereal-based diets. This volume.

Clark, J.H., Spires, H.R. and Davis, C.L. (1978). Uptake and metabolism of nitrogenous components by the lactating mammary gland. Fed. Proc., 37, 1233-1238.

Closa, S.J., Meredith, C. Rio, M.E., Gargatagli, R. and O'Donnell, A. (1977). Protein and energy requirements in infants recovering from malnutrition. Nutr. Repts. Int., 16, 557-563.

Concon, J.M. (1975). Chemical estimation of critical amino acids in cereal grains and other products. In "Protein Nutritional Quality of Foods and Feeds", Part 1, M. Friedman Ed., Dekker, New York, pp. 311-379.

Costa, P.M.A., Jensen, A.H., Harmon, B.G. and Norton, H.W. (1976). The effects of roasting and roasting temperatures on the nutritive value of corn for swine. J. Anim. Sci., 42, 365-374.

da Silveira, A.J., Teles, F.F.F., and Stull, J.W. (1978). A rapid technique for total nonstructural carbohydrate determination of plant tissue. J. Ag. Fd. Chem., 770-772.

Dreyer, J.J. (1976). Biological assessment of protein quality. Optimal essential: non-essential amino acid ratios for maintenance of certain states of nitrogen balance in young rats. SA Medical J., 50, 1521-1528.

Dvorak, Z. (1975). Comparison of the methods for the evaluation of the nutritional value of proteins. Zeszyty Problemowe Postepow Nauk Rolniczych (Polish), 167, 199-215. Article in English.

Edozien, J.C., Khan, M.A.R. and Waslien, C.I. (1976). Human protein deficiency: results of a Nigerian village study. J. Nutr., 106, 312-328.

Eggum, B.O. (1978). Protein quality of induced high lysine mutants in barley. This volume.

Eggum, B.O., Petersen, V.E., Madsen, A. and Mortensen, H.P. (1971). Nitrogen efficiency ratio (NER) determined in experiments with rats, chickens and pigs. Yearbook Kongelige Veterinaer- og Landbhojskle, Copenhagen, Denmark, pp. 177-190.

FAO (1973). "Energy and Protein Requirements", FAO Nutrition Meeting Report Series No. 52; WHO Technical Report Series No. 522, Food and Agriculture Organization of the United Nations, Rome, Italy. 118p.

FAO (1974). Handbook of Human Nutritional Requirements, FAO Nutritional Studies No. 28; WHO Monograph Series No. 61, Food and Agriculture Organization of the United Nations, Rome, Italy. 70p.

FAO (1976). Food and Nutritional Strategies in National Development, FAO Nutrition Meetings Report Series No. 56; WHO Technical Report Series No. 584, Food and Agriculture Organization of the United Nations, Rome, Italy, 64p.

Fenderson, C.L. and Bergen, W.G. (1975). An assessment of essential amino acid requirements of growing steers. J. Anim. Sci., 41, 1759-1766.

Ferguson, K.A. (1975). The protection of dietary proteins and amino acids against microbial fermentation in the rumen. In "Digestion and Metabolism in the Ruminant", I.W. McDonald and A.C.I. Warner, Eds., University New England Press, Armidale,

Australia, pp. 448-463.

Finley, J.W. and Friedman, M. (1973). Chemical methods for available lysine. Cereal Chem., 50, 101-105.

Finot, P.A., Bujard, E., Mottu, F. and Mauron, J. (1977). Availability of the true Schiff's bases of lysine. Chemical evaluation of the Schiff's bases between lysine and lactose in milk. In "Protein Crosslinking: Nutritional and Medical Consequences", M. Friedman, Ed., Plenum, New York, pp. 343-365.

Fisher, S., Hendricks, D.G. and Mahoney, A.W. (1978). Nutritional assessment of senior rural Utahns by biochemical and physical measurements. Am. J. Clin. Nutr., 31, 667-672.

Fitzhugh, H.A. (1976). Sheep and goats as food and fiber resources- current and future. In "The Role of Sheep and Goats in Agricultural Development", Winrock International Center, Morrilton, Arkansas. pp. 35-41.

Ford, J.E. (1972). A microbiological method for assessing the nutritional value of proteins. 2. The measurement of available methionine, leucine, isoleucine, arginine, histidine, tryptophan, and valine. Brit. J. Nutr., 16, 409-425.

Friedman, M. (1977a). Crosslinking amino acids—sterochemistry and nomenclature. In "Protein Crosslinking: Nutritional and Medical Consequences", M. Friedman, Ed., Plenum, New York, pp. 1-27.

Friedman, M. (1977b). Effects of lysine modification on chemical, physical, nutritive, and functional properties of proteins. In "Food Proteins", edited by J.R. Whitaker and S.R. Tannenbaum. Avi, Westport, Connecticut, pp 446-483.

Friedman, M., Ed., (1975). "Protein Nutritional Quality of Foods and Feeds", Marcel Dekker, New York, Part 1, p. 597; Part 2, pp. 635-636.

Friedman, M. (1967). Solvent effects in reactions of amino groups in amino acids, peptides, and proteins with α,β-unsaturated compounds. J. Am. Chem. Soc., 89, 4709-4713.

Friedman, M. and Broderick, G.A. (1977). Protected proteins in ruminal nutrition. In vitro evaluation of casein derivatives. In "Protein Crosslinking: Nutritional and Medical Consequences", M. Friedman, Ed., Plenum Press, New York, pp. 545-558.

Friedman, M., and Finley, J.W. (1975a). Reactions of proteins with ethyl vinyl sulfone. Int. J. Peptide Protein Res., 7, 481-486.

Friedman, M., and Finley, J.W. (1975b). Vinyl compounds as reagents for available lysine. In "Protein Nutritional Quality of Foods and Feeds," Part 1, M. Friedman, ed., Dekker, New York, pp. 503-520.

Friedman, M. and Orracah-Tetteh, R. (1978). Hair as an index of protein malnutrition. This volume.

Friedman, M. and Wall, J.S. (1966). Additive linear free energy relationships in reaction kinetics of amino groups with α,β-unsaturated compounds. J. Org. Chem. 31, 2888-2894.

Fuchs, R.J., Clarence, M.S., Theis, F., and Lancaster, M.C. (1978). A nomogram to predict lean body mass in man. Am. J. Clin. Nutr., 31, 673–678.

Gaby, A.R. and Chawala, R.K. (1976). Efficiency of phenylpyruvic acid and phenyllactic acids as substitutes for phenylalanine in the diet of the growing rat. J. Nutr., 106, 158–168.

Garling, D.L. and Wislon, R.P. (1976). Optimum dietary protein to energy ratio for channel catfish fingerlings, Ictalurus punctatus. J. Nutr., 106, 1368–1375.

Garrett, W.N., Yang, Y.T., Dunkley, W.L. and Smith, L.M. (1976). Energy utilization, feedlot performance and fatty acid composition of beef steers fed protein encapsulated tallow or vegetable oils. J. Anim. Sci., 42, 1522–1533.

Garza, C., Scrimshaw, N.S. and Young, V.R. (1977). Human protein requirements: a long-term metabolic nitrogen balance study in young men to evaluate the 1973 FAO/WHO safe level of egg protein intake. J. Nutr., 107, 335–352.

Garza, C., Scrimshaw, N.S. and Young, V.R. (1978). Human protein requirements: interrelationships between energy intake and nitrogen balance in young men consuming the 1973 FAO/WHO safe level of egg protein with added non-essential amino acids. J. Nutr., 108, 90–96.

Gjøen, A.U. and Njaa, L.R. (1977). Methionine sulphoxide as a source of sulphur-containing amino acids for the young rat. Br. J. Nutr. 37, 93–105.

Gutcho, M.H. (1977). "Textured Protein Products", Noyes Data Corporation, Park Ridge, New Jersey. p. 15.

Hackler, L.R. (1977). Methods for measuring protein quality: a review of bioassay procedures. Cereal Chem., 54, 984–995.

Hansen, N.G. (1975). Comparison of chemical methods of protein evaluation with biological value determined on rats. Z. Tierphysiol. Futtermittelkunde, 35, 302–310.

Hansen, N.G. and Eggum, B.O. (1973). The biological value of proteins estimated from amino acid analyses. Acta Agric. Scand., 23, 247–251.

Happich, M.L., Swift, C.E. and Naghski, J. (1975). Equations for Predicting PER from amino acid analysis–A review and current scope of application. In "Protein Nutritional Quality of Foods and Feeds, Part 1, Assay Methods–Biological, Biochemical and Chemical," M. Friedman, Ed., Dekker, New York pp. 125–135.

Harper, A.E. (1974). Basic concepts. In "Improvement of Protein Nutriture", National Academy of Sciences, Washington, D.C., 1–22.

Hegsted, D.M. (1974). Assessment of protein quality. In "Improvement of Protein Nutriture", National Academy of Sciences, Washington, D.C., pp. 64–88.

Hegsted, D.M. (1976). Balance studies, J. Nutr., 106, 307–311.

Hegsted, D.M. and Juliano, B.O. (1974). Difficulties in assessing the nutritional quality of rice protein. J. Nutr., 104, 772–781.

Heidelbaugh, N.D. Huber, C.S., Bednarczyk, J.F., Smith, M.J., Rambaut, P.C. and Wheeler, H.O. (1975). Comparison of three methods for calculating protein content of foods. J. Ag. Fd. Chem., 23, 611-613.

Heiman, V., Carver, J.S. and Cook, J.W. (1939). A method for determining the gross value of protein concentrates. Poultry Science, 18, 464-474.

Higgons, R.A. (1959). Nutritional needs of the aged. In "Protein and Amino Acid Nutrition", A.A. Albenese, Ed., Academic Press, New York, pp. 507-552.

Holmes, E.G. (1962). Human adult protein requirements. World Rev. Nutr. Diet. 3, 197-215.

Hötzel, D. (1958). Zur Problematik der Ermittelung der Eiweisswertigkeit. Z. Tierphsyiol. Tiernahrung und Futtermittel-kunde, 13, 193-200 (German).

Hurrell, R.F. and Carpenter, K.J. (1977). Nutritional significance of cross-link formation during food processing. In "Protein Crosslinking: Nutritional and Medical Consequences", M. Friedman, Ed., Plenum, New York, pp. 225-238.

Hurt, H.D., Forsythe, R.H. and Krieger, C.H. (1975). Factors which influence the biological evaluation of protein quality by the protein efficiency ratio method. In "Protein Nutritional Quality of Foods and Feeds", Part 1, M. Friedman Ed., Marcel Dekker, New York pp. 87-112.

Itokawa, Y., Inoue, K., Sasagawa, S. and Fujiwara, M. (1973). Effect of S-methylcysteine sulfoxide, S-allylcysteine sulfoxide and related sulfur-containing amino acids on lipid metabolism of experimental hypocholesteremic rats. J. Nutr., 103, 88-92.

Jacquot, R. and Peret, J. (1972). Protein efficiency ratio and related methods. In "Protein and Amino Acid Functions", E.J. Bigwood, Ed., Pergamon, Oxford, pp. 317-346.

Jansen, G.R. and Verburg, D.T. (1977). Amino acid fortification of wheat diets fed at varying levels of energy intake to rats. J. Nutr., 107, 289-299.

Kaba, H. and Pellett, P.L. (1975). Prediction of true limiting amino acids using available protein scoring systems. Ecology of Food and Nutrition, 4, 109-116.

Kabadi, U.M. Eisenstein, A.B. and Strack, I. (1976). Decreased plasma insulin but normal glucagon in rats fed low protein diets. J. Nutr., 106, 1247-1253.

Kamat, V.B., Graham, G.E. and Davis, M.A. (1978). Vegetable protein lipid interactions. Cereal Chem., 55, 295-307.

Kies, C. and Fox, H.M. (1971). Comparison of the protein nutritional value of TVP, methionine enriched TVP and beef at two levels of intake for human adults. J. Fd. Sci., 36, 841-845.

Kies, C. and Fox, H.M. (1978). Urea as a dietary supplement for humans. This volume.

Kies, C., Fox, H.M., Mattern, P.J., Johnson, V.A. and Schmidt, J.W. (1978). Comparative protein quality as measured by human and small animal bioassays of three lines of winter wheat. This volume.

Knipfel, J.E. (1977). Protein interrelationships in roughages as affecting ruminant dietary protein efficiency. In "Protein Crosslinking: Nutritional and Medical Consequences", M. Friedman, Ed., Plenum Press, New York, pp. 559–578.

Knipfel, J.E., Botting, H.G. and McLaughlan, J.M. (1975). Nutritional quality of several proteins as affected by heating in the presence of carbohydrates. In "Protein Nutritional Quality of Foods and Feeds", Part 2, M. Friedman, Ed., Dekker, New York, pp. 375–391.

Kofranyi, E. (1972). Protein and amino acid requirements. A. Nitrogen balance in adults. In "Protein and Amino Acid Functions", E.J. Bigwood, Ed., Pergamon, Oxford, England, pp. 1–39.

Kofranyi, E. (1973). Evaluation of traditional hypotheses on the biological value of proteins. Nutr. Repts. Int., 7, 45–50.

Labuza, T.P., Warren, R.M. and Warmbier, H.C. (1977). The physical aspects with respect to water and non-enzymatic browning. In "Protein Crosslinking: Nutritional and Medical Consequences", M. Friedman, Ed., Plenum, New York, pp. 379–418.

Lachance, P.A., Bressani, R. and Elias, L.G. Shorter protein bioassays. Nutr. Repts. Int., 16, 179–186.

Laditan, A.A.O. and Reeds, P.J. (1976). A study of the age of onset, diet and the importance of infection in the pattern of severe protein-energy malnutrition in Ibadan, Nigeria. Brit. J. Nutr., 36, 411–419.

Lalasidis, G., Boström, S. and Sjöberg, L.B. (1978). Low molecular weight enzymatic fish protein hydrolysates: chemical composition and nutritive value. J. Ag. Fd. Chem., 26, 751–756.

Landers, R.E. (1975). Relationship between protein efficiency ratio of foods and relative nutritive value measured by Tetrahymena pyriformis W bioassay technique. In "Protein Nutritional Quality of Foods and Feeds", Part 1, M. Friedman, Ed., Dekker, New York, pp. 185–202.

Lautzenheiser, M. and Pellet, P.L. (1977). Prediction of human nitrogen balance from food intake data. Am. J. Clin. Nutr., 30, 1382–1389.

Liener, I.E. (1975). Effect of anti-nutritional factors on the quality and utilization of legume proteins. In "Protein Nutritional Quality of Foods and Feeds", Part 2, M. Friedman, Ed., Dekker, New York, pp. 523–550.

Long, C.L., Schiller, W.R., Blakemore, W.S., Geiger, J.W., O'Dell, M. and Henderson, K. (1977). Muscle protein catabolism in the septic patient as measured by 3-methylhistidine excretion. Am. J. Clin. Nutr., 30, 1349–1352.

Longenecker, J.B. and Hause, N.L. (1961). Relationship between plasma amino acids and composition of the ingested protein. II. A shortened procedure to determine plasma amino acid (PAA) ratios. Am. J. Clin. Nutr., 9, 356–362.

Lyman, C.M., Chang, W.Y. and Couch, J.R. (1953). Evaluation of protein quality in cottonseed meals by chick growth and by a chemical index method. J. Nutr., 49, 679–690.

Maclean, W. C., Jr., Palcko, R.P. and Graham, G.G. (1976). Plasma free amino acids of children consuming a diet with uneven distribution of protein relative to energy. J. Nutr., 106, 241-248.

Markakis, P. (1975). The nutritive value of potato protein. In "Protein Nutritional Quality of Foods and Feeds", Part 2, M. Friedman, Ed., Dekker, New York, pp. 471-487.

Martinez, W.H. and Hopkins, D.T. (1975). Cottonseed protein products: variation in protein quality with product and process. In "Protein Nutritional Quality of Foods and Feeds", Part 2, M. Friedman, Ed., Dekker, New York, pp. 355-374.

Mata, L.J., Kromal, R.A., Urrutia, J. and Garcia, B. (1977). Effect of infection on food intake and the nutritional state: perspectives as viewed from the village. Am. J. Clin. Nutr., 30, 1215-1227.

McLaughlan, J.M. (1978). The problem of curvature in slope assays for protein quality. This volume.

McLaughlan, M.J. and Campbell, J.A. (1969). Methodology of protein evaluation. In "Mammalian Protein Metabolism", H.N. Munro, Ed., Academic Press, New York, Vol. III, pp. 391-422.

Merril, O.L. and Watt, B.K. (1955). Handbook No. 74, ARS, USDA, Washington, D.C.

Millard, M.M. and Friedman, M. (1976). X-ray photoelectron spectroscopy of BSA and ethyl vinyl sulfone modified BSA. Biochem. Biophys. Res. Commun. 70, 451-458.

Miller, D.S. and Bender, A.E. (1955). The determination of the net utilization of proteins by a shortened method. Brit. J. Nutr., 9, 382-388.

Miller, D.S. and Naismith, D.J. (1958). A correlation between sulfur content and net dietary-protein value. Nature, 182, 1786-1787.

Miller, D.S. and Payne, P.R. (1962). Weight maintenance and food intake, J. Nutr., 78, 255-262.

Miller, E.L. (1973). Evaluation of foods as sources of nitrogen and amino acids. Proc. Nutr. Soc., 32, 79-84.

Miller, S.A. (1969). Protein metabolism during growth and development. In "Mammalian Protein Metabolism", H.N. Munro, Ed., Academic Press, New York, pp. 183-233.

Mitchell, H.H. (1922). The net protein value of feed and food materials. Am. Soc. Animal Production, 55-58.

Mitchell, H.H. (1923). A method for determining the biological value of protein. J. Biol. Chem., 58, 873-903.

Munro, H.N. (1978). Nutritional consequences of excess amino acid intake. This volume.

NAS (1963). "Evaluation of Protein Quality". National Academy of Sciences-National Research Council Publication 1100, Washington, D.C., pp. 61-68.

Navarrete, D.A., Loureiro de Daqui, V.A., Eliaz, L.G., Lachance, P.A. and Bressani, R. (1977). The nutritive value of egg protein as determined by the nitrogen blance index (NBI). Nutr. Repts. Int., 16, 695-703.

Nicolosi, R.J., Herrera, M.G., el Lozy, M. and Hayes, K.C. (1976). Effect of dietary fat on hepatic metabolism of C^{14}-oleic acid and very low density lipoprotein triglyceride in the gerbil. J. Nutr., 106, 1279-1285.

Nitsan, Z. and Nir, I. (1977). A comparative study of the nutritional and physiological significance of raw and heated soya bean in chicks and goslings. Br. J. Nutr., 37, 81-91.

Offer, N.W., Evans, R.A. and Axford, R.F.E. (1976). A comparative study of non-protein nitrogen supplements for sheep. J. Agric. Sci., 87, 567-572.

Okumura, J. and Tasaki, I. (1973). Digestibility, biological value and 'available' lysine content of some protein concentrates for poultry. Japan Poultry Sci., 10, 37-40.

Oldfield, J.E. (1977). Cattle and chemistry. CHEMTECH, 290-294.

Osborne, Th. B. and Mendel, L.B. (1917). The use of soy bean as a food. J. Biol. Chem., 32, 369-386.

Oser, B.L. (1951). Method for integrating essential amino acid content in the nutritional evaluation of protein. J. Amer. Dietetic Assoc. 27, 396-402.

Oser, B.L. (1959). An integrated essential amino acid index for predicting the biological value of proteins. In "Protein and Amino Acid Nutrition", A.A. Albanese, Ed., Academic Press, New York, pp. 281-295.

Ostrowski, H.T. (1978). Analysis for availability of amino acid supplements in foods and feeds: Biochemical and nutritional implications. This volume.

Otterburn, M., Healy, M. and Sinclair, W. (1977). The formation, isolation and importance of isopeptides in heated proteins. In "Protein Crosslinking: Nutritional and Medical Consequences", M. Friedman, Ed., Plenum, New York, pp. 239-262.

Payne, P.R. (1972). Evaluation of protein quality of diets. In "Protein and Amino Acid Functions", E.J. Bigwood, Ed., Pergamon, Oxford, England, pp. 363-380.

Pelaez, R., Phillips, D.D. and Walker, D.M. (1978). Amino acid supplementation of isolated soybean protein in milk replacers for preruminant lambs. This volume.

Pellet, P.L. (1973). Methods of protein evaluation with rats. "Proteins in Human Nutrition", J.W.G. Porter and B.A. Rolls, Eds., Academic Press, London and New York, pp. 225-244.

Platt, B.S. and Miller, D.S. (1959). The net dietary-protein value (N.D.-P.V.) of mixtures of foods-its definition, determination and application. Proc. Nutr. Soc., 18, vii-ix.

Pomeranz, Y. and Moore, R.B. (1975). Reliability of several methods for protein determination in wheat. Bakers Digest, 49, 44-48, 58.

Ranawana, S.S.E. and Kellaway, R.C. (1977). Response to postruminal infusions of graded levels of casein in lactating goats. Br. J. Nutr., 37, 67-79.

Rangeley, W.R.D. and Lawrie, R.A. (1977). Methylated amino acids as indices in meat products. II. Further examination of protein sources and the practical application of methylamino acid titres in predicting meat content. J. Fd. Technol., 12, 9-26.

Rao, H.D. and Naidu, A.N. (1977). Nutritional Supplementation-whom does it benefit most. Am. J. Clin. Nutr., 30, 1612-1616.

Reis, P.J. and Tunks, D.A. (1976). The influence of abomasal supplements of zein and some amino acids on wool growth rate and plasma amino acids. J. Agric. Sci., Camb., 86, 475-482.

Reutlinger, S. and Selowsky, M. (1976). "Malnutrition and Poverty: Magnitude and Policy Options", Johns Hopkins, University Press, Baltimore, Maryland, 82p.

Rosenberg, H.R. (1959). Amino acid supplementation of foods and feeds In "Protein and Amino Acid Nutrition", A.A. Labanese, Ed., Academic Press, New York, pp. 381-416.

Rufeger, H. (1972). Proteinbewertung und Berechnung exogener und endogener Grossen des N-Stoffwechsels monogastrischer Organismen mit Hilfe einer N-Bilanzfunktion. Zentralblatt für Veterinarmedizine, A19, 713-725.

Sarwar, G., Sosulski, F.W., Bell, J.M. and Bowland, J.P. (1978). Nutritional evaluation of oilseeds and legumes as protein supplements to cereals. This volume.

Satterlee, L.D., Kendrick, J.G. and Miller, G.A. (1977). Rapid in vitro assays for estimating protein quality. Nutr. Repts. Int., 16, 187-199.

Schaffert, R.E., Lechtenberg, V.L., Oswalt, D.L., Axtell, J.D., Pickett. R.C. and Rhykerd, C.L. (1974). Effect of tannin on in vitro dry matter and protein disappearance in sorghum grain. Crop Sci., 14, 640-643.

Schelling, G.T. (1975). An efficient procedure for the complete evaluation of dietary proteins. In "Protein Nutritional Quality of Foods and Feeds", Part 1, M. Friedman, Ed., Dekker, New York, pp. 137-163.

Schwenke, K.D., Prahl, L., Ender, B., Bersukow, M.G., Belikow, W.M., Freimuth, U., Charatjan, S.G. and Wolnowa, A.J. (1975). Modifizierung von Proteinen durch Reaktion mit Carbonylverbindungen. Die Nahrung, 19, 921-927 (German).

Schwerdfeger, E. and Schuphan, W. (1976). Protein and amino acids in food plants. Qual. Plant., 26, 29-70.

Scrimshaw, N.S. and Young, V.R. (1972). Clinical methods for the evaluation of protein quality. In "Protein and Amino Acid Functions", E.J. Bigwood, Ed., Pergamon, Oxford, England, pp. 363-380.

Sherbon, J.W., Mickle, J.B. and Ward, W.D. (1978). Total solids in nonfat dry milk by atmospheric drying in forced air oven. J. Ass. Off. Anal. Chem., 61, 550-557.

Simell, O., Perheentupa, J., Rapola, J., Visakorpi, J.K. and Eskelin, L.E. (1975). Lysinuric protein intolerance. Am. J. Medicine, 59, 229-240.

Slump, P. and van Beek, L. (1975). Amino acids in feces related to digestibility of food proteins. In "Protein Nutritional Quality of Foods and Feeds", Part 1, M. Friedman, Ed., Dekker, New York, pp. 67-78.

Stahmann, M.A. and Woldegiorgis, G. (1975). Enzymatic methods
    for protein quality determination. In "Protein Nutritional
    Quality of Foods and Feeds", M. Friedman, Ed., Dekker, New York,
    pp. 211-234.
Steinke, F.H. (1977). Protein efficiency ratio pitfalls and causes
    of variability: a review. Cereal Chem., 54, 949-957.
Struthers, B.J., Hopkins, D.T., and Dahlgren, R.R. (1978).
    Reversibility of nephrocytomegaly in rats caused by lysino-
    alanine. J. Fd. Sci., 43, 616-618.
Stucki, W.P. and Harper, A.E. (1962). Effects of altering the
    ratio of indispensable to dispensable amino acids in diets
    for rats. J. Nutr., 78, 278-286.
Swenseid, M.E., Villalobos, J. and Fridrich, V. (1963). Ratios
    of essential-to-nonessential amino acids in plasma from rats
    fed different kinds and amounts of proteins and amino acids.
    J. Nutr., 80, 99-102.
Tamminga, S. (1975). Observation on protein digestion in the
    digestive tract of dairy cows. Z. Tierphysiol. Tiernahr. u.
    Futtermittelkunde, 35, 337-346.
Tanaka, M., Kimiagar, M. Lee, T. C. and Chichester, C.O. (1977).
    Effect of the Maillard browning reaction on nutritional quality
    of protein, In "Protein Crosslinking: Nutritional and Medical
    Consequences", M. Friedman, Ed., Plenum Press, New York,
    pp. 321-341.
Tews, J.K. and Harper, A.E. (1976). α-Aminoisobutyric acid trans-
    port in liver slices from rats fed low protein meals. J. Nutr.,
    106, 1497-1506.
Thomas, K. (1909). Arch. Anat. Physiol. Leipzig, Physiol. Abstr.,
    219.
Uauy, R., Scrimshaw, N.S., Rand, W.M. and Young, V.R. (1978).
    Human protein requirements: obligatory urinary and fecal nitrogen
    losses and the factorial estimation of protein needs in elderly
    males. J. Nutr., 108, 97-103.
Vaughn, D.A., Womack, M. and McClain, P.E. (1977). Plasma free
    amino acid levels in human subjects after meals containing
    lactalbumin, heated lactalbumin, or no protein. Am. J. Clin.
    Nutr., 30, 1709-1712.
Venkataswamy, G., Glover, J. Cobby, M. and Pirie, A. (1977).
    Retinol-binding protein in serum of xerophtalmic, malnourished
    children before and after treatment at a nutrition center.
    Am. J. Clin. Nutr., 30, 1968-1973.
Vilstrup, H. and Keiding, S. (1976). Effect of dietary protein
    depletion on the galactose elimination capacity in intact rats.
    J. Nutr., 106, 1492-1496.
von der Decken, A., Omstedt, P.T., Walger, B., and Walger, J. (1975).
    Nutritional evaluation of proteins as estimated by in vitro pro-
    tein synthesis: Comparison with conventional techniques. In
    "Protein Nutritional Quality of Foods and Feeds", Part 1.
    M. Friedman, Ed., Dekker, New York, pp. 165-184.

Waterlow, J.C. (1969). The assessment of protein nutrition and
    metabolism in the whole animal, with special reference to man.
    In "Mammalian Protein Metabolism", H.N. Munro, Ed., Academic
    Press, New York, pp. 325-390.
Williams, P.C., Stevenson, S.G., Starkey, P.M. and Hawtin, G.C.
    (1978). The application of near infrared reflectance spectro-
    scopy to protein-testing in pulse breeding programmes. J. Sci.
    Fd. Agric., 29, 285-292.
Womack, M., Vaughn, D.A. and Bodwell, C.E. (1975). A modified PER
    method for estimating changes in the bioavailability of
    individual essential amino acids In "Protein Nutritional Quality
    of Foods and Feeds", Part 1, M. Friedman, Ed., Dekker, New York,
    pp. 113-123.
Woodham,. A.A. (1978). The nutritive value of mixed protein.
    This volume.
Yadav, N.R. and Liener, I.E. (1978). Nutritional evaluation of
    dry-roasted navy bean flour and mixtures with cereal proteins.
    This volume.
Young, V.R., Rand, W.M. and Scrimshaw, N.S. (1977). Measuring
    protein quality in humans: a review and proposed method.
    Cereal Chem., 54, 929-948.
Young, V.R. and Scrimshaw, N.S. (1972). The nutritional signifi-
    cance of plasma and urinary amino acids. In "Protein and Amino
    Acid Functions", E.J. Bigwood, Ed., Pergamanon, Oxford, England
    pp. 541-568.
Yudkin, J. (1978). Dietary factors in arteriosclerosis: sucrose.
    Lipids, 13, 370-372.
Zezulka, A.Y. and Calloway, D.H. (1976). Nitrogen retention in men
    fed isolated soybean protein supplemented with L-methionine,
    D-methionine, and N-acetyl-L-methionine, or inorganic sulfate.
    J. Nutr., 106, 1286-1291.